Human Papillomavirus and Diseases: Clinical Theory

Edited by **Joe Becker**

FOSTER ACADEMICS

New Jersey

Published by Foster Academics,
61 Van Reypen Street,
Jersey City, NJ 07306, USA
www.fosteracademics.com

Human Papillomavirus and Diseases: Clinical Theory
Edited by Joe Becker

International Standard Book Number: 978-1-63242-236-1 (Hardback)

Printed in China.

Contents

Preface

The world is advancing at a fast pace like never before. Therefore, the need is to keep up with the latest developments. This book was an idea that came to fruition when the specialists in the area realized the need to coordinate together and document essential themes in the subject. That's when I was requested to be the editor. Editing this book has been an honour as it brings together diverse authors researching on different streams of the field. The book collates essential materials contributed by veterans in the area which can be utilized by students and researchers alike.

This book encompasses a detailed clinical theory regarding the human papillomavirus and the related diseases. Cervical cancer is the second most widespread cancer amongst women globally, and Human Papilloma Virus (HPV) infection has been identified as the main cause of this condition. The natural history of cervical cancer is distinguished by slow disease progression, making it realistically preventable and even treatable if diagnosed in early stages. Pap smear and the newly proposed prophylactic vaccines are the most commonly practiced prevention options, but regardless of the availability of these primary and secondary screening techniques, the worldwide burden of this disease continues to be unfortunately very high. This book lays emphasis on the clinical conditions of HPV and associated disease, highlighting the current advancements in this area.

Each chapter is a sole-standing publication that reflects each author´s interpretation. Thus, the book displays a multi-facetted picture of our current understanding of application, resources and aspects of the field. I would like to thank the contributors of this book and my family for their endless support.

Editor

Part 1

Clinical Aspects of Human Papillomavirus Related Diseases

1

Human Papillomavirus: Biology and Pathogenesis

José Veríssimo Fernandes[1] and
Thales Allyrio Araújo de Medeiros Fernandes[2]
[1]Federal University of Rio Grande do Norte
[2]University of Rio Grande do Norte State
Brazil

1. Introduction

The human papillomavirus (HPV) is one of the most common causes of sexually transmitted disease in both men and women around the world, especially in developing countries, where the prevalence of asymptomatic infection varies from 2 to 44%, depending on the population and studied region (Sanjosé et al., 2007). Most HPV infection is transient and some studies show that the majority of sexually active individuals are exposed to and acquire infection from this virus at some phase in their lives (Baseman and Koutsky, 2005; Trottier and Franco, 2006). HPV infection is more prevalent in young adults, at the beginning of their sexual activity, with a subsequent decline in the prevalence rate with increasing age, likely as a result of development of an immune response against the virus and reduction of sexual activity (Castle et al., 2005; Fernandes et al., 2009; Chan et al., 2010).

HPV can infect basal epithelial cells of the skin or inner-lining tissues and are categorized as cutaneous types or mucosal types. Cutaneous types are epidermotropic and infect the keratinized surface of the skin, targeting the skin of the hands and feet. Mucosal types infect the lining of the mouth, throat, respiratory, or anogenital tract epithelium (Burd, 2003). Some HPVs are associated with warts while others have been well established as the main risk factor of invasive cervical cancers and their associated pre-cancerous lesions (Clifford et al., 2005; Zekri et al., 2006; Muñoz et al., 2006). However, only few HPV-infected individuals progress to invasive cervical cancer (Burd, 2003). Most infected individuals eliminate the virus without developing recognized clinical manifestation. (Bosch et al., 2008).

Today, more than 150 different HPV types have been cataloged and about 40 can infect the epithelial lining of the anogenital tract and other mucosal areas of the human body. Based on their association with cervical cancer and precursor lesions, HPVs can also be classified as high-risk (HR-HPV) and low-risk (LR-HPV) oncogenic types. LR-HPV types, such as HPV 6 and 11, can cause common genital warts or benign hyperproliferative lesions with very limited tendency to malignant progression, while infection with HR-HPV types, highlighting HPV 16 and 18, is associated with the occurrence of pre-malignant and malignant cervical lesions (Muñoz et al., 2003; Bosch et al., 2002; Bosch et al., 2008). HR-HPV types are also associated with many penile, vulvar, anal, and head and neck carcinomas, and contribute to over 40% of oral cancers (Stanley, 2010).

Persistent infection with HR-HPV is unequivocally established as a necessary cause of cervival cancer (Trottier & Franco, 2006). The critical molecules for initiation and progression of this cancer are the oncoproteins E5, E6, and E7, that act largely by overcoming negative growth regulation by host cell proteins and by inducing genomic instability, a hallmark of HPV-associated cancers (Munger et al., 2004; Moody & Laimins, 2010).

Once HPV transmission to the genital tract occurs through sexual contact, the risk factors for the infection and cervical lesions, including cervical cancer, are the same classic risk factors for other sexually transmitted diseases. The number of sexual partners is the risk factor more consistently associated with genital HPV infection and therefore with cervical cancer. In addition, other indicators of sexual behavior and reproductive activities, heredity, immune and nutritional status, and smoking can contribute in some way to the development of cervical cancer (Tarkowski et al., 2004; Muñoz, 2006; Fernandes et al., 2010).

In this chapter we will discuss the biology and pathogenesis of human papillomavirus, analyzing some specific aspects of their interactions with the infected host and specific host cell components.

2. Biologic properties of HPV

2.1 Structure of viral particle and regulation of gene expression

The human papillomavirus (HPV) is a relatively small non-enveloped virus that contains a double-stranded closed circular DNA genome, associated with histone-like proteins and protected by a capsid formed by two late proteins, L1 and L2. Each capsid is composed of 72 capsomeres, each of which is composed of five monomeric of 55kDa units that join to form a pentamer corresponding to the major protein capsid, L1. The L1 pentamers are distributed forming a network of intra- and interpentameric disulfide interactions which serve to stabilize the capsid (Sapp et al., 1995). In addition to L1, minor capsid proteins with approximately 75kDa exist within the virion and are called the L2 protein. To assemble the viral capsid, the pentamers join to copies of L2 that occludes the center of each pentavalent capsomere. (Jo & Kim 2005; Buck et al., 2008; Conway & Meyers, 2009). Thus, each virion contains 72 copies of the L1, the major component of the capsid, and a variable number of copies of L2, a secondary component of the viral capsid, forming a particle with icosahedra symmetry and approximately 50 to 60 nm in diameter (Burd, 2003; Longworth & Laimins, 2004; zur Hausen, 2009).

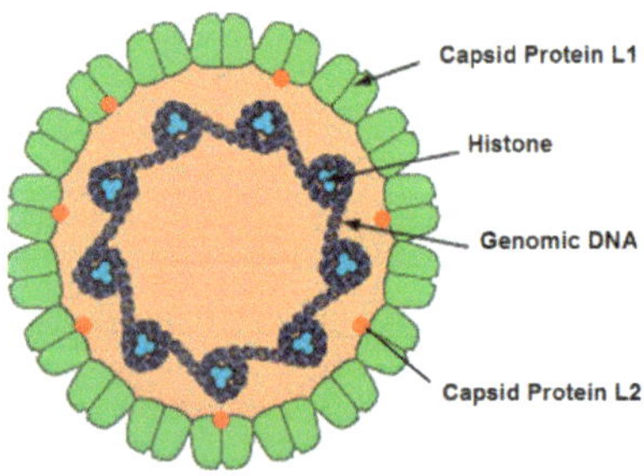

Fig. 1. The structure of HPV. (Adapted from Swiss Institute of Bioinformatics, Viral Zone. - Available in http://viralzone.expasy.org/all_by_species/5.html)

The viral genome of the HPV consists of a single molecule of double-stranded and circular DNA, containing approximately 8000 base pairs and harboring an average of 8 open reading frames (ORFs) (Jo & Kim 2005; Zheng & Baker, 2006). In a functional point of view, the HPV genome is divided into three regions. The first is a noncoding upstream regulatory region (URR) or long control region (LCR) that has regulatory function of the transcription of the E6 and E7 viral genes; The second is an early region (E), consisting of six ORFs: E1, E2, E4, E5, E6, and E7, which encodes no structural proteins involved in viral replication and oncogenesis. The third is a late (L) region that encodes the L1 and L2 structural proteins. The LCR region of the anogenital HPVs ranges in size between 800-900 pb, representing about 10% of the genome, and varies substantially in nucleotide composition between individual HPV types (Fehrmann & Laimins, 2003; Jo & Kim, 2005).

Only one strand of the double-stranded DNA serves as the template for viral gene expression, coding for a number of polycistronic mRNA transcripts. (Stanley et al., 2007). The regulation of viral gene expression is complex and controlled by cellular and viral transcription factors. Most of these regulations occur within the LCR region, which contains cis-active element transcription regulators. These sequences are bound by a number of cellular factors as well as the viral E2 product (zur Hausen, 1996). A large number of cellular transcription factors have been identified and the dysfunction of some of them appears to play a significant role in papillomavirus-linked carcinogenesis (Thierry et al., 1992; Hamid & Gaston, 2009).

The transcription start sites of viral promoters differ depending on the virus type, but, in all types, promoter usage is keratinocyte differentiation-dependent (Smith et al., 2007). The replication origin and many transcriptional regulatory elements are found in the upstream LCR region. The virus early promoter, differentiation-dependent late promoter, and two polyadenylation signals define three general groups of viral genes that are coordinately regulated during host cell differentiation. The E6 and E7 genes maintain replication competence. E1 E2, E4, E5, and E8 are involved in virus DNA replication, transcriptional control, beyond other late functions and L1 and L2, responsible for the assembly of viral particles (Bodily & Laimins, 2011).

The regulation of expression of the late genes in genital HPVs is not well understood. However, it has been shown that the second, or later, promoter is initiated in a differentiation-dependent manner, and thus is activated only when cells are grown in the host's stratifying/differentiating tissue. Once activated, the later promoter directs transcription from a heterogeneous set of start sites and will serve to produce a set of transcripts that facilitate the translation of L1 and L2 proteins (Smith et al., 2007; Conway & Meyers, 2009). Activation of the later promoter is accompanied by acceleration of viral DNA replication and by high levels of viral protein expression. As a result, virus copy-number amplifies from 50 copies to several thousands of copies per cell. So when a late promoter is activated, the expression of genes will occur, encoding the structural proteins L1 and L2, which join to assemble the capsids and to form virions (Stanley et al., 2007).

2.2 Functions of viral proteins

E1 Protein

The E1 protein represents one of the the most conserved proteins among different HPV types. It has DNA-binding functions and a binding site in the origin of replication localized in the LCR region. It assembles into a hexameric complex, supported by the E2 protein, and the resultant complex has helicase activity and initiates DNA bidirectional unwinding, constituting a prerequisite for viral DNA replication (Wilson et al., 2002; Frattini & Laimins, 1994). The carboxyl terminal domain of E1 has an ATPase/helicase activity and is necessary and sufficient for oligomerization. This domain also interacts with the E2 protein and subunit p70 of DNA polymerase α, but is not sufficient to support replication (Amin et al., 2000). A segment of approximately 160 amino acid residues upstream of the ATPase/helicase domain is the DNA-binding domain (Titolo et al., 2003). A stretch of about 50 amino acids within the amino terminus of E1 acts as a localization regulatory region (LCR) and contains a dominant nuclear export sequence (NES) and a nuclear localization signal (NSL), which are regulated by phosphorylation (Deng et al., 2004).

E2 protein

The E2 open reading frame of HPV gives rise to multiple gene products by alternative RNA splicing. The proteins derived from the E2 gene are involved in the control of viral transcription, DNA replication, and segregation of viral genomes (McPhillips et al., 2006; Kadaja et al., 2009). These different E2 types represent the major intragenomic regulators (Bouvard et al., 1994).

The E2 protein can bind to factors on mitotic chromatin and join the virus genome to host cell chromosomes during mitosis; it contributes to coordinating the HPV DNA replication with host cell chromosome duplication, allowing the viral genomes to be distributed to the daughter cell. This constitutes an important requirement for the persistence of virus DNA in undifferentiated basal cells (McPhillips et al., 2006). Furthermore, the E2 protein interacts with E1 and stimulates viral DNA replication, favoring the binding of E1 to the origin of replication (Seo et al., 1993; Chow et al., 1994).

In lesions containing HPV episomes, the E2 protein directly represses the expression of early genes as a mechanism to regulate the copy number. In addition, it has been reported that HPV E2 proteins are able to repress telomerase promoter activity mediated by the HPV E6 protein (Hamid et al., 2009). Integration of the HPV genome in the host cell chromosome usually disrupts E2 expression, causing a deregulated expression of early viral genes, including E6 and E7, and this event can favor the transformation of human cells and the transition into a malignant state (Romanczuk & Howley, 1992)

In addition to the full-length E2 protein, the infected cells can express an E8^E2C transcript, in which the small E8 domain is fused to the C-terminal domain of E2 (E2C). The full-length E2 protein forms heterodimers with repressor forms of E2, and these E2 heterodimers serve as activators of transcription and replication during the viral cycle. The single-chain E2 heterodimer in the HPV 18 genome initiates genome replication, but is not sufficient for long-term replication of the HPV 18 genome. This is due to the capacity of HPV18 in encoding the repressor E8/E2, which acts as a negative regulator of HPV18 genome replication (Kurg et al., 2010). Moreover, it has been shown that inactivation of E2 in the HPV16 genome increases E6/E7 transcription (Soeda et al., 2006), and that mutation of E8^E2C in the HPV31 or HPV16 genome increases the genome copy number and the E6/E7 transcription, suggesting that the transcriptional repressing by E8^E2C has an important role in viral replication (Lace et al., 2008). It was also noted that the E2C domain not only mediates specific DNA binding but has also an additional role in transcriptional repression by recruitment of co-repressors, such as the CHD6 protein. This suggests that repression of the E6/E7 promoter by E2 and E8^E2C involves multiple interactions with host cell proteins through different protein domains (Fertey et al., 2010).

E4 protein

Despite being considered an early protein, E4 is exclusively located in the differentiated layers of the infected epithelium (zur Hausen, 1996). Although its expression occurs in highly differentiated cells that express the capsid genes and synthesize new progeny virions, and coincides with the onset of vegetative viral DNA replication, E4 is not found in virion particles. The role of this protein in the virus life cycle has not yet been determined, but E4 is not required for transformation or episomal persistence of viral DNA, but interacts with the keratin networks and causes their collapse (Doorbar et al., 1991).

It has been suggested that E4 may have an important role in favoring and supporting the HPV genome amplification, besides regulating the expression of late genes, controlling the virus maturation, and facilitating the release of virions (Londgworth & Laimins 2004). E4 also interacts with and disrupts the organization of intermediate filaments. The role of E4 in providing the release of virus is supported by the association of E4 with the cornified cell envelope (CCE), a highly resistant structure under the plasmatic membrane of differentiated keratinocytes in the stratum corneum. Furthermore, E4 may play role in regulating gene expression and has been shown to induce G2 arrest in a variety of cell types (Londgworth & Laimins 2004).

E5 protein

The E5 protein is a small hydrophobic peptide, approximately 83 amino acids in size that localizes primarily to the endoplasmic reticulum. When expressed alone, HPV E5 has weak oncogenic properties. But in tissue culture assays, HPV E5 can enhance the transforming activity of E6 and E7, suggesting that it may have a supportive role in tumor progression. The localization of E5 to the endoplasmic reticulum suggests its activity may be related to the trafficking of cytoplasmic membrane proteins through this cellular compartment. E5 has also been reported to alter the activity of the epidermal growth factor receptor (EGFR), in addition to reducing the surface levels of major histocompatibility complex (MHC) class I proteins, modulating the MAPK pathway and altering the levels of caveolin 1 (Moody & Laimins, 2010).

The E5 protein varies in length and primary amino acid sequence among the different papillomaviruses, but maintains its hydrophobic nature that promotes fusion between cells (Hu et al., 2009). HPV16 E5 has all the characteristics of fusogenic proteins, including localization in plasma membrane, high level of hydrophobicity, and the ability for dimmers. Moreover, HPV16 E5 has been identified to be necessary and sufficient to induce cell-cell fusion with formation of tetraploid cell and cytokinesis failure (Hu et al., 2009).

The fusogenic activity of the HR-HPV E5 protein contributes to fusion among cells generating aneuploidy with tetraploid cells and chromosomal instability. These events seem to precede and favor integration of HPV genomes, which in turn, leads to expression of viral-cellular fusion transcripts and further enhances expression of the E6-E7 genes, rendering transformed cells strong growth advantages (Ziegert et al., 2003). Thus, the cell fusion HR-HPV E5-induced and cell cycle deregulation seems to have an important role in the early stages of the transformation process. This suggests that HR-HPV E5-induced cell fusion can be a critical event in the early stage of the development of HPV-associated cervical cancer (Gao and Zheng et al., 2010).

As the E5 gene is frequently deleted in cervical cancers, it is believed that the E5 protein may play a role in the early stages of the process of cellular transformation, but is dispensable for the maintenance of malignant transformation (zur Hausen, 1996).

E6 protein

The HPV E6 protein is formed by approximately 150 amino acids and contains two zinc-like fingers joined by an interdomain linker of 36 amino acids, flanked by short amino (N) and carboxy (C) terminal domains of variable lengths (Howie et al., 2009). The best known property of the E6 proteins of HR-HPVs is the ability to bind and degrade the tumor-suppressor protein p53, through the recruitment of the E6-associated protein (E6-AP), a cellular E3 ligase that does not bind to p53 in the absence of E6. Both E6 proteins from HR-HPV and LR-HPV bind to p53, but the interaction is stronger in HR-HPV (Lechner et al., 1994).

The E6 protein can overcome the cell arrest and proapoptotic activities of p53 by targeting p53 for degradation, inactivating the Mdm2 pathway. E6 can also inhibit the transcriptional activities of p53 independently of E6-AP (Thomas et al., 2005). Three different mechanisms have been proposed to explain this p53 inactivation: The first is inhibiting the binding of p53 to its target sequence in the genome; second, E6 may be able to inhibit p53 signaling by maintaining it in cytoplasm; and third, the mechanism employed by E6 to inhibit p53 activity is the abrogation of the transactivation of p53 responsive genes via interaction with either the CBP/p300 or hADA3 histone acetyltransferases. The E6 proteins have been shown to bind to p300, and this interaction inhibits p35 acetylation at p53 dependent sites, leading to decreased expression from p53. However, unlike p300, E6 interaction with hADA3 results in hADA3 degradation (Kumar et al., 2002). E6 may also inhibit p53 activation by blocking the p14/ARF pathway. Thus, E6 is able to modulate transcription of p53-dependent genes by both degradation of p53 and by interaction with the p300 and hADA3 transactivators (Shamanin et al., 2008).

The degradation or blocking of the p53 function inhibit apoptotic signaling that would eliminate the HPV infection cell. There are two major apoptotic pathways that can be triggered by different stresses: the extrinsic and intrinsic pathways. The E6 protein is able to disrupt both pathways to facilitate a cytoprotective environment and prevent cell death (Howie et al., 2009).

In addition, E6 is able to modulate transcription from other cellular signaling pathways as well as potentiating its ability to act as a diverse modulator of host cell signaling. It has been shown that E6 interact with three different proteins, such as a novel protein termed E6-targeted protein 1 (E6TP1) in an E6-AP dependent manner (Wooldridge et al., 2007), beyond another protein with GAP activity, tuberin, that can also be bound and degraded by E6 (Zeng et al. 2008). Furthermore, HR-HPV E6 has been shown to interact with two proteins that are part of the innate immune response to viral infection: interferon regulatory factor-3 (IFR-3) and toll-like receptor 9 (TLR9) (Hasan et al., 2007). Exogenous expression of HPV16 E6/E7 has been shown to inhibit TLR9 transcription, leading to a functional loss of TLR9 signaling pathways within the cell (Hasan et al., 2007).

HR-HPV E6 is also able to interact with members of the PDZ family of proteins, promoting its proteasome-mediated degradation, an activity that seems to be required for induction of cervical cancer (Shai et al., 2007). HR-HPV E6 PDZ binding can mediate suprabasal cell proliferation and this is thought to occur by uncoupling the cell proliferation and polarity control that exist in a differentiated epithelium (Sterlinko et al., 2004). LR-HPV E6 does not contain the PDZ-binding motif and therefore cannot target these proteins. Degradation of PDZ proteins results in cellular transformation due to loss of cell-cell contact and loss of cell polarity (Storrs and Silverstein, 2007). In addition, it has been demonstrated that the degradation of phosphatase PTPN13 by E6 results in anchorage-independent growth and a Ras-dependent invasive phenotype (Spanos et al., 2008).

Another function of the HR-HPV E6 protein that is important for immortalization is their ability to activate the expression of the catalytic subunit of telomerase (hTERT). Thus, the E6 protein is able to promote the maintanance of the telomere, through the action of telomerase. Interestingly, over-expression of hTERT in conjunction with E7 is sufficient to immortalize human primary keratinocytes. The HPV E2 proteins are reported to repress hTERT promoter activity, but the interplay of E6 and E2 during the regulation of this promoter has not been investigated (Hamid et al., 2009).

E7 protein

The E7 protein has around 100 amino acids in length and contains three conserved regions: CR1, CR2, and CR3 (Münger and Howley, 2002). It will induce cellular proliferation by binding to several cellular factors. The best characterized of these interactions is with the RB tumor suppressor and the related family members p107 and p130. The binding of high-risk E7 to pRB disrupts the interaction between pRB and E2F, a family of transcription factors, resulting in the constitutive expression of E2F-responsive genes, such as cyclin A and cyclin E, and promotes premature S phase entry, DNA synthesis, and the progression of cell cycle (Zerfass et al., 1995). Thus, in cells overexpressing the HPV E7 protein, this checkpoint control at G1/S transition is lost and the cells will continue their cell cycle, causing an uncontrolled cellular proliferation. Moreover, E7 induces the degradation of pRb via the proteasome-dependent pathway, using a mechanism that involves association with and reprogramming of the cullin 2 ubiquitin ligase complex (Jo & Kim, 2005; Huh et al., 2007).

HPV E7 can also associate directly with cdk2/cyclin A and cylin E complexes, resulting in an increased cdk2 activity (Nguyen & Münger, 2008). Another action of E7 that contributes to cellular immortalization is its interaction with the CDK inhibitors (CKI) p21 and p27, efficiently neutralizing their inhibitory effects on CDK2 activities, an important factor for G1 to S phase entry and progression (Moody & Laimins, 2010). The ability of E7 to inactivate these CKIs may contribute to its capacity to abrogate TGF-β mediated growth inhibition. Moreover, TGF-β also induces a cdk4/cdk6 specific CKI, P15Inkb, and p15Inkb-induced growth suppression, and these actions may require functional pRB, which is targeted for degradation by E7 (McLaughlin-Drubin & Münger, 2009). High-risk E7 has further been shown to increase the levels of the CDC25A phosphatase, which can induce tyrosine dephosphorylation of CDK2, promoting its activation (Moody & Laimins, 2010).

E7 also affects the expression of S phase genes by directly interacting with E2F factors and with histone deacetylases (HDAC): E7-E2F6 interaction prevents repression of gene expression by E2F6, maintaining a S phase environment conductive for viral replication

(McLaughlin-Drubin et al., 2008), and E7-HDAC binding facilitates HDAC removal at promoters to activate transcription (Longworth & Laimins, 2004).

Another major apoptotic pathway targeted by HPV proteins is anoikis, a form of apoptosis that is triggered when normal cells attempt to divide in the absence of a matrix (Tasaki et al., 2005). E6 and E7 interact with some factors involved with anoikis, such as paxillin, fibulin 1, and p600 (Huh et al., 2005), promoting the prevention of anoikis.

Furthermore, E6 and E7 interfere with the effects of various growth inhibitory cytokines that are induced following infection. High-risk HPV proteins repress the transcription of many IFN-inducible genes (Chang & Laimins, 2000; Kanodia et al., 2007; Tindle, 2002) and block apoptosis binding to TNF receptor 1, inhibiting the formation of the death-inducing signaling complex and consequent transduction of apoptotic signals (Filippova et al., 2002). The exsposure to E7 in a non-inflammatory epithelial environment can also be sufficient to induce a peripheral tolerance to E7 in the cytotoxic T lymphocytes population (Tindle, 2002).

E6 also interacts with the adaptor protein FAS-associated protein with death domain (FADD) and caspase 8 to block cell death in response to FAS and TRAIl. Also, E6 can interfere with induction of the extrinsic and intrinsic (mitochondrial) apoptotic pathways through interactions with the pro-apoptotic Bcl2 members BAK and BAX, as well as by upregulation of the inhibitors of apoptosis such as the inhibitor of apoptosis protein 2 (IAP2, also known as BIRC2) and survivin (also known as BIRC5) (Garnett & Duerksen-Huges, 2006).

L1 protein

The L1 gene corresponds to a sequence of about 1200 base pairs, which encodes a structural protein highly conserved among different HPV types, the (Xu et al., 2006). The L1 protein is formed by five monomeric units of 55kDa that join to form a pentameric structure, totaling 72 per each capsid (Buck et al., 2008). The L1 protein is highly immunogenic and has conformational epitopes that induce the production of neutralizing type-specific antibodies against the virus, which prevent the infection (Carter et al., 2003), making it the target of prophylactic vaccines (Villa et al., 2007; D'Andrilli et al., 2010).

Comparison among L1 sequences of different papillomaviruses suggests a conserved heparin-binding domain at the C-terminus, and the cleavage of this domain from L1 prevents binding to both heparin and human keratinocytes (Culp et al., 2006; Selinka et al., 2007). Thus, it is believed that the L1 major capsid protein contains the major determinant required for initial attachment of the viral particles to cell surface receptors, HSPGs, and therefore has an important role in infection (Schiller et al., 2010).

L2 protein

L2 is a secondary component of viral capsid and it is present in a variable number of copies per each capsid, being located on the inner surface in the central cavity below the pentamers of L1, where they are arranged to form the capsid (Buck et al., 2008). Despite the paucity of L2 in the virion, this protein has recently been shown to have many more functions than a simple structural role. L2 contributes to the binding of virion in the cell receptor, favoring its uptake, transport to the nucleus, and delivery of viral DNA to replication centers. Besides, E2 helps the packaging of viral DNA into capsids and, due to the presence of a usual neutralization epitope in L2 proteins of many papillomaviruses, it may be instrumental in conferring immunity across different types of HPV. L2 also contributes to the interaction of virion in the cell surface. Two distinct regions in the N-terminal protein of L2 interact with the cell surface, and this interaction occurs after an initial low-specificity interaction between L1 and the cell surface. After this, a conformational switch occurs in the capsid, exposing the L2 epitopes and promoting interactions with a more specific secondary receptor. The cleavage of the N-terminus of L2 is necessary for the binding of L1 to the secondary receptor, an indication that L2 has an important role in HPV infection (Schiller et al., 2010) .

Protein	Functions
E1	Viral DNA replication
E2	Control of viral transcription, DNA replication, and segregation of viral genomes.
E4	Favor and support the HPV genome amplification, besides regulating the expression of late genes, controlling the virus maturation, and facilitating the release of virions
E5	Enhance the transforming activity of E6 and E7; Promotes fusion between cells, generating aneuploidy and chromosomal instability; Contribute to immune response evasion.
E6	Bind and degrade the tumor-suppressor protein p53, inhibiting apoptosis; Interact with proteins of the innate immune response, contributing to immune evasion and persistence of virus;Activate the expression of telomerase.
E7	Bind and degrade the tumor-suppressor protein pRB; Increase cdk activity; Affects the expression of S phase genes by directly interacting with E2F factors and with histone deacetylases; Induce a peripheral tolerance in cytotoxic T lymphocytes (CTL) and Downregulate the expression of TLR9, contributing to immune response evasion
L1	Major capsid protein; contains the major determinant required for attachment to cell surface receptors. It is highly immunogenic and has conformational epitopes that induce the production of neutralizing type-specific antibodies against the virus.
L2	Minor capsid protein; L2 contributes to the binding of virion in the cell receptor, favoring its uptake, transport to the nucleus, and delivery of viral DNA to replication centers. Besides, E2 helps the packaging of viral DNA into capsids.

Table 1. The HPV proteins and functions

3. HPV Infection

The HR-HPVs have the ability to infect several types of epithelial cells, but they can cause cancer more frequently in the uterine cervix (Timmons et al., 2010). The cervical cancer arises preferentially in the cervical transformation zone (TZ), located in the boundary between the squamous epithelium of ectocervix and the columnar epithelium of endocervix. Basal cells in the TZ retain the ability to differentiate, a property required for virion production (Crum & McKeon, 2010). The basal cells in TZ are more susceptible to HPV infection in that there are fewer overlying layers than in other locations. In addition, the presence of hormones, such as estrogen and progesterone, that orchestrate cervical changes during menstruation and childbirth, can help both HPV infection and cancer development (Timmons et al., 2010; Roberts et al., 2007; Chung et al., 2008).

It has been reported that two types of cells are present in the basal layer of cervix. The first type comprises the transit amplifying (TA) cells, which are proliferating cells that are able to undergo terminal differentiation. TA cells divide and differentiate, representing the majority of cells in the suprabasal layers. The second class of basal cells is the stem cells, which have unlimited proliferation potential but divide only rarely in order to replenish the TA pool, serving as reserve cells to enable long-term maintenance of the tissue. Only one daughter cell of a stem cell division goes on to become a TA cell, while the other remains a stem cell. It is unclear which cells in the basal layer are the target of HPV infection, and perhaps both cell classes can be infected. If this is true, infection of stem cells could lead to one long-term persistent infection, whereas infection of TA cells could lead to short-term infections, followed by a cure (Jones et al., 2007).

Studies in vitro and in vivo revealed that the L1 major capsid protein contains the major determinant required to the initial attachment of the viral particles to the cell surface receptor, the heparan sulfate proteoglycans (HSPGs). Laminin-5 can also contribute to the binding of viral capsids to the extracellular matrix (ECM) in the epithelial cell lines (Culp et al., 2006; Selinka et al., 2007).

In vivo, the viral particles bound efficiently to regions of the basement membrane (BM) only after these regions had been exposed by mechanical or chemical trauma of the epithelium. The L1 capsid protein binds to HSPGs in segments of the BM exposed after epithelial trauma. After this, L1 undergoes a conformational change that exposes the N-terminus of the L2 minor capsid protein, which is cleaved by furin or the closely related protein convertase (PC) 5 and 6 (Richards et al., 2006). L2 proteolisis exposes a previously occluded surface of L1 that binds to an undetermined cell surface receptor on keratinocytes that have migrated over the BM to close the wound. This receptor is still unknown, but in vitro studies indicate the α6-integrin as a possible candidate (Kines et al., 2009). The cleavage of L2 may be necessary due to the fact that the surface intact of the epithelia apparently contains sulfation patterns that do not bind capsids. Binding to the BM may promote the preferential interaction with basal keratinocytes that are migrating over the exposed BM to close the wound. Thus, papillomaviruses (PV) are the only viruses that initiate the infectious process at an extracellular site (Schiller et al., 2010).

The capsids are internalized via the keratinocytes-surface receptor and subsequently surf toward the cell body. The first phase in infection is the internalization, which usually occurs 2-4 h after cell surface binding (Culp et al., 2004). The pathway involved in internalization and intracellular trafficking is still unclear, but it seems to occur slowly and asynchronously over a span of several hours (Schiller et al., 2010). Clatrin-mediated endocytosis has been pointed out to be like the endocytic pathway for the majority of HPV types. However, some studies suggest that they can enter through a caveolae-mediated pathway and not via clatrin-mediated endocytosis (Smith et al., 2007). On the other hand, it has been proposed that HPV-16 initially enters via clatrin-coated pits but the traffic occurs through caveosomes to eventually reach the endoplasmic reticulum (Hindmarsh et al., 2007; Laniosz et al., 2008). Moreover, it has been suggested that the capsids might be internalized via a novel pathway involving tetraspanin-enriched microdomains (Spoden et al., 2008).

The uncoating is not observed until 8-12 h after cell surface binding, and it seems that L2 has a critical role in the endosome escape (Kamper et al., 2006). The cytoplasm transport along microtubules is mediated by protein complex, and L2 has been found to interact with the microtubule network via the motor protein dynein during infectious entry (Florin et al., 2006). After the entry of the viral genome into the nucleus, the complexes predominantly localize in distinct punctate nuclear domains designated as ND10 bodies or promyelotic leukemia (PML) oncogenic domains (PODs). There is evidence that cell division is required for establishment and expression of the viral genome in the nucleus (Pyeon et al., 2009).

4. Life cycle of HPV

The HPV life cycle begins with infection of stem cells in the basal layer of the epithelium. After the entry in the cells, the virus requires the expression of E1 and E2 genes to maintain a low number of copies of genome. These proteins bind to the viral origin of replication and recruit cellular DNA polymerases and other proteins necessary for DNA replication (Hamid et al., 2009). In the suprabasal layer, the expression of genes E1, E2, E5, E6 and E7 contributes to the maintenance of the viral genome and induces cell proliferation , increasing the number of HPV-infected cells in the epithelium, resulting in a higher number of cells that will eventually produce infectious virions (Hamid & Gston, 2009; Lazarczyk et al., 2009). In the more differentiated cells of this same layer of the epithelium occurs the activation of differentiation-dependent promoter and maintenance of gene expression E1, E2, E6 and E7. Furthermore, there will be activation of the expression of E4 gene, whose product will induce amplification of the viral genome replication, greatly increasing the number of virus copies per cell, at the same time that occurs the expression of genes L1 and L2 (Nakahara et al., 2005; Lazarczyk et al., 2009). In the granular layer, the products of late genes, the major and minor proteins of the viral capsid, L1 and L2 respectively, gather to assembly of the viral capsids and formations of virions, which reach cornified layer of the epithelium and are released (Lazarczyk et al., 2009).

For a better understanding, the life cycle of HPV was divided into two parts: a maintenance phase and differentiation-dependent phase (Bodily & Laimins, 2011).

4.1 Maintenance phase

HPV virions infect cells in the basal epithelial layer that become exposed through microlesions. The viral capsid binds initially to the basal cell layer and infection occurs when activated keratinocytes move into the wound, to the upper layers of the epithelium (Kines et al., 2009). HPV genomes replicate in the nucleus of the basal cell layer, where the viral replication is considered nonproductive and the virus establishes itself as a low-copy-number episome by using the host DNA replication machinery (Moody & Laimins, 2010). In this way, viral proteins are expressed at very low levels in undifferentiated cells, and this contributes to immune avasion and persistence (Bodily & Laimins, 2011).

The maintenance of the viral episome in basal cells is the basic function of the early or maintenance phase of the viral cycle. The expression of E6, E7, E1, and E2 are necessary for continued episomal maintenance. E1 and E2 cooperate to initiate viral DNA replication, whereas E6 and E7 modulate cell-cycle regulators to maintain long-term replication competence (Conger et al., 1999). The E2 protein is probably a major regulator of this process because it is able to make both positive and negative control of the early viral promoter that regulates expression of E6, E7, and E1 as well as E2 itself (Steger et al., 1997).

Following this establishment phase, viral DNA is replicated coordinately with host cell chromosomes, and virus genomes are distributed to the daughter cells. However, in the differentiated keratinocytes of the suprabasal layers of the epithelium, the virus switches to a rolling-circle mode of DNA replication, amplifying its DNA to a high copy number, synthesizing capsid proteins, and assembling the viral particle (Flores et al., 1999).

HPV replication begins when the host cell factors interact with the LCR region of the HPV genome and begin the transcription of the early viral genes, highlighting the E6 and E7. The viral E6 and E7 gene products deregulate the cell cycle, subverting the cell growth-regulatory pathways and modifying the cellular environment in order to faclitate viral replication in a cell that is terminally differentiated and has exited the cell cycle (Syrjânen & Syrjânen, 1999)

4.2 Differentiation-dependent phase

During the maintenance phase in undifferentiated cells, viral proteins are expressed in extremely low levels. However, when HPV-infected cells leave the basal layer, they undergo differentiation and high levels of viral proteins synthesis are induced. This restriction of viral protein synthesis to highly differentiated cells delays the expression of viral antigens to locations less susceptible to the host immune response (Frazer, 2009).

This compartimentalization of gene expression by HPVs constitutes an important strategy to sustain long-term infection, but it creates some problems for the virus. To solve this, the virus forces the cell to remain active in the cell cycle, enabling productive replication in differentiating cells. The viral protein E7 is responsible for maintaining the replication competence in differentiated cells and this is accomplished in part by inactivation of pRB family members (Münger et al., 2004). The activation of the late viral promoter in response to host-cell differentiation occurs in the vicinity of the spinous epithelial layer and is responsible for high levels of viral protein expression. As a result, the virus copy-number amplifies from 50-200 copies to several thousands of copies per cell (Bedell et al., 1991).

The viral proteins E1, E4, and E5 contribute to the activation of late viral functions upon differentiation (Wilson et al., 2005; Fehrmann et al., 2003). The E2-mediated down-regulation of E6 and E7 transcription results in the release of the p53 and pRB cellular proteins, and allows the normal differentiation process of the host cell. Then, a putative late promoter activates the capsid genes, L1 and L2. Finally, the viral particles are assembled in the nucleus, and the complete virions are released when the cornified layers of the epithelium are shed. The virions are shed in an environment with desquamated cells in the absence of lysis or necrosis, and this further contributes to virus persitence because it avoids inflammation (Stanley, 2008).

Most women infected with a specific HPV type will not show evidence of that same type after 6-12 months. It is not known whether the HR-HPV can be detected for periods similar to those for LR-HPV. Some studies show similar duration (Richardson et al., 2003), but others reveal longer durations of infection for HR-HPV types (Franco et al., 1999; Ho et al., 1998). It appears that HR-HPV, particularly HPV16, has a longer time to clearance and is more likely to develop persistent infection (Richardson et al., 2003).

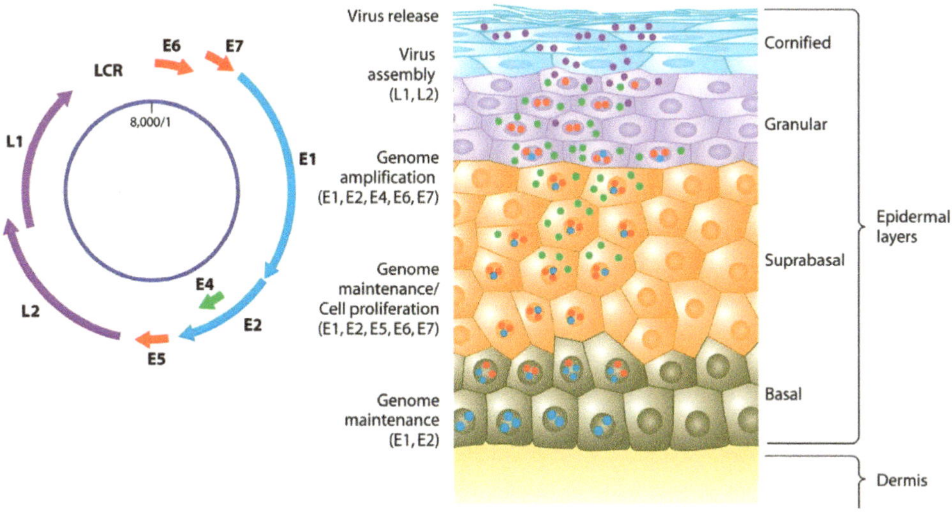

Fig. 2. HPV Cycle life (copied from Lazarczyk et al., 2009, with permission of the author).

5. Pathogenesis

5.1 Persistence x clearance

The infection with HR-HPV typically lasts from 12 -18 months and is eventually cleared by the immune system (Richardson et al., 2003). However, approximately 10% of women fail to clear HPV infections, resulting in a persistent infection. The main consequence of persistent infection with HR-HPV is the development of lesions that may progress to malignancy, and this constitutes the most important risk factor for the development of cervical cancer (Stanley, 2008; Bodily & Laimins; Moody & Laimins, 2010;).

Details about the immune response that results in clearance of HPV infection are still unknown. HPV clearance seems to result in long-term humoral and/or cellular protection against re-infection by the same HPV type; whether the protection is lifelong is not known (Stanley, 2006). Although the term clearance is used when an HPV infection can no longer be detected using sensitive test methods, the HPV presence might not be completely discarded because the latent state of HPV is still poorly understood. Reappearance of HPV from latency even in the absence of definite immunosuppression is common, but most cases are probably benign (Gonzalez et al., 2010). By contrast to HPV infections that clear, the risk of cancer increases dramatically in persistent HPV infections (Schiffman et al., 2010).

It is important to remember that it is not easy to characterize a persistent HPV infection and differentiate persistent infection from healing followed by re-infection, although re-infection with the same HPV type appears to be uncommon. Many studies classify HPV infection as persistent if the HPV was detected in two consecutive follow-up visits 4-6 months apart. However, because the interval between follow-up visits varies among studies and there are many unknown questions regarding the natural history of HPV, it is complicated to distinguish persistent and transience infections. Furthermore, an undetectable HPV infection could be a period of viral latency, in which the HPV levels are below the detectable threshold of current HPV DNA assays, instead of representing a cleared host (Baseman and Koutsky, 2005).

The persistent nature of HPV infection and DNA viral integration into the genome of the cell contributes to increasing the risk of high-grade and malignant lesions because of genomic instability generated. E6 and E7 can induce centrosomal abnormalities resulting in abnormal centrosome reduplication, leading to abnormal numbers of centrosomes Furthermore, abrogation of cell-cycle checkpoints through the targeting of p53 and pRB family members allows retention of cells with chromosomal abnormalities (Münger et al., 2004). This can result in genetic changes that accumulate over an extended period of time until resulting in a combination of genetic abnormalities, allowing cancer development (Bodily & Laimins, 2011).

In benign and malignant HPV lesions, the cellular proliferation increases the demand for nutrients, generating a competition for nutrients and oxygen. To overcome this constraint, both HR-HPV and LR-HPV E7 proteins enhance the levels of the transcription factor Hypoxia-inducible factor-1 (HIF-1), as well as induce the increased expression of HIF-1 target genes under hypoxia conditions (Nakamura et al., 2009). The enhancement of HIF-1 activity results in an increased transcription of a subset of genes that favor angiogenesis, and this induction of angiogenesis is crucial to both persistence and growth of HPV lesions (Bodily & Laimins, 2011).

5.2 Mechanism of immune evasion

HPV infections are chronic, exclusively local and intraepithelial in which the virus remains in the host for many months, even years, during which the mechanisms of host defense apparently remains ignorant of the pathogen for long period of time Stanley, 2009b). So, the immune response to HPV infection is often insufficient to eliminate the virus so that the infected individuals do not heal but develop persistent infection. The main reason for this is an ingenious strategy developed by this virus in which viral DNA replication and virus assembly occur in a cell that will be terminally differentiated and die by natural causes (Staney, 2008). To achieve this lifestyle, HPV must avoid the host defense sytem, and the key to understanding how this occurs is the virus replication cycle which itself is an immune evasion mechanism that inhibits the host´s detection of the virus. The infection and vegetative HPV growth are absulotely dependent upon a complete program of keratinocyte differentiation (Doorbar, 2005).

Papillomavirus late genes also contain codons that mammalian cells rarely use, implying that production of abundant papillomavirus capsid proteins is inhibited in mammalina basal-epithelial cells by the restricted availability of the appropriated tRNAs. The early viral proteins localize mainly to the nucleus, and they are produced in insufficient quantities and/or are not aceesible for immune recognition (Tindle, 2002). Besides, there is viral-induced cytolysis or necrosis, and therefore no inflammation. For most of the duration of the

HPV infectious cycle, there is little or no release into the local milieu of pro-infammatory cytokines, which are important for antigen presenting cell (APC) activation and migration. This way, the central signals to kickstart the immune response in squamous epithelia are absent (Stanley, 2006).

Even in the absence of cellular changes such as cytolysis, necrosis, or cell death, HPV-infected keratinocytes should activate to the production of type 1 interferons, a powerful, generic antiviral and innate immune defense system. The type 1 Interferons, IFN-α and IFN-β, have antiviral, antiproliferative, antiangiogenic, and immunostimulatory properties that act as a bridge between innate and adaptative immunity, activating immature DCs (Le Bon & Tough, 2002). High-risk HPV types actively inhibit the endogenous interferon response, down-regulate toll-like receptors and this combined with the low levels of viral protein generated during the infectious cycle and absence of infammation leads to inefficient activation of the innate immune response, with the consequent ineffectiveness of the adaptive immune response. Thus, the milieu becomes operationally HPV antigen-tolerant and host defences become irrevocably compromised. HPV antigen-specific effector cells are both poorly recruited to the focus and their activity is down-regulated (Stanley, 2009b).

It was demonstrated that infection with HR-HPV, especially HPV 16, downregulates IFN-α inducible gene expression, through E6 and E7 proteins that directly interact with components of the interferon signaling pathways (Konodia et al., 2007). Infected cells with episomal HPV are cleared after exposure to IFN-β, but cells with integrated HPV-DNA are resistant to this antiviral effect (Pett et al., 2006). T-cell response to E2 and E6 are lost or reduced in CIN 3 and carcinoma invasive. Thus, even if HPV antigen-specific cytotoxic T-cells have been generated, regulatory T-cells increasingly dominate the lesion and abrogate the killer defense response (Kobayashi et al., 2004). High-risk HPV infected cervical keratinocytes expressing high level risk of E6 and E7 oncoproteins are not killed in this immunosuppressive tolerante mileu, nad progression to high-grade disease and cancer can result (Stanley, 2009b).

As HPV infections are exclusively intraepithelial, theoretically, an HPV attack would be detected by the professional APC cells of squamous epithelia, the Lanherhans cells (LCs), which are the intraepithelial dendritic cells (DCs). Virus capsid entry is usually an activating signal for CDs, but there is evidence that LCs are not activated by the uptake of HPV capsids. The life cycle of HPV is organized to form a limited viral antigen synthesis in undifferentiated cells, and high-expression is restricted to highly differentiated cells.

HPV replication and release does not cause cell death and inflammation since the differentiating keratinocyte is already programmed to die and this death by natural causes does not act as a danger signal in the infected site (Staley, 2009b). Besides, the absence of viremia, cell lysis, necrosis, or any other signals to trigger an inflammatory response reduces the possibility of an effective immune response in this site (Stanley, 2009a). Thus, the virus becomes pratically invisible to the host who remains indifferent to infection for long periods of time, facilitating the viral persistence (Staley, 2009b)

The healing of the HPV-induced lesions is dependent on the mechanisms of the cell-mediated immune response and is accompanied by interaction of CD8+ and CD4+ limphocytic. Langerhans cells (LCs) are the major dendritic cells (DCs) found in squamous epithelia, and these are probably responsible for triggering an anti-HPV immune response.

The function of LCs is disrupted by HPV at several levels. It has been shown that the infiltration of HPV-infected tissue by LCs and DCs is inhibited by HPV-induced changes in the pattern of cytokine expression (Stanley, 2008). The HPV L2 protein is able to suppress maturation, migration, and cytokine secretion by LCs. Furthermore, the interaction between LCs and keratinocytes can be disrupted by the reduction of E-caderin levels induced by the E6 HPV protein (Ghittoni et al., 2010).

In immunosuppressed patients, HPV infection frequently leads to the appearance of abundant HPV-induced lesions, indicating that the immune system acts to limit HPV infection (Scott et al., 2001). Therefore, in order to persist, HPV must actively suppress both innate and adaptative immune response. One important mechanism of the innate pathway targeted by HPV acting in multiple ways is the interferon response (Samuel, 2001; Stanley, 2008). Keratinocytes constitutively express a low level of interferon-inducible genes in absence of interferon. The cells infected with HR-HPV express E6 and E7, which repress the transcription of many interferon target genes including Stat-1, a transcriptional activator of Interferon-inducible genes (Nees et al., 2001). E6 can bind to and block the action of IRF-3, a regulator of the interferon pathway and also blocks activation of protein kinase R (PKR) as well as the activity of kinase Tyk2, responsible for activating Stat-1, while E7 can bind to IRF-1, that is also a regulator of the interferon pathway (Hebner et al., 2006; Stanley, 2009b). Both E6 and E7 can inhibit expression of the toll-like receptor (TLR9), which is important for sensing doubled-stranded DNA (Hasan et al., 2007).

It is well known that keratinocytes constitutively express low levels of several cytokines that are upregulated following virus infection (Ghittoni et al., 2010). When these cells are infected with HPV show significantly reduced expression of the wide range of inlammatory cytokines including IL-1, IL-6, TNF-α, and TGF-β, at the same time, expression of the anti-inflammatory cytokine IL-10 is increased (Alcocer-Gonzalez et al., 2006; Ghittoni et al., 2010). Thus, HPV infection induces alteration in cytokine production, reducing the ability of immune cells to infiltrate the infected tissue. Keratinocytes constitutively express low levels of interferons α, β, and κ. The expression of interferon κ is suppressed in HPV positive cells and this could contribute to the inhibition of expression of interferon-inducible genes (Rincon-Orozco et al., 2009).

Development of HPV-specific T-cell response is repressed or delayed in HPV-infected patients, this effect being more pronounced in HR-HPV compared with LR-HPV infections (van der Burg and Palefsky, 2009). One reason for this impairment is probably the downregulation of major histocompatribiliy complex (MHC) I expression, probably due to interactions occuring between the viral proteins E6, E7, and E5 and the host cell. Furthermore E7 has been reported to downregulate the transporter associated with antigen processing (ATP), thereby interfering with presentation of antigens via the MHC I pathway (Ghittoni et al., 2010).

The expression of HPV E7 in epithelial cells does not directly impair, but rather slightly increase, MHC clase I expression. E7 expression is nevertheless associated with impairment of IFN-gama-induced enhancement of presentation of endogenous antigen to cytotoxic T lymphocytes (Zhou et al., 2011). Further mechanism of HPV-mediated immune escape involve viral proteins: HPV E7 has high and widespread similarity to several humans proteins, causing a limited immunogenicity (Natale et al., 2000); E6 can downregulate IL-18 expression (Cho et al., 2001); E5 mediate acidification of endossomes, affecting antigen processing and presentation in antigen presentation cells (Straight et al., 1995); E5 also downregulate CD1d, a MHC I-like glycoprotein that presents self or microbial lipid antigen to natural killer - the downregulation of this molecule is utilized by a variety of microbes to evade immune detection (Miura et al., 2010). Finally, natural killer (NK) cell activity is also reduced in patients with HR-HPV infection (Stanley, 2009a; O´Brien and Campos, 2002).

5.3 The role of the physiology of the cervical epithelium

The cervical and anal transformation or transition zones (TZs) are dynamic areas of a few millimeters in size, in which a columnar glandular epithelium coexists with a squamous epithelium, and result from an adaptive process called metaplasia (Mukonoweshuro et al., 2005). These metaplastic conversions are influenced by the acidification of vaginal pH and by trauma such as that resulting from receptive anal intercourse, and can be considered as a stepwise progression of changes. Although these adaptive responses frequently occur at the cervical and anal squamocolumnar junctions, the molecular mechanism underlying the development and the maintenance of the metapastic epithelium are still not completely understood (Herfs et al., 2011).

It is believed that this phenomenon could result from the reprogramming of adult stem cells and that the metaplastic epithelium is associated with a deregulated production of receptors, adhesion molecules, and soluble mediators of the inflammatory response, such as cytokines, chemokines, prostaglandins, and growth factors. These molecules might not only exercise influence epithelial differentiation but also alter the local antiviral immune response, favoring HPV infections. Importantly, a substantial majority of cervical and anal pre-neoplastic lesions develop within the metaplastic microenvironment of TZs (Bodily & Lamins, 2010). This implies that exogenous or endogenous factors specific to the anatomical milieu of squamocolumnar junctions could be conducive to persistent HPV infection (Herfs et al., 2011)

In contrast to normal squamous epithelium, metaplastic epithelia have an altered maturation characterized by a weak expression of several keratin intermediate filaments and cell envelope components such as involucrin and loricrin (Herfs et al., 2008). The primary function of keratins and other cytoskeletal proteins is to provide resistance to mechanical and non-mechanical stresses that can cause cell rupture and death. Thus, because of their immature state, keratinocytes of the squamocolumnar junctions could be more vulnerable to the trauma required for HPV infection (Gu & Colombe, 2007). Therefore, the increased sensitivity of anal and cervical TZs to pre-neoplastic lesions can be attributed to the fact that both the basement membrane and the target actively dividing basal cells for HPV infection could be more accessible in metaplastic areas in which monostratified glandular and pluristratified squamous coexist (Herfs et al., 2011).

Cervical TZs with squamous metaplasia have a higher density of estrogen and progesterone receptor-positive cells compared with normal squamous epithelia. Besides, the cervical TZs are more sensitive to the induction of squamous cell carcinogenesis by estrogen. Among the possible mechanisms by which sex hormones could facilitate HPV-induced carcinogenesis would be the stimulation of expression of E6 and E7 HPV genes, directly and/or indirectly through steroid response elements in the viral genome or still stimulating cellular proliferation (Bhattacharya et al., 1997; Yuan et al., 1999).

It is also possible that hormones sensitize the TZs to persistent HPV infection by altering the local immune microenvironment (Herfs et al., 2011). It has been observed that 17β estradiol can both reduce the migration and/or functional capacity of antigen-presenting cells and promotes the initiation of Th2 immune response, which is generally associated with the progression of the disease (Uemura et al., 2008). Together with these observations, the topography of the cervical TZs is affected by the hormonal status of women, suggesting that sex hormones might not only be involved in the development and maintenance of the metaplastic epithelium but might also be implicated in the high sensivity of TZs to HPV infection and cancer progression (Herfs et al., 2011).

Also observed was a reduction of secretion of soluble factors of innate immune response involved in antiviral defense in the anal and cervical squamocolumnar junctions (Herfs et al., 2010). The β-defensin 2 is weakly expressed in cervical TZs and pre-neoplastic lesions compared with normal exocervical (Hubert et al., 2007). Furthermore, the density of Langerin-positive Langerhans cells (LCs) and their function are significantly altered in the anal and cervical TZs compared with the normal squamous epithelia (Herfs et al., 2008; Giannini et al., 2002) suggesting that keratinocyte-LC interaction could play an important role in the establishment of HPV infection in these regions (Herfs et al., 2011). It was also suggested that a Th2 immunoderivation of immune response could participate in the immunological escape of virus-infected cells (Herfs et al., 2011).

Altering the local immune response, metaplastic cells might not only promote viral infections but might also be involved in the HPV-induced development of cervical and anal carcinoma in the TZs. This could explain, at least in part, why HPV-associated lesions located elsewhere in the anogenital tract outside the TZs, such as the vagina and vulva, are less likely to progress to cancer than those that develop within the TZs. Therefore, the anatomical, histological, physiological, and immunological features of TZs might not only promote the mucosal entry of HPV but also be involved in the HPV-induced development of cervical and anal carcinoma (Herfs et al., 2010).

5.4 The oncogenics activities of HPV

5.4.1 The role of the E5 protein

The hydrophobic E5 protein is mainly found within the Golgi apparatus, as well as in the plasma membranes of HPV-infected cells. The E5 protein has weak oncogenic properties, which results in the increasing expression for the epidermal growth factor receptor (EGFR) (Tsai & Chen, 2003) and in the inhibition of the expression of the major histocompatibility complex (MHC) class I on the plasma membrane modulating the MAPK pathway and altering the levels of caveolin 1 (Moody & Laimins, 2010).

The virus-induced cell fusion mediated by oncogenic viruses is a well-known event among human oncogenic viruses, including HPV, and it seems that this phenomenon plays an important role in the carcinogenesis process (Duelli et al., 2007; Hu et al., 2009). HPV16 E5 has all the characteristics of fusogenic proteins, including the localization of the plasma membrane, the high level of hydrophobicity, and the ability for dimmers. More recently, HPV16 E5 has been identified as necessary and sufficient to induce cell-cell fusion with the formation of the tetraploid cell (Hu et al., 2009).

Aneuploidy with the presence of tetraploid cells is frequently found in precancerous lesions associated with HPV infection. It is reported that expression of either HPV E6 or E7 alone is sufficient to deregulate cytokinesis and consequently produce the tetraploid cell (Heilman et al., 2009). However, it was demonstrated that the formation of these cells is primarily attributed to E5-induced cell fusion, rather than E6, E7, and cytokinesis failure (Ho et al., 2009). Tetraploid cells formed by accident cannot undergo normal mitosis which would trigger p53-dependent cell cycle arrest or apoptosis, whereas oncogenic virus-induced cell fusion is sufficient to induce chromosomal instability when fusion occurs concomitantly with expression of viral oncoproteins capable of perturbing p53 or apoptosis (Duelli et al., 2007).

In vivo and clinical studies reveal that chromosomal instability and aneuploidization seem to precede and favor integration of HPV genomes, which in turn leads to expression of viral-cellular fusion transcripts and further enhances expression of the E6-E7 genes, which renders the strong growth advantages of transformed cells (Ziegert et al., 2003). The cell fusion HR-HPVE5-induced and cell cycle deregulation are two key events for initiation of transformation. This suggests that HR-HPVE5-induced cell fusion can be a critical event in the early stage of development HPV-associated cervical cancer (Gao & Zheng, 2010). As the open reading frame coding E5 is frequently deleted in cervical cancer, it is possible that this viral protein is not required for tumor maintenance, but that it can play a critical role in the early stage of HPV-associated cervical cancer.

5.4.2 The role of the E6 protein

The E6 HPV protein binds not only to cellular p53 and E6-AP but also to a wide range of other cellular proteins, being known a more complete compendium of cellular factors that can interact with this viral oncoprotein. Among the other cellular proteins that interact with E6, the following may be cited: transcription factors such as p300, myc, interferon regulatory (IRF3), autocrine motility factor 1 (AMF-1/gPS2); factors that determine adhesion, cytoskeleton and polarity, such as paxillin, the human homologue of Drosophila disk-large tumor-suppressor gene product (DGL), and membrane-associated guanylate inverted-1 (MAGI-1); apoptosis factors such as the pro-apoptotic Bcl2 and Bak; replication factors and DNA repair factors such as mcm7 and XRCC1; and other cellular proteins such as E6 target protein 1 (E6TP1). In addition, E6 induces telomerase activity by inducing the expression of human telomerase reverse transcriptase (hTERT) (reviewed in IARC, 2007).

HR-HPV E6 proteins have a motif designated as S/TXV at their C-terminal which mediates binding to specific domains on cellular proteins known as PDZ proteins. PDZ domains are approximately 90 amino acid stretches found in a wide variety of cellular proteins. The importance of p53 in the orchestration of the cellular response to damage suffered by DNA as a result of exposure to cytotoxic agents becomes quite evident by the fact that approximately one-half of all human cancers present mutations in the p53 gene (Howie et al., 2009). Normally, p53 protein levels are regulated by the Mdm2 E3 ubiquitin ligase. However, Mdm2-mediated degradation of p53 is inhibited during viral infection and other stress conditions, allowing for stabilization of p53 protein levels and subsequent activation. In contrast, during an HR-HPV infection E6 induces p53 degradation by forming a complex with another E3 ubiquitin ligase, E6-AP. Only E6 HR-HPV is capable of binding to the core region of p53 and this binding of the core region is required for p53 degradation mediated by E6.

Three other mechanisms have been proposed to explain the interaction of the viral E6 protein with p53. The first is by inhibiting the binding of p53 to its site-specific DNA sequence. In the second mechanism, E6 may be able to inhibit p53 signaling independent of protein degradation by means of the sequestration of p53 in the cytoplasm. The third mechanism employed by E6 to inhibit p53 activity is its abrogation of the transactivation of p53 responsive genes via interaction with either the CBP/p300 or hADA3 histone acetyltransferases. The E6 proteins have been shown to bind to p300, and this interaction inhibits p35 acetylation at p53 dependent sites, leading to decreased expression from a p53 (Zimmermann et al., 2000). However, unlike with p300, E6 interaction with hADA3 results in hADA3 degradation (Kumar et al., 2002). E6 may also inhibit p53 activation by blocking the p14/ARF pathway (Shamanin et al., 2008).

Thus, E6 is able to modulate transcription of p53-dependent genes by both degradation of p53 and by interaction with the p300 and hADA3 transactivators. In addition, E6 is able to modulate transcription from other cellular signaling pathways as well as potentiate its ability to act as a diverse modulator of host cell signaling. With respect to G-protein signaling, E6 has been shown to interact with three different proteins, such as a novel protein termed E6-targeted protein 1 (E6TP1), in an E6-AP dependent manner (Lee et al., 2007), beyond another protein with GAP activity, tuberin, which also can be bound and degraded by E6 (Zeng et al., 2008).

High-risk E6 has been shown to interact with two proteins that are part of the innate immune response to viral infection: interferon regulatory factor-3 (IFR-3) and toll-like receptor 9 (TLR9) (Hasan et al., 2007). IRF-3 becomes activated by dsRNA or viral infection, and this activation leads to the transcription of interferon-beta (IFN-β) (Hiscott, 2007). TLR9 becomes activated by viral or bacterial dsDNA derived CpG motifs, and induces cytokine production as a means to defend the cell against the invading organism (Müller et al., 2008). Exogenous expression of HPV16 E6/E7 has been shown to inhibit TLR9 transcription, leading to a functional loss of TLR9 signaling pathways within the cell (Hasan et al., 2007).

The p53 degradation or blocking of its function mediated by E6 has, as a consequence, the inhibition of apoptotic signaling that would otherwise eliminate the HPV infected cell. There are two major apoptotic pathways that can be triggered by different stresses: the extrinsic and the intrinsic pathways. The E6 protein is able to disrupt both pathways to facilitate a cytoprotective environment and prevent cell death, thus highlighting the critical signaling events that a cell undergoes following exogenous or endogenous stress (Howie et al., 2009).

E6 is able to inhibit extrinsic apoptotic signaling at each of the stages, by interacting with TNFR-1, FADD, and caspase-8. It was shown that E6 is able to bind directly to the death receptor TNFR-1 and blocked TNFR-1 DD mediated apoptosis (Filippova et al., 2002). In addition to the TNF pathway, E6 is capable of inhibiting apoptosis stimulated by both Fas and TRAIL pathways. This inhibition is mediated by E6 binding to and degradation of both the FADD adapter protein and the effector caspase-8 (Garnett et al., 2006). As the binding of FADD is not dependent on the conserved PDZ domain of high-risk E6, but rather by a new domain (Tungteakkhun et al., 2008), it is possible that other E6 proteins may inhibit these extrinsic pathways.

HPV E6 proteins have been shown to inhibit intrinsic apoptotic pathway binding to Bak and to induce its proteasomal-dependent degradation (Underbrink et al., 2008). While E6-AP has been shown to play a role in Bak degradation, it has also been proposed that this may not be a universal mechanism for all of the HPV types (Simmonds & Story, 2008). Evidence has shown that Bak degradation is not constitutive, but rather occurs only after apoptotic signals have been initiated, indicating that a Bak conformational change and/or dissociation from its anti-apoptotic partner MCL-1 may be necessary for its interaction with E6 and E6-AP (Underbrink et al., 2008)

Another important effect of E6 in the development of genital cancer is the activation of telomerase reverse transcriptase (hTERT) (Howie et al., 2009). HPV E6 induces histone acetylation at the hTERT promoter, and this acetylation depends on E6-AP (James et al., 2006; Xu et al., 2008). To induce hTERT expression and telomerase activity in keratinocytes, HPV E6/E6-AP requires expression of NFX1-123 (Katzenellenbogen et al., 2007).

In addition to increasing the expression of hTERT, E6 also interacts with other proteins involved in maintaining chromosomal stability within the HPV-infected cell, for example, the minichromosome maintenance 7 (hMCM7) proteins. As MCM7 is involved in licensing DNA replication to ensure a single-round replication per cell cycle, it is thought that E6 interaction with and/or degradation of MCM7 may lead to chromosomal abnormalities in the HPV-infected cell. E6 can also interact with two proteins involved in single-strand DNA break repair: XRCC1 and O(6)-metylguanine-DNA methane transferase (MGMT). XRCC1 to be bound E6; this interaction reduces the ability of XRCC1 to repair metyl metane sulfate (MMS) induced DNA damage (Iftner et al., 2002). E6 interaction with MGMT induces its proteasomal-mediated degradation via E6-AP, which has been hypothesized to sensitize HPV-infected cells to alkylating DNA damage (Srivenugopal & Ali-Osman, 2002). Finally, high-risk E6 mediated p53 loss inactivates the G1 checkpoint. Prolonged proliferation in the absence pf p53 can lead to the loss of the G2 checkpoint, which can result in aneuplody. Together, these interactions may lead to increased genomic instability and accelerate the progression to carcinogenesis (Howie et al., 2009).

Another major apoptotic pathway targeted by HPV proteins is anoikis, a form of apoptosis that is triggered when normal cells attempt to divide in the absence of a matrix (Tasaki et al., 2005). E6 has been shown to bind to paxilin and zyxin, adhesion molecules involved in tethering the cellular cytoskeleton to the extra cellular matrix (ECM) and transmitting signals along the actin network from the ECM to the nucleus. This interaction results in the disruption of actin fibers and a failure to maintain proper cell structure (Howie et al., 2009). HR-HPVE6 proteins also bind to hScrib, a protein involved in epithelial tight junctions, mediating the adhesion of basal cells to the ECM, and at least in some cell types it has been shown that E6 mediates hScrib degradation (Nakagawa & Huibregtse, 2000). Recently, it has been demonstrated that PTPN3, a membrane-bound tyrosine phosphatase that regulates growth factor receptors, is also a PDZ protein that binds and is disrupted by E6 (Jing et al., 2007; Spanos et al., 2008).

5.4.3 The role of the E7 protein

HR-HPVE7 proteins destabilize pRb through its proteosomal degradation via a mechanism that involves association with and reprogramming of the cullin 2 ubiquitin ligase complex by HPV E7 (Huh et al., 2007). The induction of the pRB degradation by HR-HPVE7 proteins and the resulting activation of E2F-mediated transcription represent an important mechanism by which these viruses achieve and maintain S-phase competence in differentiated epithelial cells. HR-HPVE7 proteins, in addition to targeting pRb proteasomal degradation, also contribute to cell cycle deregulation through several additional mechanisms involving cyclin-dependent kinases (cdks), motors that drive the cell division cycle (Zerfass et al., 1995).

HPV16 E7 has been shown to interact with and abrogate the growth-inhibitory activities of the cyclin-dependent kinase inhibitors (CKIs) $p21^{CIP1}$ (Jones et al., 1997) and $p27^{KIP1}$ (Zerfass et al., 1996), which are induced by anti-proliferative signals, including growth factor withdrawal and loss of cellular adhesion (Fang et al., 1996). The ability of HPV E7 to abrogate CKIs, together with its ability to disrupt the pRB/E2F complex, which results in increased cyclin E and A levels, retains differentiating keratinocytes in a DNA synthesis competent state. HPV E7 can also directly associate with cdk2/cyclin A and cylin E complexes, resulting in increased cdk2 activity (Nguyen & Münger, 2008).

It was demonstrated that HPV16 E7 induces pRb degradation, but the mechanism of cell death depends on the integrity of the p53 tumor suppressor pathway; it does not involve transcriptional activation of canonical p53 transcriptional targets. Intriguingly, E7 expression generally interferes with the transcriptional activity of p53 (Eichten et al., 2002). Furthermore, the mechanism of cell death triggered by HPV16 E7 expression appears to be distinct from classic apoptosis; although caspases are active and DNA is degraded, cell death is mostly caspase independent (Eichten et al., 2004). Although HPV E7 signaling pathways have not yet been molecularly analyzed, HPV 16 E7 expression causes normal human epithelial cells to undergo cell death in response to growth factor deprivation (Zhou & Münger, 2009).

High- and low-risk HPV E7 proteins are associated with the 600 KD retinoblastoma protein-associated factor, p600 (DeMasi et al., 2005; Huh et al.,2005). Although its biological functions have not been fully elucidated in mammalian cells, p600 is implicated as a regulator of anoikis, a form of apoptosis that is triggered when normal cells attempt to divide in the absence of a matrix (Tasaki et al., 2005). Therefore, the interaction between E7 and p600 may deregulate anoikis and protect detached cells from apoptosis, thereby contributing to viral transformation (DeMasi et al., 2007; Huh et al., 2005). Consistent with this idea, HPV16 E7 associates with p600 through the CR1 domain, which is necessary for the transformation capability of HPV16 E7 (DeMasi et al., 2007).

It is known that HPV16 E7 can directly bind to E2F1 and enhance E2F1-mediated transcriptional. E2F1, which plays a role in mediating the transcriptional control of the E2F6 gene, which is unregulated at the G1/S-phase transition, to exert an opposing effect on the activities of E2F-responsive promoters, thereby directing appropriate cell cycle exit and differentiation (Lyons et al., 2006). Interestingly, HPV E7 associates with E2F6 and abrogates its ability to function as a transcriptional repressor (McLaughlin-Drubin et al., 2008), suggesting that the functional deregulation of E2F6 by HPV E7 is needed to counterbalance the up-regulation of E2F6 as a consequence of the activation of E2F1 by E7, thus ensuring that the cells remain in an S-phase-competent state, which is necessary for the viral cycle (McLaughlin-Drubin & Münger, 2009).

Malignant progression mediated by HR-HPVoncogene expression of these cells occurs after prolonged passages in culture or when additional oncogenes, such as *ras* or *fos*, are expressed (Pei et al., 1993). This is comparable to the extended period of time between initial HPV infection and the development of invasive cervical carcinoma. Thus, while the expression of the HPV oncogenes is necessary and sufficient for initiation of cervical carcinogenesis, additional host genome mutations are needed for malignant progression. Indeed, cervical cancer cells have accumulated a wide range of numerical and structural chromosomal abnormalities (Mitelman et al., 2007).

The presence of DNA repairs foci seen in HPV16 E7-expressing cells indicate that E7 may induce double-strand DNA breaks or interfere with break repair. This may facilitate viral genome integration. Consequently, E7 may be a driving force for integration of HR-HPVgenomes into host cellular chromosomes, an event that frequently accompanies malignant progression of high-risk HPV-associated lesions. This may result in double-stranded HPV DNA fragments breaking off of the circular genome and being integrated into the host genome via the endogenous DNA double-strand break (DSB) repair machinery. If the upstream regulatory region is integrated into the host DNA, it may be the site of continued "onion skin" replication as long as the viral E1 and E2 replication proteins are expressed (Kadaja et al., 2007).

Fanconi anemia (FA) patients have an increased incidence of squamous cell carcinomas at sites that are infected by HPVs, and oral cancers arising in FA patients are HPV positive at a significantly higher rate than in the general population. The possible contribution of HPV infection to the increase in incidence of cancer in these patients was reinforced by the demonstration that the FA pathway is activated by HPV16 E7 expression and that the capacity of HPV16 E7 to induce DNA repair foci is enhanced in the FA patient-derived cell lines (Spardy et al., 2007).

Transforming growth factor β (TGF-β) is a potent inhibitor of epithelial cell growth, and acquisition of TGF-β resistance is the hallmark of epithelial tumor cervical carcinoma cell lines. Ectopic HPV16 E7 expression abrogates TGF-β-mediated growth inhibition. Acquisition of TGF-β resistance is a multi-step process, where TGF-β can repress HPV16 E6/E7 expression, which has been correlated to Ski overexpession, but the exact mechanism of this is not yet known (Baldawin et al., 2004). Both $p21^{CIP1}$ and $p27^{KIP1}$ have been implicated in TGF-β-mediated growth inhibition (Datto et al., 1995); and HPV16 E7 ability to inactivate these CKIs may contribute to its ability to abrogate TGF-β-mediated growth inhibition. TGF-β also induces a cdk4/cdk6-specific CKI, P15Inkb, and p15INKB-induced growth suppression may require functional pRB, which is targeted for degradation by HPV16 E7 (MaLac & Münger, 2009).

The tumor necrosis factor- α (TNF-α) is an important part of the immune response mediator that is produced by the cytotoxic T cell in response to a viral infection normal in keratinocytes undergoing G1 growth arrest and cellular differentiation in response to tumor necrosis factor (TNF). HPV E7 also compromises interferon (IFN) signaling through association with and inhibition of the IFN-α-induced nuclear translocation of p48, the DNA-binding component of ISGF-3. Besides, HPV E7 can interfere with interferon regulatory factors (IRFs) associated with IRF-1 and impair its transcriptional activity (Park et al., 2000). Moreover, IFN-γ has been shown to inhibit HPV16 E7 expression, and the IFN-γ-induced suppressor of cytokine signaling-1 (SOCS-1)/JAB can associate with and induce the ubiquitin-mediated degradation of E7 (Kamio et al., 2004). HPV16 E7 may also interfere with insulin-like growth factor (IGF) signaling, which regulates cell survival. HPV16 E7 can associate with IGFP3 and accelerate its proteosome-mediated degradation (Santer et al., 2007).

E7 proteins are also associated with histone modifying enzymes and associated transcriptional co-factors (Bernat et al., 2003). HPV E7 interacts with class I histone deactylases (HDACs), which act as a transcriptional co-repressor by including chromatin remodeling by reversing acetyl of lysin residues on histone. The association between E7 and HDACs results in increased levels of E2F-mediated transcription in differentiating cells possibly influencing S-phase progression. (Longworth et al., 2005). E7 is also associated, directly or indirectly, with histone acetyl transferases (HATs) including p300, pCAF, and SRC1, and has been shown to abrogate SRC1-associated HAT activity (Baldwin et al., 2006). Moreover, the histone methyl transferase, enhancer of zeste homologue 2 (EZH2), has been identified as a transcriptional target of the HPV E7 protein (Holland et al., 2008).

6. Conclusion

HPV is a non-enveloped virus with double-stranded circular DNA genome, protected by an icosahedra capsid forming a particle with about 55 nm. HPV genome is divided into three regions: a long control region (LCR), an early region (E), consisting of six ORFs: E1, E2, E4, E5, E6, and E7, which encodes no structural proteins involved in viral replication and oncogenesis and a late region (L) that encodes the L1 and L2 structural proteins of the viral capsid. The regulation of viral gene expression is controlled by cellular and viral transcription factors. Most of these regulations occur within the LCR region. The virus early promoter, differentiation-dependent late promoter, and two polyadenylation signals define three general groups of viral genes that are coordinately regulated during host cell differentiation. The E6 and E7 genes maintain replication competence, E1 E2, E4, E5, and E8 are involved in virus DNA replication, transcriptional control, beyond other functions. The products of the late genes L1 and L2 are responsible for the assembly of viral particles The HPV life cycle begins with infection of stem cells in the basal layer of the epithelium. After entering the cells, the virus requires the expression of genes E1 and E2 to maintain a low number of genome copies. The expression of E6, E7, E1, and E2 are required for episomal maintenance continued. E1 and E2 act together to initiate replication of viral DNA, while E6 and E7 modulate cell cycle regulators to maintain replication competency in the long-term. The activation of differentiation-dependent promoter leads to an increased production of proteins E1, E2, E5, E6 and E7, resulting in increased cell proliferation and therefore in the number of cells infected with HPV, as well as the number of viral genome copies per cell. Then there is the E4 gene expression that induces genome amplification, at the same time that occurs the expression of genes L1 and L2 and assembly of viral particles. Among the mechanisms that allow the persistence of the virus include a specific differentiation during of the life cycle of the virus, the mechanisms for keeping the number of copies of the genome in undifferentiated cells, angiogenesis, and strategies to evade of both innate and adaptive immune surveillance. In most cases, host defenses prevail and HPV infections resolve themselves. In some cases, however, infections persist for longer periods, allowing the accumulation of additional cellular changes leading to cancer.

The ingenious strategy developed by HPV, in which viral DNA replication and assembly occur only in in terminally differentiated cell and the fact that a local infection and intraepithelial, allows the virus to remain in host for many months, even years, invisible to the host defense mechanism. The HPV achieve this enviable lifestyle through a combination of abilities that contribute to avoid immune response. The viral infectious cycle is confined to the epithelial compartment, there is no viremia or blood-borne spread, and virus particles are eliminated from the mucosal surfaces far from vascular and lymphatic channels. As a result, there is little access to proteins of viruses and virus to the lymph nodes where adaptive immune responses are initiated. Besides, there is no necrosis or cell death virus-induced, and the proinflammatory cytokines that activate APCs in the epithelium are absent. In addition, HPV downregulate interferon responses and disable epithelial LCs. This allows for long uninterrupted periods of viral replication in the epithelium in the absence of host defense mechanisms.This is a high risk strategy for the host when the infection is caused by oncogenic genital HPVs, it increases the risk that the host immune system may become tolerant or unresponsive to viral proteins.

The development of cervical cancer involves a coordinated targeting of multiple pathways involving the HPV oncoproteins, where each one has a distinct role in malignant progression by interacting with many cellular proteins. The oncoproteíns of high-risk HPV usurp or disrupt multiple signaling pathways to maintain the proliferative state in infected cells to facilitate viral replication and persistence. One consequence of this, however, is the accumulation of mutations in cellular genes and increased genomic instability, which results in full transformation. The major viral factors responsible for altering these pathways and mediating the progression to malignancy are the E5, E6 and E7 proteins. The efficient interruption of the functions of p53 and pRb by E6 and E7 is essential for this process. Recent studies have identified other important cellular targets, including telomerase, members of the pathway of DNA damage and important factors for centrosome duplication and signaling proteins. HPV promotes cell proliferation by multiple pathways in the absence of active cellular mechanisms of defense. The new appreciation of the role of other viral proteins, such as E5, in the progression of HPV-induced disease is also emerging. Although the recently introduced vaccines are effective in preventing initial infections caused by the high risk HPV types comprised in the vaccine, they have no effect on existing lesions and cancer, nor will it protect against diseases caused by other HPV types.

7. References

Alcocer-Gonzalez, JM., Berumen, J., Tamez-Guerra, R., Bermudez-Morales, V., Peralta-Zaragoza, O., Hernandez-Pando, R., Moreno, J., Gariglio, P. & Madrid-Marina, V. In vivo expression of immunosuppressive cytokines in human papillomavirus-transformed cervical cancer cells. *Viral Immunology*, Vol. 19, No. 3, (Jun 2006), pp. 481-491, ISSN 0882-8245.

Baldwin, A., Pirisi, L. & Creek, KE. (2004). NFI-Ski Interactions Mediate Transforming Growth Factor ß Modulation of Human Papillomavirus Type 16 Early Gene Expression. *Journal of Virology*, Vol. 78, No. 8, (April 2004), pp. 3953-3964, ISSN 0022-538X.

Baldwin, A., Huh, K-W., & Münger, K. (2006). Human Papillomavirus E7 Oncoprotein Dysregulates Steroid Receptor Coactivator 1 Localization and Function. *Journal of Virology*, Vol. 80, No. 13, (Jul 2006), pp. 6669 - 6677, ISSN 0022-538X.
Baseman, JG., & Koutsky LA. (2005). The epidemiology of human papillomavirus infections. *Journal of Clinical Virology*, Vol. 32, No.4 - Suppl 1, (Mar 2005), pp. S16-S24, ISSN 1386-6532.
Bernat, A., Avvakumov, N., Mymryk, JS. & Banks, L. (2003). Interaction between the HPV E7 oncoprotein and the transcriptional coactivator p300. *Oncogene*, Vol. 22, No. 39, (Sep 2003), pp. 7871-7881, ISSN 0950-9232.
Bhattacharya, D., Redkar, A., Mittra, I., Sutaria, U. & MacRae KD. (1997). Oestrogen increases S-phase fraction and oestrogen and progesterone receptors in human cervical cancer in vivo. *British Journal of Cancer*, Vol. 75, No. 4, (Jan 1997), pp. 554-558, ISSN 0007-0920.
Black, CM., Papp,JR., Markowitz, L., Unger, ER. Tarkowski, TA., Koumans, EH., Sawyer, M & Pierce, A. (2004). Epidemiology of human papillomavirus infection and abnormal cytologic test results in an urban adolescent population. *The Journal of Infectious Disease*, Vol. 189, No. 1, (Jan 2004), pp. 46-50, ISSN 0022-1899.
Bodily J. & Laimins, LA. (2011). Persistence of human papillomavirus infection: keys to malignant progression. *Trends in Microbiology*, Vol. 19, No. 1, (Jan 2011), pp. 33-39, ISSN 0966-842X.
Bodily, M., Beglin, Kyo, S., Inoue, M. & Laimins, LA. (2009). Hypoxia-specific stabilization of HIF-1alpha by human papillomaviruses. *Virology*, Vol. 387, No. 2, (May 2009), pp. 442-448, ISSN 0042-6822
Bosch, FX., de Sanjosé, S. & Castellsagué, X. (2008). Chapter 4 HPV and genital cancer: the essential epidemiology. *Vaccines for the Prevention of Cervical Cancer*, (Jan 2008); 1: med-9780199543458-chapter-4. DOI: 10.1093/med/9780199543458.003.0004.
Bosch, FX., Lorincz, A., Muñoz, N., Meijer, CJLM. & Shah, KV. (2002). The causal relation between human papillomavirus and cervical cancer. *Journal of Clinical Pathology*, Vol. 55, No. 4, (Apr 2002), pp. 244-265, ISSN 0021-9746.
Bouvard, V., Storey, A., Pim, D. & Banks, L. (1994). Characterization of the human papillomavirus E2 protein: evidence of trans-activation and trans-repression in cervical keratinocytes. *EMBO Journal*, Vol. 13, No. 22, (Nov 1994), pp. 5451-5459, ISSN 0261-4189.
Bryan JT & Brown DR. (2000). Association of the human papillomavirus type 11 E1()E4 protein with cornified cell envelopes derived from infected genital epithelium. *Virology*, Vol. 277, No. 2, (Nov 2000), pp. 262-269, ISSN 0042-6822.
Buck CB, Cheng N, Thompson CD, Lowy DR, Steven AC, Schiller JT, Trus BL. (2008). Arrangement of L2 within the papillomavirus capsid. *Journal of Virology*, Vol. 82, No. 11, (Mar 2008), pp. 5190-5197, ISSN 0022-538X.
Burd, EM. (2003). Human papillomavirus and cervical cancer. *Clinical Microbiology Reviews*. Vol. 16, No. 1, (Jan 2003), pp. 1-17, ISSN 1098-6618.
Caberg, J-HD., Hubert, PM., Begon, DY., Herfs, MF., Roncarati, PJ., Boniver, JJ. & Delvenne, PO. (2008). Silencing of E7 oncogene restores functional E-cadherin expression in human papillomavirus 16-transformed keratinocytes. *Carcinogenesis*, Vol. 29, No. 7, (Jul 2008), pp, 1441-1447, ISSN 0143-3334.
Carter, JJ., Wipf, GC., Benki, SF., Christensen, ND. & Galloway DA. (2003). Identification of a human papillomavirus type 16-specific epitope on the C-terminal arm of the major capsid protein L1. *Virology*, Vol. 77, No. 21, (Nov 2003), pp. 11625 -11632, ISSN 0042-6822.

Chan, PK., Chang, AR., Yu, MY., Li, WH., Chan, MY., Yeung, AC., Cheung, TH., Yau, TN., Wong, SM., Yau, CW..& Ng HK. (2010). Age distribution of human papillomavirus infection and cervical neoplasia reflects caveats of cervical screening policies. *International Journal of Cancer*, Vol. 126, No. 1, (Jan 2010), pp. 297-301, ISSN 0020-7136.

Cho, YS., Kang, JW., Cho, M., Cho, CW., Lee, S., Choe, YK., Kim, Y., Choi, I., Park, SN., Kim, S., Dinarello, CA. & Yoon, DY. Down modulation of IL-18 experssion by human papillomavirus type 16 E6 oncogene via binding to Il-18. *FEBS Letters*, Vol. 501, No 2-3, pp. 139-145, ISSN 0014-5793.

Chow LT & Broker TR. (1994). Papillomavirus DNA replication. *Intervirology*, Vol. 37, No. 4, (Jan 1994), pp. 150-158, ISSN 0300-5526.

Chung, S-H., Wiedmeyer, K., Shai, A., Korach, KS. & Lambert, PF. (2008). Requirement for estrogen receptor α in a mouse model for human papillomavirus–associated cervical cancer. *Cancer Research*, Vol. 68, No. 23, (Dec 2008), pp. 9928-9934, ISSN 0008-5472.

Clifford, GM., Rana, RK., Franceschi, S., Smith, JS., Gough, G. & Pimenta, JM. (2005). Human papillomavirus genotype distribution in low-grade cervical lesions: comparison by geographic region and with cervical cancer. *Cancer Epidemiology, Biomarkers & Prevention*, Vol. 14, No. 5, (May 2005), pp. 1157-1164, ISSN 1055-9965.

Conger, KL., Liu, J-S., Kuo, S-R., Chow, LT & Wang, TS-F. (1999). Human papillomavirus DNA replication. interactions between the Viral E1 protein and two subunits of human DNA polymerase α/primase. *the Journal Biological Chemistry*, Vol. 274, N. 5, (Jan 1999), pp. 2696-2705, ISSN 0021-9258.

Conway, MJ. & Meyers, C. (2009). Replication and assembly of human papillomaviruses *Journal of Dental Research*, Vol. 88, N. 4, (Apr 2009), pp 307-317, ISSN 0022-0345.

Crum CP & McKeon FD (2010). p63 in epithelial survival, germ cell surveillance, and neoplasia. *Annual Review of Pathology*, Vol. 5, (Febr 2010), pp. 349-371, ISSN 1553-4006.

Culp, TD., Budgeon, LR. & Christensen ND. (2006). Human papillomaviruses bind a basal extracellular matrix component secreted by keratinocytes which is distinct from a membrane-associated receptor. *Virology*, Vol. 34, No. 1, (Mar 2006), pp,147-159, ISSN 0042-6822.

Culp, TD., Budgeon, LR., Marinkovich, MP., Meneguzzi, G. & Christensen, ND. (2006). Keratinocyte-secreted laminin 5 can function as a transient receptor for human papillomaviruses by binding virions and transferring them to adjacent cells. *Journal of Virology*, Vol. 80, No. 18, (Sep 2006), pp, 8940–8950, ISSN 0022-0345.

D'Andrilli, G., Bovicelli, A., Giordano A. (2010). HPV vaccines: state of the art. *Journal of Cellular Physiology*, Vol. 224, No. 3, (Sep 2010), pp. 567–847, ISSN 0021-9541

Datto, MB., Yu, Y. & Wang, X-F. (1995). Functional Analysis of the Transforming Growth Factor β Responsive Elements in the WAF1/Cip1/p21 Promoter. *The Journal of Biological Chemistry*, Vol. 270, No. 48, (Dec 1995), pp. 28623-28628, ISSN 0021-9258.

DeMasi, J., Huh, K-W., Nakatani, Y. Münger, K. & Howley, PM. (2005). Bovine papillomavirus E7 transformation function correlates with cellular p600 protein binding. *PNAS*, Vol. 102, No. 32, (Aug 2005), pp. 11486 - 11491 ISSN 0027-8424.

DeMasi, J., Chao, MC., Kumar, AS. & Howley PM. (2007). Bovine Papillomavirus E7 Oncoprotein Inhibits Anoikis. *Journal of Virology*, Vol. 81, No. 17, (Sep 2007), pp. 9419 - 9425, ISSN 0022-538X.

De Sanjose, S., Diaz, M., Castellsague, X., Clifford., G., Bruni, L., Munoz, N., & Bosch, FX. (2007). Worldwide prevalence and genotype distribution of cervical human papillomavirus DNA in women with normal cytology: a meta-analysis. *Lancet Infectious Diseases*, Vol. 7, No. 7, (Jul 2007), pp. 453-459, ISSN 1473-3099.

Deng, S-J., Pearce, KH., Kelly, EP., Hartley, A., Stanley, TB., Lobe, DC., Garvey, EP., Kost, TA., Petty, RL., Rocque, WJ., Alexander, KA. & Underwood, MK. (2004). Identification of peptides that inhibit the dna binding, trans-activator, and dna replication functions of the human papillomavirus type 11 E2 protein. *Journal of Virology*, Vol. 78, No. 5, (Mar 2004),pp 2637-2641, ISSN 0022-538X.

DiMaio D,& Mattoon D (2001). Mechanisms of cell transformation by papillomavirus E5 proteins. *Oncogene*. Vol. 20, No. 54, (Nov 2001), pp. 7866-7873, ISSN 0950-9232.

Doorbar, J., Ely, S. Sterling, J., McLean, C. & Crawford, L. (1991). Specific interaction between HPV-16 E1-E4 and cytokeratins results in collapse of the epithelial cell intermediate filament network. *Nature*, Vol. 352, No. 6368, (Aug 1991), pp. 824-827, ISSN 0028-0836.

Duelli, DM., Padilla-Nash, HM., Berman, D., Murphy, KM., Ried, T. & Lazebnik, Y. (2007). A virus causes cancer by inducing massive chromosomal instability through cell fusion. *Current Biology*, Vol. 17, No. 5 (Mar 2007), pp. 431-437, ISSN 0960-9822.

Duesing, S. & Munger, K. (2004). Mechanisms of genomic instability in human cancer: insights from studies with human papillomavirus oncoproteins. *International Journal of Cancer*, Vol. 109, No. 2, (Mar 2004), pp. 157-162, ISSN 0020-7136.

Eichten, A., Westfall, M., Pietenpol, JA. & Munger, K. (2002). Stabilization and functional impairment of the tumor suppressor p53 by the human papillomavirus type 16 E7 oncoprotein. *Virology*, Vol. 295, No. 1 (Mar 2002), pp. 74-85, ISSN 0042-6822.

Eichten, A., Rud, DS., Grace, M., Piboonniyom, SO., Zacny, V. & Munger, K. (2004). Molecular pathways executing the "trophic sentinel" response in HPV-16 E7-expressing normal human diploid fibroblasts upon growth factor deprivation. *Virology*, Vol. 319, No. 1. (Feb 2004), pp. 81-93, ISSN 0042-6822.

Filippova, M., Song, H. Connolly, JL., Dermody, TS. & Duerksen-Hughes, PJ. (2002). The Human Papillomavirus 16 E6 Protein Binds to Tumor Necrosis Factor (TNF) R1 and Protects Cells from TNF-induced Apoptosis. *The Journal Biological Chemistry*, Vol. 277, No. 24, (Jun 2002), pp. 21730 - 21739, ISSN 0021-9258.

Fehrmann F. & Laimins, LA. Human papillomaviruses: targeting differentiating epithelial cells for malignant transformation. *Oncogene*, Vol. 22, No. 33, (Aug 2003), pp. 5201-5207, ISSN 0950-9232.

Fehrmann, F., Klumpp, DJ. & Laimins, LA. (2003). Human papillomavirus type 31 E5 protein supports cell cycle progression and activates late viral functions upon epithelial differentiation. *Journal of Virology*, Vol. 77, No. 5, (Mar 2003), pp. 2819-2831, ISSN 0022-538X.

Fernandes, JV., Meissner, RV., Carvalho, MG., Fernandes, TAAM., Azevedo, PR., Sobrinho, JS., Prado, JC. & Villa, LL. (2010). Prevalence of human papillomavirus in archival samples obtained from patients with cervical pre-malignant and malignant lesions from Northeast Brazil. *BMC Research Notes*, Vol. 3, No. 1, (Jan 2010), pp. 96, ISSN 1756-0500.

Fernandes, JV., Meissner, RV., de Carvalho, MG., Fernandes, TAAM., de Azevedo, PR & Villa, LL. (2009). Prevalence of HPV infection by cervical cytologic status in Brazil. *International Journal of Gynaecology and Obstetrics*, Vol. 105, No. 1, (Apr 2009), pp. 21-24, ISSN 0020-7292.

Fertey, J., Ammermann, I., Winkler, M., Stöger, R., Iftner, T. & Stubenrauch, F. (2010). Interaction of the papillomavirus E8 E2C protein with the cellular CHD6 protein contributes to transcriptional repression. *Journal of Virology*, Vol. 84, No. 18, (Sep 2010), pp. 9505-9515, ISSN 0022-538X.

Filippova, M., Song, H., Connolly, JL., Dermody, TS & Duerksen-Hughes, PJ. (2002). Interaction of the papillomavirus E8 E2C protein with the cellular CHD6 protein contributes to transcriptional repression. *The Journal of Biological Chemistry*, Vol. 277, No. 18, (Jun 2002), pp. 21730-21739, ISSN 0021-9258.

Flores, ER., Allen-Hoffmann, BL., Lee, D., Sattler, CA. & Lambert PF. (1999). Establishment of the human papillomavirus type 16 (HPV-16) life cycle in an immortalized human foreskin keratinocyte cell line. *Virology*, Vol. 262, No. 2, (Sep 1999), pp, 344-354, ISSN 0042-6822.

Florin, L., Becker, ka., Lambert, c., Nowak, T., Sapp, C., Strand, D., Streeck, RE. & Sapp, M. (2006). Identification of a dynein interacting domain in the papillomavirus minor capsid protein L2. *Journal of Virology*, Vol. 80, No. 13, (Jul 2006), pp. 6691-6696, ISSN 0022-538X.

Franco, EL., Villa, LL., Sobrinho, JP., Prado, JM., Rousseau, M-C., Désy, M. & Rohan, TE. (1999). Epidemiology of acquisition and clearance of cervical human papillomavirus infection in women from a high-risk area for cervical cancer. *The Journal of Infectious Disease*, Vol. 180, No. 5, (Nov 1999), pp, 1415-1423, ISSN 0022-1899.

Frazer, IH. (2009). Interaction of human papillomaviruses with the host immune system: a well evolved relationship.*Virology*, Vol. 384, No 2, (Feb 2009), pp. 410-414, ISSN 0042-6822.

Gao, P. & Zheng, J. (2010). High-risk HPV E5-induced cell fusion: a critical initiating event in the early stage of HPV-associated cervical cancer. *Virology Journal*, Vol.7, No 238, (Jan 2010), pp. 1-3, ISSN 1743-422X.

Garnett, TO & Duerksen-Hughes PJ. (2006). Modulation of apoptosis by human papillomavirus (HPV) oncoproteins. *Archives of Virology*, Vol. 151, No. 12, (Dec 2006), pp. 2321-2335, ISSN 0304-8608.

Ghittoni, R. Accardi, R. Hasan, U., Gheit, T., Sylla, B. & Tommasino, M.(2010). The biological properties of E6 and E7 oncoproteins from human papillomaviruses. *Virus Genes*, Vol. 40, No. 1, (Feb 2010), pp. 1-13, ISSN 0920-8569.

Giannini, SL., Hubert, P., Doyen, J., Boniver, J. & Delvenne, P. (2002). Influence of the mucosal epithelium microenvironment on Langerhans cells: implications for the development of squamous intraepithelial lesions of the cervix. *International Journal of Cancer*, Vol. 97, No. 5, (Feb 2002), pp. 654-659, ISSN 0020-7136.

González, P., Hildesheim, A., Rodríguez, AC., Schiffman, M., Porras, CP., Wacholder, S., Piñeres, AG., Pinto, LA., Burk, RD & Herrero, R. (2010). Behavioral/lifestyle and immunologic factors associated with HPV infection among women older than 45 years. *Cancer Epidemiology. Biomarkers & Prevention*, Vol. 19, No. 12, (Dec 2010), pp, 3044-3054, ISSN 1055-1065.

Gu, LH & Coulombe, PA. (2007). Keratin function in skin epithelia: a broadening palette with surprising shades. *Current Opinion in Cell Biology*, Vol. 19, No. 1, (Feb 2007), pp.13-23, ISSN 0955-0674.

Hamid, NA., Brown, C. & Gaston K. (2009).The regulation of cell proliferation by the papillomavirus early proteins. *Cellular and Molecular Life Science*, Vol. 66, No. 10, (May 2009), pp. 1700-1717, ISSN 1420-682X.

Hasan, U.A., Bates, E., Takeshita, F., Biliato, A., Accardi, R., Bouvard, V., Mansour, M., Vincent, I., Gissmann, L., Iftner, T., Sideri, M., Stubenrauch, F., Tommasino, M., 2007. TLR9 expression and function is abolished by the cervical cancer-associated human papillomavirus type 16. *Journal of Immunology*, Vol. 178, No. 5, (Mar 2007), pp. 3186-3197, ISSN 1550-6606.

Hasan, UA., Caux, C., Perrot, I., Doffin, A-C., Menetrier-Caux, C. Trinchieri, G., Tommasino, M. & Vlach, J. (2007). Cell proliferation and survival induced by Toll-like receptors is antagonized by type I IFNs. *PNAS*, Vol. 104, No. 19, (May 2007), pp. 8047-8052, ISSN 0027-8424.

Hebner, CM. & Laimins, LA. (2006). Human papillomaviruses: basic mechanisms of pathogenesis and oncogenicity. *Reviews in Medical Virology*, Vol. 16, No 2, (Mar 2006), pp. 83-97, ISSN 1052-9276.

Heilman, SA., Nordberg, JJ., Liu, Y., Sluder, G. & Chen, JJ. Abrogation of the Postmitotic Checkpoint Contributes to Polyploidization in Human Papillomavirus E7-Expressing Cells. *Journal of Virology*, Vol. 83, No. 6, (Mar 2009), pp. 2756 - 2764, ISSN 0022-538X.

Herfs, M., Hubert, P., Kholod, N., Caberg,JH., Gilles, C.,Berx, G., Savagner, P.,Boniver, J. & Delvenne, P. (2008).Transforming growth factor-β1-mediated slug and snail Transcription factor up-regulation reduces the density of langerhans vells in epithelial metaplasia by affecting E-cadherin expression. *American Journal of Pathology*. Vol. 172, No. 5, (May 2008), pp 1391-1402, ISSN 0002-9440.

Herfs, M., Hubert, P., Moutschen, M. & Delvenne, P. (2011). Mucosal junctions: open doors to HPV and HIV infections? *Trends in Microbiology*, Vol. 19, No 3, (Mar 2011), pp. 114-120, ISSN 0966-842X.

Hindmarsh, PL. & Laimins, LA.(2007). Mechanisms regulating expression of the HPV 31 L1 and L2 capsid proteins and pseudovirion entry. *Virology Journal*, Vol. 4. (Feb 2007), pp. 1-12, ISSN 1743-422X

Hiscott, J. (2007).Triggering the Innate Antiviral Response through IRF-3 Activation. *The Journal of Biological Chemistry*, Vol.282, No. 21, (May 2007), pp. 15325-15329, ISSN 0021-9258.

Ho, GY., Bierman, R., Beardsley, L., Chang, CJ. & Burk, RD. (1998). Natural history of cervicovaginal papillomavirus infection in young women. *The New England Journal of Medicine*, Vol. 338, No. 7, (Feb 1998), pp, 423-428, ISSN 0028-4793.

Holland, D., Hoppe-Seyler, K., Schuller, B., Lohrey, C., Maroldt, J., Dürst, M. & Hoppe-Seyler, F. (2008). Activation of the Enhancer of Zeste Homologue 2 Gene by the Human Papillomavirus E7 Oncoprotein. *Cancer Research*, Vol. 68, No. 23, (Dec 2008), pp. 9964 - 9972, ISSN 0008-5472.

Howie, HL., Katzenellenbogen, RA. & Galloway DA. (2009). Papillomavirus E6 proteins. *Virology*, Vol. 384, No. 2, (Feb 2009), pp. 324-334, ISSN 0042-6822

Hu, L., Plafker, K., Vorozhko, V., Zuna, RE., Hanigan, Gorbsky, GJ., Plafker, SM., Angeletti, PC. & Ceresa, PB. (2009). Human papillomavirus 16 E5 induces bi-nucleated cell formation by cell-cell fusion. *Virology*, Vol. 384, No. 1, (Feb 2009), pp. 125-134, ISSN 0042-6822.

Huh, KW., DeMasi, J., Ogawa, H., Nakatani, Y., Howley, PM & Münger, K. (2005). Association of the human papillomavirus type 16 E7 oncoprotein with the 600-kDa retinoblastoma protein-associated factor, p600. *PNAS*, Vol. 102, No. 32, (Aug 2005), pp, 11492-11497, ISSN 0027-8424 .

Huh, KW., Zhou, X., Hayakawa, H., Cho, J-Y., Libermann, TA., Jin, J., Harper, JW. & Munger, K. (2007). Human papillomavirus type 16 E7 oncoprotein associates with the cullin 2 ubiquitin ligase complex, which contributes to degradation of the retinoblastoma tumor suppressor. *Journal of Virology*, Vol. 81, No. 18 (Sep 2007), pp. 9737-9747, ISSN 0022-538X.

Iftner, T., Elbel, M., Schopp, B., Hiller, T., Loizou, JI., Caldecott, KW. & Stubenrauch, F. (2002). Interference of papillomavirus E6 protein with single-strand break repair by interaction with XRCC1. *EMBO Journal*, Vol. 21, No. 17 (Sep 2002), pp. 4741-4748. ISSN 0261-4189.

International Agency for Research on Cancer (IARC). (2007). *IARC Monograph on the evaluation of carcinogenics risks to human - Human Papillomavirus*, World Health Organization, ISBN 978-92-832-1290-4, Lyon, France.

James, MA., Lee, JH. & Klingelhutz, AJ. (2006). HPV16-E6 associated hTERT promoter acetylation is E6AP dependent, increased in later passage cells and enhanced by loss of p300. *International Journal of Cancer*, Vol. 119, No. 8, (Oct 2006), pp. 1878-1885, ISSN 0020-7136.

Jing, M., Bohl, J., Brimer, N., Kinter, M. & Vande Pol, SB. (2007). Degradation of Tyrosine Phosphatase PTPN3 (PTPH1) by Association with Oncogenic Human Papillomavirus E6 Proteins. *Journal of Virology*, Vol. 81, No.5, (Mar 2007), pp.2231-2239, ISSN 0022-538X.

Jo, H. & Kim, JW. (2005). Implications of HPV infection in uterine cervical cancer. *Cancer Therapy*, Vol. 3, (July 2005), pp 419-434, ISSN 1543-9135.

Jones, DL., Thompson, DA. & Munger K. (1997).Destabilization of the RB tumor suppressor protein and stabilization of p53 contribute to HPV type 16 E7-induced apoptosis. *Virology*, Vol. 239, No. 1, (Dec 1997), pp. 97-107, ISSN 0042-6822.

Jones, PH., Simons, BD. & Watt, FM. (2007) Sic transit gloria: farewell to the epidermal transit amplifying cell? *Cell Stem Cell*, Vol. 1, No. 4, (Oct 2007), pp. 371-381, ISSN 1934-5909.

Kadaja, M., Sumerina, A., Verst, T., Ojarand, M., Ustav, E. & Ustav, M. (2007). Genomic instability of the host cell induced by the human papillomavirus replication machinery. *EMBO Journal*, Vol. 26, No. 8, (Apr 2007) 2180-2191, ISSN 0261-4189.

Kadaja, M., Silla MT., Ustav E.& Ustav, M. (2009). Papillomavirus DNA replication from initiation to genomic instability. *Virology*, Vol. 384, No. 2, (Apr 2009), pp. 360-368, ISSN 0042-6822.

Kamio, M., Yoshida, T., Ogata, H., Douchi, T., Nagata, Y., Inoue, M., Hasegawa, M., Yonemitsu, Y. & Yoshimura, A. (2004). SOCS1 [corrected] inhibits HPV-E7-mediated transformation by inducing degradation of E7 protein. *Oncogene*, Vol. 23, No. 17, (Apr 2004), pp. 3107-3115, ISSN 0950-9232.

Kämper, N., Day, PM., Nowak, T., Selinka, H-C., Florin, L., Lydia, JB. John, H., Schiller, JT & Sapp, M. (2006). A membrane-destabilizing peptide in capsid protein L2 is required for egress of papillomavirus genomes from endosomes. *Journal of Virology*, Vol. 80, No. 2, (Jan 2006), pp. 759-768, ISSN 0022-538X.

Kanodia S, Fahey LM, Kast WM. Mechanisms used by human papillomaviruses to escape the host immune response. *Current Cancer Drug Targets*. Vol. 7, No. 1 (Feb 2007), pp. 79-89, ISSN 1568-0096.

Kines, RC., Thompson, CDE., Lowy, DR., Schiller, JT & Day, PM (2009). The initial steps leading to papillomavirus infection occur on the basement membrane prior to cell surface binding. *PNAS*, Vol. 106, No. 48, (Dec 2009), pp. 20458-20463, ISSN 0027-8424.

Kobayashi, N., Takata, H., Yokota S., & Takiguchi, M. (2004). Down-regulation of CXCR4 expression on human CD8+ T cells during peripheral differentiation. *European Journal of Immunology*, Vol. 34, No. 12, (Dec 2004), pp 3370-3378, ISSN 0014-2980.

Katzenellenbogen, RA., Egelkrout, EM., Vliet-Gregg, P., Gewin, LC., Gafken, PR & Galloway, DA. (2007). NFX1-123 and Poly(A) Binding Proteins Synergistically

Augment Activation of Telomerase in Human Papillomavirus Type 16 E6-Expressing Cells. *Journal of Virology*, Vol. 81, No. 8, (Apr 2007), pp. 3786-3796, ISSN 0022-538X.

Kumar, A., Zhao, Y., Meng, G., Zeng, M., Srinivasan, S., Delmolino, LM., Gao, Q., Dimri, G., Weber, GF., Wazer, DE., Band, H. & Band, V. (2002). Human papillomavirus oncoprotein E6 inactivates the transcriptional coactivator human ADA3. *Molecular and Cellular Biolology*, Vol. 22, No.16, (Aug 2002), pp. 5801-5812, ISSN 0270-7306.

Kurg,R., Uusen, P., Vosa, L. & Ustav, M. (2010). Human papillomavirus E2 protein with single activation domain initiates HPV18 genome replication, but is not sufficient for long-term maintenance of virus genome. *Virology*, Vol. 408, No. 2, (Dec 2010), pp. 159-166, ISSN 0042-6822.

Lace, MJ., Anson, JR., Thomas, GS., Turek, LP. and Haugen TH. (2008). The E8∧E2 gene product of human papillomavirus type 16 represses early transcription and replication but is dispensable for viral plasmid persistence in keratinocytes. *Journal of Virology*, Vol. 82, No. 21, (Nov 2008), pp. 10841-10853, ISSN 0022-538X.

Laniosz, V., Nguyen, KC. & Meneses, PI. (2007). Bovine papillomavirus type 1 infection is mediated by SNARE syntaxin 18. *Journal of Virology*, Vol. 81, No. 14, (Jul 2007), pp, 7435 - 7448. ISSN 0022-538X.

Lazarczyk, M., Cassonnet, P., Pons, C., Jacob, Y. & Favre, M. (2009). The EVER proteins as a natural barrier against papillomaviruses: a new insight into the pathogenesis of human papillomavirus infections. *Microbiology and Molecular Biology Reviews*, Vol. 73, No. 2, (June 2009), pp. 348-370, ISSN 092-2172.

Le Bon A. & Tough, DF. Links between innate and adaptive immunity via type I interferon. *Current Opinion in Immunology*, Vol. 14, No 4, (August 2002), pp. 432-436, ISSN 0952-7915.

Lechner MS. & Laimins LA. (1994). Inhibition of p53 DNA binding by human papillomavirus E6 proteins. *Journal of Virology*, Vol. 68, No. 7, (Jul 1994), pp. 4262-4273, ISSN 0022-538X.

Lee, C. Wooldridge, TR. & Laimins, LA. (2007). Analysis of the roles of E6 binding to E6TP1 and nuclear localization in the human papillomavirus type 31 life cycle. Virology, Vol. 358, No. 1, (Feb 2007), pp. 201-1210, ISSN 0042-6822.

Longworth, MS.& Laimins, LA. (2004). Pathogenesis of human papillomaviruses in differentiating epithelia. *microbiology and molecular Biology Reviews*, Vol. 68, No. 2, (Jun 2004), pp. 362 - 372, ISSN 1092-2172 .

Longworth, MS., Wilson, R. & Laimins, LA. (2005). HPV31 E7 facilitates replication by activating E2F2 transcription through its interaction with HDACs. *EMBO Journal*, Vol. 24, No. 10, (May 2005), pp. 1821-30, ISSN 0261-4189.

Lyons, TE. Salih, M. & Tuana, BS. (2006). Activating E2Fs mediate transcriptional regulation of human E2F6 repressor. *American Journal Physiology Cell Physiology*, Vol. 290, No. 1, (Jan 2006), pp. C189 - C199, ISSN 0363-6143.

Mark Schiffman, M. Wentzensen, N., Wacholder, S., Kinney, W., Gage, JC. & Castle, PE. (2011). Human papillomavirus testing in the prevention of cervical cancer. *Journal of the National Cancer Institute*, Vol. 103, No. 5, (Jan 2011), pp. 368-383, ISSN 0027-8874.

McLaughlin-Drubin, ME & Munger, K. (2009). Oncogenic activities of human papillomaviruses. *Virus Research*, Vol. 143, No 2, (Aug 2009), pp 195-208, ISSN 0168-1702

McLaughlin-Drubin, ME., Huh, KW. & Munger, K . (2008). Human papillomavirus type 16 E7 oncoprotein associates with E2F6. *Journal of Virology*, Vol. 82, No. 17, (Sep 2008), pp. 82: 8695 - 8705, ISSN 0022-538X.

McPhillips, MG., Oliveira, JG., Spindler, JE., Mitra, R. & McBride AA. (2006). Brd4 Is required for E2-mediated transcriptional activation but not genome partitioning of all papillomaviruses. *Journal of Virology*, Vol. 80, No. 19, (Oct 2006), pp. 9530-9543, ISSN 0168-1702.

Miura, S., Kawana, K., Schust, DJ., Fujii, T., Yokoyama, T., Iwasawa, Y., Nagamatsu, T., Adachi, K., Tomio, A., Tomio K., Kojima, S., Yasugi, T., Kozuma, S. & Taketani Y. (2010). CD1d, a sentinel molecule bridging innate and adaptative immunity, is downregulated by the human papillomavirus (HPV) E5 protein: a possible mechanism for immune evasion by HPV. *Journal of Virology*, Vol 84, No 22, (Nov 2010), pp. 1114-11623, ISSN 0168-1702.

Mei Xu, M., Luo, W., Elzi, DJ., Grandori,C. & Galloway, DA. (2008). NFX1 Interacts with mSin3A/Histone Deacetylase To Repress hTERT Transcription in Keratinocytes. *Molecular and Cellular Biology*, Vol. 28, No. 15, (August 2008), pp. 4819-4828, ISSN 0270-7306.

Mitelman, F., Johansson, B. & F Mertens, F. (2007). The impact of translocations and gene fusions on cancer causation. *Nature Reviews Cancer*, Vol. 7, No. 4, (Apr 2007), pp. 233-245, ISSN 1474-175X

Moody, CA. & Laimins, LA. (2010). Human papillomavirus oncoproteins: pathways to transformation. *Nature Reviews Cancer*, Vol. 10, No. 8, pp. 550-560, ISSN 1474-175X.

Mukonoweshuro, P., Oriowolo A. & Smith M. (2005). Audit of the histological definition of cervical transformation zone. *Journal of Clinical Pathologv*, Vol. 58, No. 6, (Jun *2005)*, pp. 670-672, ISSN 0021-9746.

Münger, K. & Peter M. Howley, PM. (2002). Human papillomavirus immortalization and transformation functions. *Virus Research*, Vol. 89, No. 2, (Nov 2002), pp. 213-228, ISSN 0168-1702

Münger, K., Baldwin, A., Edwards, KM., Hayakawa, H., Nguyen, CL., Owens, M., Grace, M. & Huh, K. (2004). Mechanisms of human papillomavirus-induced oncogenesis. *Journal of Virology*, Vol. 78, No. 21, (Nov 2004), pp. 11451-11460, ISSN 0022-538X.

Munõz, N., Bosch, FX., de Sanjosé, S., Herrero, R., Castellsagué, X., Shah, KV., Snijders, PJF., Chris, JLM. & Meijer, MD. (2003). Epidemilogic classification of human papillomavirus types associated with cervical cancer. *The New England Journal Medicine*, Vol. 348, No 6, (Feb 2003), pp. 518-527, ISSN 0028-4793.

Muñoz, N., Castellsagué, X., de González, AB., Gissmann, L. (2006). Chapter 1: HPV in the etiology of human cancer. *Vaccine*, Vol. 24, Suppl 3, (Aug 2006), pp. 1-10, ISSN 0264-410X..

Nakahara, T., Peh, WL., Doorbar, J., Lee, D. & Lambert, PF. (2005). Human papillomavirus type 16 E1∧E4 contributes to multiple facets of the papillomavirus life cycle. *Journal of Virology*, Vol. 79, No. 20, (Oct 2005), pp. 13150-13165, ISSN 0022-538X.

Natale, C., Giannini, T., Lucchese , A., Kanduc, D. (2000).Computer-assisted analysis of molecular mimicry between human papillomavirus 16 E7 oncoprotein and human protein sequences. *Immunology Cell Biology, Vol.* 78, No. 6 (Dec 2000), pp. 580-585, ISSN 0818-9641.

Nees, M., Geoghegan, JM., Hyman, T., Frank, S., Miller, L. & Woodworth, CD. (2001). Papillomavirus type 16 oncogenes downregulate expression of interferon-responsive genes and upregulate proliferation-associated and INF- B-responsive genes in cervical keratinocytes. *Journal of Virology*, Vol. 75, No. 9, (May 2001), pp. 4283-4296, ISSN 0022-538X.

Nguyen, CL. & Munger, K. (2008). Direct association of the HPV16 E7 oncoprotein with cyclin A/CDK2 and cyclin E/CDK2 complexes. *Virology*, Vol. 380, No 1 (Oct 2008), pp. 21-25, ISSN 0042-6822.

O'Brien, PM & Campos, MS. (2002). Evasion of host immunity directed by papillomavirus-encoded proteins. *Virus Research*, Vol. 88, No. 2, (Sep 2002), pp.103-117, ISSN 0168-1702.

Park, J-S., Kim, E-J., Kwon, H-J., Hwang, E-S., Namkoong, S-E. & Um, S-J. (2000). Inactivation of Interferon Regulatory Factor-1 Tumor Suppressor Protein by HPV E7 Oncoprotein. Implication for the E7-mediated immune evasion mechanism in cervical carcinogenesis. *The Journal Biological Chemistry*, Vol. 275, No. (Mar 2000), pp. 6764 - 6769, ISSN 0021-9258.

Pei, XF., Meck, JM., Greenhalgh, D. & Schlegel, R. (1993). Cotransfection of HPV-18 and v-fos DNA induces tumorigenicity of primary human keratinocytes. *Virology*, Vol. 196, No. 2, (Oct 1993), pp. 855-860, ISSN 0042-6822.

Pett, MK., Herdman, MT., Palmer, RD., Yeo, GSH., Shivji,MK., Stanley, MA. & Coleman, N. (2006). Selection of cervical keratinocytes containing integrated HPV16 associates with episome loss and an endogenous antiviral response. *PNAS*, Vol. 103, No. 10, (Mar 2006), pp. 3822-3827, ISSN 0027-8424.

Philip E Castle, PE., Schiffman, M., Herrero, R., Hildesheim, A., Rodriguez, AC., Bratti, MC., Sherman, EM., Wacholder, S., Tarone, R. & Burk, RD. (2005). A prospective study of age trends in cervical Human Papillomavirus acquisition and persistence in Guanacaste, Costa Rica. *The Journal of Infectious Disease*, Vol.191, No. 11, (Jun 2005), pp. 1808-1816, ISSN 0022-1899.

Pyeon, D., Pearce, SM., Lank, SM., Ahlquist, P. & Lambert, PF. (2009). Establishment of human papillomavirus infection requires cell cycle progression. *PLoS Pathogens*, Vol. 5, No. 2, (Feb 2009), pp. 1-9, ISSN 1553-7366.

Richards, RM., Lowy, DR., Schiller, JT. & Day, PM. (2006). Cleavage of the papillomavirus minor capsid protein, L2, at a furin consensus site is necessary for infection. *PNAS*, Vol. 103, No. 5, (Jan 2006), pp.1522-1527, ISSN 0027-8424.

Richardson, H., Kelsall, G., Tellier, P., Voyer, H., Abrahamowicz, M., Ferenczy, A., Coutlée, F. & Franco, EL. (2003). The natural history of type-specific human papillomavirus infections in female university students. *Cancer Epidemiology, Biomarkers & Prevention*, Vol. 12, No. 6, (Jun 2003), pp. 485-490, ISSN 1055-9965.

Rincon-Orozco, B., Halec, G., Rosenberger, S., Muschik, D., Nindl, I., Bachmann, A., Ritter, TM., Dondog, B., Ly, R., Bosch, FX., Zawatzky, R. & Rösl, F. (2009). Epigenetic silencing of interferon-κ in human papillomavirus type 16–positive cells. *Cancer Research*, Vol. 69, No. 22, (Nov 2009), pp. 8718-8725, ISSN 0008-5472.

Roberts, JN., Buck, CB., Thompson, CD., Kines, R., Bernardo, M., Choyke, PL., Lowy, DR. & Schiller, JT. (2007). Genital transmission of HPV in a mouse model is potentiated by nonoxynol-9 and inhibited by carrageenan. *Nature Medicine*, Vol. 13, No. 7, (Jul 2007), pp. 857-861, ISSN 1078-8956.

Romanczuk, H. & Howley, PM. (1992). Disruption of either the E1 or the E2 regulatory gene of human papillomavirus type 16 increases viral immortalization capacity. PNAS, Vol. 89, No. 7, (Apr 1992), pp 3159-3163, ISSN 0027-8424.

Samuel, CE. (2001). Antiviral actions of interferons. *Clinical Microbiology Reviews*, Vol. 14, No. 4, (Oct 2001), pp. 778-809, ISSN 1098-6618.

Santer, FR., Moser, B., Spoden, GA., Jansen-Dürr, P. & Zwerschke, W. (2007). Human papillomavirus type 16 E7 oncoprotein inhibits apoptosis mediated by nuclear insulin-like growth factor-binding protein-3 by enhancing its ubiquitin/ proteasome-dependent degradation. *Carcinogenesis*, Vol. 28, No. 12, (Dec 2007), pp. 2511 - 2520, ISSN 0143-3334.

Sapp, M., Volpers, C., Müller, M. & Streeck, RE. (1995). Organization of the major and minor capsid proteins in human papillomavirus type 33 virus-like particles. *Journal of General Virology*, Vol. 76, No. 9, (Sep 1995), pp. 2407-2412, ISSN 0022-1317.

Schiller, JT., Day, PM. & Kines, RC. (2010).Current understanding of the mechanism of HPV infection. *Gynecologic Oncology*, Vol. 118 (Jun 2010), Suppl 1, S12-17, ISSN 0090-8258.

Scott, M., Nakagawa, M. & Moscicki, AB. (2001). Cell-mediated immune response to human papillomavirus infection. *Clinical and Diagnostic Laboratory Immunology*, Vol. 8, No. 2, (Mar 2001), p. 209 -220, ISSN 1071-412X.

Selinka, H-C., Florin, L., Patel, HD., Freitag, K., Vadim, MS., Makarov, A. & Sapp, M. (2007). Inhibition of transfer to secondary receptors by heparan sulfate-binding drug or antibody induces noninfectious uptake of human papillomavirus. *Journal of Virology*, Vol. 81, No. 20, (Oct 2007), pp. 10970-10980, ISSN 0022-538X.

Seo, YS, Müller, F., Lusky, M., Gibbs, E., Kim, HY., Phillips, B & Hurwitz J. (1993). Bovine papilloma virus (BPV)-encoded E2 protein enhances binding of E1 protein to the BPV replication origin. *PNAS*, Vol. 90, No. 7, (Apr 1993), pp. 2865-2869, ISSN 0027-8424.

Shai, A., Nguyen, ML., Wagstaff, J., Jiang,YH. & Lambert PF. (2007). HPV16 E6 confers p53-dependent and p53-independent phenotypes in the epidermis of mice deficient for E6AP. *Oncogene*, Vol. 26, No 23, (May 2007), pp. 3321-3338, ISSN 0950-9232.

Shamanin, VA., Sekaric, P. & Androphy, EJ. (2008). hAda3 degradation by papillomavirus type 16 e6 correlates with abrogation of the p14arf-p53 pathway and efficient immortalization of human mammary epithelial cells. *Journal of Virology*, Vol. 82, No. 8, (Apr 2008), pp. 3912-3920, ISSN 0022-538X.

Shunsuke Nakagawa, S. & Huibregtse, JM. (2000). Human Scribble (Vartul) Is Targeted for Ubiquitin-Mediated Degradation by the High-Risk Papillomavirus E6 Proteins and the E6AP Ubiquitin-Protein Ligase. *Molecular Cellular Biology*, Vol. 20, No.21, (Nov 2000), pp. 8244- 8253, ISSN 0270-7306.

Simmonds, M. & Storey, A. (2008). Identification of the regions of the HPV 5 E6 protein involved in Bak degradation and inhibition of apoptosis. *International Journal of Cancer*, Vol. 123, No. 10, (Nov 2008), pp. 2260-2266, ISSN 0020-7136.

Smith, JL., Campos, SK. & Ozbun, MA. (2007). Human papillomavirus type 31 uses a caveolin 1- and dynamin 2-mediated entry pathway for infection of human keratinocytes. *Journal of Virology*, Vol. 81, No. 18, (Sep 2007), pp. 9922-9931, ISSN 0022-538X.

Spanos, WC., Hoover, A., Harris, GF., Wu, S. Strand, GL., Anderson, ME., Klingelhutz, AJ., Hendriks, W., Bossler, AD. & Lee JH. (2008). The PDZ binding motif of Human Papillomavirus type 16 E6 induces PTPN13 loss, which allows anchorage-independent growth and synergizes with Ras for invasive growth. *Journal of Virology*, Vol. 82, No. 5, (Mar 2008), pp. 2493-2500, ISSN 0022-538X.

Spardy, N., Duensing, A., Charles, D., Haines, N., Nakahara, T., Lambert, PF. & Duensing, S. (2007). The Human Papillomavirus Type 16 E7 Oncoprotein Activates the Fanconi Anemia (FA) Pathway and Causes Accelerated Chromosomal Instability in FA Cells. *Journal of Virology*, Vol. 81, No. (Dec 2007), pp.13265 - 13270, ISSN 0022-538X.

Spoden, G.,Freitag, K., Husmann, M., Boller, K., Sapp, M., Lambert, C. & Florin L. (2008). Clathrin- and caveolin-independent entry of human papillomavirus type 16--involvement of tetraspanin-enriched microdomains (TEMs). *PLoS One*, Vol. 3, No. 10, (Jan 2008), pp. e-3313, ISSN 1932-6203.

Srivenugopal, KS. & Ali-Osman, F. (2002). The DNA repair protein, O(6)-methylguanine-DNA methyltransferase is a proteolytic target for the E6 human papillomavirus oncoprotein. *Oncogene,* Vol. 21, No. 38, (Aug 2002) 5940-5945, ISSN 0950-9232.

Stanley, MA. (2006). Immune responses to human papillomavirus. *Vaccine,* Vol. 24, Suppl 1, (Mar 2006), pp. S16-22, ISSN 0264-410X.

Stanley, M., Lowy, DR. & Frazer, I. (2006). Chapter 12: Prophylactic HPV vaccines: underlying mechanisms. *Vaccine,* Vol. 24, Suppl 3, (Aug 2006), pp. S106-113, ISSN 0264-410X.

Stanley, MA., Pett, MR. & Coleman, N. (2007). HPV: from infection to cancer. *Biochemical Society Transactions,* Vol. 53, No 6, (Dec 2007), pp. 1456-1460, ISSN 0300-5127.

Stanley, MA. (2008). Immunobiology of HPV and HPV vaccines. *Ginecologic Oncology,* Vol. 109, Suppl 2, (Feb 2008), pp. S15–21, ISSN 0090-8258

Stanley, MA. (2009a). Immune responses to human papilloma viruses. Indian Journal Medicine Research, Vol. 130, No. 3, (Sep 2009), pp. 266-276, ISSN 0971-5916.

Stanley, MA. (2009b). Immunobiology of genital HPV infection. *CME Journal of Gynecologic Oncology,* Vol. 14, pp. 36-43, ISSN 1219-9087.

Stanley MA. (2010). Pathology and epidemiology of HPV infection in females. *Gynecologic Oncology,* Vol. 117, Suppl 2, (May 2010), pp. S5-10, ISSN 0090-8258.

Steger, G & Corbach, S. (1997). Dose-dependent regulation of the early promoter of human papillomavirus type 18 by the viral E2 protein. *Journal of Virology,* Vol. 71, No. 1, (Jan 1997), pp. 50-58, ISSN 0022-538X.

Sterlinko GH, Weber M, Elston R, McIntosh P, Griffin H, Banks L & Doorbar J.(2004). Inhibition of E6-induced degradation of its cellular substrates by novel blocking peptides. *Journal of Molecular Biology.* Vol. 335, No. 4, (Jan.2004), pp 971-985, ISSN 0022-2836.

Storrs, CH. & Silverstein SJ. (2007) PATJ, a tight junction-associated PDZ protein, is a novel degradation target of high-risk human papillomavirus E6 and the alternatively spliced isoform 18 E6. *Journal of Virology.* Vol. 81, No. 8, (Apr 2007), pp. 4080-4090, ISSN 0022-538X.

Straight, SW., Herman, B. & McCance, DJ. (1995). The E5 oncoprotein of human papillomavirus type 16 inhibits the acidification of endosomes in human keratinocytes. *Journal of Virology,* Vol. 69, No.5 (May 1995), pp. 3185 - 3192, ISSN 0022-538X.

Stubenrauch, F., Colbert, AME.& Laimins, LA. (1998). Transactivation by the E2 protein of oncogenic human papillomavirus type 31 is not essential for early and late viral functions. *Journal of Virology,* Vol. 72, No. 10, (Oct 1998), pp. 8115-8123, ISSN 0022-538X.

Syrjänen SM. & Syrjänen KJ. (1999). New concepts on the role of human papillomavirus in cell cycle regulation. *Annals of Medicine,* Vol. 31, No 3, (Jun 1999), pp.175-187, ISSN 0785-3890.

Tasaki, T., Mulder, LCF., Iwamatsu, A., Lee, MJ., Davydov, IV., Varshavsky, A., Muesing, M & Kwon YT. (2005). A family of mammalian E3 ubiquitin ligases that contain the UBR box motif and recognize N-degrons. *Molecular and Celularl Biology,* Vol. 25, No. 16, (Aug 2005), pp. 7120-7136, ISSN 0270-7306.

Thierry, F., Spyrou, G., Yaniv, M. & Howley, P. (1992). Two AP1 sites binding JunB are essential for human papillomavirus type 18 transcription in keratinocytes. *Journal of Virology*, Vol. 66, No. 6, (Jun 1992), pp. 3740-3748, ISSN 0022-538X.

Thomas, MC. & Chiang, CM. (2005). E6 oncoprotein represses p53-dependent gene activation via inhibition of protein acetylation independently of inducing p53 degradation. *Molecular Cell*, Vol. 17, No 2, (Jan 2005), pp, 251-264. ISSN 1097-2765

Timmons, B., Akins, M. & Mahendroo, M. (2010). Cervical remodeling during pregnancy and parturition. *Trends in Endocrinology Metabolism*. Vol. 21, No 6, (June 2010), pp. 353-361, ISSN 1043-2760.

Tindle, RW. (2002). Immune evasion in human papillomavirus-associated cervical cancer. *Nature Reviews Cancer*, Vol. 2, No. , (January 2002), pp. 1-7, ISSN 1474-175X

Trottier, H & Franco, EL. (2006). The epidemiology of genital human papillomavirus infection. *Vaccine*, Vol. 24, Suppl 1, (Mar 2006), pp. S1-15, ISSN 0264-410X.

Tsai, TC. & Chen, SL. (2003) The biochemical and biological functions of human papillomavirus type 16 E5 protein. *Archives Virology*, Vol. 148, No. 8, (Aug 2003), pp.1445-1453, ISSN 0304-8608.

Tungteakkhun, SS., Filippova, M., Neidigh, JW., Fodor, N., & Penelope J. Duerksen-Hughes, PJ. (2008). The Interaction between Human Papillomavirus Type 16 and FADD Is Mediated by a Novel E6 Binding Domain. *Journal of Virology*, Vol. 82, No. 19, (Oct 2008), pp. 9600 - 9614, ISSN 0022-538X.

Uemura, Y., Liu, T-Y. Narita, Y., Suzuki M. & Matsushita, S. (2008). 17β-Estradiol (E2) plus tumor necrosis factor-α induces a distorted maturation of human monocyte-derived dendritic cells and promotes their capacity to initiate T-helper 2 responses. *Human Immunology*, Vol. 69, No. 3, (March 2008), pp. 149-157, ISSN 0198-8859.

Underbrink, MP., Howie, HL., Bedard, KM., Koop, JI. & Galloway, DA. (2008). E6 Proteins from Multiple Human Betapapillomavirus Types Degrade Bak and Protect Keratinocytes from Apoptosis after UVB Irradiation. *Journal of Virology*, Vol. 82, No. 21, (Nov 2008), pp.10408 - 10417, ISSN. 0022-538X.

van der Burg, SH. & Palefsky, JM. (2009) Human immunodeficiency virus and human papilloma virus - why HPV-induced lesions do not spontaneously resolve and why therapeutic vaccination can be successful. *Journal of Translational Medicine*, Vol. 7, No 108 (Jan 2009), pp. 1-8, ISSN 1479-5876.

Villa, LL. (2007). Overview of the clinical development and results of a quadrivalent HPV (types 6, 11, 16, 18) vaccine. *International Journal of Infectious Diseases*, Vol.11, Suppl 2, (Nov 2007), pp. S17-25, ISSN 1201-9712.

White, PW., Titolo, S., Brault, K., Thauvette, L., Pelletier, A., Welchner, E., Bourgon, L., Doyon, L., Ogilvie, WW., Yoakim, C., Cordingley, MG.& Archambault, J. (2003). Inhibition of human papillomavirus DNA replication by small molecule antagonists of the E1-E2 protein interaction. *The Journal of Biological Chemistry*. Vol. 278, No. 29, (Jul 2003), pp. 26765-26772, ISSN 0021-9258

Wilson, R., Fehrmann, F. & Laimins, LA. (2005). Role of the E1^E4 protein in the differentiation-dependent life cycle of human papillomavirus type 31. *Journal of Virology*, Vol. 79, No.11, (Jun 2005), pp. 6732-6740, ISSN 0022-538X.

Xu, YF, Zhang, YQ., Xu, XM. & Song, GX. (2006). Papillomavirus virus-like particles as vehicles for the delivery of epitopes or genes. *Archives of Virology*, Vol. 151, No. 11, (Nov 2006), pp. 2133-2148, ISSN 0304-8608.

Yuan, F., Auborn, K. & James C. (1999). Altered growth and viral gene expression in human papillomavirus type 16-containing cancer cell lines treated with progesterone. *Cancer Investigation*, Vol. 17, No. 1, (Jan 1999), pp. 19-29, ISSN 0735-7907.

Zekri, AR., Bahnassy, AA., Seif-Eldin, WM., Alam El-Din, HM., Madbouly, MS., Zidan, AZ., El-Hoshy, K., El-Ramly, A. & Abdel-Hamid, NA. (2006). Role of human papilloma virus (HPV) in common and genital warts and its relation to P53 expression. *Journal of the Egyptian National Cancer Institute*, Vol. 18, No 2, (Jun 2006), pp. 117-124, ISSN 1110-0362..

Zerfass, K., Schulze, A., Spitkovsky, D., Friedman, V., Henglein, B. & P Jansen-Durr, P. (1995). Sequential activation of cyclin E and cyclin A gene expression by human papillomavirus type 16 E7 through sequences necessary for transformation. *Journal of Virology*, Vol. 69, No. 10, (Oct 1995), pp. 6389-6399, ISSN 0022-538X.

Zerfass-Thome, K., Zwerschke, W., Mannhardt, B., Tindle, R., Botz, JW. & Jansen-Durr, P. (1996). Inactivation of the cdk inhibitor p27KIP1 by the human papillomavirus type 16 E7 oncoprotein. *Oncogene*, Vol. 13, No. 11, (Dec 1996), pp. 2323-2330, ISSN 0950-9232.

Zheng, L., Ding, H., Lu, Z., Li, Y., Pan, Y., Ning, T. & Ke, Y. (2008). E3 ubiquitin ligase E6AP-mediated TSC2 turnover in the presence and absence of HPV16 E6. Genes to cells : devoted to molecular & cellular mechanisms, Vol.13, No. 3, (Mar 2008), pp. 285–294, ISSN 1356-9597.

Zheng, ZM & Baker, CC. (2006). Papillomavirus genome structure, expression, and post-transcriptional regulation. *Frontiers in Bioscience*. Vol. 11, (Jan 2006), pp. 2286-2302. ISSN 1945-0494.

Zhou, X. & Munger, K. (2009) Expression of the human papillomavirus type 16 E7 oncoprotein induces an autophagy-related process and sensitizes normal human keratinocytes to cell death in response to growth factor deprivation. *Virology*, Vol. 385, No. 1, (Mar 2009), pp. 192-197, ISSN 0042-6822.

Zhou, F., Legaatt, GR & Frazer IH. (2011). Human papillomavirus 16 E7 protein inhibit inteferon-γ-mediated enhancement of keratinocyte antigen processing and T-cell lysis. *FEBS Journal*, Vol. 278, No 6, (Apr 2011), pp. 955-963. ISSN 1742-464X.

Ziegert, C., Wentzensen, N., Vinokurova, S., Kisseljov, F., Einenkel, J., Hoeckel, M. & Doeberitz MK. (2003). A comprehensive analysis of HPV integration loci in anogenital lesions combining transcript and genome-based amplification techniques. *Oncogene*, Vol. 22, No. 25, (Jun 2003), pp. 3977-3984, ISSN 0950-9232.

Zimmermann, H., Koh, C-H., Degenkolbe, R., O'Connor, MJ., Müller, A., Steger, G., Jason J., Lui, CY., Androphy, E. & Bernard, H-U. (2000). Interaction with CBP/p300 enables the bovine papillomavirus type 1 E6 oncoprotein to downregulate CBP/p300-mediated transactivation by p53. *Journal of General Virology*, Vol. 8, No. 11, (Nov 2000), pp. 2617-2623, ISSN 0022-1317.

zur Hausen, H. (1996). Papillomavirus infections - a major cause of human cancers. *Biochimica et Biophysica Acta*, Vol. 1288, No. 2, (Oct 1996), pp. 55-78, ISSN 0006-3002.

zur Hausen, H. (2009). Papillomaviruses in the causation of human cancers - a brief historical account. *Virology*, Vol. 384, No. 2, (Feb 2009), pp 260-265, ISSN 0042-6822.

2

Screening Methods in Prevention of Cervical Cancer

Robert Koiss
St. Stephen's Hospital, Obstetrics & Gynecology-Gynecology-Oncology Department, Budapest Hungary

1. Introduction

In this chapter I present the evidence about the performance of existing cervical cancer prevention technologies and discuss how HPV testing can be integrated. All screening and diagnostic test, including HPV DNA, and biomolecular tests, cervical cytology, colposcopy are the markers of risk of cervical cancer.

A summary and update of recently published meta-analyses and systemic reviews on clinical applications of HPV DNA testing is provided in this chapter.

1. triage of women with equivocal or low grade cytological alterations.
2. follow-up of women with abnormal screening results who are negative at biopsy
3. prediction of the therapeutic treatment of CIN
4. primary screening HPV test, lonely and combination with traditional Pap smear to detect the precancer lesions.

2. Screening

Screening is a public health activity to detect disease among people thought a priori to be well. In the United States, the major cervical screening target is treatable CIN3 (or, to be especially cautious, CIN2), not invasive cervical cancer, for which treatment causes far more morbidity and is less certain to succeed. Therefore, cervical screening distinguishes between the few women who might become patients because they are at highest risk of cancer and the overwhelming majority of women who are at far lower risk. Screening that targets the common, minor, and typically benign cytological and histological evidence of acute HPV infection cannot be cost-effective because the risk of invasive cancer is so low However, finding a woman with CIN3 is considered a screening success because she has a high risk of invasive cancer and can be treated before cancer develops.demonstrated in Nordic countries and in the United Kingdom (Bulkmans et al., 2005; Sasieni & Adams, 1999.)

2.1 Cytological screening

Since the development of cytology-based cervical in the mid-20th century screening using Pap smear test the mortality of cervical cancer has decreased substantially. In the US rates have fallen by 75 % or more since 1960s. The key aspects of the cervical screening programs based on cytology are the exfoliated cervical cells which are examined to predict the underlying risk of cervical cancer.

The consistently observed substantial reduction of cervical cancer incidence after introduction of cytology screening and the marked difference in cervical cancer incidence between countries with and without screening programs indicates that Pap testing does prevent cervical cancer. (Gustafsson et al., 1997)

Papanicolaou originally introduced cervical cytology with morphological classifications that were based on probability of underlying cancer. However, the current US cytology classification—the Bethesda system—incorporates a view of cervical carcinogenesis that is explicitly based on the natural history of HPV.

For example, the classification of low-grade squamous intraepithelial lesion (LSIL) is based on microscopic signs of an acute HPV infection, whereas high-grade squamous intraepithelial lesion (HSIL) suggests the possibility of an underlying CIN3 (or the more uncertain precancer diagnosis, CIN2) (Smith et al., 2007) The great majority of HSIL and approximately two-thirds of LSIL are associated with carcinogenic HPV types. (Clifford et al., 2005) Very common and equivocal cytological changes, which are classified as atypical squamous cells of undetermined significance (ASC-US), form the boundary between normal and abnormal cytological interpretations; roughly half of changes classified as ASC-US are positive for carcinogenic HPV. In the United States, ASC-US is more common than all other abnormalities combined. Because this finding is common and some represent true abnormalities, a sizeable fraction of CIN3+ cases are detected by ASC-US cytology, despite poor interobserver reproducibility.(Kinney et al., 1998)

With some noteworthy exceptions (Hutchinson et al., 1999; Kitchener et al., 2009) typically a single cervical cytological screen is insensitive for detecting CIN3; sensitivity estimates as low as 50%–60% have been reported in various settings. (Nanda et al., 2000.)

Although a single negative high-quality Papanicolaou test does indicate a substantially lowered risk of cervical cancer lasting multiple years, stronger reassurance of safety (ie, a high negative predictive value) requires repeated rounds of screening to detect growing CIN3 lesions. (Wright et al., 2007.)

In many countries, conventional Papanicolaou smears are still the standard of care. In the United States and a few other countries, liquid-based cytology techniques that create more uniform slides and computer-assisted cytology evaluation systems have been adopted to achieve greater laboratory productivity, but there is no evidence that they detect CIN3 more accurately than conventional cytology (Ronco et al., 2007; Siebers et al., 2009.); therefore, we do not distinguish among cytological techniques when considering the new role of HPV testing.

In Central and South America, coverage may be high in places, but the quality of the cytology programmes and access to treatment are typically poor, and rates of cervical cancer remain some of the highest documented in the world. A notable exception is Chile, where high quality cytology-based screening has had a substantial impact on cancer incidence and mortality. (Sepulveda & Prado., 2005)

Cytology is a subjective test and in programmes without quality control/quality assurance it is virtually impossible to achieve and maintain the clinical performance of cytology.

Cytology is labour intensive and to date has been refractory to high-throughput automated screening. Despite the low cost of consumables and because of the three reasons cited above, high-quality cytology is expensive in absolute terms and may not necessarily be the most cost-effective option for screening. (Goldie et al.,2005) Liquid-based cytology has logistical and operational advantages (interpretation at higher speed, lower rate of unsatisfactory smears and possibility of ancillary molecular testing using remnant fluid), but is more expensive and is neither more sensitive nor more specific than conventional cytology with respect to detection of histologically confirmed high-grade CIN. (Arbyn et al., 2008) We must continue to recognise both the strengths and limitations of cytology for cervical cancer screening. In populations vaccinated against HPV-16/18 we should anticipate that the positive predictive value (PPV) of cervical screening will be reduced because there will be fewer high-grade lesions amongwomen with cytological abnormalities. It is therefore rational to develop multiple, viable modalities for cervical cancer prevention, including methods that achieve similar or better screening performance than cytology alone but also meet the demands of underserved populations, suchas lowcost, the need for fewer than three visits (cytology, diagnostic colposcopy and treatment) in each intervention (screening) cycle and/or fewer interventions in a lifetime due to a greater negative reassurance of a single intervention. It is naive to think that one modality, whether it be cytology-based screening, visual inspection with acetic acid (VIA), HPV DNA testing or HPV vaccination will meet the demands of all populations throughout the world. Importantly, each screening method must be validated for its technical performance and must be cost-effective within the capacity of the region in which it is to be adopted. In other words, the cost-utility of one method *versus* another must be evaluated within the limits of acceptable expenditures and available resources in different settings. Papanicolaou (Pap) test originally introduced cervical cytology with morphological classifications of the cervical cells. However, the current cytology classification, the Bethesda system, incorporated a view of cervical carcinogenesis that is based on the way of HPV infection.

2.2 HPV DNA test

Human papillomavirus (HPV) infection is very common in young women after the onset of sexual activity and, when it persists, the viral oncoproteins produce perturbation of the cell-cycle controls resulting in cervical intraepithelial neoplasia (CIN). At their mildest (CIN1), these lesions are generally no more than manifestations of HPV infection, but at their most severe (CIN3) the risk of progression to cancer is higher if not detected and treated. Fortunately, the transition to cancer usually takes years or decades, thus allowing the opportunity for detection by exfoliative cytology. The peak incidence of HPV infection occurs at about age 20, the peak incidence/detection of CIN3 occurs at about age 30, and the peak incidence of cancer occurs in the 40 s. It is estimated that without secondary prevention, cervical cancer would occur in around 3–5% of women who acquire a high-risk HPV infection, although for every cancer that occurs a far larger number of CIN lesions develop, of which the majority will spontaneously regress. Most of the pre-malignant and malignant lesions are of the squamous type, but around 15% are of the glandular type. HPV types -16 and 18 are the dominant oncotypes in squamous lesions but type -18 is relatively more important in glandular lesions. The recognition of the strong causal relationship between persistent infection of the genital tract with high-risk HPV types and occurrence of cervical cancer has resulted in the development of a number of HPV DNA or RNA detection systems for screening.

Here I briefly summarize the update results of the meta-analysis trials.

There is now overwhelming evidence from randomized clinical trials that high risk HPV DNA screening is more sensitive than cytological screening for detecting histological proved CIN3. (Cuzick et al., 2008.)

Based on the central role of persistent infections with carcinogenic human papillomavirus (HPV) in cervical cancer, DNA testing for carcinogenic genotypes of HPV has recently been introduced into cervical cancer screening. HPV testing is more reliable (Carozzi et al., 2005; Castle et al., 2004.) and more sensitive but less specific than routinely performed cytology for detection of cervical intraepithelial neoplasia grade III and cancer (grade III+) or grade II+. (Arbyn et al., 2006; Bulkmans et al., 2007; Cuzick et al.,2006; Mayrand et al., 2007; Naucler et al., 2007.) HPV testing might soon be widely accepted as an alternative to routine cytology for cervical cancer screening.

In Castle's trial the aim was to evaluate the cumulative incidence of cervical intraepithelial neoplasia II or worse (grade II+) or cervical intraepithelial neoplasia grade III+ after short term persistence of prevalently detected carcinogenic human papillomavirus (HPV) (Castle et al., 2009).

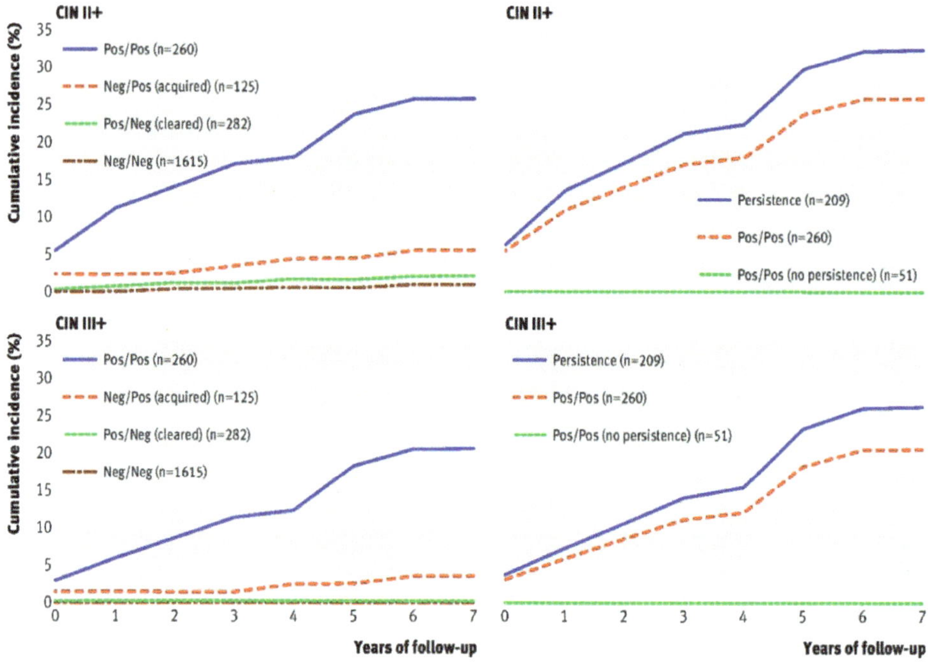

Fig. 1. Cumulative incidence of cervical intraepithelial neoplasia (CIN) grade II or worse (II+) and grade III+ after repeat measurements of carcinogenic human papillomavirus (HPV) at about one year (Castle et al., 2009)

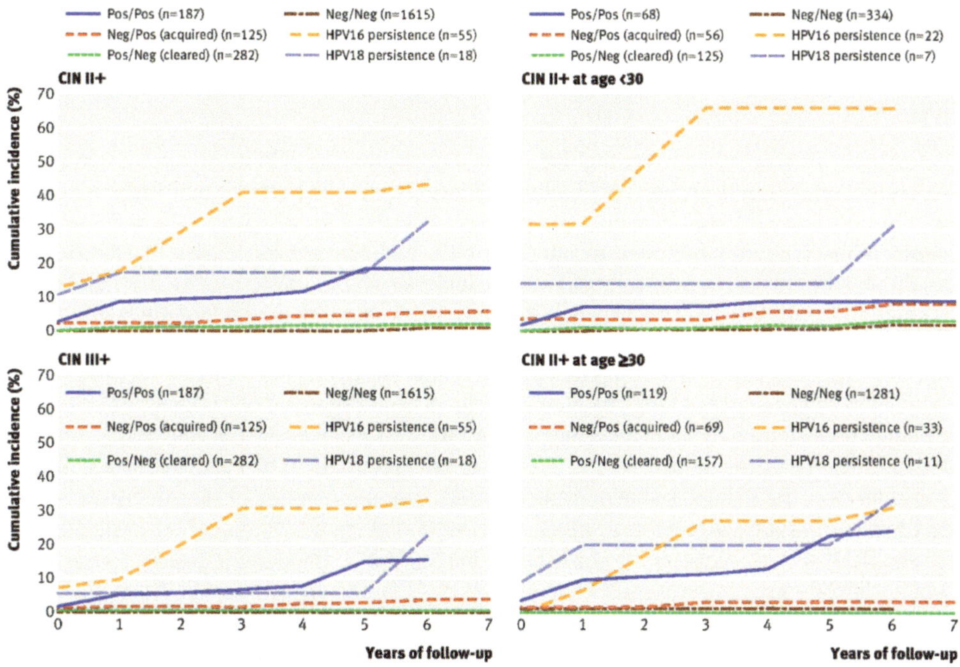

Fig. 2. In figure 2 The cumulative incidence of cervical intraepithelial neoplasia (CIN) grade II or more severe (grade II+) or grade III+ after repeat measurements of human papillomavirus (HPV) at about one year interval (9-21 months) in women who had persistent HPV 16, had persistent HPV 18, tested positive for carcinogenic HPV twice (Pos/Pos), tested positive for carcinogenic HPV at enrolment but negative at follow-up ("cleared"), tested carcinogenic HPV negative at enrolment but positive at follow-up ("acquired"), and tested negative at both time points (Neg/Neg). In right panels same groups are stratified by age. Time 0* indicates start time of analysis, 9-21 months after enrolment (Castle et al., 2009)

Among women aged <30, short term persistence of HPV 16 was highly predictive of a subsequent diagnosis of cervical intraepithelial neoplasia grade II+ (CIN2+), with a three (and five) year risk of 65.9% (40.4% to 91.5%). By comparison, among women aged ≥30, the three (and five) year risk after short term HPV 16 persistence was 27.2% (11.1% to 43.3%). There was no significant difference in the intensity of follow-up (median number of days between visits) by HPV status, although women who were in higher risk HPV groups (such as persistent HPV 16) naturally had fewer follow-up visits on average because of censoring treatments for diagnoses of grade 2+. In the summarise of Castle's trial I can allocate that women who tested positive twice for carcinogenic HPV had an increased risk of CIN2+ and CIN3+, while the risk in women who test negative for carcinogenic HPV at either or both time points was low. They did not observe any appreciable differences in the risks between those women with a shorter and longer time intervals between the enrolment and follow-up visit, suggesting that these findings are robust to variability in which women return for follow-up testing. Among those who tested positive twice for carcinogenic HPV, all subsequent diagnoses of cervical intraepithelial neoplasia grade II+ were linked to persistence of a specific HPV genotype. With the exception of HPV 16 and possibly HPV 18, however, detection of persistence of a specific genotype did not differentiate women at risk for CIN2+ qualitatively better than repeated detection of an aggregate of carcinogenic HPV types (Castle et al., 2009).

Some trials' results, which were highlighted at a press briefing held in advance of the annual meeting of the American Society of Clinical Oncology (ASCO), confirmed that for women with a negative HPV test and normal cytology, a 3-year follow-up appears to be safe and appropriate. Women who tested negative for HPV had a 5-year cancer risk that was similar to those who tested negative for HPV and had normal cytology (3.8 vs 3.2 per 100,000 women per year; $P = .8$). This was half the cancer risk of women who had a negative result on Pap testing only (3.8 vs 7.5 per 100,000 women per year; $P = .3$). Concurrent HPV testing and cervical cytology (cotesting) is an approved and promising alternative to cytology alone in women 30 years and older. Screening guidelines from organizations such as the American College of Obstetricians and Gynecologists and the American Cancer Society have endorsed the use of cotesting in this age group as a safe alternative to Pap testing alone. The summarize of the results is shown at the 1. table. (Annual Meeting of the American Society of Clinical Oncology, 2011).

Test Results	**5-Year Risk (%)**	**Excess Risk (%)**
HPV positive	7.6	7.4
HPV negative	0.2	
Pap positive	4.7	4.3
Pap negative	0.4	
HPV positive/Pap positive	12.0	
HPV positive/Pap negative	6.0	
HPV negative/Pap positive	0.9	
HPV negative/Pap negative	0.2	

Table 1. 5-Year Risk for Cancer/Precancer by Test Results

3. HPV DNA screening in triage of women with equivocal or low grade cytological alterations

In seven studies, where also repeat Pap smear was taken, the sensitivity of HPV DNA test was on average 14 % higher than repeat cytology, considering ASCUS or worse as a positive result for detection of CIN2+. The HPV DNA test and cytology triage showed similar specificity(Cuzick et al., 2008). The sensitivity of HC2 triage of women with an index smear showing low-grade squamous intraepithelial lesions (LSIL) was very high: 97.2% (95% CI: 95.6-98.8%), pooled from 11 studies for the outcome of CIN2+ and 97.1% (95% CI: 94.0-100%), pooled from six studies for CIN3+ (Cuzick et al., 2008; Kulasingam et al., 2002; Sherman et al., 2002; Schneider et al., 2000). However its specificity was very low: 30.6% (95% CI: 22.7-38.6%) for CIN2+ and 26.1% (95% CI: 15.1-37.1%) for CIN3+. Histologically confirmed CIN2+ and CIN3+ were present in respectively 17.6% (95% CI: 11.8-23.3%) and 7.4% (95% CI: 2.9-12.0%). The very large majority of women with LSIL had a positive HC2 result: pooled estimate of 74.4% (95% CI: 67.0–81.9%; range: 58–85%). However, Cuzick's overview trial found that for women aged 35 or more, the HPV positivity rate was much lower than for younger women and that the potential value of HPV DNA testing as an adjunct to cytology in this group was substantially better than for younger women (Ronco et al., 2007). Similar observations were made in the HPV in Addition to Routine Testing (HART) study (Cuzick et al., 2003). However, another study found a high rate of HPV positivity in women older than 35 with only a small decreasing gradient with age, suggesting that specificity may not be improved very much in this group by using HPV DNA testing before referring to colposcopy (Moss et al., 2006). Furtherwork is needed to synthesise all the data on HPV triage of LSIL according to age. Even more important, a negative HPV test provides long- term risk stratification: 5-10 years of reassurance, due to the high negative predictive value of the HPV DNA test, of not developing CIN3 and even more stronger reassurance of not developing invasive cancer among HPV DNA negative women. Because the vast majority of HPV infections represented acute HPV infection what are disappeared without causing cancer, HPV DNA testing has mediocre specificity and positive predictive value for cervical cancer screening. (Figure 3.)

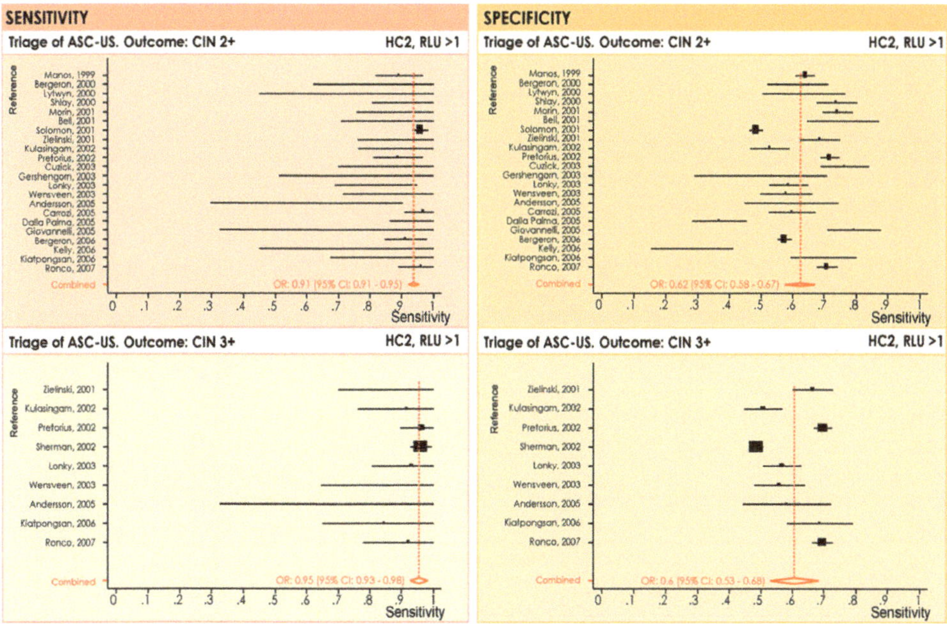

Fig. 3. Meta-analyses of the sensitivity (left) and specificity (right) of triage of women with cytological findings of ASC-US using the Hybrid Capture® 2 assay (RLU > 1) for identifying underlying CIN2 or worse (upper) or CIN3 or worse (lower). ASC-US: abnormal squamous cells of undetermined significance; CI: confidence interval; CIN2+: CIN grade 2 orworse; CIN3+: CIN grade 3 orworse; HC2: Hybrid Capture® 2 (Qiagen Gaithersburg, Inc. MD, USA (previously Digene Corp.); OR: odds ratio; RLU: relative light unit.(Castle et al., 2009; Pretorius et al., 2002)

4. Primary screening HPV test, lonely and combination with traditional Pap smear to detect the precancer lesions

Successful risk stratification based on HPV screening depends on whether the infection found are persistent (high risk for CIN) or new (low risk for CIN), especially in elderly women.

Women aged 30 years or older, who test positive for high risk HPV DNA, especially the first time they are tested (when the infections might already be persistent), are at sufficiently high risk of CIN3+ to merit intensified follow-up.

There is now overwhelming evidence from randomized clinical trials that carcinogenic HPV DNA screening is more sensitive than cytological screening for detecting histological CIN3 (Mayrand et al., 2007; Ronco et al., 2010). Even more important, a negative HPV test provides long-term risk stratification: 5–10 years of reassurance (ie, a high negative predictive value) of not developing CIN3 and even stronger reassurance of not developing invasive cancer among HPV DNA–negative women. High negative predictive value permits safe and cost-effective lengthening of the cervical screening interval when HPV testing is used (Dillner et al., 2008; Khan et al., 2005) (Figure 4).

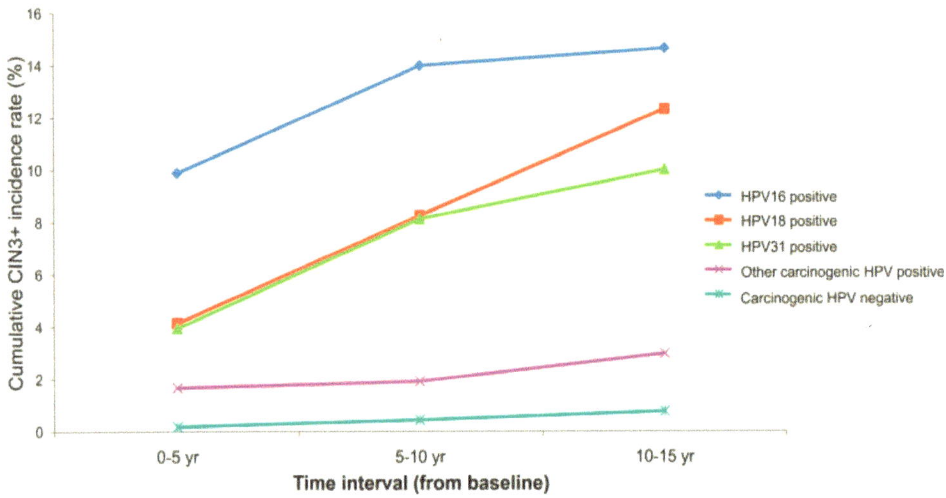

Fig. 4. Cumulative incidence rate of cervical intraepithelial neoplasia grade 3 or invasive cervical cancer (CIN3+) over 15 years following a single human papillomavirus (HPV) test. A cohort of 20 000 women from Kaiser Permanente (Portland, OR) was followed up by conventional cytology screening for approximately 15 years (78). Archived cervical specimens obtained from the women at enrollment (baseline) were tested for carcinogenic HPV types. The risk estimates, adjusted for loss to follow-up, show primarily that in this older cohort (average age approximately 35 years), a negative HPV test predicts very low risk of subsequent CIN3+. Baseline test positivity for HPV16, HPV18, or HPV31 was most strongly linked to subsequent CIN3+. (Schiffman et al., 2011)

Overall, the sensitivity of HC2 for finding underlying high-grade intraepithelial neoplasia was 89.7% (95% CI: 86.4-93.0%)) but varied over a large range between 50% (Clavel et al., 2001; Sankaranarayanan et al., 2004) and 100%. In North America and Europe, the pooled specificity was higher: 91.7% (95% CI: 90.3-93.1%; range: 85-95%).

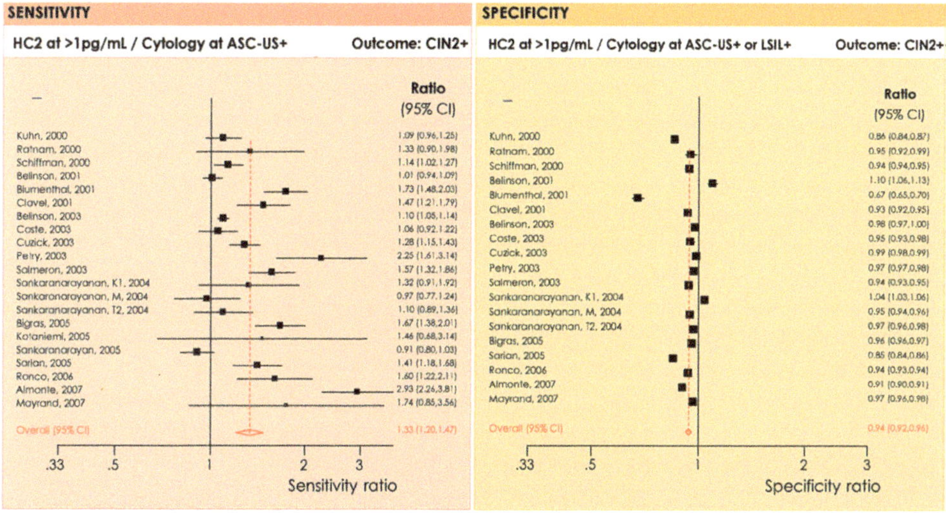

Fig. 5. Relative sensitivity (left) and specificity (right) of HPV testing using the Hybrid Capture® 2 assay compared to cytology in primary screening studies. ASC-US: abnormal squamous cells of undetermined significance; CI: confidence interval; CIN2+: CIN grade 2 or worse; HC2: Hybrid Capture® 2 (Qiagen Gaithersburg, Inc. MD, USA (previouslyDigene Corp.); LSIL: low-grade squamous intraepithelial lesion (Cuzick et al., 2008).

Because the vast majority of HPV infections represent acute HPV infections that are destined to clear without causing cancer, HPV testing has mediocre specificity and positive predictive value for cervical cancer screening. The women who test HPV positive 3 years after a negative HPV test [the current recommendation for cotesting are at much lower risk of CIN2 or CIN3+ than women who are HPV positive at their first screen and, therefore, may already have a persistent infection (Schiffman et al., 2011).

This important fact mandates much longer HPV screening intervals than current cytology screening intervals of every 2 years and suggests that the current 3-year interval for cotesting will still be too frequent. The corollary of high sensitivity of HPV testing for incipient as well as prevalent CIN3+ is a high negative predictive value that lasts for years (Schiffman et al., 2011). Several studies have shown that HPV negativity alone or in combination with negative cytology signifies a longer disease free interval against CIN2+ than being negative for cytology alone.

Early studies measured HPV retrospectively and did not use it for management. Sherman ME et al. followed 20,810 women for 10 years and found that in cytologically negative women lesions were diagnosed much more rapidly in those who were HPV-positive compared to women who were HPV-negative (Sherman et al., 2003). In two Danish cohorts of women aged 22–32 years and 40–50 years HPV DNA was measured retrospectively and again not used for triage. The authors concluded that HPV DNA testing at five-yearly intervals offers protection similar to cytology testing at three-yearly intervals (Kjaer et al., 2002). Clavel C et al. reported that 5 of 4,401 women with negative cytology and HPV DNA tests and followed-up for a median of 34 months developed high-grade lesions, compared to 29 of 501 women who were initially cytology-negative but HPV-positive and concluded that a screening interval of three to five years was safe in double negative women (Clavel et al., 2004). Similar conclusions were obtained by Bulkmans NW et al. in a cohort of 2,810 cytology-negative women followed for five years, where 4 of 62 HPV-positive women developed CIN3+ compared to 1 of 2,175 HPV-negative women (Bulkmans et al., 2005). Long-term follow-up of the Hammersmith cohort and two large recent randomised trials in Sweden and The Netherlands have all shown that the higher detection rate for CIN2+, when HPV DNA testing was used as part of the initial screening process, led to lower rates of CIN3+ at the subsequent screening round and indicates that HPV DNA tests are highly sensitive to detect prevalent cases(Cuzick et al., 2008; Naucler et al., 2007). In the Hammersmith study, the cumulative proportion of CIN2+ within five-years after a negative HPV DNA test, when most women would have had at least one routine repeat smear was about half as high as for women who were originally cytology negative (0.6% versus 1.2%), and only after six or more years do the CIN2+ rates in women originally HPV-negative approach those seen after three years in women who were originally cytology-negative. In the Swedish study of women aged 32–38, the detection rate for CIN2+ associated with the addition of HPV DNA testing was increased 51% percent at the initial screen, but 42% lower in the follow-up period (mean: 4.1 years). For the Dutch study, the detection rate of CIN3+ was 70% higher initially but 55% lower in the 6.5 year mean follow-up period. The fact that the higher detection rate for CIN2+ when HPV DNA testing was used as part of the initial screening process led to lower rates of disease at the subsequent screening round (Bulkmans et al., 2007; Naucler et al., 2007). It also suggests that there is minimal over-diagnosis for women aged over 30, as the cumulative CIN2+ rates over two rounds were similar in all three studies, and also that the screening interval can be safely extended to at least 6 years with HPV DNA testing.

Although the ability to lengthen screening intervals is a great advance, it poses a major challenge for transitioning from cervical screening programs that are based on repeated cytology. In particular, in the United States, the considerable general reluctance to move to long-interval screening is due at least in part to reasons unrelated to theoretical best public health practice. By contrast, in some European settings, where cervical cancer screening practices are dictated more directly by public health considerations, detailed planning is underway for a transition to long-interval HPV testing (Naucler et al.,2009).

The limited data on follow-up beyond six to seven years does not allow evaluation of longer screening intervals at this time and further work is needed to see if even longer intervals might be safe, particularly for women with two or more negative HPV tests (Cuzick et al., 2008).

Some professional organizations now recommend the routine use of HPV DNA testing for screening women aged 30 years and older.

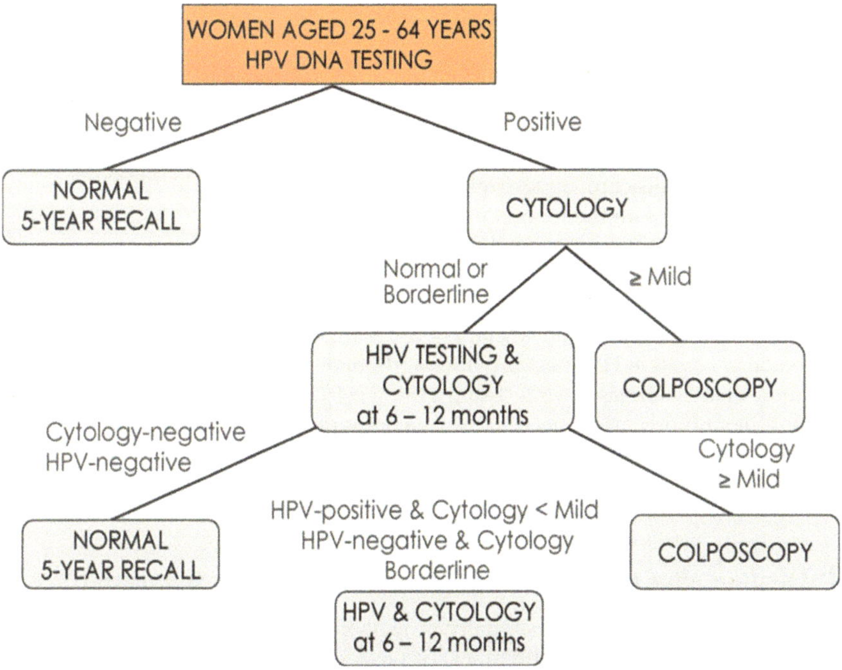

Fig. 6. Proposed new screening algorithm which employs HPV DNA testing as the primary screening test and uses cytology to triage HPV positive women (Cuzick et al., 2008).

5. HPV screening with triage by novel biomarkers

Most of the biomarkers identified thus far are markers of HPV related transformation , which reveals HPV infection. These biomarkers are more prevalent in CIN3 than in acute HPV infection.

Currently developed and used biomarkers can be shared as follow:

a. markers of increased HPV oncogene expression, such as HPV mRNA,
b. markers of increased cell proliferation, such as Ki-67, p16
c. markers of chromosomal instability, such as HPV DNA integration

At present, the most promising candidate as a biomarker for triage after a positive HPV test is immunocytochemical staining of cytology slides for p16 (Denton et al., 2010; Tsoumpou et al., 2009; Wentzensen et al., 2007).

The p16 overexpression is associated with the disruption of the retinoblastoma cell cycle pathway by HPV E7 (Denton et al., 2010; Tsoumpou et al., 2009). A combined stain for p16 and Ki-67 that was recently introduced into the diagnostics market can highlight rare transformed cells (Denton et al., 2010). Because its sensitivity for CIN3 is far higher than cytology's and almost equal to that of HPV testing and its specificity is comparable to cytology's, this stain could be used as a triage following primary HPV testing if it proves reliable and the cost for routine use is low (Denton et al., 2010).

6. HPV DNA test as a subsequent management after negative biopsy and/or colposcopy

Historically, colposcopically directed biopsies have been the clinical reference standard for diagnosing and grading pre-cancer into CIN1, 2, or 3. However, the choice of biopsy site and the histopathological diagnosis of resultant biopsies tend to be variable and subjective. Clinicians rely on colposcopy to determine the presence or absence of epithelial lesions, find the area of the cervix with the highest degree of the lesion and direct biopsy for histological diagnosis. Unfortunately well -trained gynecologists have false negative colposcopy rates as high as 20-40 % in patients with histological diagnosed pre-cancer lesion(Schiffmanet al., 2007).The use of HPV DNA testing related to triage is in women who are referred for colposcopy, because of alteration smear, but no visible lesion on colposcopy allowable. For these women, a negative HPV test provides additional reassurance, that there is unlikely to be any undetectable disease, while being HPV positive (especially for types -16 and 18), indicates a continuing risk needing for short-term repeat testing(Gravittet al.,2008). Especially for type -18, the possibility of an adenocarcinoma or its precursor lesion, adenocarcinoma in situ, should be excluded by careful examination of the endocervical canal.

7. HPV testing after treatment of cervical intraepithelial neoplasia

CIN is a very common disease especially in women of reproductive age and a balance is needed to maximize the prevention of cervical carcinoma and the same time avoid overtreatment. Management strategies of CIN include decision-making regarding the appropriateness of conservative approach versus treatment. Conservative strategies are appropriate for women with low-grade CIN, particularly in the younger age range. High-grade CIN (CIN2 or CIN3) should be treated. Conservative methods reduce overtreatment as low-grade CIN lesions may regress spontaneously. When HG-CIN is detected the treatment is mandatory. CIN 3 which is the true precursor of cervical cancer will progress to cancer if left untreated at a rate of around 30 % over 2 years (Kitchener& Stern,2008). CIN 1 has been reported to progress to CIN 2/3 at a rate of 15 % over 2 years but some of these cases may harbour undetected CIN2/3 (Castellsague et al., 2006; Kitchener& Stern,2008). Screening programs that exploit the extra sensitivity for CIN3+ conferred by HPV testing must still minimize treatment of women that is unnecessary on both public health and individual grounds. In the United States, the predominant mode of treatment for CIN2 or CIN3 is the excision of the transformation zone using a wire loop cautery, commonly known as loop electrosurgical excision procedure (LEEP) or large loop excision of the transformation zone. This office-based procedure has two advantages: it can be performed under local anesthesia and it produces a tissue specimen. The concern over the risk of premature delivery following this treatment motivates recent efforts to reduce overscreening and overtreatment, especially among young women(Kyrgiou et al.,2006). However, the societal trade-offs that come from trying to prevent every case of cervical cancer, vs the desire to prevent overtreatment of many women , should and will be debated. HPV testing following treatment with LEEP can identify women who remain at high risk of recurrence (Kreimer et al., 2006). Successful treatment of the transformation zone often leads to HPV negativity in cervicovaginal specimens for the causative HPV type (Kreimer et al., 2007)., although HPV infects the vagina (and vulva and anogenital skin) and not just the cervix. The reason for viral clearance even when the excision heals, thus creating a new transformation zone, is not certain. The pre-reconisation HPV testing might be useful in reducing the number of reconisations in those cases where high-risk HPV test is either negative or does not confirm the same HPV type, as before (Koiss et al., 2001). Nonetheless, negative HPV tests after LEEP predict a high probability of cure (Kreimer et al., 2006). The HPV test can be useful to replace cytology for the follow up due to the high negative predictive value.

8. Conclusions

In conclusion, much has been achieved during the last 10 years from research on prevention of cervical cancer through vaccination and screening. It is imperative that planning for future prevention guidelines does not address vaccination and screening separately. Implementation of all components of an organized prevention would increase the efficiency of the process. Increased coverage of prevention activities, both vaccination and screening, will be of utmost importance (Koiss et al., 2010). It is abundantly clear that HPV DNA testing is substantially more sensitive than cytology at detecting high-grade CIN. However, HPV testing is somewhat less specific than cytology due primarily to the detection of transient infections that have not produced cytologic alterations. Basic principles suggest that in such circumstances the more sensitive test should be applied first (i.e., HPV DNA testing) and the more specific test (i.e., cytology) should then be used only for HPV-positive women to determine management. Management of HPV-positive, cytology-negative women presents a new challenge. Management of HPV-positive, cytology-negative women presents a new challenge. Results from the HART, Swedish and the Amsterdam (POBASCAM) studies suggest they can safely be managed by repeating the testing with both cytology and HPV after one year and this is being further explored in several ongoing studies (Bulkmans et al., 2007; Cuzick et al., 2003; Naucler et al., 2007). Women double negative at that time could be returned to routine screening while positives could be referred to colposcopy. This approach of using HPV DNA testing as the sole primary screening modality has several advantages: HPV DNA detection assays provide an automated, objective and very sensitive test. Implementation projects of the HPV/Pap triage screening strategy to demonstrate what could be acceptably safe intervals for both vaccinated and unvaccinated women should be initiated. We will also need to determine the best follow-up algorithms for HPV-positive/Pap-negative women. Genotyping tests, which specify the exact HPV types present on the cervix, and molecular markers of HPV targeting oncogene mRNA or proteins associated with deregulation of the cell cycle may prove to be useful for this purpose. If second-generation HPV vaccines targeting most hrHPV types are included in vaccination programs, screening activities will need to be reevaluated and algorithms modified. These prospects provide hope for a further decrease in cervical cancer incidence and mortality in the coming decades.

9. References

Annual Meeting of the American Society of Clinical Oncology. *Abstract 1508.* June 6, 2011

Arbyn M,Sasieni P, Meijer CJ, Clavel C, Koliopoulos G, Dillner J.(2006) Clinical applications of HPV testing: a summary of meta-analyses. *Vaccine Chapter 9*: Vol.24(suppl 3):S78-89

Arbyn M, Bergeron C, Klinkhamer P, Martin-Hirsch P, Siebers AG, Bulten J. (2008) Liquid compared with conventional cervical cytology: a systematic review and metaanalysis. *Obstetrics Gynecology* Vol.111,No.1,(January),pp:167-77.

Bulkmans NW,Rozendaal L, Voorhorst FJ, Snijders PJ,Meijer CJ.(2005) Long-term protective effect of high-risk human papillomavirus testing in population-based cervical screening. *British Journal of Cancer* Vol.92,No.9,(May),pp.1800-2.

Bulkmans N,Berkhof J, Rozendaal L, van Kemenade FJ, Boeke A, Bulk S.(2007) Human papillomavirus DNA testing for the detection of cervical intraepithelial neoplasia grade 3 and cancer: 5-year follow-up of a randomised controlled implementation trial. *Lancet*, Vol.370,No.24 (November),pp.1764-72.

Carozzi FM, Del Mistro A, Confortini M, Sani C, Puliti D, Trevisan R, (2005) Reproducibility of HPV DNA testing by hybrid capture 2 in a screening setting. *American Journal of Clinical Pathology*, Vol. 24,No.5,(November),pp.716-21.

Castellsague X, Diaz M, de Sanjose S, et al (2006) Worldwide human papillomavirus etiology of cervical adenocarcinoma and its cofactors: implications for screening and prevention. *Journal of the National Cancer Institute.*Vol.98,No.5,(March),pp.303-315

Castle PE, Wheeler CM, Solomon D, Schiffman M, Peyton CL.(2004) Interlaboratory reliability of hybrid capture 2. *American Journal of Clinical Pathology* Vol.122,No.:2,(Augustus),pp.238-45.

Castle PE, Rodríguez AC, Burk RD, Herrero R, Wacholder S, Alfaro M, Morales J, Guillen D, Sherman ME, Solomon D, Schiffman M;(2009) Proyecto Epidemiológico Guanacaste (PEG) Group, Short term persistence of human papillomavirus and risk of cervical precancer and cancer: population based cohort study. *British Medical Journal.* Vol.28,No.339 (July),*pp:b2569. Doi: 10.1136/bmj.b2569.*

Clavel C, Masure M, Bory JP, Putaud I, Mangeonjean C, Lorenzato M, Nazeyrollas P, Gabriel R, Quereux C, Birembaut P.(2001) Human papillomavirus testing in primary screening for the detection of high-grade cervical lesions: a study of 7932 women. *British Journal of Cancer* Vol.84,No.12.(June),pp.1616-23.

Clavel C, Cucherousset J, Lorenzato M, Caudroy S, Nou JM, Nazeyrollas P, Polette M, Bory JP, Gabriel R, Quereux C, Birembaut P. (2004) Negative human papillomavirus testing in normal smears selects a population at low risk for developing high-grade cervical lesions. *British Journal of Cancer* Vol.90,No.9 (May),pp.1803-8.

Clifford GM, Rana RK, Franceschi S, Smith JS, Gough G, Pimenta JM. (2005) Human papillomavirus genotype distribution in low-grade cervical lesions: comparison by geographic region and with cervical cancer. *Cancer Epidemiology & Biomarkers Prevention* Vol.14,No.5,(May),pp.1157-1164

Cuzick J, Szarewski A, Cubie H, Hulman G, Kitchener H, Luesley D, McGoogan E, Menon U, Terry G, Edwards R, Brooks C, Desai M, Gie C, Ho L, Jacobs I, Pickles C, Sasieni P. (2003) Management ofwomen who test positive for high-risk types of human papillomavirus: the HART study. *Lancet* Vol.362, No.9399,(December),pp.1871-6.

Cuzick J, Clavel C, Petry KU, Meijer CJ, Hoyer H, Ratnam S, Szarewski A, Birembaut P, Kulasingam S, Sasieni P, Iftner T. (2006) Overview of the European and North American studies on HPV testing in primary cervical cancer screening. *International Journal of Cancer* Vol.119,No.5,(September),pp.1095-101.

Cuzick J, Arbyn M, Sankaranarayanan R, Tsu V, Ronco G, Mayrand MH, Dillner J, Meijer CJ.(2008) Overview of Human Papillomavirus-Based and Other Novel Options for

Cervical Cancer Screening in Developed and Developing Countries. *Vaccine* 26S Vol.26, Suppl 10,(Augustus),K29-41

Cuzick J,Szarewski A, Mesher D, Cadman L, Austin J, Perryman K, Ho L, Terry G, Sasieni P, Dina R, Soutter WP. (2008) Long-term follow-up of cervical abnormalities among women screened by HPV testing and cytology-Results from the Hammersmith study. *International Journal of Cancer* Vol.122,No.10(May) pp.2294-300.

Denton KJ, Bergeron C, Klement P, Trunk MJ, Keller T, Ridder R; European CINtec Cytology Study Group. (2010)The sensitivity and specificity of p16(INK4a) cytology vs HPV testing for detecting high-grade cervical disease in the triage of ASC-US and LSIL pap cytology results. *American Journal of Clinical Pathology* Vol.134,No.1(July),pp.12-21.

Dillner J, Rebolj M, Birembaut P, Petry KU, Szarewski A, Munk C, de Sanjose S, Naucler P, Lloveras B, Kjaer S, Cuzick J, van Ballegooijen M, Clavel C, Iftner T; Joint European Cohort Study. (2008) Long term predictive values of cytology and human papillomavirus testing in cervical cancer screening: joint European cohort study. *British Medical Journal* Vol.337,No.1754, (October), *doi: 10.1136/bmj.a1754.*

Gravitt P, Coutlée F, Iftner T, Sellors J, Quint W, Wheeler CM. (2008) New Technologies in Cervical Cancer Screening. *Vaccine* Vol.26,Suppl. 10(Augustus)pp.K42-52.

Goldie SJ, Gaffikin L, Goldhaber-Fiebert JD, Gordillo-Tobar A, Levin C, Mahé C, Wright TC; Alliance for Cervical Cancer Prevention Cost Working Group (2005)Cost-effectiveness of cervical-cancer screening in five developing countries *The New England Journal of Medicine* Vol.353,No.20,(November),pp.2158-68.

Gustafsson L, Pontén J, Bergström R, Adami HO.(1997) International incidence rates of invasive cervical cancer before cytological screening. *International Journal of Cancer* Vol.71,No.2, (April),pp.159-165.

Hutchinson ML, Zahniser DJ, Sherman ME, Herrero R, Alfaro M, Bratti MC, Hildesheim A, Lorincz AT, Greenberg MD, Morales J, Schiffman M. (1999) Utility of liquid-based cytology for cervical carcinoma screening: results of a population-based study conducted in a region of Costa Rica with a high incidence of cervical carcinoma. *Cancer* Vol.87,No.2,(April),pp.48-55.

Khan MJ, Castle PE, Lorincz AT, Wacholder S, Sherman M, Scott DR, Rush BB, Glass AG, Schiffman M. (2005) The elevated 10-year risk of cer¬vical precancer and cancer in women with human papillomavirus (HPV) type 16 or 18 and the possible utility of type-specific HPV testing in clinical practice. *Journal of the National Cancer Institute* Vol.97,No.14,(July)pp.1072-1079.

Kinney WK, Manos MM, Hurley LB, Ransley JE.(1998) Where's the high-grade cervical neoplasia? The importance of minimally abnormal Papanicolaou diagnoses. *Obstetrics Gynecology*. Vol.91,No.6,(June),pp.973-976.

Kitchener HC, Almonte M, Thomson C, Wheeler P, Sargent A, Stoykova B, Gilham C, Baysson H, Roberts C, Dowie R, Desai M, Mather J, Bailey A, Turner A, Moss S, Peto J. (2009) HPV testing in combination with liquid-based cytology in primary cervical screening (ARTISTIC): a randomised controlled trial. *Lancet Oncology* Vol.10,No.7,(July),pp.672-682.

Kjaer SK, van den Brule AJ, Paull G, Svare EI, Sherman ME, Thomsen BL, Suntum M, Bock JE, Poll PA, Meijer CJ. (2002) Type specific persistence of high risk human papillomavirus (HPV) as indicator of high grade cervical squamous intraepithelial lesions in young women:population based prospective follow up study. *British Medical Journal* Vol.325,No.7364,(September),pp.572.

Koiss R., Siklós P.(2010): Relationship between human papillomavirus infection and cervical carcinoma. *Lege Artis Medicine*, Vol.20,No.2(April),pp.96-102 (Hungarian)

Koiss R, Babarczi E,Jenei C,Gőcze P.Horányi L,Siklós P.(2011) Reconisation or repeated HPV test? *P6-21 EUROGIN* 2011 Lisbon Portugal, 8-11., May, 2011

Kreimer AR, Guido RS, Solomon D,Schiffman M, Wacholder S, Jeronimo J, Wheeler CM, Castle PE. (2006) Human papillomavirus testing following loop electrosurgical excision procedure identifies women at risk for posttreatment cervical intraepithelial neoplasia grade 2 or 3 disease. *Cancer Epidemiology & Biomarkers Prevention* Vol.15,No.5,(May),pp.908–914

Kreimer AR, Katki HA, Schiffman M, Wheeler CM, Castle PE; ASCUS-LSIL; Triage Study Group (2007) Viral determinants of human papillomavirus persistence following loop electrical excision procedure treatment for cervical intraepithelial neoplasia grade 2 or 3. *Cancer Epidemiology & Biomarkers Prevention* Vol.16,No.1,(January) pp.11–16.

Kulasingam SL, Hughes JP, Kiviat NB, Mao C, Weiss NS, Kuypers JM, Koutsky LA.(2002) Evaluation of human papillomavirus testing in primary screening for cervical abnormalities: comparison of sensitivity, specificity, and frequency of referral. *The Journal of the American Medical Association* Vol.288,No.14,(October),pp.1749-57.

Kyrgiou M, Koliopoulos G, Martin-Hirsch P,Arbyn M, Prendiville W, Paraskevaidis E. (2006) Obstetric outcomes after conservative treatment for intraepithelial or early invasive cervical lesions: systematic review and meta-analysis. *Lancet* Vol,367,No.9509,(February),pp.489–498.

Mayrand MH, Duarte-Franco E, Rodrigues I, Walter SD, Hanley J, Ferenczy A, Ratnam S, Coutlée F, Franco EL; Canadian Cervical Cancer Screening Trial Study Group. (2007) Human papillomavirus DNA versus Papanicolaou screening tests for cervical cancer. *The New England Journal of Medicine* Vol.357,No.16,(October), pp.1579-88.

Moss S, Gray A, Legood R, Vessey M, Patnick J, Kitchener H.; Liquid Based Cytology/Human Papillomavirus Cervical Pilot Studies Group. (2006) Effect of testing for human papillomavirus as a triage during screening for cervical cancer: observational before and after study. *British Medical Journal* Vol.332,No.7533, (January),pp.83–5.

Nanda K, Macrory DC, Myers ER, Bastian LA, Hasselblad V, Hickey JD, Matchar DB. (2000) Accuracy of the Papanicolaou test in screening for and follow-up of cervical cytologic abnormalities: a systematic review. *Annals of Internal Medicine* Vol.132, No.10,(May),pp.810–819.

Naucler P, Ryd W, Tornberg S, Strand A, Wadell G, Elfgren K, Rådberg T, Strander B, Johansson B, Forslund O, Hansson BG, Rylander E, Dillner J. (2007) Human papillomavirus and Papanicolaou tests to screen for cervical cancer. *The New England Journal of Medicine* Vol.357,No.16,(October),pp.1589-97.

Naucler P,Ryd W, Tornberg S, Strand A, Wadell G, Elfgren K, Rådberg T, Strander B, Forslund O, Hansson BG, Hagmar B, Johansson B, Rylander E, Dillner J. (2009) Efficacy of HPV DNA testing with cytology triage and/or repeat HPV DNA testing in primary cervical cancer screening. *Journal of the National Cancer Institute* Vol.101,No.2,(January),pp.88–99.

Pretorius RG, Peterson P, Novak S, Azizi F, Sadeghi M, Lorincz AT. (2002) Comparison of two signal-amplification DNA tests for high-risk HPV as an aid to colposcopy. *The Journal of Reproductive Medicine* Vol.47,No.4,(April),pp.290-6.

Ronco G, Cuzick J, Pierotti P,Cariaggi MP, Dalla Palma P, Naldoni C, Ghiringhello B, Giorgi-Rossi P, Minucci D, Parisio F, Pojer A, Schiboni ML, Sintoni C, Zorzi M, Segnan N, Confortini M. (2007)Accuracy of liquid based versus con¬ventional cytology: overall results of new technologies for cervical cancer screening: randomised controlled trial. *British Medical Journal.* Vol.335,No.7609,(July),pp.28–31.

Ronco G, Cuzick J, Segnan N, Brezzi S, Carozzi F, Folicaldi S, Dalla Palma P, Del Mistro A, Gillio-Tos A, Giubilato P, Naldoni C, Polla E, Iossa A, Zorzi M, Confortini M, Giorgi-Rossi P; NTCC working group. (2007)HPV triage for low grade (L-SIL) cytology is appropriate for women over 35 in mass cervical cancer screening using liquid based cytology. *European Journal of Cancer* Vol.43,No.3,(February),pp.476–80.

Ronco G, Giorgi-Rossi P, Carozzi F, Confortini M, Dalla Palma P, Del Mistro A, Ghiringhello B, Girlando S, Gillio-Tos A, De Marco L, Naldoni C, Pierotti P, Rizzolo R, Schincaglia P, Zorzi M, Zappa M, Segnan N, Cuzick J; New Technologies for Cervical Cancer screening (NTCC) Working Group. (2010) Efficacy of human papillomavirus testing for the detection of invasive cervical cancers and cervical intraepithelial neoplasia: a randomised controlled trial. *Lancet Oncology* Vol.11,No.3,(March),pp.249–257.

Sankaranarayanan R, Chatterji R, Shastri SS, Wesley RS, Basu P, Mahe C, Muwonge R, Seigneurin D, Somanathan T, Roy C, Kelkar R, Chinoy R, Dinshaw K, Mandal R, Amin G, Goswami S, Pal S, Patil S, Dhakad N, Frappart L, Fontaniere B. (2004) Accuracy of human papillomavirus testing in primary screening of cervical neoplasia: results from a multicenter study in India. *International Journal of Cancer.* Vol.112,No.2,(November),pp.341-7.

Sasieni P, Adams J. Effect of screening on cervical cancer mortality in England and Wales: analysis of trends with an age period cohort model. *British Medical Journal* Vol.318,No.7193,(May),pp.1244–5.

Schiffman M, Castle PE, Jeronimo J, Rodriguez AC, Wacholder S. (2007)Human papillomavirus and cervical cancer. *Lancet* Vol.370,No.9590,(September),pp.890–907.

Schiffman M, Wentzensen N, Wacholder S, Kinney W, Gage JC, Castle PE.(2011) Human papillomavirus testing in the prevention of cervical cancer. *Journal of the National Cancer Institute* Vol.103,No.5,(March),pp.:368-83.

Schneider A, Hoyer H, Lotz B, Leistritza S, Kühne-Heid R, Nindl I, Müller B, Haerting J, Dürst M.(2000) Screening for high-grade cervical intra-epithelial neoplasia and cancer by testing for high-risk HPV, routine cytology or colposcopy. *International Journal of Cancer.* Vol.89,No.6,(November),pp.529-34.

Screening for squamous cervical cancer: duration of low risk after negative results of cervical cytology and its implication for screening policies. IARCWorking Group on evaluation of cervical cancer screening programmes. *British Medical Journal* (clinres Ed) 1986; Vol.293,No.6548,(September),pp.659-64

Sepulveda C, Prado R.(2005) Effective cervical cytology screening programmes in middle-income countries: the Chilean experience. *Cancer Detection and Prevention* Vol.29,No.5,(September),pp.405–11.

Sherman ME,Schiffman M, Cox JT (2002); Atypical Squamous Cells of Undetermined Significance/Low-Grade Squamous Intraepithelial Lesion Triage Study Group. Effects of age and human papilloma viral load on colposcopy triage: data from the randomized Atypical Squamous Cells of Undetermined Significance/Low-Grade Squamous Intraepithelial Lesion Triage Study (ALTS) *Journal of the National Cancer Institute* Vol.94,No.2,(January),pp.102-7.

Sherman ME, Lorincz AT, Scott DR,Wacholder S, Castle PE, Glass AG,Mielzynska-Lohnas I, Rush BB, Schiffman M. (2003) Baseline cytology, human papillomavirus testing, and risk for cervical neoplasia: a 10-year cohort analysis. *Journal of the National Cancer Institute* Vol.95,No.1,(January),pp.46–52.

Siebers AG,Klinkhamer PJ, Grefte JM, Massuger LF, Vedder JE, Beijers-Broos A, Bulten J, Arbyn M. (2009) Comparison of liquid-based cytology with conventional cytology for detection of cervical cancer precursors: a randomized controlled trial. *The Journal of the American Medical Association* Vol.302,No.16,(October),pp.1757–1764.

Smith JS, Lindsay L, Hoots B, Keys J, Franceschi S, Winer R, Clifford GM. (2007) Human papillomavirus type distribution in invasive cervical cancer and high-grade cervical lesions: a meta-analysis update. *International Journal of Cancer.* Vol.121,No.3,(Augustus),pp.621–632.

Stern P.L.; Kitchener H.C.: Vaccines for the Prevention of cervical Cancer 2008 *OOL*, ISBN 978-0-19-954345-8,Oxford

Tsoumpou I, Arbyn M, Kyrgiou M,Wentzensen N, Koliopoulos G, Martin-Hirsch P, Malamou-Mitsi V, Paraskevaidis E. (2009) P16(INK4a) immunostaining in cytological and histological specimens from the uterine cervix: a system¬atic review and meta-analysis. *Cancer Treatment Reviews* Vol.35,No3,(May),pp.210–220.

Wentzensen N, Bergeron C, Cas F, Vinokurova S, von Knebel Doeberitz M.(2007) Triage of women with ASCUS and LSIL cytology: use of qualitative assessment of p16ink4a positive cells to identify patients with high-grade cervical intraepithelial neoplasia. *Cancer* Vol.111,No.1,(February),pp.58–66.

Wright TC Jr., Massad LS, Dunton CJ, Spitzer M, Wilkinson EJ, Solomon D; (2007) 2006 consensus guidelines for the management of women with abnormal cervical cancer screening tests. *American Journal of Obstetrics& Gynecology* Vol.197,No.4,(February), pp.346–355.23

Zielinski G, Snijders PJ, Rozendaal L, Voorhorst FJ, Runsink AP, de Schipper FA, Meijer CJ(2001) High-risk HPV testing in women with borderline and mild dyskaryosis: long-term follow-up data and clinical relevance. *The Journal of Pathology.* Vol.195,No.3,(October), pp.300-6.

3

Immunohistochemistry in the Diagnosis of Squamous Intraepithelial Lesions of the Uterine Cervix

Evanthia A. Kostopoulou and George Koukoulis
University of Thessaly
Greece

1. Introduction

During the last few decades accumulated epidemiological, clinical, and experimental evidence has revealed the important role of human papillomavirus (HPV) in the development of cervical carcinomas, an association almost unique in cancer epidemiology. Several important questions have been answered and a large number of scientific studies have paved the way for the introduction of new and effective vaccines, which will hopefully diminish the incidence of HPV-related carcinomas and precursor lesions in forthcoming years (Crum et al., 2003; zur Hausen, 1977, 2008). However, the exact recognition and proper treatment of clinically important lesions often poses problems both to pathologists and gynecologists.

Morphology remains the gold standard for lesion diagnosis, despite the fact that it can be hampered by inter- and intra-observer variability. Additionally, the contribution of morphology in the field of human papillomavirus research cannot be overemphasized, since cytologic and/or histologic examination allow the recognition of viral cytopathic effects, and, with the aid of immunohistochemical and other *in situ* techniques, may reveal the exact cells, in which some main interactions take place. Thus, the correlation of cellular alterations with new sensitive methods of detection either for human papillomavirus nucleic acids or for HPV-related intracellular interactions might lead both to the identification of different groups of lesions according to their clinical significance, as well as to the correct application of current morphological criteria.

The following chapter will focus on those immunohistochemical methods that can facilitate or confirm the detection of intraepithelial lesions of cervical squamous epithelium (SILs) in biopsy specimens, additionally presenting in brief some data concerning the mechanisms by which these specific cellular targets are related to important actions of HPV oncoproteins. Finally, a short comment concerning the application in diagnosis of methods other than immunohistochemistry has been added.

1.1 HPV in carcinogenesis

In the last three decades a large number of scientific studies have focused on the subject of cervical carcinogenesis. These resulted in the accumulation of data linking several types of human papillomavirus to the development of cervical cancer (Bosch et al., 2002; Bosch et al., 2006; Crum et al., 1984; zur Hausen, 1977, 2009). The revealed strong association led to the suggestion that HPV is not only the main cause of cervical cancer, but also a necessary cause (Walboomers et al., 1999). Human papillomavirus is associated with more than 99% of all cervical cancer cases. In addition, a significant percentage of vulvar, vaginal, penile, anal and perianal carcinomas are HPV-positive (Fuste et al., 2010; Gross & Pfister, 2004; Insinga et al., 2008; Munoz et al., 2006), often containing HPV 16 DNA (zur Hausen, 2009), while a fraction of carcinomas in other sites of the human body has also been linked to high-risk (HR) HPV infections. Percentages of HPV positivity observed in carcinomas of the anogenital region are presented in Table 1.

Human papillomavirus is estimated to comprise a causal agent in 5% of human cancers and is associated with more human cancers than any other virus (Bergonzini *et al., 2010).* Among them, cervical cancer represents a well-studied prototype of a human tumor related to a viral infection.

Vaginal carcinomas	60-91%
Vulvar carcinomas	50%
Penile carcinomas	30-50%
Anal and perianal carcinomas	60-94%

Table 1. Percentage of HPV detection in carcinomas of the anogenital region other than cervical carcinoma (Munoz et al., 2006; zur Hausen, 2009).

The most common viral types detected in cervical carcinomas include HPV 16, 18, 45, 31, 33, 52, 58, and 35 (Clifford et al., 2003; Munoz et al., 2003). The fraction of squamous cell carcinomas or adenocarcinomas attributable to HPV16 and HPV18, which comprise the two most common types, is 70% and 86%, respectively. The paradox is that, although infection with oncogenic types of HPV is very common, malignancy is a rare outcome. This difference in incidence between infection and cancer development reveals the significance of complex interactions between viral, environmental and host-related factors (Frazer, 2009; Moscicki et al., 2006; Snijders et al., 2006; Whiteside et al., 2008; zur Hausen, 2008). Viral persistence is an important determinant in this sequence of events, while immune status, viral integration into the host DNA, and infection with multiple HPV genotypes have significant roles. These multiple interactions are reflected in the long interval between infection and invasive carcinoma detection, often spanning a period of 15 to 25 years (zur Hausen 2008). Other factors that may modify the risk for HPV DNA-positive women include smoking, the use of oral contraceptives, and previous exposure to other sexually transmitted diseases (Bosch et al., 2006; Collins et al., 2010; Luie et al., 2011; Munoz et al., 2006).

In recent years a large number of scientific studies have resulted in the introduction of effective vaccines, which are expected to diminish the incidence of HPV-related carcinomas of the uterine cervix and other organs (Bogaardts et al., 2011; Frazer, 2009; Stanley, 2010; The FUTURE I/II Study Group, 2010; zur Hausen, 2008). Moreover, they are expected to reduce the incidence of intraepithelial HPV-related lesions. A large number of the latter are caused by non-carcinogenic HPV types and do not constitute precancerous lesions, but still may be the cause of significant anxiety and distress for the patients. Furthermore, in rare instances they can give rise to life-threatening conditions, like recurrent respiratory papillomatosis.

Another main result of human papilloma virus research was the introduction in clinical practice of new diagnostic techniques (Cuzick et al., 2006; Gravitt et al., 2008; Poljak & Kocjan, 2010; Snijders et al., 2010). These allow for a more precise evaluation of the following: a) the presence of HPV in biologic specimens and the viral type present, b) the viral load, and c) the presence of an HPV-associated lesion demanding further therapeutic measures in cytological or biopsy material.

Finally, an important aspect of human papilloma virus research is the fact that the complex interactions between HPV oncoproteins and their multiple cellular targets offer to investigators the opportunity to study important cellular pathways related to the carcinogenic process in general.

1.2 Interactions between HPV oncoproteins and cellular pathways

High-risk mucosal HPVs encode three transforming proteins: E5, E6 and E7. Their multiple biological activities have been extensively studied in the last few decades; however, several aspects remain to be elucidated (McLaughlin-Drubin M & Münger K, 2009a).

HPV E5 is able to transform mouse fibroblasts and keratinocytes in culture (Straight et al., 1993). It is believed to contribute to early stages of carcinogenesis and works in concert with E6 and E7 (Talbert-Slagle & DiMaio, 2009; Hu et al., 2009). The latter proteins are necessary for the induction and maintenance of the transformed phenotype. They inhibit the function of tumor suppressors p53 and pRb, respectively, whereas their expression enables cells to bypass normal cell cycle checkpoints.

One of the main actions of HPV E7 proteins is the interaction with the retinoblastoma tumor suppressor protein, pRB, which controls S-phase entry through association with E2F transcription factor family members. They also interact with the related pocket proteins, p107 and p130. High-risk HPV E7 targets pRB for proteasomal degradation, while low-risk HPV E7 binds pRB with lower efficiency (approximately 10-fold lower) than HR- HPV E7 (McLaughlin-Drubin M & Münger K, 2009a; Munger et al., 1991). E7 proteins cause aberrant activation of cdk2 (cyclin dependent kinase 2), which is associated with cyclins E and A, as well as cdk inhibitors, mainly $p21^{CIP1}$ and $p27^{KIP1}$. E7 expression results in dysregulated expression of cyclins E and A (McLaughlin-Drubin M & Münger K, 2009b; Zerfass et al., 1995). It also results in retaining differentiating keratinocytes in a DNA synthesis competent state.

High-risk HPV E6 proteins target p53 for proteasomal degradation through association with the cellular ubiquitin ligase E6AP (McLaughlin-Drubin M & Münger K, 2009b; Scheffner et al., 1990). Low-risk HPV E6 proteins can also associate with E6AP; however, high-risk HPV proteins target p53 for ubiquitination.

Furthermore, HR-HPV E6 and E7 proteins cooperate to generate mitotic defects and aneuploidy through induction of supernumerary centrosomes and multipolar mitoses in epithelial cells (Duensing et al., 2000), while genomic instability results in the addition of molecular alterations. The detection of abnormal mitoses is a useful morphologic indicator of high-risk HPV-associated lesions (Crum et al. 1984).

Finally, integration of HPV genome into host chromosomes is an important event in cervical carcinogenesis (Hopman et al., 2006; Pett & Coleman, 2007), which occurs frequently during malignant progression and may result in dysregulation of E6/E7 expression due to disruption of E2, with associated loss of the inhibitory E2 action.

2. Immunohistochemical stains in the diagnosis of Squamous Intraepithelial Lesions (SIL)

Clinical management of preinvasive cervical disease consists of confirmation of SIL diagnosis by histopathological examination, followed by treatment or careful follow-up of certain lesions, according to the current guidelines. Histopathological diagnosis of CIN is based on well-defined criteria. However, in certain cases distinguishing both low- and high-grade lesions from their mimics may pose problems (Crum & Rose, 2006; Kostopoulou et al., 2001; Kurman et al., 1992), even to experienced gynecologic pathologists. The distinction of florid reactive changes, immature metaplastic patterns, and atrophic changes from HPV-induced alterations may cause difficulties. Attempts have been made to redefine the traditional criteria for lesion diagnosis, while other efforts aimed at the adoption of new, more objective methods, which might support the former (Bollmann et al., 2005; Cho et al., 2005; Guillaud et al., 2005; Prasad et al., 1994; Salvia et al., 2004; Scheurer et al., 2007). However, studies attempting to correlate HPV presence and replication to certain cytohistologic alterations are becoming less frequent and/or fruitful.

In recent years molecular studies have revealed several markers that might be of utility in the diagnosis of squamous intraepithelial lesions, including cellular proteins targeted directly by viral oncoproteins, and markers related to the cell cycle, which is disturbed by multiple actions of the virus, as summarized in the above paragraphs. The immunohistochemical stains that are currently in use in several laboratories worldwide, as well as some new promising markers are presented in the following text. The terms low grade squamous intraepithelial lesion (LSIL) and high grade squamous intraepithelial lesion (HSIL) will be used interchangeably with CIN1 and CIN2/3, respectively.

2.1 p16

One extensively studied marker is p16 INK4A (hereafter referred to as p16), a cyclin-dependent kinase inhibitor. p16 decelerates the cell cycle and functions as a tumor suppressor, while having a role in cellular senescence. p16 affects pRb-mediated regulation of the G1/S transition (Lukas et al., 1995; Ohtani et al., 2004; Quelle et al., 1995; Serrano, 1997; Sano et al., 1998).

The expression of p16 is altered in several human tumors by deletions, mutations, or methylation (Cohen & Geradts, 1997; Nakashima et al., 1999; O'Neill & McCluggage, 2006; Ruas & Peters 1998) and has also been altered in cervical carcinoma cases. However, increased expression is often observed in HPV-related intraepithelial lesions and this is mainly attributed to the presence of a feedback loop, which depends on the status of retinoblastoma protein (pRb) and the potential of high-risk HPV E7 protein to inactivate the latter (Lukas et al., 1995; Giarre et al., 2001; McLaughlin-Drubin & Münger, 2009b). Correlation has been reported between HR-HPV oncogene expression and high scores of p16 positivity (Andersson et al., 2006), and enhancement of p16 RNA level has been observed in vitro after immortalization by high-risk HPV types (Nakao et al., 1997). Despite the presence of high levels of p16 in SILs, its suppressor function is not normally exerted.

Several groups of investigators have examined immunohistochemically the expression of p16 in cervical squamous intraepithelial lesions (reviewed by Kostopoulou et al., 2011) and its possible correlation with HR-HPV types and/or lesion "progression". Indeed, p16 is one of the best studied markers in gynaecologic pathology. However, percentages of immunohistochemical positivity vary among different studies, as presented in Table 2. In the latter, studies published in the last ten years and including more than 100 cases of squamous intraepithelial lesions in histopathologic specimens are summarized, and the reported percentages of p16 immunopositivity are presented, together with the criteria and the antibodies used by the authors. Importantly, different criteria have been used for p16 immunoreactivity evaluation, with some authors focusing only on diffuse immunopositivity, some reporting any type of immunostaining, and others reporting nuclear and cytoplasmic staining separately. It should be also noted that some authors interpret focal positivity as a false-positive reaction. Positivity in the studies presented below varied from 5.6% to 100% for low-grade lesions and from 45.2% to 100% for high-grade lesions (Table 2). The percentage of immunopositivity observed in non-neoplastic epithelia also varied between 0% and 32.7%.

In a recent study (Kostopoulou et al., 2011) the two basic patterns of immunoreactivity, that is focal and diffuse, were further subdivided into groups as following: Focal positivity was subdivided into cases with occasional positive cells, dispersed or in small groups, observed mainly in the lower epithelial layers, and cases with occasional positive cells, dispersed or in small groups, commonly above the parabasal layer. Diffuse positivity (Figure 1) in the horizontal plane involved either all epithelial layers, or only the basal, parabasal and intermediate layers, without extending to the upper third of the epithelium. In HSIL, only diffuse positivity was encountered, observed in 24/25 cases (96%). In LSIL 41/55 cases (74.5%) showed some type of positivity, most commonly focal/sporadic (Figures 2 and 3). Interestingly, three out of eight LSILs showing diffuse immunoreactivity were characterized by markedly increased nuclear dimensions in the upper epithelial layers in comparison to other lesions characterized as low-grade. Another interesting finding of the above study was the different HPV type distribution observed between the two patterns of sporadic/focal positivity, involving lower *vs* intermediate/upper epithelial layers, and probably reflecting an earlier sporadic expression of E7 in certain lesions (Kostopoulou et al., 2011). The percentage of high-risk or probable high-risk HPV associated LSILs positive for p16 was 71.4% (25/35). This was not significantly different from immunopositivity observed in low-risk HPV associated lesions. Moreover, study of the pertinent literature revealed that a significant percentage of LSILs testing positive for HR-HPV by PCR or HC2 does not exhibit any p16 immunopositivity. The percentage of p16 positivity reported for HR-HPV positive LSILs varied from 32.4% to 94.4% (Ishikawa et al. 2006; Kalof et al., 2005; Kostopoulou et al., 2011).

Reference	Number of SILs examined	LSIL positivity	HSIL positivity	Non-neoplastic epithelia	Evaluation of staining	Antibody used in the study
Agoff et al., 2003	269	56.6%	84.5%	11.5%	N and C ≥5% cells	E6H4 (MTM)
Branca et al., 2004	137	35%	81.2%	0%	N and/or C	Polyclonal (Abcam)
Negri et al., 2004	127	74.7%	100%	ND	N and C ≥5% cells in lower third	CINtec p16 Histology Kit (DakoCytomation)
Volgareva et, al. 2004	113	37.2%	45.2%	3.2%	N and/or C	E6H4 (MTM)
Wang et al., 2004	113	72%	94.7%	32.7%	Any reactivity	E6H4 (MTM)
Dray et al., 2005	104	74.1%	96.1%	7.0%	N and/or C	JC8 (Biocare Medical)
Murphy et al., 2005	117	100%	98.7%	0%	N or C	p16 (Pharmingen)
Ishikawa et al., 2006	141	24.5%	87.5%	0%	Moderate and strong	E6H4 (MTM)
Focchi et al., 2007	153	90.9%	100%	7.9%	C and N ≥5% cells	Ab7 16PO7 (Neomarkers)
Hariri & Oster, 2007	140	71.4%	100%	6%	Continuous basal and parabasal	p16 Histology Kit (Dako)
Van Niekerk et al., 2007	184	57.1%	96.9%	22.9%	N and C ≥5% cells in each layer	E6H4 (DakoCytomation)
Godoy et al. 2008	115	50%	96.2%	0%	C and N	CINtec p16 Kit (Dako)
Dijkstra et al., 2010	406	5.6%	96.7%	ND	Diffuse, >1/3 of epithelium	Ab-4, 16P04 (Lab Vision)
Tan et al., 2010	129	26.7%	79.7%	0%	N and C ≥5% cells	p16 (NeoMarkers)

LSIL: low-grade squamous intraepithelial lesion; HSIL: high-grade squamous intraepithelial lesion; N: nuclear; C: cytoplasmic; ND: no data

[a] Only studies including more than 100 cases of squamous intraepithelial lesions in histopathologic specimens and published in the last ten years are presented.

Table 2. p16 immunopositivity in low- and high- grade squamous intraepithelial lesions reported in the literature[a]

The results of the above studies point towards the use of p16 immunostain in conjunction with histopathologic evaluation. Addition of a consecutive p16-stained slide to the HE-stained slides has been shown to improve significantly interobserver agreement for both punch and cone biopsies (Bergeron et al., 2010; Dijkstra et al., 2010; Horn et al., 2008), and to help in the identification of occult lesions (Ordi et al., 2008). The differential diagnosis from non-neoplastic alterations can be facilitated, especially in conjunction with other immunostains, as presented below. Moreover, lesion grading can be faster, especially concerning aggressive-appearing low-grade lesions, which otherwise might be upgraded (Dijkstra et al., 2010). Awareness of the different patterns of immunoreactivity might allow for a most proper use in certain clinicopathological settings. However, significant variability remains in the reported percentage of cases that stain positively for p16 and several unresolved technical issues remain, underlining the need for standardization of sample preparation and evaluation protocols (Mulvany et al., 2008; Tsoumpou et al., 2009).

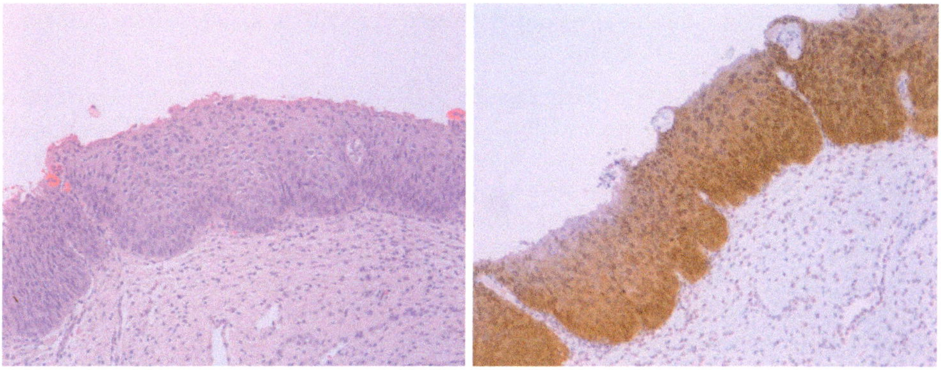

(a) (b)

Fig. 1. (a,b). High-grade squamous intraepithelial lesion (HSIL-CIN2): (a) Hematoxylin and eosin staining, (b) p16 immunostain showing diffuse positivity.

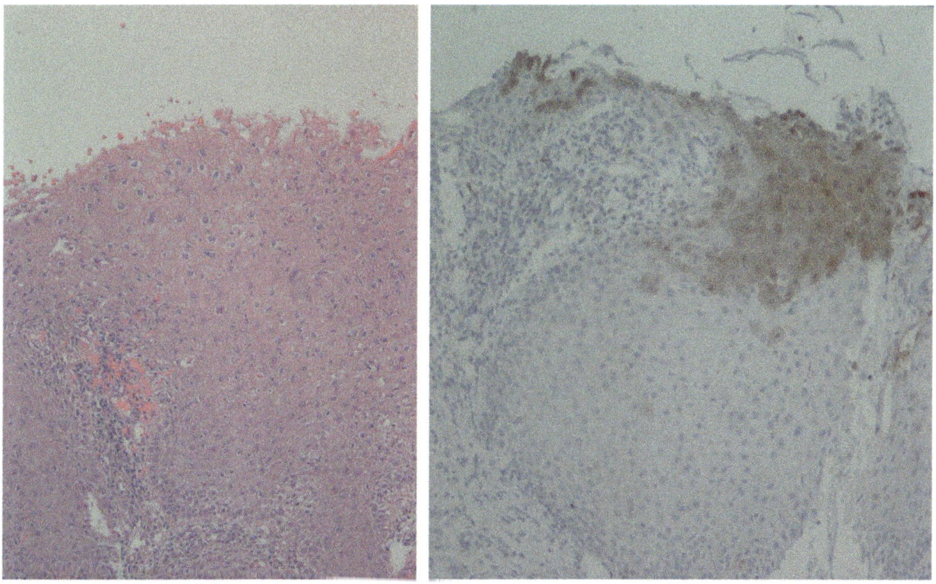

(a) (b)

Fig. 2. (a,b). Low-grade squamous intraepithelial lesion: (a) Hematoxylin and eosin staining, (b) p16 immunostain showing focal positivity.

It is of note that: (a) in several studies, especially with increasing number of cases, there often appears a small group of HSILs that do not show any immunoreactivity, and (b) a significant percentage of LSILs associated with HR-HPV, as detected by PCR or HC2, does not exhibit p16 immunopositivity (Kostopoulou et al., 2011). The above observations lead to the conclusion that a negative or equivocal p16 immunostain should be carefully evaluated in conjunction with the histopathologic findings and should not be used as the main criterion for diagnosis. However, p16 may also be of use in evaluating cauterized cervical resection margins, since the positive staining pattern of HGSIL is not affected by diathermy in LLETZ biopsies (Dray et al., 2005).

Finally, another aspect of p16 immunostaining is the possibility of correlation with lesion "progression". It has been suggested that certain phases of a given HR-HPV-associated neoplastic process may have different indices of p16 expression (Keating et al., 2001). Although the detailed examination of this subject is not included in the aim of the present text, it should be mentioned that in an interesting study by Hariri and Oster (2007) 25/26 low-grade lesions with negative p16 staining (concerning diffuse staining) and a minimum follow-up period of five years had a benign or normal outcome, revealing a negative predictive value of p16 in predicting the outcome of CIN 1 cases as high as 96%. In a study including conization specimens with coexisting CIN1 and CIN3 areas, all CIN1 were p16 positive (Negri et al., 2008), while p16 staining did not predict persistence or clearance of HR-HPV after treatment for CIN in a study by Branca et al. (2004).

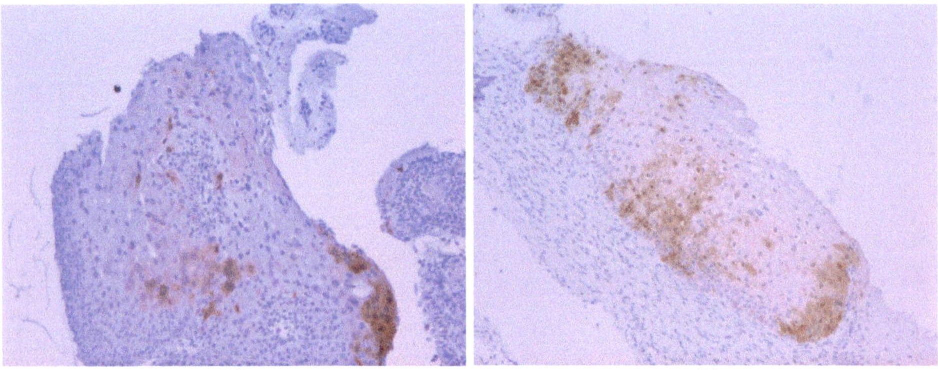

(a) (b)

Fig. 3. (a,b). Common patterns of p16 positivity in low-grade lesions

2.2 Cyclins

Cyclins have been reported to be of help in the evaluation of cervical biopsies. Cyclin E is uncommonly expressed in epithelia not infected by HPV and its conspicuous immunopositivity may facilitate the recognition of SIL (Keating et al., 2001). In addition, cyclin B1 immunoreactivity above the basal/parabasal cells correlates significantly with HPV detection and could be a marker of HPV presence (Kostopoulou et al., 2008a). Cyclins D and A have been also studied as possible markers of HPV-related lesions.

2.2.1 Cyclin B1

It has been reported that E6/E7 oncoproteins of HPV type 18 induced changes in the expression of cell cycle regulatory proteins very early and before immortalization (Pei, 1996). Significantly increased expression was noted for cyclin B and its transcriptional activation was documented. In 2000, Southern et al. demonstrated increased cyclin B1 expression in HGSILs. In their study cyclin B protein was up-regulated and persisted into the upper epithelial layers in parallel with cyclin A expression in high-grade squamous intraepithelial lesions.

In a study performed in our laboratory cyclin B1 immunostaining above the basal/parabasal layers was observed in all cases of HSIL (100%), most often involving the superficial layers as well (Kostopoulou et al., 2008a). Furthermore, increased cyclin B1 immunopositivity was observed in 51/52 low-grade lesions (98.07%) (Figure 4), and in seven of 15 biopsies (46.6%) characterized as atypia of unknown significance (AUS). Six of these seven cases tested HPV-positive by PCR.

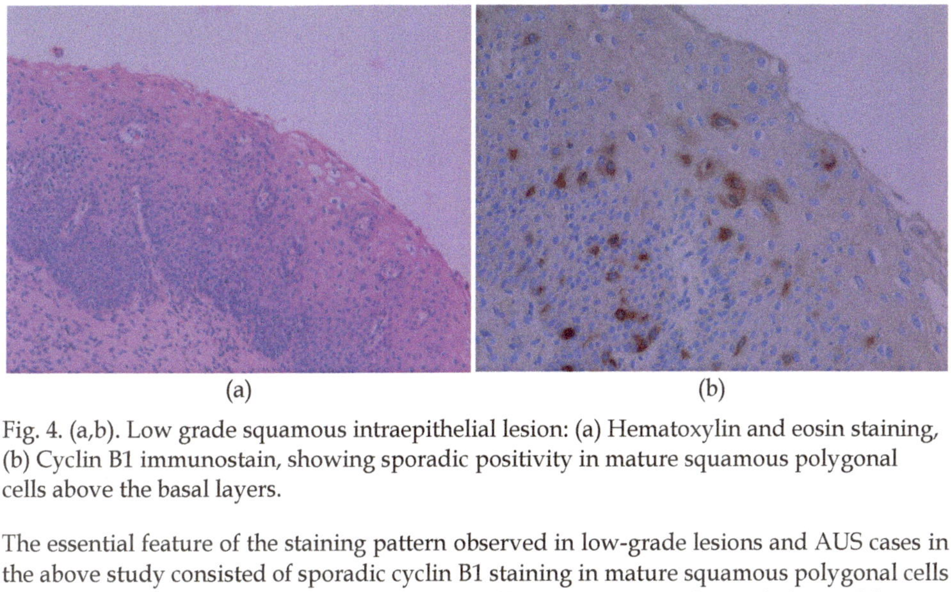

(a) (b)

Fig. 4. (a,b). Low grade squamous intraepithelial lesion: (a) Hematoxylin and eosin staining, (b) Cyclin B1 immunostain, showing sporadic positivity in mature squamous polygonal cells above the basal layers.

The essential feature of the staining pattern observed in low-grade lesions and AUS cases in the above study consisted of sporadic cyclin B1 staining in mature squamous polygonal cells often just above the basal layers, with slight differences between flat and elevated lesions. This pattern of immunoreactivity was seen in 52 of 55 cases with HPV infection detected by PCR, whereas it was seen in only 5 cases without PCR-proven HPV infection. In 4 of the latter cases, however, p16 immunopositivity was detected, suggesting that HPV could be present though not detected by PCR.

The pattern of immunoreactivity observed in low-grade lesions and AUS cases could be perceived as cytoplasmic accumulation or retention of cyclin B1 in suprabasal squamous cells. Several mechanisms could be related to this reaction (Kostopoulou et al., 2008a), while this pattern might reflect early events in the inhibition of G2-to-M transition, a well-known phenomenon during HPV infection in vitro. The possibility was suggested that these cyclin

B1-positive cells could be viewed as a type of "prekoilocytes", whose eventual progression to koilocytes would depend on several parameters related to the intricacies of HPV infection.

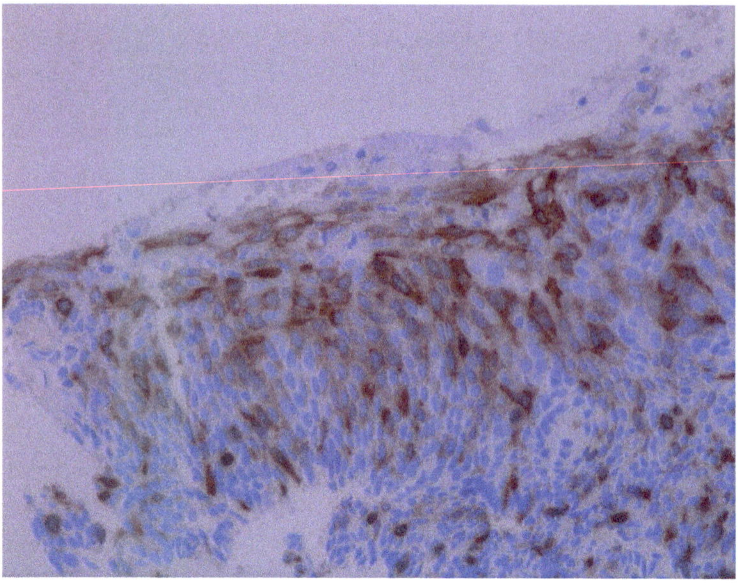

Fig. 5. Cyclin B1 positivity in an HSIL.

In conclusion, cyclin B1 positivity above the basal/parabasal layers correlates significantly with HPV detection and could be a marker of HPV presence. Thus, it might constitute a helpful finding in difficult to diagnose cases. Immunopositivity in a specimen showing non-diagnostic atypia should prompt reevaluation and/or HPV testing, as it is likely that the case could represent a genuine low-grade intraepithelial lesion.

2.2.2 Cyclin E

Cyclin E, another important cell cycle regulator, which promotes G1 transition, has been reported to exhibit increased expression in squamous intraepithelial lesions and invasive cervical carcinomas, although the exact mechanisms are not clear (Keating et al., 2001).

In a study by Keating et al., (2001) moderate to strong immunopositivity for cyclin E was observed in 92.6% and in 91.6% of low-grade and high-grade intraepithelial lesions, respectively, being positive in 38/41 HR-HPV positive cases. Furthermore, in a group of nondiagnostic squamous atypias cyclin E positivity was associated with HPV positivity.

In a study by Bahnassy et al. (2007), cyclin E staining increased from CIN1 to invasive carcinoma (16.7% to 88.4%, respectively), while gene amplification was detected in 11.1% of CIN1 cases and in 88.4% of carcinoma cases.

In conclusion, although cyclin E staining is not useful in the distinction of low-grade from high-grade lesions, it could be used to discriminate reactive from neoplastic epithelium (Crum & Rose, 2006), especially in conjunction with other markers, as discussed in other parts of the present text. As is the case with the other immunostains examined in this text, standardization of staining and evaluation protocols are important for the appropriate application of these markers in certain diagnostic dilemmas.

2.3 Other proliferation/cell cycle markers

2.3.1 Ki-67

Ki-67, an antigen expressed in the nuclei of proliferating cells, has also been studied as an indicator of CIN. Ki-67 is expressed in the nucleus during the whole cell cycle, except for the G0 and G1 early phases. Although positivity is observed under normal conditions in the lower compartments of the multilayered squamous epithelium, staining of the middle and upper layers is indicative of an intraepithelial lesion (Figure 6).

Immunopositivity for Ki-67 increases as a function of increasing lesion grade (Arafa et2008; *Conesa-Zamora* et al., 2009; Carreras et al., 2007; Keating et al., 2001; Mimica et al., 2010; Pinto et al., 2008), but immunostains should be interpreted with caution, since reactive and inflammatory lesions may result in increased epithelial proliferation. It is well-known to pathologists that reactive and reparative changes may pose a problem in the examination of proliferation markers and in the case of Ki-67 immunostaining positive nuclei may extend through most of the epithelium. However, Ki-67 immunostaining can be used as an adjunct to other markers, as already discussed.

It should be noted that Ki-67 immunohistochemical stain may be especially helpful in differentiating atrophic epithelial changes from high-grade lesions (Crum & Rose, 2006).

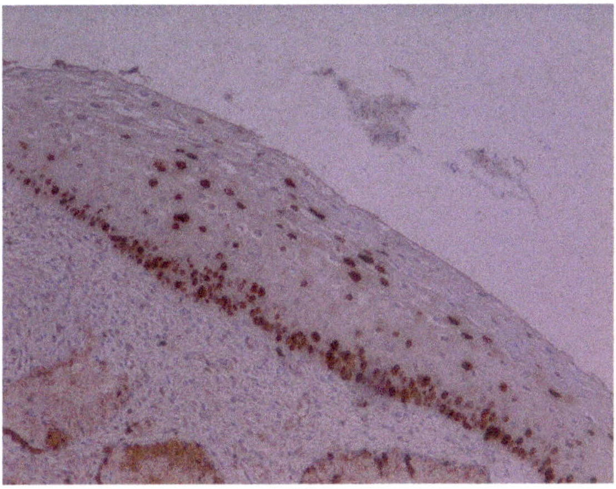

(a)

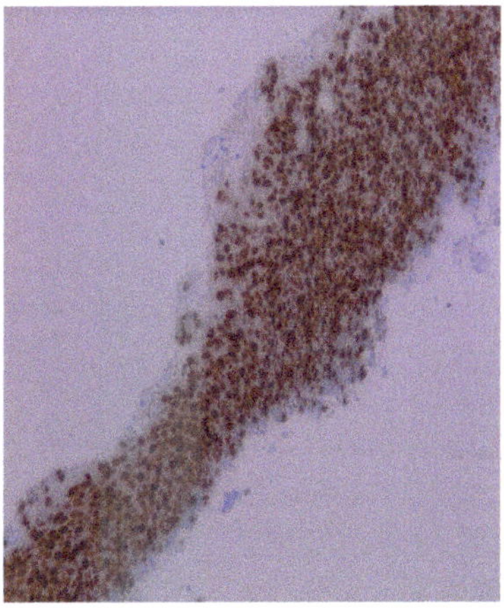

(b)

Fig. 6. (a,b). Ki-67positivity in (a) a low- and (b) a high-grade intraepithelial lesion.

2.3.2 Aberrant S-phase

Two relatively new biomarkers include the minichromosome maintenance protein 2 (MCM2) and DNA topoisomerase IIa (TOP2A) (Pinto et al., 2008). These two proteins have a significant role in the regulation of DNA replication during S-phase. They are overexpressed when S-phase induction is aberrant and have been shown to be overexpressed in CINs and cervical carcinomas (Badr et al., 2008; Pinto et al., 2008; Shi et al., 2007). TOP2A is a nuclear enzyme that regulates the enzymatic unlinking of DNA strands during chromosome replication. MCM2 functions also during DNA replication by loading the pre-replication complex onto DNA and unwinding the latter through helicase activity to permit synthesis. ProEx C (Tambouret et al., 2008) is a recently developed immunohistochemical assay that targets these two proteins and appears to be efficient in distinguishing reactive epithelial changes from squamous lesions, alone or in conjunction with p16.

According to Shi et al. (2007), ProEXC is a better marker than p16 for the detection of LSILs, showing positivity in 94% of the cases in a series of 34 LSILs. In a study by Badr et al. (2008) strong positive staining for ProEx C involving the lower and upper halves of the epithelium was observed in 92% of high-grade squamous intraepithelial lesions. Condylomas and CIN I showed greater variability in patterns of staining, with immunopositivity extending into the upper half of the epithelium in 48% of cases.

Pinto et al. (2008) included in their study cases with the differential diagnosis of HSIL *vs* reactive epithelial changes. ProEx C showed 87% sensitivity and 71% specificity for SIL in biopsy material. The authors reported a larger number of cells stained by ProEx C in comparison to MiB-1 in both HSIL and LSIL cases. In addition, the combination of p16 and ProEx C predicted more NoSIL (including normal, reactive, and/or atrophic epithelia) than p16 and MiB-1 (61% vs 43%). These observations suggested that ProEx C could be more useful in the distinction of reactive epithelial changes from SILs than MiB-1, providing a lower false positive rate relative to the latter.

In a study by Sanati et al. (2010) sensitivity, specificity, positive and negative predictive value of ProExC in distinguishing high-grade squamous intraepithelial lesion from squamous metaplasia were 89%, 100%, 100%, and 82%, respectively. In a recent study by Guo et al., (2011) diffuse positivity for ProExC significantly increased from benign cervix/CIN 1 to CIN 2 or 3/carcinoma, while the highest specificity for CIN 2+ and CIN3+ (100% and 93%, respectively) was achieved when immunostaining was positive for both ProExC and p16, suggesting that it is advantageous to use these two markers together in order to distinguish high-grade lesions from their mimics.

Walts and Bose (2009) suggested as cost saving strategy the use of two markers initially, p16 and ProExC, followed by Ki-67 immunostaining in discordant cases. According to the above authors, performing the two above stains initially and adding Ki-67 only when p16 and ProExC yield discordant results provided the same diagnostic accuracy while reducing the cost, since only one third of the cases required performance of the third stain.

2.4 Other markers and applications

In the present text an effort has been made to cover the immunohistochemical markers, which are currently most useful from a diagnostic point of view, and have been evaluated in several studies and laboratories.

In addition to the above biomarkers, which are in use in many pathology departments worldwide, a large number of other markers have been examined for their potential utility in the diagnosis and/or prognosis of cervical precursor lesions and in resolving problematic cases (Galgano et al., 2010; Khan et al., 2008; Kostopoulou et al., 2008b). The results of these studies have been described in detail in the pertinent literature. In addition, image analysis methods have been used in an attempt to bring more objectivity to the interpretation of biopsy specimens. Furthermore, although the detection of SILs in cytology material and the evaluation of screening strategies are beyond the scope of the present text, it should be mentioned that the contribution of the above markers is important in this context, as presented in brief in the following (Carozzi et al., 2008; Depuydt et al., 2011; Tsoumpou et al., 2009).

2.4.1 L1 capsid protein

One recently studied marker, which has been examined repeatedly in cytologic material, is L1. Nuclear positivity for HPV L1 capsid protein, the major structural protein of human papillomavirus, is mainly observed in productive lesions and is gradually lost in high grade lesions and carcinomas.

It has been suggested that combined L1/p16 immunostaining may be helpful for clinical management, especially in cases in which the grade of the lesion is difficult to assess (Negri et al., 2008).

In a study by Galgano et al. (2010), this protein, which should be highly correlated with a productive viral infection, was neither sensitive nor specific for any group of cervical neoplasia in biopsy material. This was attributed to the complexity of the temporal evolution of the HPV virion production which may be quite transient. It is interesting that L1 positive cases with a negative consensus diagnosis in this study had commonly at least 1 reviewer diagnosis of CIN1, revealing once again the difficulties in the distinction of SIL *vs* negative for SIL and the importance of a panel of immunostains in this specific context.

2.4.2 In situ hybridization techniques

Detection of papillomavirus nucleic acids is currently performed by methods that can be broadly subdivided into methods based on target amplification and those based on signal amplification (Snijders et al., 2010). In addition to several existing liquid phase techniques, in situ hybridization (ISH) methods have been developed for cytological and histological specimens. Both fluorescent detection and coloured substrate deposition followed by bright-field microscopy can be used, and can be combined with tyramide signal amplification. ISH assays can also be automated along the same lines as immunohistochemistry. Finally, except for HPV nucleic acids, other applications of in situ hybridization include the detection of amplification of the gene coding for the telomerase RNA component (TERC) at 3q26 (Hopman et al., 2006; Zheng et al., 2010).

Issues concerning sensitivity of the above techniques in comparison to PCR have been repeatedly raised. However, ISH techniques are becoming increasingly sensitive and can now detect low copy numbers of HPV DNA (Kelesidis et al., 2011; Montag et al., 2011). In addition, their important contribution to HPV research is the fact that they allow concurrent morphological evaluation of the areas examined, mainly in the case of histological specimens. Furthermore, the signal patterns observed in HPV ISH have been reported to be associated with the physical status of viral DNA in the cells examined, that is episomal or integrated. Specifically, the punctate pattern of positivity has been linked to the presence of integrated viral forms in the host genome (Cooper et al., 1991; Evans et al., 2002; Hopman et al., 2005).

In a study by Guo et al. (2008) ISH and PCR had fair to good agreement in detecting HPV DNA across CIN categories, but ISH detected significantly fewer HPV-positive cases in carcinomas than PCR did, probably as a result of lower copy numbers of episomal as compared to integrated HPV DNA in the latter. In addition, although the pure punctate pattern of HPV indicated a high level of viral integration, the level of HPV integration could not be accurately determined in cases with mixed signal patterns, probably due to a variation in the percentage of the two patterns in these cases. Recently, Ho et al. (2011) reported a punctate pattern in 8.7% of CIN1 lesions *vs* 34.0% of CIN3 lesions in cytology material, while Alameda et al. (2011) reported a correlation of the punctate pattern with lesion persistence in cytology specimens.

According to Kong et al. (2007), in cases of atypical squamous metaplasia, p16 reactivity (focal strong and diffuse strong) was significantly more sensitive than ISH in correlating with the presence of human papillomavirus as detected by polymerase chain reaction. In a more recent study by Kelesidis et al. (2011), ISH exhibited a sensitivity of 89.5% for the detection of CIN2+ lesions, while PCR showed sensitivity of 94.7% for these lesions. A percentage of ISH-positive cases was not detected by PCR (performed on liquid-based sample media), emphasizing the technical problems and limitations of the techniques.

Voss et al. (2009) compared a fluorescence in situ hybridization (FISH) HR-HPV assay to Hybrid Capture 2 (HC2) and polymerase chain reaction (PCR) for the detection of HR-HPV subtypes in cervical cytology specimens. FISH was concordant with HC2 and PCR in 85% and 82% of the specimens, respectively, while HC2 and PCR were concordant in 84% of the specimens.

It is apparent from the above results that the applications of HPV ISH are partly dependent on the sensitivity of the assay and its sufficiency to carry a high negative predictive value (Crum & Rose 2006). This is especially important if clinical decisions are based on a negative result. However, ISH represents a useful tool for ancillary molecular HPV testing in cervical specimens, and may be important in certain clinicopathologic situations.

2.4.3 Applications in cytology

The preceding text focused mainly on the application of immunohistochemistry in SIL diagnosis in histopathology specimens. However, several of the above markers have been applied in cytopathology material, as presented in brief in the following paragraphs. The introduction of liquid-based techniques, which has been one of the most important advances in this field, has facilitated relevant applications.

The most studied marker in cytology is p16. Positivity has been observed in 10%-86% of LSIL and in 42%-100% of HSIL, as reviewed by Tsoumpou et al. (2009). The lack of general consensus regarding threshold values for p16 positivity is especially important in cervical cytology specimens. Several authors have used both quantitative and qualitative criteria, evaluating the number of positive cells as well as cell morphology, recognizing the fact that p16 overexpression may be often detected in nondysplastic cells. In the contrary, other investigators used only quantitative criteria.

It has been suggested that p16 immunocytochemical testing can be used as a reflex test in conjunction with liquid-based cytology following a cytologic result of ASC-US or LSIL, or be used on destained conventional or liquid-based cytology specimens (Denton et al., 2010). p16 in conjunction with Ki-67 provide high sensitivity for the detection of CIN2+ lesions (Schmidt et al., 2011; Yu et al., 2010).

The prognostic utility of L1 immunocytochemistry, especially in association with p16 in cytology, has been reported by several authors (Griesser et al., 2004; Sarmadi et al., 2011; Yoshida et al., 2008).

The use of HPV in situ hybridization has already been discussed in the previous section. It is of note that, in a recent study, prior knowledge of HPV status resulted in significantly higher detection rate of CIN2+ in cytology specimens compared to screening blinded to HPV status, with limited loss of specificity (Benoy et al., 2011). This raises several important questions, although more research is needed to study the significance of this type of knowledge provided prior to cytological reading.

3. Conclusion

Although histopathology remains the "gold standard" for the diagnosis of SIL, both low- and high-grade, certain biomarkers have emerged as helpful adjuncts. Their combined use may assist in the histopathologic classification of preinvasive lesions and facilitate the distinction from non-HPV induced alterations. It is clear from the above that the diagnosis of a squamous intraepithelial lesion in a diagnostically challenging case cannot at present be based solely on any particular marker, but rather on a combination of markers with careful morphological evaluation, the latter comprising the most important part of the diagnostic procedure. Standardization of protocols and familiarity with the patterns of immunostaining, especially in nonneoplastic cervical tissue, are important requirements for the proper use of the above markers. Awareness of the strengths and limitations of each particular technique cannot be overemphasized. In addition, the performance of several markers and methods in the detection of lesions related to HPV types other than those addressed by the current vaccines remains to be carefully evaluated.

4. References

Agoff, SN., Lin, P., Morihara, J., Mao, C., Kiviat, N.B. & Koutsky, L.A. (2003). p $^{16(INK4a)}$ expression correlates with degree of cervical neoplasia: a comparison with Ki-67 expression and detection of high-risk HPV types. *Modern Pathology*, Vol.16, pp.665-673

Alameda, F., Mariñoso, M.L., Bellosillo, B., Muset, M., Pairet, S., Soler, I., Romero, E., Larrazabal, F., Carreras, R. & Serrano, S. (2011). Detection of HPV by in situ hybridization in thin-layer (ThinPrep) cervicovaginal samples. *Tumour Biology*, Vol.32, No.3, pp.603-609, Epub 2011 Feb 8

Andersson, S., Hansson, B., Norman, I., Gaberi, V., Mints, M., Hjerpe, A., et al. (2006). Expression of E6/E7 mRNA from 'high risk' human papillomavirus in relation to

CIN grade, viral load and p16INK4a. *International Journal of Oncology*, Vol. 29, No.3, pp. 705-711

Arafa, M., Boniver, J & Delvenne P. (2008). Detection of HPV-induced cervical (pre) neoplastic lesions: a tissue microarray (TMA) study. *Applied Immunohistochemistry and Molecular Morphology*, Vol.16, No.5, pp.422-432

Badr, R.E., Walts, A.E., Chung, F. & Bose, S. (2008). BD ProEx C: a sensitive and specific marker of HPV-associated squamous lesions of the cervix. *American Journal of Surgical Pathology*, Vol.32, pp.899-906

Bahnassy, A., Zekri, A., Saleh, M., Lotayef, M., Moneir, M. & Shawki, O. (2007). The possible role of cell cycle regulators in multistep process of HPV-associated cervical carcinoma. *BMC Clinical Pathology*, Vol.7, pp.4

Benoy, I., Vanden Broeck, D., Ruymbeke, M., Sahebali, S., Arbyn, M., Bogers, J., Temmerman, M. & Depuydt, C. Prior knowledge of HPV status improves detection of CIN2+ by cytology screening. *American Journal of Obstetrics and Gynecology*, in press.

Bergeron, C., Ordi, J., Schmidt, D., Trunk, M., Keller, T. & Ridder, R., for the European CINtec Histology Study Group. (2010). Conjunctive p16INK4a Testing Significantly Increases Accuracy in Diagnosing High-Grade Cervical Intraepithelial Neoplasia. *American Journal of Clinical Pathology*, Vol.133, pp.395-406

Bergonzini, V., Salata, C., Calistri, A., Parolin, C. & Palu, G. (2010). View and review on viral oncology research. *Infectious Agents and Cancer*, Vol.5:, pp.11

Bogaards, J.A., Coupé, V.M., Xiridou, M., Meijer, C.J., Wallinga, J. & Berkhof, J. (2011). Long-term Impact of Human Papillomavirus Vaccination on Infection Rates, Cervical Abnormalities, and Cancer Incidence. *Epidemiology*, Vol.22, No.4, pp.505-515

Bollmann, M., Bankfalvi, A., Trosic, A., Speich, N., Schmitt, C. & Bollmann, R. (2005). Can we detect cervical human papillomavirus (HPV) infection by cytomorphology alone? Diagnostic value of non-classic cytological signs of HPV effect in minimally abnormal Pap tests. *Cytopathology*, Vol.16, pp.13–21

Bosch, F.X., Lorincz, A., Munoz, N., Meijer, C.J. & Shah, K.V. (2002). The causal relation between human papillomavirus and cervical cancer. *Journal of Clinical Pathology.*, Vol.55, pp.244-265

Bosch, F.X., Qiao, Y. & Castellsague, X. (2006). The epidemiology of human papillomavirus infection and its association with cervical cancer. *International Journal of Gynecology and Obstetrics*, Vol.94(Supplement 1), pp.S8---S21

Branca, M., Ciotti, M., Santini, D., Di Bonito, L., Giorgi, C., Benedetto, A., et al. (2004). $p16^{INK4a}$ expression is related to grade of CIN and high-risk human papillomavirus but does not predict virus clearance after conization or disease outcome. *International Journal of Gynecological Pathology*, Vol. 23, pp.354-365

Carozzi, F., Confortini, M., Dalla Palma, P., Del Mistro, A., Gillio-Tos, A., De Marco, L., Giorgi-Rossi, P., Pontenani, G., Rosso, S., Sani, C., Sintoni, C., Segnan, N., Zorzi, M., Cuzick, J., Rizzolo, R., Ronco, G.; New Technologies for Cervival Cancer Screening (NTCC) Working Group. (2008). Use of p16-INK4A overexpression to increase the specificity of human papillomavirus testing: a nested substudy of the NTCC randomised controlled trial. *Lancet Oncology*, Vol.9, No.10, pp.937-945, Epub 2008 Sep 8.

Carreras, R., Alameda, F., Mancebo, G., García-Moreno, P., Mariñoso, M.L., Costa, C., Fusté, P., Baró, T. & Serrano, S. (2007). A study of Ki-67, c-erbB2 and cyclin D-1 expression in CIN-I, CIN-III and squamous cell carcinoma of the cervix. *Histology and Histopathology*, Vol.22, No.6, pp.587-592

Cho, N.H., Kang, S., Hong, S., Jeong, G.B., Choi, I.W., Choi, H.J. & Choi, H.K. (2005). Multinucleation of koilocytes is in fact multilobation and is related to aberration of the G2 checkpoint. *Journal of Clinical Pathology*, Vol.58, pp.576–582

Clifford, G.M., Smith, J.S., Plummer, M., Munoz, N. & Franceschi, S. (2003). Human papillomavirus types in invasive cervical cancer worldwide: a metaanalysis. *British Journal of Cancer*, Vol.88, No.1, pp.63–73

Cohen, J.A. & Geradts, J. (1997). Loss of Rb and MTS1/CDKN2 (P16) expression in human sarcomas. *Human Pathology*, Vol.28, pp.893–898

Collins, S., Rollason, T., Young, L. & Woodman C. (2010). Cigarette smoking is an independent risk factor for cervical intraepithelial neoplasia in young women: A longitudinal study. *European Journal of Cancer*, Vol. 46, No.2, pp.405–411

Conesa-Zamora, P., Domenech-Peris, A., Orantes-Casado, F., Ortiz-Reina, S., Sahuquillo-Frias, L., Acosta-Ortega, J., Garcia-Solano, J. & Perez-Guillermo, M. (2009). Effect of Human Papillomavirus on Cell Cycle–Related Proteins p16, Ki-67, Cyclin D1, p53, and ProEx C in Precursor Lesions of Cervical Carcinoma. *American Journal of Clinical Pathology*, Vol.132, pp.378-390

Cooper, K., Herrington, C.S., Stickland, J.E., Evans, M.F. & McGee J.O.. (1991). Episomal and integrated human papillomavirus in cervical neoplasia shown by non-isotopic in situ hybridization. *Journal of Clinical Pathology*, Vol.44, pp.990–996

Crum, C.P., Ikenberg, H., Richart, R.M. & Gissmann, L. (1984). Human papillomavirus type 16 and early cervical neoplasia. *New England Journal of Medicine*, Vol.310, pp.880–883

Crum, C.P. Contemporary theories of cervical carcinogenesis: the virus, the host, and the stem cell. (2000). *Modern Pathology*, Vol.13, pp.243–251

Crum, C.P., Abbott, D.W. & Quade, B.J. (2003). Cervical cancer screening: from the Papanicolaou smear to the vaccine era. *Journal of Clinical Oncology*, Vol. 21(10 Suppl), pp.224–230

Crum, C.P. & Rose, P. (2006). Cervical squamous neoplasia. In: *Diagnostic Gynecologic and Obstetric Pathology*. C.P. Crum & K.R. Lee, (Eds.), 267-354, Elsevier

Cuzick, J., Mayrand, M., Ronco, G., Snijders, P. & Wardle, J. (2006). Chapter 10: New dimensions in cervical cancer screening. *Vaccine*, Vol.24(S3), pp.S90-97

Denton, K., Bergeron, C., Klement, P., Trunk, M., Keller, T. & Ridder, R., for the European CINtec Cytology Study Group. (2010). The Sensitivity and Specificity of p16INK4a Cytology vs HPV Testing for Detecting High-Grade Cervical Disease in the Triage of ASC-US and LSIL Pap Cytology Results. *American Journal of Clinical Pathology*, Vol.134, pp.12-21

Depuydt, C.E., Makar, A.P., Ruymbeke, M.J., Benoy, I.H., Vereecken, A.J. & Bogers, J.J. (2011). BD-ProExC as adjunct molecular marker for improved detection of CIN2+ after HPV primary screening. *Cancer Epidemiology, Biomarkers and Prevention*, Vol.20, No.4, pp.628-637, Epub 2011 Feb 4

Dijkstra, M.G., Heideman, D.A., de Roy, S.C., Rozendaal, L., Berkhof, J., van Krimpen, K., van Groningen, K., Snijders, P.J., Meijer, C.J. & van Kemenade, F.J. (2010).

p16(INK4a) immunostaining as an alternative to histology review for reliable grading of cervical intraepithelial lesions. *Journal of Clinical Pathology*, Vol.63(, No.11, pp.972-927, Epub 2010 Oct 5

Dray, M., Russell, P., Dalrymple, C., Wallman, N., Angus, G., Leong, A. et al. (2005). p16^{INK4a} as a complementary marker of high-grade intraepithelial lesions of the uterine cervix. I: Experience with squamous lesions in 189 consecutive cervical biopsies. *Pathology*, Vol. 37, No.2, pp.112-124

Duensing, S., Lee, L.Y., Duensing, A., Basile, J., Piboonniyom, S., Gonzalez, S., Crum, C.P. & Munger, K. (2000). The human papillomavirus type 16 E6 and E7 oncoproteins cooperate to induce mitotic defects and genomic instability by uncoupling centrosome duplication from the cell division cycle. *Proceedings of the National Academy of Sciences*, Vol.97, pp.10002-10007

Evans, M.F., Mount, S.L., Beatty, B.G. & Cooper, K. (2002). Biotinyltyramide-based in situ hybridization signal patterns distinguish human papillomavirus type and grade of cervical intraepithelial neoplasia. *Modern Pathology*,Vol.15, pp.1339-1347

Focchi, G., Silva, I., Nogueira-de-Souza, N., Dobo, C., Oshima, C. & Stavale, J. (2007). Immunohistochemical Expression of p16(INK4A) in Normal Uterine Cervix, Nonneoplastic Epithelial Lesions, and Low-grade Squamous Intraepithelial Lesions. *Journal of Lower Genital Tract Disease*, Vol.11, pp.98-104

Frazer, I. (2009). Interaction of human papillomaviruses with the host immune system: A well evolved relationship. *Virology*, Vol.384, pp.410-414

Fuste, V., del Pino, M., Perez, A., Garcia, A., Torne, A., Pahisa, J. & Ordi, J. (2010). Primary squamous cell carcinoma of the vagina: human papillomavirus detection, p16INK4A overexpression and clinicopathological correlations. *Histopathology*, Vol.57, pp.907-916

Giarrè, M., Caldeira, S., Malanchi, I., Ciccolini, F., Leão, M.J. & Tommasino, M. (2001). Induction of pRb degradation by the human papillomavirus type 16 E7 protein is essential to efficiently overcome p16INK4a-imposed G1 cell cycle arrest. *Journal of Virology*, Vol. 75, No.10, pp.4705-4712

Godoy, A., Mandelli, J., Oliveira, F., Calegari, S., Moura, L. & Serafini, E. (2008). p16INK4 expression in precursor lesions of squamous cell cervical cancer related to the presence of HPV-DNA. *Brazilian Journal of Medical and Biological Research*, Vol.41, pp.583-588

Gravitt, P.E., Coutlье, F., Iftner, T., Sellors, J.W., Quint, W.G. & Wheeler, C.M. (2008). New technologies in cervical cancer screening. *Vaccine*, Vol.26, No.Suppl.10, pp.42-52

Griesser, H., Sander, H., Hilfrich, R., Moser, B. & Schenck U. (2004). Correlation of immunochemical detection of HPV L1 capsid protein in pap smears with regression of high-risk HPV positive mild/moderate dysplasia. *Analytical and Quantitative Cytology and Histology*, Vol.26, No.5, pp.241-245

Gross, G. & Pfister, H. (2004). Role of human papillomavirus in penile cancer, penile intraepithelial squamous cell neoplasias and in genital warts. *Medical Microbiology and Immunology*, Vol.193:, pp.35-44

Guillaud, M., Adler-Storthz, K., Malpica, A., Staerkel, G., Matisic, J., Van Niekirk, D., Cox, D., Poulin, N., Follen, M. & MacAulay, C. (2005). Subvisual chromatin changes in cervical epithelium measured by texture image analysis and correlated with HPV. *Gynecologic Oncology*, Vol.99, No.3suppl 1), pp.16-23

Guo, M., Baruch, A.C., Silva, E.G., Jan, Y.J., Lin, E., Sneige, N. & Deavers M.T. (2011). Efficacy of p16 and ProExC immunostaining in the detection of high-grade cervical intraepithelial neoplasia and cervical carcinoma. *American Journal of Clinical Pathology*, Vol.135, No.2, pp.212-220

Guo, M., Gong, Y., Deavers, M., Silva, E.G., Jan, Y.J., Cogdell, D.E., Luthra, R., Lin, E., Lai, H.C., Zhang, W. & Sneige, N. (2008). Evaluation of a commercialized in situ hybridization assay for detecting human papillomavirus DNA in tissue specimens from patients with cervical intraepithelial neoplasia and cervical carcinoma. *Journal of Clinical Microbiology*, Vol.46, No.1, pp.274-280, Epub 2007 Oct 31

Hariri, J. & Oster, A. (2007). The Negative Predictive Value of p16INK4a to Assess the Outcome of Cervical Intraepithelial Neoplasia 1 in the Uterine Cervix. *International Journal of Gynecological Pathology*, Vol.26, pp.223–228

Ho, C.M., Lee, B.H., Chang, S.F., Chien, T.Y., Huang S.H., Yan, C.C. & Cheng, W.F. (2011). Clinical significance of signal pattern of high-risk human papillomavirus using a novel fluorescence in situ hybridization assay in cervical cytology. *Clinical Microbiology and Infection*, Vol.17, No.3, pp.386-394

Hopman, A. H., Kamps, M. A., Smedts, F., Speel E. J., Herrington, C. S., & Ramaekers, F. C.. (2005). HPV in situ hybridization: impact of different protocols on the detection of integrated HPV. *International Journal of Cancer*, Vol.115, pp.419–428

Hopman, A.H.,Theelen, W., Hommelberg, P.P., Kamps, M.A., Herrington, C.S., Morrison, L.E., Speel, E.J., Smedts, F. & Ramaekers, F.C. (2006). Genomic integration of oncogenic HPV and gain of the human telomerase gene TERC at 3q26 are strongly associated events in the progression of uterine cervical dysplasia to invasive cancer. *Journal of Pathology*, Vol.210, No.4, pp.412-419

Horn, L., Reichert, A., Oster, A., Arndal, S., Trunk, M., Ridder, R., et al. (2008). Immunostaining for p16INK4a Used as a Conjunctive Tool Improves Interobserver Agreement of the Histologic Diagnosis of Cervical Intraepithelial Neoplasia. *American Journal of Surgical Pathology*, Vol. 32, pp.502–12

Hu, L., Plafker, K., Vorozhoko, V., Zuna, R., Hanigan, M., Gorbsky, G., Plafker, S., Angeletti, P. & Ceresa, B. (2009). Human Papillomavirus 16 E5 Induces Bi-Nucleated Cell Formation By Cell-Cell Fusion. *Virology*, Vol.384, No.1, pp.125–134

Insinga, R., Liaw, K., Johnson, L., & Madeleine, M. (2008). A Systematic Review of the Prevalence and Attribution of Human Papillomavirus Types Among Cervical, Vaginal and Vulvar Precancers and Cancers in the United States. *Cancer Epidemiology Biomarkers and Prevention*. Vol. 17, No.7, pp.1611–1622

Ishikawa, M., Fujii, T., Saito, M., Nindl, I., Ono, A., Kubushiro, K., et al. (2006). Overexpression of $p16^{INK4a}$ as an indicator for human papillomavirus oncogenic activity in cervical squamous neoplasia. *International Journal of Gynecological Cancer*, Vol.16, No.1, pp.347–353

Kalof, A.N., Evans, M.F., Simmons-Arnold, L., Beatty, B. & Kumarasen, C. (2005). p16INK4A immunoexpression and HPV in situ hybridization signal patterns: potential markers of high-grade cervical intraepithelial neoplasia. *American Journal of Surgical Pathology*, Vol.29, pp.674–679

Keating, J.T., Cviko, A., Riethdorf, S., Riethdorf, L., Quade, B.J., Sun, D., et al. (2001). Ki-67, cyclin E, and p16INK4 are complimentary surrogate biomarkers for human papilloma virus-related cervical neoplasia. *American Journal of Surgical Pathology,* Vol. 25, pp.884–891

Kelesidis, T., Aish, L., Steller, M.A., Aish, I.S., Shen, J., Foukas, P., Panayiotides, J., Petrikkos, G., Karakitsos, P. & Tsiodras, S. (2011). Human Papillomavirus (HPV) Detection Using In Situ Hybridization in Histologic Samples: Correlations With Cytologic Changes and Polymerase Chain Reaction HPV Detection. *American Journal of Clinical Pathology,* Vol.136, No.1, pp.119-127

Khan, A.M. & Singer, A. (2008). Biomarkers in cervical precancer management: the new frontiers. *Future Oncology,* Vol.4, No.4, pp.515-524

Kong, C.S., Balzer, B.L., Troxell, M.L., Patterson, B.K. & Longacre, T.A. (2007). p16INK4A immunohistochemistry is superior to HPV in situ hybridization for the detection of high-risk HPV in atypical squamous metaplasia. *American Journal of Surgical Pathology,* Vol.31, No.1, pp.33-43

Kostopoulou, E., Keating, J.T. & Crum, C.P. (2001). Pathology. In: *American Cancer Society Atlas of Clinical Oncology. Cancer of the female lower genital tract.* P.J. Eifel, C. Levenback, (Eds), 9-36, BC Decker, Hamilton, London

Kostopoulou, E., Samara, M., Kollia, P., Zacharouli, K., Mademtzis, I., Daponte, A., Messinis, I.E. &, Koukoulis, G. (2008a). Correlation Between Cyclin B1 Immunostaining in Cervical Biopsies and HPV Detection by PCR. *Applied Immunohistochemistry and Molecular Morphology,* Vol.17, No.2, pp.115-120, Epub Oct 28; 2008a.

Kostopoulou, E., Samara, M., Kollia, P., Zacharouli, K.& Koukoulis, G. (2008b). INCENP, cyclin B1 and ERK1 immunopositivity in cervical biopsies. *Histopathology,* Vol.53, No.438Sp.Iss., pp.192-193

Kostopoulou, E., Samara, M., Kollia, P., Zacharouli, K., Mademtzis, I., Daponte, A., Messinis, I.E. & Koukoulis, G. (2011). Different patterns of p16 immunoreactivity in cervical biopsies: Correlation to lesion grade and HPV detection, with review of the literature. *European Journal of Gynaecological Oncology,* Vol.32, No.1, pp.54-61

Kurman, R., Norris, H. & Wilkinson, E. (1992). *Tumors of the cervix, vagina and vulva. A.F.I.P. Atlas of tumor Pathology, 3rd series.* A.F.I.P., Washington

Louie, K.S., Castellsague, X., de Sanjose, S., Herrero, R., Meijer, C.J., Shah, K., Munoz, N., Bosch, F.X.; for the International Agency for Research on Cancer Multicenter Cervical Cancer Study Group. (2011). Smoking and Passive Smoking in Cervical Cancer Risk: Pooled Analysis of Couples from the IARC Multicentric Case-Control Studies. *Cancer Epidemiology, Biomarkers and Prevention.* Vol.20, No.7, pp.1379-1390, Epub 2011 May 24.

Lukas, J., Parry, D., Aagaard, L., Mann, D. J., Bartkova, J., Strauss, M., et al. (1995). Retinoblastoma-protein-dependent cell-cycle inhibition by the tumour suppressor p16. *Nature,* Vol.375, pp.503–506

McLaughlin-Drubin, M. & Münger, K. (2009a). The Human Papillomavirus E7 Oncoprotein. *Virology,* Vol.384, No.2, pp.335–344

McLaughlin-Drubin, M. & Münger, K. (2009b). Oncogenic Activities of Human Papillomaviruses. *Virus Research,* Vol.143, No.2, pp. 195–208

Mimica, M., Tomić, S., Kardum, G., Hofman, I.D., Kaliterna, V. & Pejković, L. (2010). Ki-67 quantitative evaluation as a marker of cervical intraepithelial neoplasia and human papillomavirus infection. *International Journal of Gynecological Cancer,* Vol.20, No.1, pp.116-119

Montag, M., Blankenstein, T., Shabani, N., Bru¨ning, A. & Mylonas, I. (2011) Evaluation of two commercialised in situ hybridisation assays for detecting HPV-DNA in formalin-fixed, paraffin-embedded Tissue. *Archives of Gynecology and Obstetrics,* Vol.284, pp.999–1005

Moscicki, A., Schiffman, M., Kjaer, S. & Villa, L. (2006) Chapter 5: Updating the natural history of HPV and anogenital cancer. *Vaccine,* Vol.24, No.S3, pp.42-51

Mulvany, N.J., Allen, D.G.& Wilson, S.M. (2008). Diagnostic utility of p16INK4a: a reappraisal of its use in cervical biopsies. *Pathology,* Vol.40, No.4, pp.335-344

Münger, K., Yee, C.L., Phelps, W.C., Pietenpol, J.A., Moses, H.L. & Howley, P.M. (1991). Biochemical and biological differences between E7 oncoproteins of the high- and low risk human papillomavirus types are determined by amino-terminal sequences. *Journal of Virology,* Vol.65, pp.3943–3948

Munoz, N., Bosch, F.X., de Sanjose, S., Herrero, R., Castellsague, X., Shah, K.V., et al. (2003). Epidemiologic classification of human papillomavirus types associated with cervical cancer. *New England Journal of Medicine,* Vol.348, pp.518–527

Munoz, N., Castellsague, X., Berrington de Gonzalez, A. & Gissmann, L. (2006) Chapter 1: HPV in the etiology of human cancer. *Vaccine,* Vol.24, No.S3, pp.1-10

Murphy, N., Ring, M., Hefron, C.C., King, B., Killalea, A., Hughes, C., et al. (2005). p16INK4A, CDC6, and MCM5: predictive biomarkers in cervical preinvasive neoplasia and cervical cancer. *Journal of Clinical Pathology,* Vol.58, pp.525–534

Nakao, Y., Yang, X., Yokoyama, M., Ferenczy, A., Tang, S.C., Pater, M.M., et al. (1997). Induction of p16 during immortalization by HPV 16 and 18 and not during malignant transformation. *British Journal of Cancer,* Vol.75, No.10, pp.1410-1416

Nakashima, R., Fujita, M., Enomoto, T., Haba, T., Yoshino, K., Wada, H., et al. (1999). Alteration of p16 and p15 genes in human uterine tumours. *British Journal of Cancer,* Vol.80, pp.458-467

Negri, G., Vittadello, F., Romano, F., Kasal, A., Rivasi, F., Girlando, S., et al. (2004). P16INK4a expression and progression risk of low-grade intraepithelial neoplasia of the cervix uteri. *Virchows Archives,* Vol.445, pp.616–20

Negri, G., Bellisano, G., Zannoni, G.F., Rivasi, F., Kasal, A., Vittadello, F., et al. (2008). P16ink4a and HPV L1 immunohistochemistry is helpful for estimating the behavior of low-grade dysplastic lesions of the cervix uterii. *American Journal of Surgical Pathology,* Vol.32, No.11, pp.1715-1720

O'Neill, C. & McCluggage, G. (2006). p16 expression in the female genital tract and its value in diagnosis. *Advances in Anatomic Pathology,* Vol.13, pp.8–15

Ohtani, N., Yamakoshi, K., Takahashi, A. & Hara, E. (2004). The p16^{INK4A}-RB pathway: molecular link between cellular senescence and tumor suppression. *Journal of Medical Investigation,* Vol.51, pp.146-153

Ordi, J., Garcia, S., del Pino, M., Landol, S., Alonso, I., Quinto,' L., & Torne,' A. (2008). p16INK4a immunostaining identifies occult CIN lesions in HPV-positive women. *International Journal of Gynecological Pathology,* Vol.28, pp.90–97

Pei, X.F. (1996). The human papillomavirus E6/E7 genes induce discordant changes in the expression of cell growth regulatory proteins. *Carcinogenesis,* Vol.17, pp.1395–1401

Pett, M. & Coleman, N. (2007). Integration of high-risk human papillomavirus: a key event in cervical carcinogenesis? *Journal of Pathology,* Vol.212:, pp.356–367

Pinto, A., Schlecht, N., Woo, T., Crum, C.P. & Cibas, E. (2008). Biomarker (ProEx C, p16INK4A, and MiB-1) distinction of high-grade squamous intraepithelial lesion from its mimics. *Modern Pathology*, Vol.21, pp.1067-1074

Poljak, M. & Kocjan, B. (2010) Commercially available assays for multiplex detection of alpha human papillomaviruses Expert Rev. *Anti Infect Therapy,* Vol.8, No.10, pp.1139-1162

Prasad, C., Genest, D. & Crum, C.P. (1994). Nondiagnostic squamous atypia of the cervix (atypical squamous epithelium of undetermined significance): histologic and molecular correlates. *International Journal of Gynecological Pathology,* Vol.13, pp.220-227

Quelle, D., Zindy, F., Ashmund, R. & Sherr, C.J. (1995). Alternative reading frames of the INK4α tumor suppressor gene encode two unrelated proteins capable of inducing cell cycle arrest. *Cell,* Vol.83, pp.993-1000

Ruas, M. & Peters, G. (1998). The p16INK4a/CDKN2A tumor suppressor and its relatives. *Biochimica et Biophysica Acta,* Vol.1378, pp.115-177

Salvia, P., Bergo, S., Bonesso-Sabadini, P., Tagliarini, E., Hackel, C. & De Angelo Andrade, L. (2004). Correlation between histological criteria and human papillomavirus presence based on PCR assay in cervical biopsies. *International Journal of Gynecological Cancer,* Vol.14, pp.126-132

Sanati, S., Huettner, P. & Ylagan, L.R. (2010). Role of ProExC: a novel immunoperoxidase marker in the evaluation of dysplastic squamous and glandular lesions in cervical specimens. *International Journal of Gynecological Pathology,* Vol.29, No.1, pp.79-87

Sano, T., Oyama, T., Kashiwabara, K., Fukuda, T. & Nakajima, T. (1998). Expression status of p16 protein is associated with human papillomavirus oncogenic potential in cervical and genital lesions *American Journal of Pathology,* Vol.153, pp.1741-1748

Sarmadi, S., Izadi-Mood, N., Pourlashkari, M., Yarandi, F. & Sanii, S. (2011). HPV L1 capsid protein expression in squamous intraepithelial lesions of cervix uteri and its relevance to disease outcome. *Archives of Gynecology and Obstetrics,* Jul 26. [Epub ahead of print]

Scheffner, M., Werness, B.A., Huibregtse, J.M., Levine, A.J. & Howley, P.M. (1990). The E6 oncoprotein encoded by human papillomavirus types 16 and 18 promotes the degradation of p53. *Cell,* Vol.63, pp.1129-1136

Scheurer, M.E., Guillaud, M., Tortolero-Luna, G., McAulay, C., Follen, M. & Adler-Storthz, K.(2007). Human papillomavirus-related cellular changes measured by cytometric analysis of DNA ploidy and chromatin texture. *Cytometry B Clinical Cytometry,* Vol.72, pp.324-331

Schmidt, D., Bergeron, C., Denton, K.J., Ridder, R.; European CINtec Cytology Study Group. (2011). p16/ki-67 dual-stain cytology in the triage of ASCUS and LSIL papanicolaou cytology: results from the European equivocal or mildly abnormal Papanicolaou cytology study. *Cancer Cytopathology,* Vol.119, No.3, pp.158-166

Serrano, M. (1997). The Tumor Suppressor Protein p16^{INK4a}. *Experimental Cell Research,* Vol.237, pp.7-13Shi, J., Liu, H., Wilkerson, M., Huang, Y., Meschter, S., Dupree, W., Schuerch, C. & Lin, F. (2007). Evaluation of p16INK4a, minichromosome maintenance protein 2, DNA topoisomerase IIalpha, ProEX C, and p16INK4a/ProEX C in cervical squamous intraepithelial lesions. *Human Pathology,* Vol.38, pp.1335-1344

Snijders, P., Steenbergen, R., Heideman, D., & Meijer, C. (2006). HPV-mediated cervical carcinogenesis: concepts and clinical implications. *Journal of Pathology,* Vol.208, pp.152–164

Snijders, P.J., Heideman, D.A. & Meijer, C.J. (2010). Methods for HPV detection in exfoliated cell and tissue specimens. *APMIS,* Vol.118, No.6-7, pp.520-528

Southern, S., McDicken, I. & Herrington, C.S. (2000). Evidence for keratinocyte immortalization in high-grade squamous intraepithelial lesions of the cervix infected with high-risk human papillomaviruses. *Laboratory Investigation,* Vol.80, pp.539–544

Stanley, M. (2010). HPV - immune response to infection and Vaccination. *Infectious Agents and Cancer,* Vol.5, pp.19

Straight, S.W., Hinkle, P.M., Jewers, R.J. & McCance, D.J. (1993). The E5 Oncoprotein of Human Papillomavirus Type 16 Transforms Fibroblasts and Effects the Downregulation of the Epidermal Growth Factor Receptor in Keratinocytes. *Journal of Virology,* Vol.67, No.8, pp.4521–4532

Talbert-Slagle, K. & DiMaio, D. (2009). The bovine papillomavirus E5 protein and the PDGF beta receptor: it takes two to tango. *Virology,* Vol.384, No.2, pp.345–351

Tambouret, R.H., Misdraji, J. & Wilbur, D.C. (2008). Longitudinal clinical evaluation of a novel antibody cocktail for detection of high-grade squamous intraepithelial lesions on cervical cytology specimens. *Archives of Pathology and Laboratory Medicine,* Vol.132, No.6, pp.918-925

Tan, G.C., Norlatiffah, S., Sharifah, N.A., Razmin, G., Shiran, M.S., Hatta, A.Z. & Paul-Ng, H.O. (2010). Immunohistochemical study of p16 ^{INK4A} and survivin expressions in cervical squamous neoplasm. *Indian Journal of Pathology and Microbiology,* Vol.53, pp.1-6

The FUTURE I/II Study Group. (2010). Four year efficacy of prophylactic human papillomavirus quadrivalent vaccine against low grade cervical, vulvar, and vaginal intraepithelial neoplasia and anogenital warts: randomised controlled trial. *BMJ,* Vol.340, pp.c3493

Tsoumpou, I., Arbyn, M., Kyrgiou, M., Wentzensen, N., Koliopoulos, G., Martin-Hirsch, P., Malamou-Mitsi, V. & Paraskevaidis, E. (2009). p16INK4a immunostaining in cytological and histological specimens from the uterine cervix: a systematic review and meta-analysis. *Cancer Treatment Reviews,* Vol.35, No.3, pp.210–220

Van Niekerk, D., Guillaud, M., Matisic, J., Benedet, J., Freeberg, J., Follen, M., et al. (2007). p16 and MIB1 improve the sensitivity and specificity of the diagnosis of high grade squamous intraepithelial lesions: Methodological issues in a report of 447 biopsies with consensus diagnosis and HPV HCII testing. *Gynecologic Oncology,* Vol.107, pp.S233–240.

Volgareva, G., Zavalishina, L., Andreeva, Y., Frank, G., Krutikova, E., Golovina, D. et al. (2004). Protein p16 as a marker of dysplastic and neoplastic alterations in cervical epithelial cells. *BMC Cancer,* Vol. 4, pp.58

Voss, J.S., Kipp, B.R., Campion, M.B., Sokolova, I.A., Henry, M.R., Halling, K.C. & Clayton, A.C.. (2009). Comparison of fluorescence in situ hybridization, hybrid capture 2 and polymerase chain reaction for the detection of high-risk human papillomavirus in cervical cytology specimens. *Analytical and Quantitative Cytology and Histology,* Vol.31, No.4, pp.208-216

Walboomers, J., Jacobs, M., Manos, M., Bosch, F.X., Kummer, J.A., Shah, K.V., Snijders, P.J.F., Peto, J., Meijer, C. & Munoz, N. (1999). Human papillomavirus is a necessary cause of invasive cervical cancer worldwide. *Journal of Pathology*, Vol.189, pp.12–19

Walts, A.E. & Bose, S. (2009). p16, Ki-67, and BD ProExC immunostaining: a practical approach for diagnosis of cervical intraepithelial neoplasia. *Human Pathology*, Vol.40, No.7, pp.957-964,Epub 2009 Mar 9

Wang, S.S., Trunk, M., Schiffman, M., Herrero, R., Sherman, M., Burk, R., et al. (2004). Validation of p16INK4a as a marker of oncogenic human papillomavirus infection in cervical biopsies from a population-based cohort in Costa Rica. *Cancer Epidemiology, Biomarkers and Prevention*, Vol. 13, pp.1355–1360

Whiteside, M., Siegel, E. & Unger, E. (2008). Human Papillomavirus and Molecular Considerations for Cancer Risk. *Cancer*, Vol.113, No.10 suppl, pp.2981–2994

Wright, T.C. (2006). Pathology of HPV infection at the cytologic and histologic levels: basis for a 2-tiered morphologic classificationsystem. *International Journal of Gynecology and Obstetrics*, Vol.94, No.suppl 1, pp.22–31

Yoshida, T., Sano, T., Kanuma, T., Owada, N., Sakurai, S., Fukuda, T. & Nakajima, T. (2008). Immunochemical analysis of HPV L1 capsid protein and p16 protein in liquid-based cytology samples from uterine cervical lesions. *Cancer*, Vol.114, No.2, pp.83-88

Yu, L., Wang, L., Zhong, J. & Chen, S. (2010). Diagnostic Value of p16INK4A, Ki-67, and Human Papillomavirus L1 Capsid Protein Immunochemical Staining on Cell Blocks From Residual Liquid-Based Gynecologic Cytology Specimens. *Cancer (Cancer Cytopathology)*, Vol.118, pp.47–55

Zerfass, K., Schulze, A., Spitkovsky, D., Friedman, V., Henglein, B. & Jansendurr P. (1995). Sequential activation of cyclin E and cyclin A gene expression by human papillomavirus type 16 E7 through sequences necessary for transformation. *Journal of General Virology*, Vol.69, pp.6389–6399

Zheng, L., Liu, A.L., Qi, T., Wang, Q., Cai, Z., Su, Y.J., Hu, Y.W., Liu, G.B. & Wei, L.H. (2010). Human telomerase RNA gene amplification detection increases the specificity of cervical intraepithelial neoplasia screening. *International Journal of Gynecological Cancer*, Vol.20, No.6, pp.912-917

zur Hausen, H. (1977). Human papilloma viruses and their possible role in squamous cell carcinomas. *Current Topics in Microbiology and Immunology*, Vol.78, pp.1–30

zur Hausen, H. (2008). Papillomaviruses—to Vaccination and Beyond. *Biochemistry (Moscow)*, Vol.73, No.5, pp.498-503

zur Hausen, H. (2009). Papillomaviruses in the causation of human cancers – a brief historical account. *Virology*, Vol.384, pp.260–265

4

Clinical Manifestations of Genital HPV Infection

Edison Natal Fedrizzi
Department of Gynecology and Obstetrics of
The Federal University of Santa Catarina, Florianópolis
Director of HPV Project Clinical Research Center University
Hospital – Federal University of Santa Catarina
Brazil

1. Introduction

The Human papillomavirus infection is the sexually transmitted infection most frequent in man and woman (Koutsky, 1997; Worda, 2005). The probability of transmission of HPV through sexual intercourse varies from 5 to 100% with an average of 40%. The probability of transmission per partner (male-female) is estimated at 60% for HPV 16 and 60% for HPV that causes genital warts. Detection of HPV DNA by the molecular biological methods, does not necessarily represent the manisfestation of a disease (Burchell et al, 2006). According to The World Health Organization (WHO), more than 630 million men and women (1 in every 10 people) are infected with HPV in the world (Ferlay et al, 2004; CDC, 2007). Clinical manifestation is present in less than 10% and the infection is often asymptomatic and can be unnoticed by the patient even though a lesion is present. It is believed, that approximately 1/3 of all women en the world have some form of clinically manifested HPV infection. Also, half of all the women of the world sexually active are infected with this virus (Snoeck, 2006).

It is believed as well that after exposure to HPV, the virus infects the entire lower genital tract epithelium (Shepherd & Bryson, 2008). The incubation period is highly variable, ranging from a few days to many years (20 to 30 years or more) (Sinal & Woods, 2005) (Figure 1). When the infection process starts, there is a proliferation phase ranging from from 3 to 6 months, when many lesions many lesions appear. After the response of B and T cells to the infection, what follows is the containment phase that also lasts for 3 to 6 months, when regression will occur to more than 80% of the lesions. The other 20% will have an active disease or recurrence after variable disease-free intervals (Franco & Steben, 2007). The clinical manifestations are variable and are associated with systemic and local immune response of each individual, with different environmental factors. Dependent on the host immune system, the course of the infection can take one of the three following forms. The most frequent is the Latent Infection, where no clinical manifestation of the infection occurs, and it is only detected by the HPV DNA detection methods. The second form is the Subclinical Infection with minimal clinical manifestation, that is usually diagnosed by colposcopy, cytology and histology. The third form, that is the least common is the Clinical Infection. In this form there is an active expression of the disease, manifested mainly by genital warts, precancerous lesions and invasive cancer (Chow et al, 2010). The different manifestations are also dependent on different types of HPV (currently more than 200 types) and also the host immune system (Bernard, 2005). The low-risk HPV will mainly produce warts (condyloma) and the high risk HPV will mainly produce an intraepithelial lesion (Trofatter, 1997).

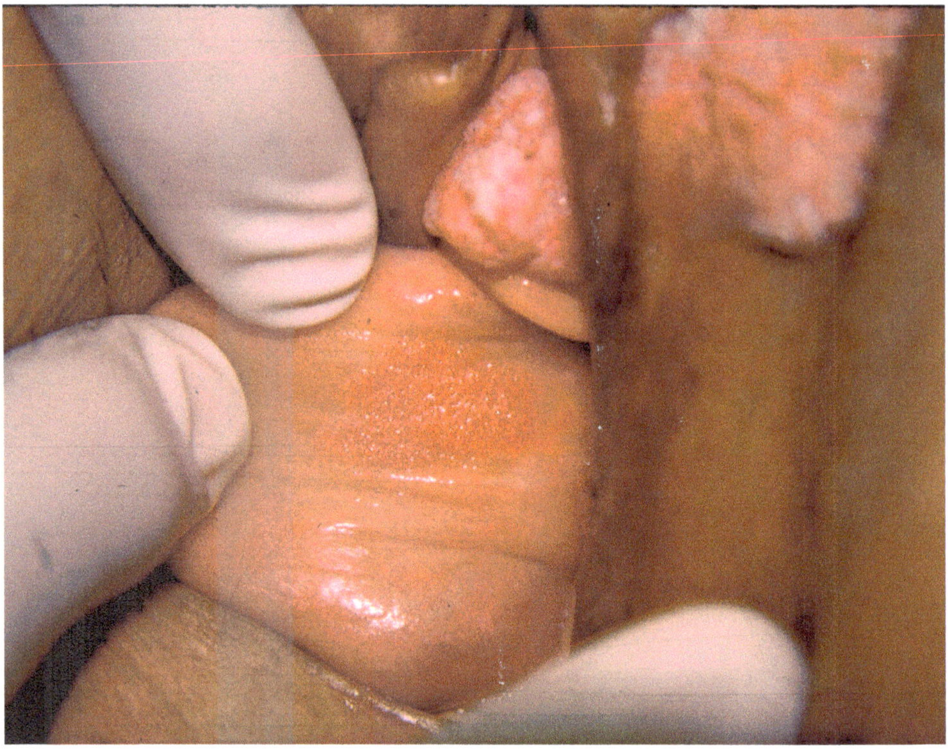

Fig. 1. A 75-year-old woman sexually inactive for 25 years showing a wart on the vulva that appeared 6 months ago. There is also a VAIN 3 and an urethral cancer HPV 16 induced.

2. Clinical lesions

Clinical lesions (only 2 to 3% of HPV infections) are mainly represented by condyloma acuminatum, Bowenoid papulosis (vulvar intraepithelial neoplasia usual type) and Buschke-Loewenstein tumor. The presence of acuminate lesions on the cervix (Figure 2) are infrequent (in 6% of the women that have vulvar condyloma) and this represents an indication of high-risk HPV infections (20% of these infections have associated an intraepithelial lesion) (Scheurer et al, 2005). Genital warts are easily recognized by papillary epithelial proliferations, often with vascular loops inside. Lesions may be single or multiple, scattered or confluent (Sadjadi et al, 2003) (Figure 3 and 4).

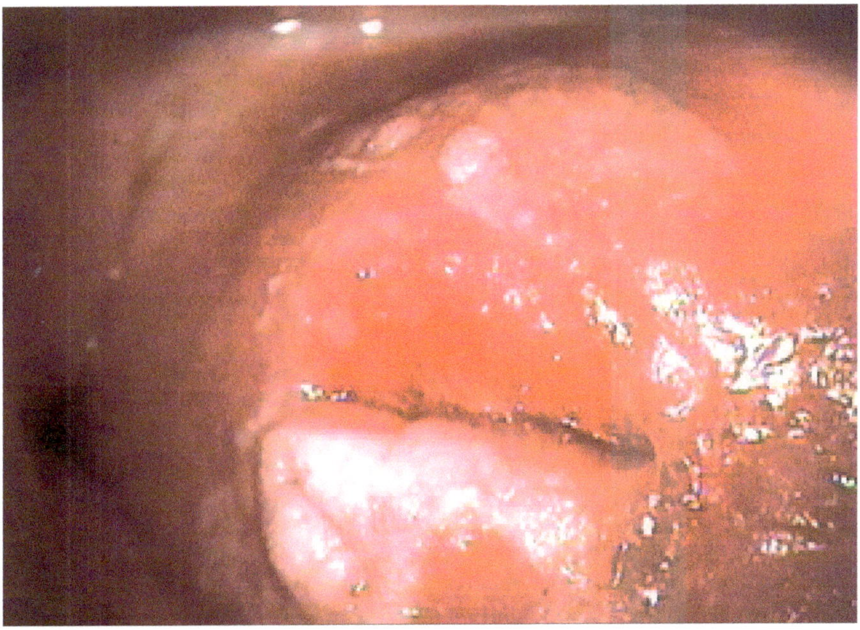

Fig. 2. Condyloma acuminata in the cervix

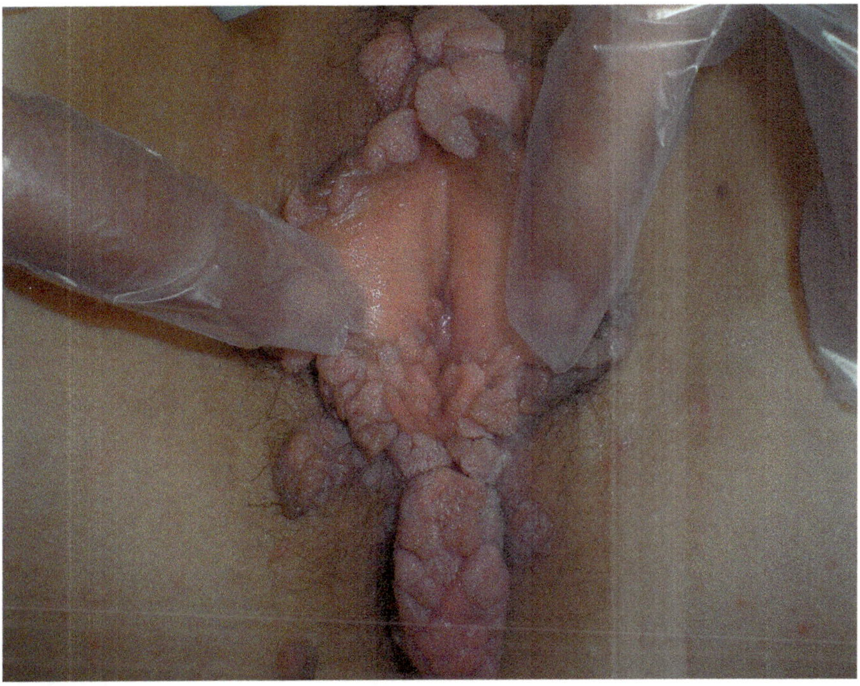

Fig. 3. Multiple condyloma acuminata on the vulva

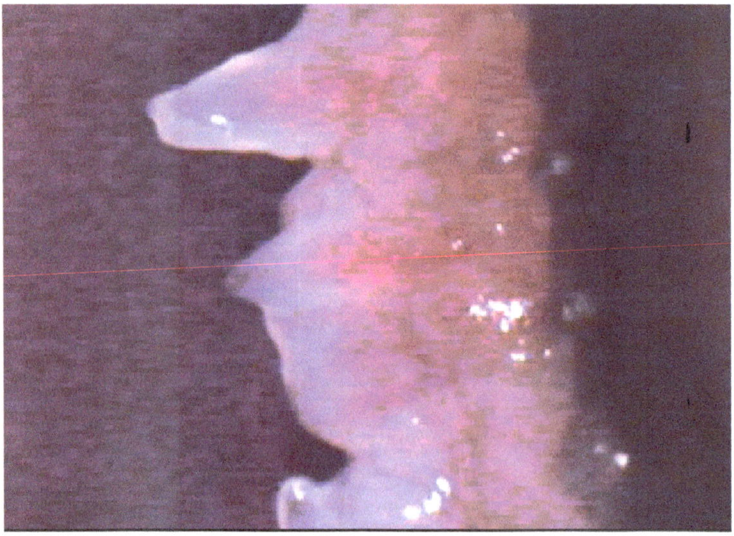

Fig. 4. Detail of a condyloma acuminatum with a characteristic central vessel.

Vaginal warts can be detected by careful examination in more than one third of the cases of women who have vulvar warts. Generally, they are usually small and multiple and can be hidden by the speculum. The lesions may involve the entire length of the vagina, but most frequentely occur in the upper and lower thirds of the vagina (Figure 5). Although vaginal warts are usually asymptomatic, vaginal discharging and itching can occur, and less often, post-coital bleeding, may be present (Row et al, 1981).

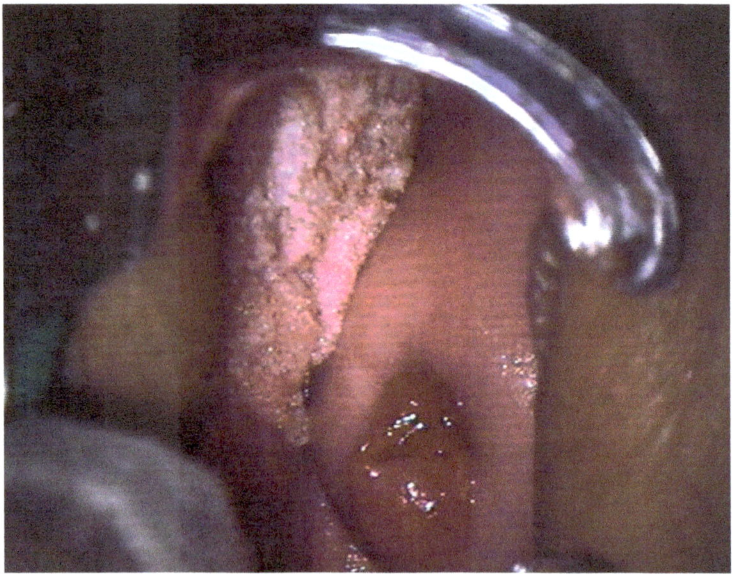

Fig. 5. Multiple vaginal warts in the upper third of the vagina

The verrucous lesions in the vulvar region have increased in numbers in recent years, affecting mainly younger women. Vulvar warts generally occur in moist areas of the skin and in places subjected mostly to trauma during intercourse.

About 25% of the women with vulvar warts have these lesions in the anal and perianal region as well, and are not necessarily associated with the practice of anal sex (Figure 3). These lesions may be sessile or pedunculated, papular, hyperkeratotic or hyperpigmented. Vulvar manifestations depend on each individual, ranging from small lesions (Figure 6) to gigantic such as in the cases of a Buschke-Loewenstein tumor (Ambriz-Gonzalez et al, 2005) (Figure 7). Papular and hypercrhromic vulvar lesions (vulvar intraepithelial neoplasia (VIN) usual type) (Figure 8) represent today, a high-grade intraepithelial neoplasia (Forcier & Musacchio, 2010).

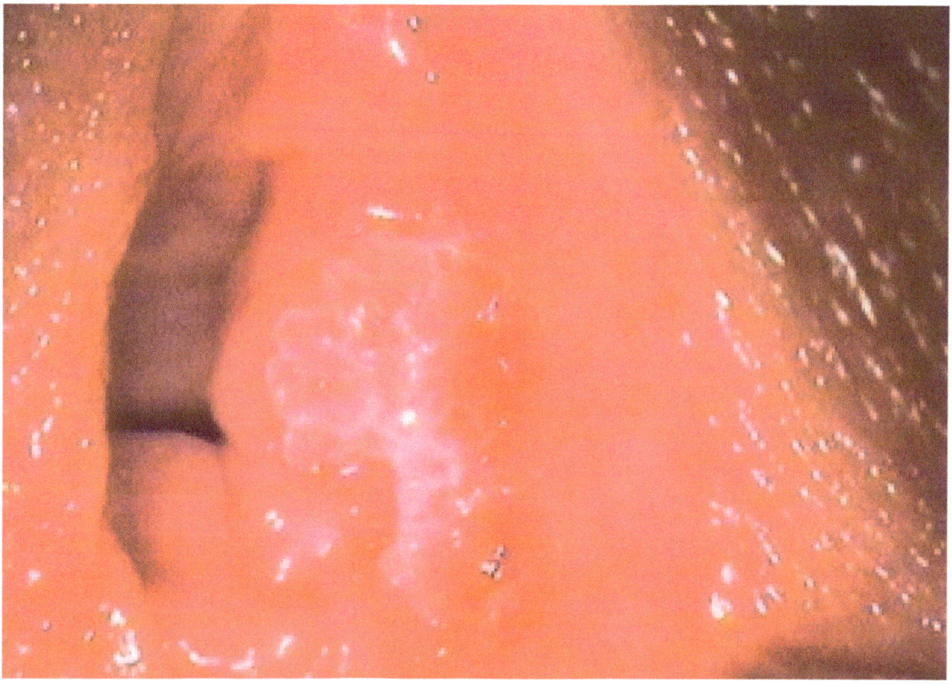

Fig. 6. Small vulvar wart

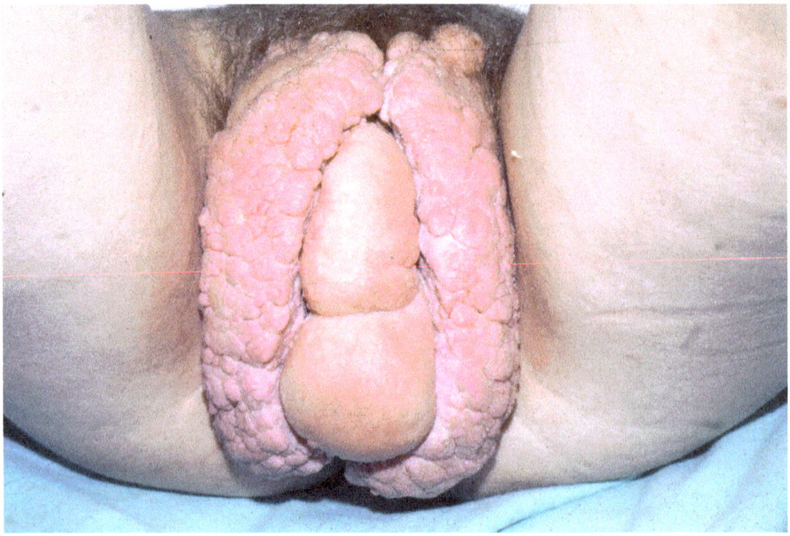

Fig. 7. Buschke-Loewenstein tumor in a woman of 18 years who begun sexual activity 6 months before with only the same partner

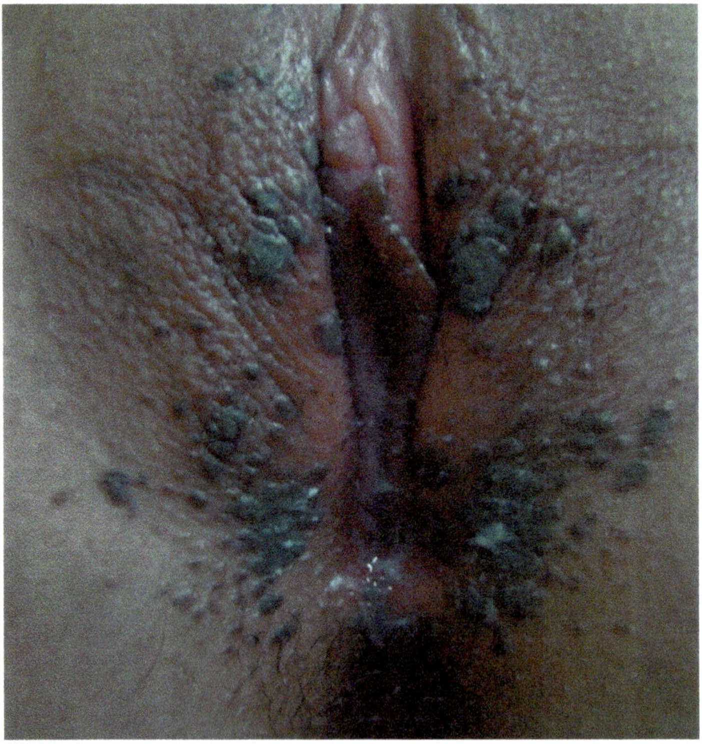

Fig. 8. A typical example of VIN usual type with hyperchromic papules coalescing

Approximately 18% of women with vulvar condyloma have anal and perianal warts as well (Figure 9). Depending on the extent of the injuries, discomfort or bleeding may occur during evacuation. In these cases, the rectal examination should also be performed, since approximately 10% of women with anal warts, exhibit rectal lesions (Nadal et al, 1999).

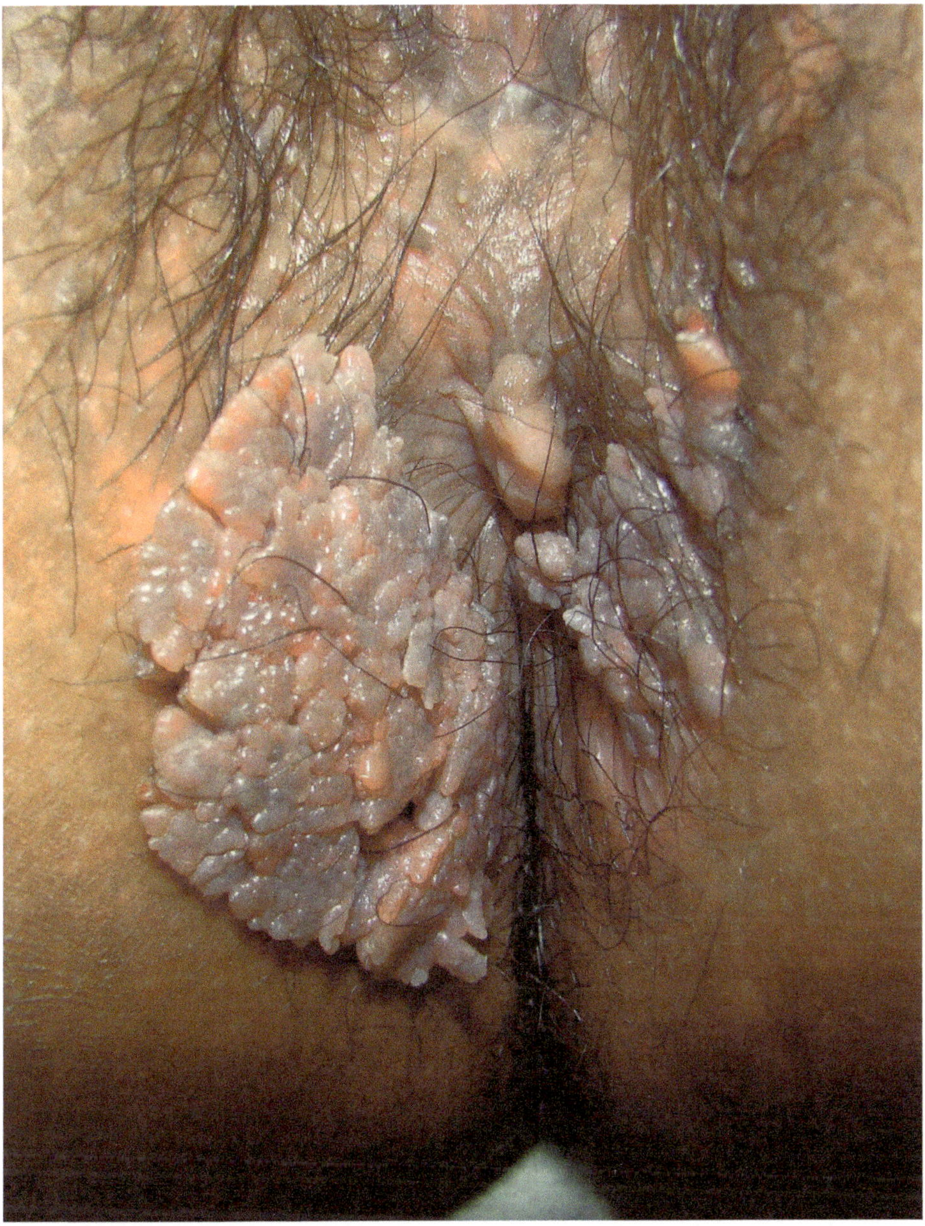

Fig. 9. Multiple condyloma acuminatum in the anal and perianal region

When evaluating male partners of women with genital disease associated with HPV, approximately 40 to 50% of them also have lesions. The lesions may manifest as penile warts, papules or papillae. The lesions appear mainly in areas of trauma, especially related to sexual activity (the penile shaft, preputial cavity, coronal sulcus and glans) (Figure 10). Urethral involvement (Figure 11) is more frequent in men than women (10 to 28% of the men with genital warts and less than 5% of the women with genital diseases associated with HPV) (Buechner, 2002).

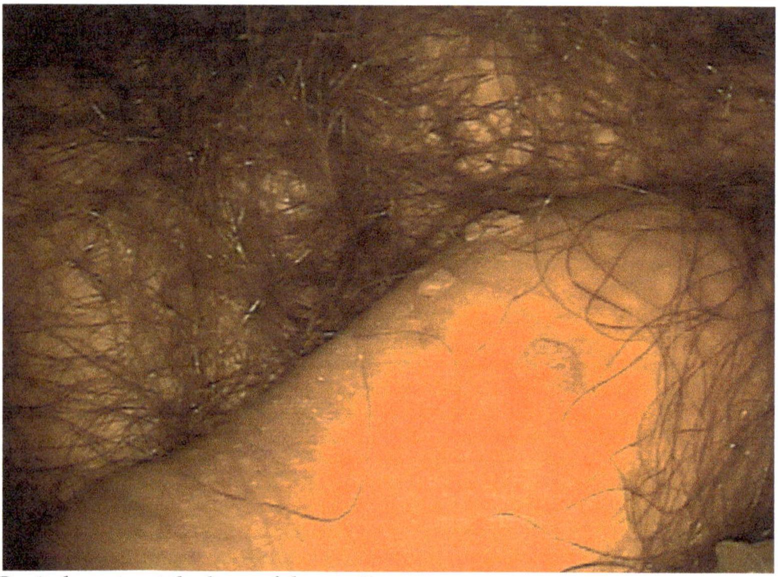

Fig. 10. Genital warts at the base of the penile

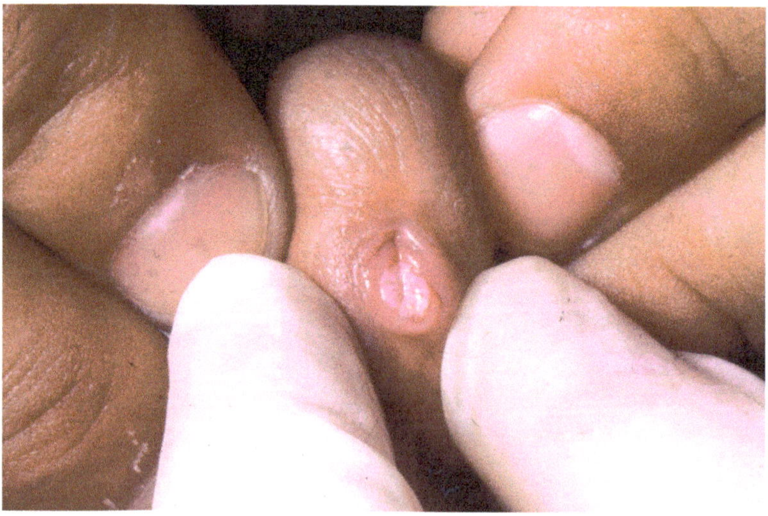

Fig. 11. Condyloma in the urethra of a young man

3. Sub-clinical lesions

Subclinical lesions represent 60% of the cases of external anogenital HPV and 95% of the cases of cervical HPV infection. The main symptoms are micropapillary, micropapular, spike, and keratotic lesions. The diagnosis of these lesions is accomplished primarily by colposcopy, cytology and histology (Forcier & Musacchio, 2010).

The cytopathic effects of HPV infection, specifically koilocytotic atypia, dyskeratosis and the cellular multinucleation are detected in 2 to 3% of routine Pap smears (Figure 12). The cytological and histological patterns of HPV-induced lesions are essentially the same (Wright, 2006) (Figure 13).

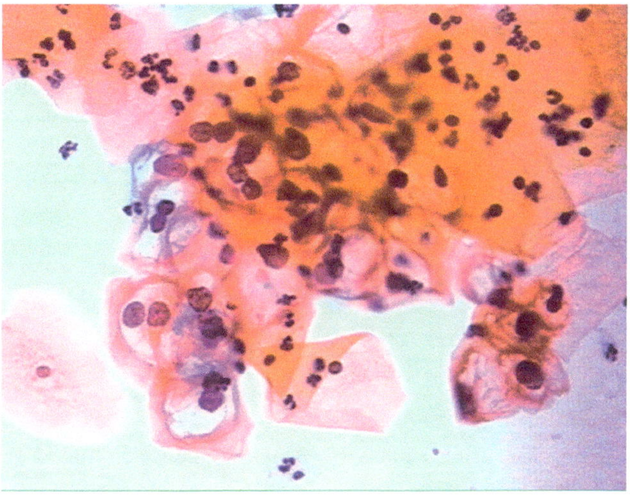

Fig. 12. Cytopathic effects of HPV infection (koilocytotic atypia)

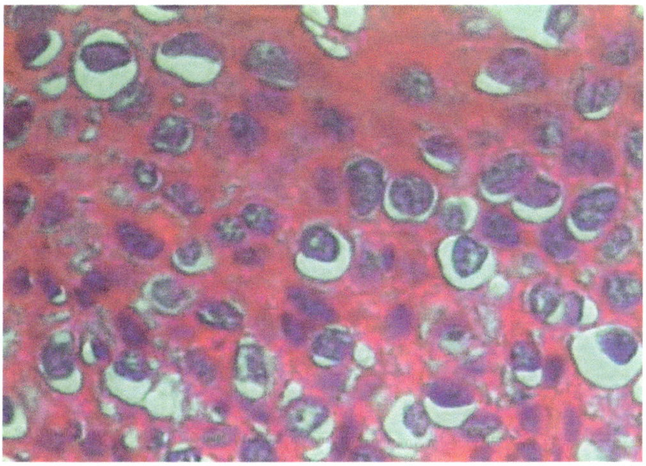

Fig. 13. Histology of a cervical intraepithelial neoplasia with cytopathic effects of HPV infection (koilocytosis)

Cervical intraepithelial neoplasia (CIN) is the most common manifestation of HPV in the cervix. These lesions are manifested by colposcopy using acetic acid that produces aceto-white epithelium, punctation or mosaic. At the colposcopic exam, the cellular changes in the low-grade squamous intraepithelial lesions (LSIL) are discrete (Figure 14) while in high-grade lesions (HSIL) are bigger (Figure 15), including an atypical vascularization. An aceto-white lesion outside the cervical transformation zone is highly suggestive of an HPV infection (Figure 16). The low-grade lesions often regress spontaneously, ranging from 25 to 60% in one year. The regression rate for high-grade lesions is much smaller (Chase et al, 2008).

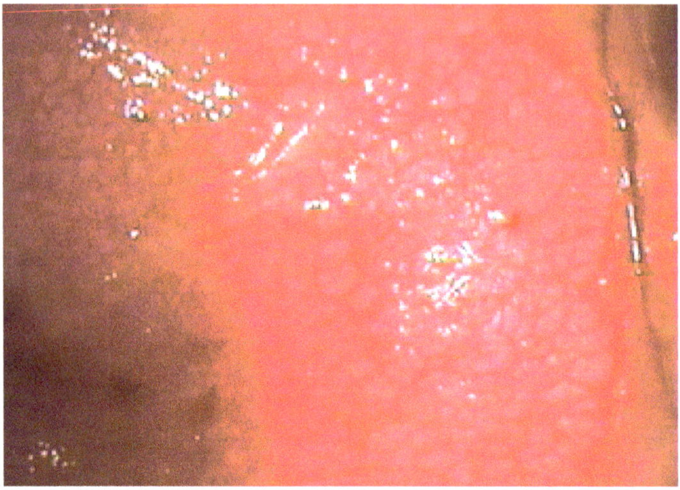

Fig. 14. Colposcopy of a low-grade squamous intraepithelial lesion caused by the HPV infection (mosaiciform lesion)

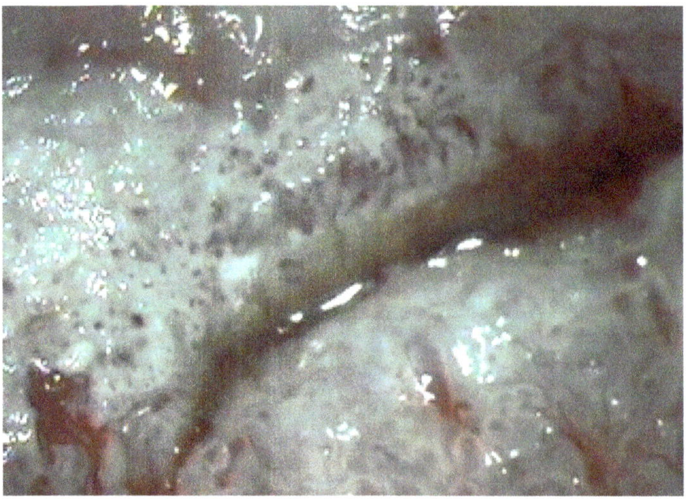

Fig. 15. Colposcopy of a high-grade squamous intraepithelial lesion caused by the HPV infection (atypical vessels)

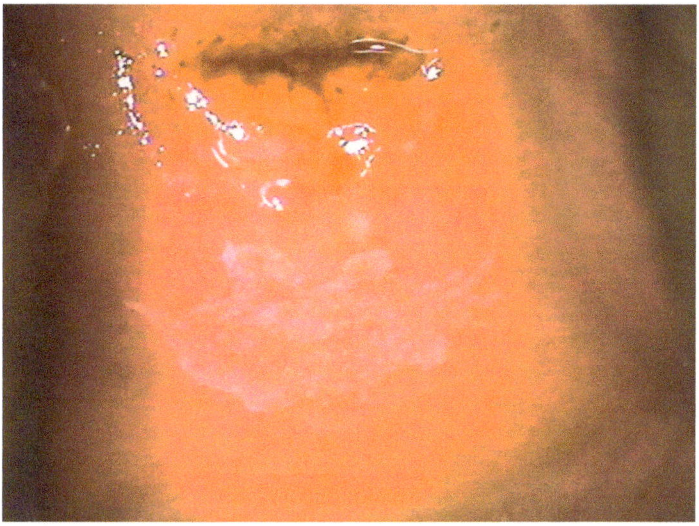

Fig. 16. Aceto-white lesion outside the cervical transformation zone due to the HPV infection

The manifestations of the HPV infection in the vagina is poor. Changes are usually aceto-white, flat or the micropapillary lesion that are visible after the application of acetic acid at 2 to 5% (Figure 17) and are better visualized after applying Lugol's iodine (Figure 18). The punctation and mosaics caused by HPV should be differentiated mainly from the congenital transformation zone and may be related to a vaginal low or high-grade intraepithelial neoplasia (Davis, 1993) . The natural history of vaginal intraepithelial neoplasia (VAIN) based on a 3-year follow-up study of no treatment suggests a regression rate of 78%, 13% persistence, and 9% progression to cancer (Aho et al, 1991).

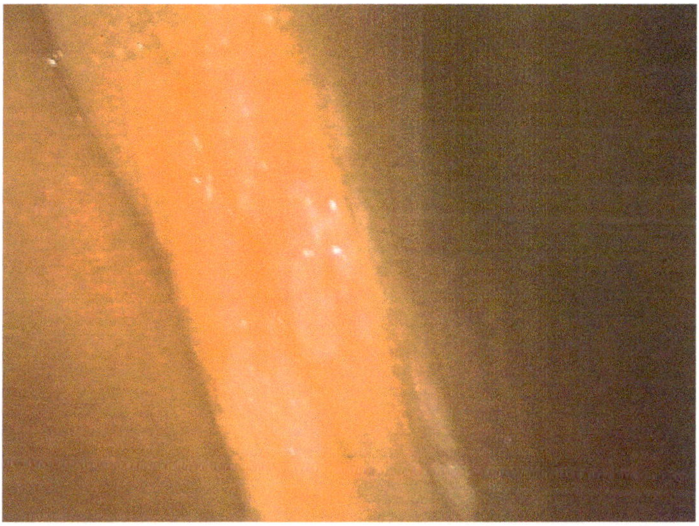

Fig. 17. Colposcopy of a vaginal intraepithelial neoplasia after applying acetic acid 2%

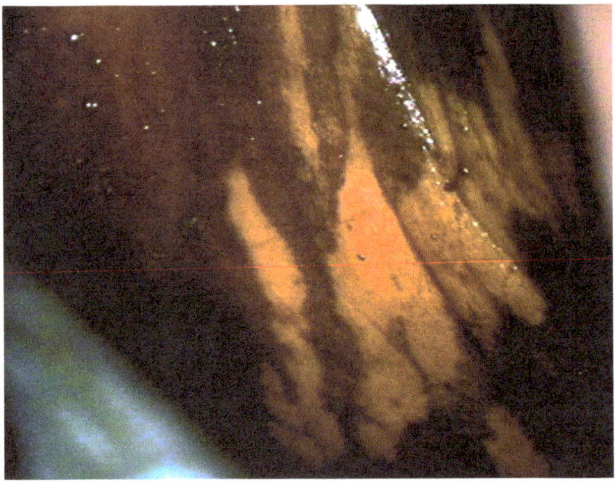

Fig. 18. The visualization of a vaginal intraepithelial neoplasia with colposcopy is better after applying Lugol's iodine solution

The colposcopic examination of the vulva after the application of acetic acid at 5% permits the identification of the minimum changes associated with HPV, usually expressed by the aceto-white epithelium. These changes are often multifocal and commonly involve the vaginal fourchette and labia minora. It is necessary, however, to have an expert colposcopist to differentiate the subclinical alterations induced by HPV from inflammatory changes (Gagné, 2008). The vulvar intraepithelial neoplasia (VIN) associated with HPV (VIN usual type) has a very small risk of progression to an invasive lesion. The most severe intraepithelial lesions (VIN differentiated type, that are not associated with HPV) tend to be multicentric and multifocal. These lesions may be associated with pruritus and local irritation (Heller, 2007).

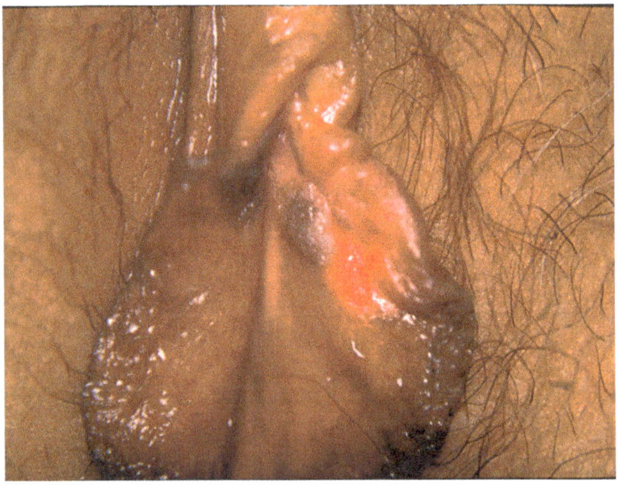

Fig. 19. A hyperpigmented and aceto-white lesion of a vulvar intraepithelial neoplasia (VIN usual type) of the minor labia observed by colposcopy after applying acetic acid 5%.

Subclinical changes in the perianal and anal area are much less frequent and pratically all are associated with an aceto-white epithelium of varying severity after the use of acetic acid at 5% (Chin-Hong & Palefsky 2002) (Figure 20).

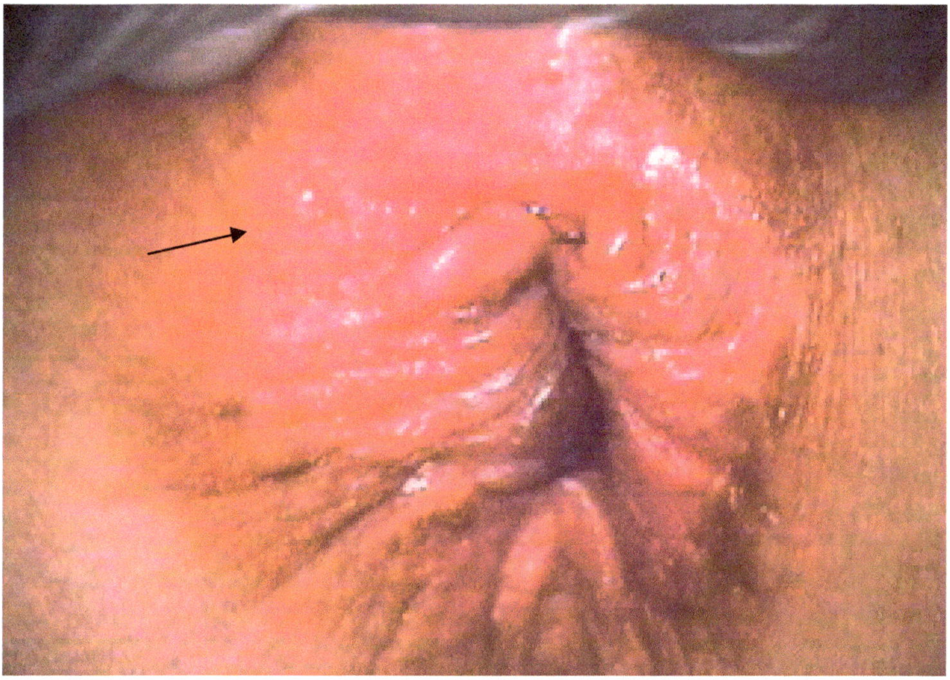

Fig. 20. Aceto-white epithelium of an anal intraepithelial neoplasia observed by colposcopy after applying acetic acid 5%

When evaluating with colposcopy (peniscopy) and acetic acid on male partners of women with genital disease associated with HPV, approximately 40 to 50% of them also have lesions associated with HPV. About 20 to 30% of partners of women with cervical intraepithelial neoplasia also have a penile intraepithelial neoplasia (PIN). Half of these lesions are subclinical. Circumcised men have a lower prevalence of subclinical disease due to the majority of the lesions being located on the foreskin. Penile intraepithelial neoplasias may also exhibit a hyperchromic (Figure 21) or reddish lesion. Rarely these lesions are symptomatic, but when this occurs, itching or burning is more frequent (Krebs & Schneider, 1987).

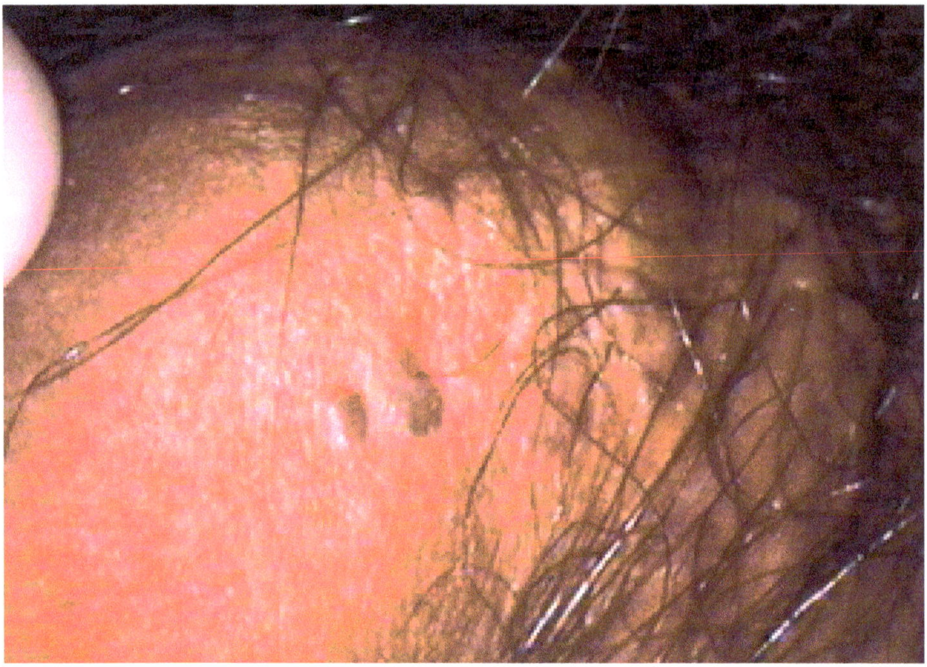

Fig. 21. Penile intraepithelial neoplasia observed by peniscopy after applying acetic acid 5% exhibiting hyperpigmented papules on the foreskin

4. Latent infection

In latent infections there are no clinical manifestation. In the general female population, the prevalence of the HPV infection ranges from 2 to 44%. Infection also occurs in approximately 8% of women who are not yet sexually active and approximately 20% in women who have had sexual activity with women only. In men, the percentage of HPV infection can reach as high as 45%, depending on the population studied. The diagnosis of latent infection is performed using molecular biology methods, especially the hybrid capture and polymerase chain reaction (PCR) methods, due to the clinical examination, colposcopy, cytology and histology are normal (Chow et al, 2010).

5. References

Aho, M.; Vesterinen, E. & Meyer, B (1991). Natural history of vaginal intraepithelial neoplasia. *Cancer*, Vol. 68, pp. 195–197.

Ambriz-Gonzalez, G.; Escobedo-Zavala, L. C.; Carrilo de La Mora, F.; Ortiz-Arriaga, A.; Cordero-Zamora, A. & Corona-Nakamura, A. (2005). Buschke-Lowenstein tumor in childhood: a case report. *J Pediatr Surg*, Vol.40, N°9, pp.25-27.

Bernard, H. U. (2005). The clinical importance of the nomenclature, evolution and taxonimy of human papillomaviruses. *J Clin Virology*, Vol.32S, pp. S1-S6.

Buechner, S. A. (2002). Common skin disorders of the penis. *Br J Urol Int*, Vol. 90, N°5, pp.498-506.

Burchell, A. N.; Winer, R. L.; de Sanjose, S. & Franco, E. L. (2006). Epidemiology and transmission dynamics of HPV infection. *Vaccine*, Vol. 24 , Suppl. 3, pp.52–56.

CDC (2007). Quadrivalent human papillomavirus vaccine: recommendations of the advisory committee on immunization practices. *MMWR*, Vol.56, pp. 1–24.

Chase, D.M.; Kalouyan, M. & Di Saia, P. J. (2009). Colposcopy to evaluate abnormal cervical cytology in 2008. *Am J Obstet Gynecol*, Vol.200, N°5, pp. 472-480.

Chin-Hong, P. V. & Palefsky, J. M. (2002). Natural history and clinical management of anal human papillomavirus disease in men and women infected with human immunodeficiency virus. *Clin Infect Dis*, Vol.35, pp.1127–1134.

Chow, L. T.; Broker, T. R.; Steinberg, B. M. (2010). The natural history of human papillomavirus infections of the mucosal epithelia. *APMIS*, Vol. 118, pp.422–449.

Davis, G. G. (1993). Colposcopic examination of vagina. *Obstet Gynecol Clin North Am*, Vol.20, pp.1-15.

Ferlay, J.; Bray, F.; Pisani, P. & Parkin, D.M. (2004). Globocan 2002 cancer incidence. Mortality and prevalence worldwide. *IARC Cancer Base*, Vol.5, pp.123-129.

Forcier, M. & Musacchio, N. (2010). An overview of human papillomavirus infection for the dermatologist: disease, diagnosis, management, and prevention. *Dermatol Therapy*, Vol. 23, pp. 458–476.

Franco, E. D. & Steben, M. (2007). Human papilomavirus infection: Epidemiology and pathophysiology. *Gynecol Oncol*, Vol.107, pp.S2-S5.

Gagné, H.M. (2008). Colposcopy of the vagina and vulva. Obstet Gynecol Clin N Am, Vol. 35, pp. 659–669.

Heller, D.S. (2007). Report of a new ISSVD classification of VIN. *J Low Genit Tract Dis*, Vol. 11, pp. 46–47.

Koutsky, L. (1997). Epidemiology of genital human papillomavirus infection. *Am J Med*, Vol.102, pp. 3-8.

Krebs, H. B. & Schneider, V. (1987). Human papillomavirus associated lesions of the penis: colposcopy, cytology, and histology. *Obstet Gynecol*, Vol.70, pp.299–304.

Nadal, S. R.; Manzione, C. R. & Galvão, V. M. (1999). Perianal diseases in HIV-positive patients compared with a seronegative population. *Dis Colon Rectum*, Vol.42, pp.649-654.

Row, M. M.; Meisels, A. & Fortier, M. (1981). Vaginal condylomata and human papillomavirus infection. *Clin Obstet Gynecol*, Vol.24, pp. 461-464.

Sadjadi, A.; Malekzadech, R.; Derakhshan, M. H.; Sephr, A.; Nouraire, M. & Sotoudeh, M. (2003). Cancer ocurrence in Ardabil: result of a populacion based cancer registry from Iran. *Int J Cancer*, Vol.107, N°1, pp.113-118.

Scheurer, M. E.; Tortolero-Luna, G. & Adler-Storthz, K. (2005). Human papillomavirus infection: biology, epidemiology and prevention. *Int J Gynecol Cancer*, Vol. 15, pp. 727-746.

Shepherd, L. J. & Bryson, S. C. (2008). Human papillomavirus – lessons from history and challenges for the future. *J Obstet Gynaecol Cancer*, Vol.30, N°11, pp.1025-1033.

Sinal, S. H. & Woods, C. R. (2005). Human papillomavirus infections of the genital and respiratory tracts in young children. *Semin Pediatr Infect Dis*, Vol. 16, N°4, pp.306-316.

Snoeck, R. (2006). Papillomavirus and treatment. *Antiviral Research*, Vol 71, pp. 181-191.

Trofatter, K. F. (1997). Diagnosis of human papillomavirus genital tract infection. *Am J Med*, Vol.102, N° 5A, pp. 21-27.

Worda, C.; Huber, A.; Hudelist, G.; Schatten, C.; Peipold, H. & Czerwenka, K. (2005). Prevalence of cervical and intrauterine Human papillomavirus infection in the third trimester in asymptomatic women. *J Soc Gynecol Invest*, Vol.12, pp.440-444.

Wright, T. C. (2006). Pathology of HPV infection at the cytologic and histologic levels: Basis for a 2-tiered morphologic classification system. Int J Gynecol Obstet, Vol. 94, Suppl.1, pp. S22-S31.

Part 2

Human Papillomavirus Vaccines

5

Development of New Human Papillomavirus Vaccines

Carmen Rodríguez-Cerdeira[1], Silvia Díez-Moreno[2], E. Sánchez[3] and Alfonso Alba[4]
[1]Department of Dermatology (CHUVI)& University of Vigo, Vigo
[2,3]Postgraduate Researcher, University of Vigo
Spanish Society of Cervical Pathology and Colposcopy &
[4]Centre for Molecular and Cellular Studies, Lugo,
Spain

1. Introduction

Over the past 35 years, we have observed a remarkable and important increase in the prevalence of HPV infection, both in its clinical forms and appearance of its condyloma acuminate. Colposcopic exploration of this area would be required, with special focus at the regions of introitus and inter-labial folds. Both genital and anal examinations (Guerra-Tapia et al., 2009) are necessary to determine the sub-clinical expression of HPV identified by cytological changes, colposcopy, and/or vulvoscopy and vaginoscopy. Clinical forms of HPV infections generally caused by LR-HPV strains (6, 11) tend to be benign. Sub-clinical forms include benign and pre-malignant lesions, and are generally caused by HR-HPV strains (16 and 18) (Fig. 1) (Rodríguez-Cerdeira C et al., 2008a, 2008b, , 2009a; Walboomers et al., 1999). In a recent study by the International Agency for Cancer Research (IACR) group in 13 areas in 11 countries including Spain, a high prevalence of HPV was seen in both Europe and Sub-Saharan Africa (International Agency for Research on Cancer [IARC], 1995; Muñoz et al., 2003). Furthermore, it was observed that HPV-16 infection was more frequent among European women. We observed the same genotype in a study involving 436 women aged between 16 and 80 years. Three samples from the cervix and vagina of each patient were cytologically examined (Rodríguez-Cerdeira C et al., 2009b).

Thus, epidemiological studies supported by molecular techniques and liquid cytology have confirmed the incidental role of certain strains of HPV in the development of cervical, vulvar, vaginal, anal, and penile cancer (Fig. 2), the risk for which is greatly increased in human immunodeficiency virus (HIV)+ patients (Rodríguez Cerdeira C et al., 2011). An international series with high-sensitivity polymerase chain reaction (PCR) has proven that HPV DNA is present in 90.7% of cervical–uterine carcinomas and is present in all the cases confirmed by exhaustive histological examination. This also occurs in the majority of intraepithelial lesions of the lower genital tract (Walboomers et., 1999).

Persistent HPV infection is considered the principal causative agent of cervical and other anogenital cancers. The finding that HPV DNA is present in practically all cases of cervical cancer has great importance in developing preventive strategies (Fig. 3) (Rodríguez Cerdeira C et al., 2007; Mougin et al., 2001; Trottier et al., 2006). Integration of the viral genome with the host cell genome does not occur in all cases of cervical cancer and may be explained by mutations in repressive areas such as the region Ying-Yang (YYI), which would maintain the continued expression of E6 and E7 or by the production of a more stable 'chimeric' RNA, thereby permitting greater synthesis of these oncoproteins (Fig. 4) (Alba et al., 2009).

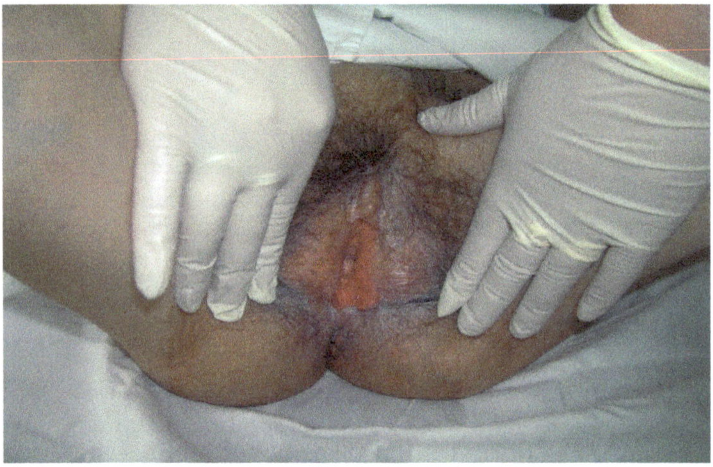

Fig. 1. High-grade vulvar intraepithelial neoplasia in a smoker

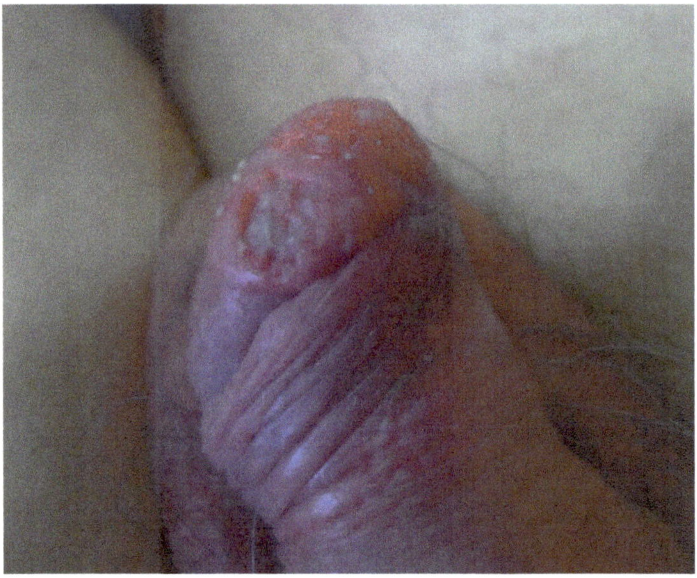

Fig. 2. Penile intraepithelial neoplasia developing into invasive carcinoma with extensive exophytic ulcerous mass that invades the gland and projects beyond the preputial-balanic fold in a human papillomavirus-positive patient

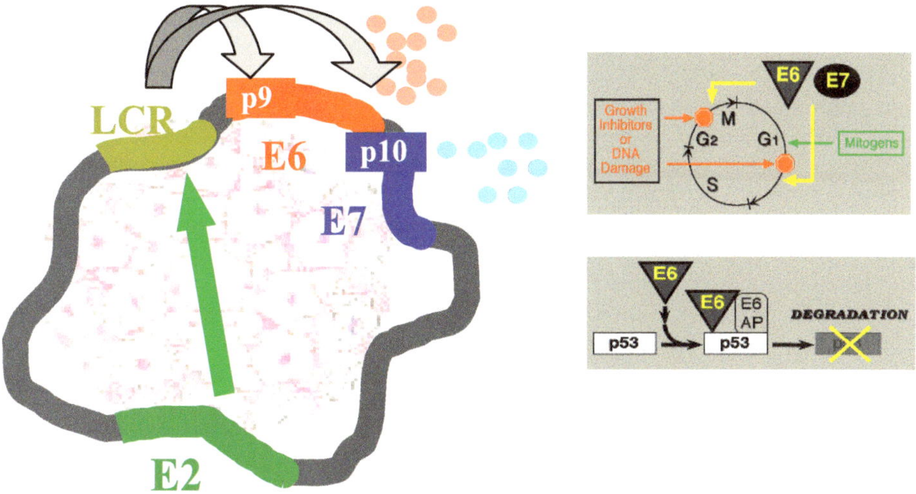

Fig. 3. Interaction between the viral protein and the cell cycle

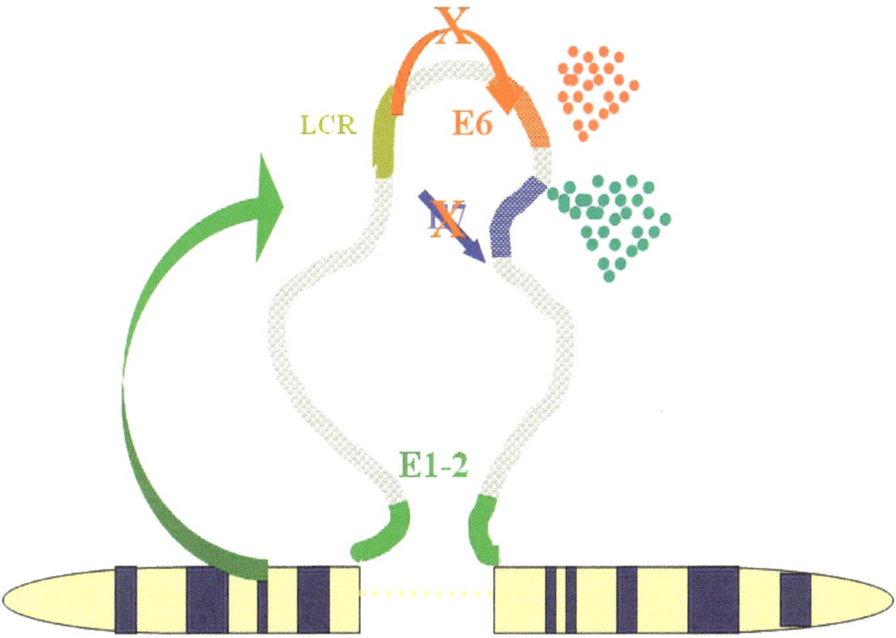

Fig. 4. Integration of human papillomavirus in the host genome

Over the recent years, the morbimortality and health costs associated with cervical, vaginal, vulvar, anal, and peneal cancers and their precursory lesions have provoked intense investigation (Kadish et al., 1992; Guerra-Tapia et al., 2009; Rodríguez-Cerdeira C et al., 2008a) to achieve vaccine-based prevention of HPV infections, which would dramatically reduce the risk of these cancers. Experiences with girls or women with current infection with 1 or more of the vaccine HPV types gained protection from the infections or diseases caused by the remaining vaccine HPV types, and they were also protected against re-infection with the same HPV type after clearance of an infection caused by a vaccine HPV type. High seroconversion rates and high levels of anti-HPV antibodies were observed in all vaccinated individuals of all age ranges from 9 to 45 years. Rechallenge with a quadrivalent HPV vaccine produced a potent anamnestic humoral immune response (Rodríguez Cerdeira C et al., 2009a, 2009b; Alba et al., 2009). The vaccine is generally well tolerated, and is projected to be cost effective in most pharmacoeconomic models. However, there are some questions that we are faced with: Does the intensity of such a humoral immune response correlate with long-term protection? Although a direct correlation between antibody levels and protection may seem intuitively obvious, it is still unclear whether differing antibody titres indicate better disease protection or longer duration of immune protection. Given that virtually all vaccinated women are seroconverted, we may deduce that until now, we do not have any immunological correlates for protection. The question still remains unanswered: Why, when the body's natural antibodies respond so poorly, do the HPV vaccines that generate serum neutralizing antibodies work? The answer is that the quality and quantity of the immune response generated by the vaccine is different from those by natural infections.

Is it stated that vaccines will induce a generation of long-lived memory immune cells that, after re-exposure to the relevant antigen, will generate a potent immune response, thus preventing HPV infections? Time is needed to suitably answer this question. In the opinion of other investigators, preventive HPV vaccination is an expensive practice, and it may be an insufficient tool to tackle cervical cancer worldwide. Therapeutic intervention is seeking for safe/effective vaccines inducing the activation of $CD8^+$ cytotoxic T lymphocytes (CTLs) that are required to clear the tumour. Linking a tumour-specific antigen (i.e. E7 oncoprotein of 'high-risk' HPVs) to molecules able to increase its immune 'visibility' represents a strategy to force the immune system to fight cancer. They focussed on plants as sources of innovative immunostimulatory sequences. Thus, a new vaccination route for systemic and mucosal immunity, and other issues will be addressed throughout this chapter.

2. HPV infection and immunity

Any viral infection requires the presence of a cellular receptor that allows for the internalisation of the viral particles. This circumstance supposes the principal barrier to entry and explains the species-specific and even organ-specific nature of viral infections. Some viruses use the major histocompatibility complexes I and II (MHC I and II) as receptors for their internalisation, while others use molecules on the cellular surface (CD4, chemokines, growth factors, and β2 microglobulin). The HPV does not have a specific cellular receptor but rather has a well-conserved surface molecule with vital cellular functions, which makes its use impossible as a target for blocking infection. As opposed to other viruses, it does not appear that the surface receptors are implied in tissue or species specificity or in HPV tropism (Alba et al., 2009).

Infection recognition by the host cell and specific tropism of each viral subgroup determine the cytopathic effects in specific tissues (Rodríguez-Cerdeira C et al., 2008a); this makes it possible to distinguish between latent infections that do not show their effects for long periods and active infections that have practically immediate cytopathic effects. Based on these parameters, it is possible to qualify the antigenic or immunogenic level of each virus to comprise the knowledge base for the manufacture of therapeutic or prophylactic vaccines (Alba et al., 2009; Rodríguez-Cerdeira et al., 2009c).

2.1 Cellular and humoral immunity to human papillomavirus

Cellular immunity is principally represented by T cells, which act at the local tissue level via close cell-cell contact. The humoral response is measured by B cells according to the instructions from T helper cells, through antibody production. The T cells recognise proteins on the surface of the HPV that are associated with the molecules from the cellular surface (human leukocyte antigen [HLA]), while the antibodies recognise both surface and soluble antigens. In the latter case, this is done with greater specificity. The T-cell receptors recognise specific sequences of small peptides presented by the MHC, while the antibodies recognise steric three-dimensional structures with determined structures. If correct presentation of the antigen is essential for inducing an immunological response, the kinetics of antigen-antibody joining and the number and distribution of these joins would be the factors determining the immunological response level.

In general, after the first infection of the cervical epithelial cells by HPV, a non-specific response is provoked, accompanied by an inflammatory process, neutrophil chemoattraction, macrophage activation, natural killer (NK) cell intervention, production of natural antibodies, and activation of the complement system, which forms the first non-specific yet defensive immunological barrier. Prolongation of the response over time and protection against future infections requires specific immunological mechanisms (Alba et al., 2009; Kadish et al., 1992; Rodríguez-Cerdeira et al., 2009c). T CD4 lymphocyte activation requires recognition of the surface molecules exposed by the presenter cell. The viral peptide along with class II HLA will be recognised in the context of T cell receptor and CD4, but requires a 'safety' mechanism for deactivation process control. Thus, it is necessary that other molecules such as CD40 and B7 that are present on the presenter cell surface be recognised by their receptors (CD40 linking and CD28, respectively) for activation to occur. Each activated T CD4 lymphocyte will be converted into a type 1 or 2 lymphocyte T helper cell depending on a series of local tissue factors fundamentally comprising antigen entry route, processing mechanism, and the presence of different interleukins. The Th1 pathway will induce T CD8+ lymphocyte maturity towards cytotoxic effector cells (Fig. 5) (Alba et al., 2009; Rodríguez-Cerdeira et al., 2009c, 2009d).

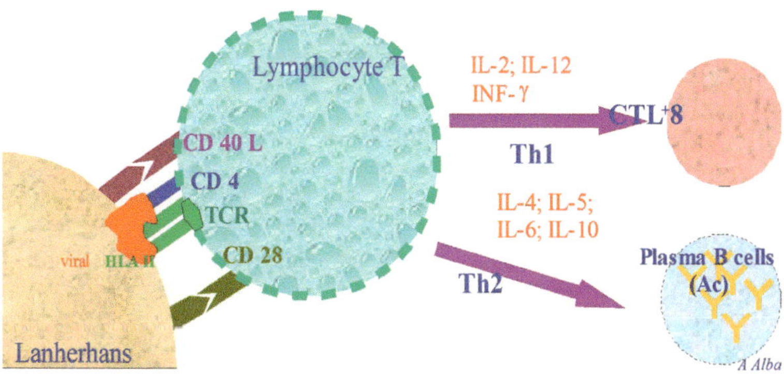

Fig. 5. Lymphocyte activation towards cytotoxic effector cells

Specific cells existing in the cervical epithelium are capable of acting as antigen presenters. Although some keratinocytes develop this ability, Langerhans reticular cells are the true antigen presentation specialists in the cervical epithelium. These cells absorb the viral particles to digest them into endosomes and start an activation process that includes presentation on the antigen surface together with the presenter cell HLA. These activated cells will be recognised by the T CD4 lymphocytes in the case that they recognise every molecule in the correct environment, after which, they evolve into lymphocyte helpers (Th) in the local context of the expression of certain interleukins (IL). Depending on IL type, it will advance to differentiation towards a Th1 pathway that will induce the activation and proliferation of T CD8+ cytotoxins with specific immunity (CTL+8) or towards a Th2 pathway that will induce the activation and expansion of B lymphocytes, which differentiate towards plasma-antibody producer cells for the viral base proteins of non-specific immunity that we could identify as prophylactic (Alba et al., 2009). CTL+8 would have the ability to act against the established viral infection, while the plasma B cells produce antibodies act against the external viral antigens that are exposed during this and successive HPV infections.

The nature of antibody responses and duration following HPV vaccination plays a key role in long-term protection against HPV infection. The importance of vigorous and prolonged immune protection is also very important. In addition, it provides maximum benefit against cervical cancer and other HPV-related cancers (Alba et al., 2009; Rodríguez-Cerdeira et al., 2008a, 2009c, 2009d). Nevertheless, it should also be highlighted that long-term protection is not fully predictable at the introduction of any vaccine, because it varies according to many variables (e.g. cohort target, coverage, acceptance, catch-up) that are not strictly related to immune response. Although some researchers have developed a model to predict long-term immunity, it remains an ongoing and challenging issue. HPV is a family of many different genotypes. Ideally, a vaccine should cover at least the majority of the genotypes that are linked to tumour development, i.e. those that are considered HR-HPV. Nevertheless, the large number of different genotypes among the HPV viruses raises the question about the number of HPV viruses that must be included in the vaccine preparation process. Thus, the possibility of developing second-generation cross-reacting vaccines covering a larger portion of the HPV family must be considered in the HPV investigation (Mariani & Venuti , 2010) biological evolution is concerned, HPV strains are successful infectious agents. They induce persistent infections without causing frequent or serious complications for the host and shed virions for transmission to other naive individuals. To achieve this lifestyle and maintain a state of equilibrium, HPV must avoid the host's defence system. Many factors contribute to evading immune pools, particularly, the following:

- Virus capsid entry is usually an activating signal for dendritic cells (DCs).
- Free virus particles are shed from the surface of the squamous epithelia with poor access to the vascular and lymphatic channels and to the lymph nodes where immune responses are initiated.
- Most DNA viruses have mechanisms for inhibiting interferon (IFN) synthesis and receptor signalling, and papillomaviruses are no exception.

Despite HPV's ability to evade the host's immune system and to down-regulate innate immunity, a primary HPV infection is cleared naturally in approximately 90% of the cases, thus indicating the central role of immunity in the resolution of cervical and anogenital

HPV-associated diseases. Innate immunity acts as the first line of non-specific defence against any pathogen (DCs, IFN-α, cytokines, neutrophils, and macrophages), and attacks by HPV should be detected by the intraepithelial DCs. There is evidence indicating that DCs are not activated by the uptake of HPV capsids, suggesting a limited role in the host's response to HPV infection (Mariani & Venuti , 2010; Fausch et al, 2002, 2003).

Other critical point is in regards to the long-term clinical significance of immunity evoked by natural infection. Certain studies have showed that some women in the placebo group developed the disease despite consuming antibodies against the offending HPV types at enrolment, thus confirming, as stated in the recent WHO position paper, that host antibodies directed against the viral L1 protein do not necessarily protect against subsequent infection by the same HPV genotype (Fausch et al, 2002; Olsson et al., 2009; World Health Organization [WHO], 2009).

3. Prophylactic vaccines against human papillomavirus

Prophylactic vaccines against HPV infection, which are currently in the advanced stage of development and evaluation, seem to give more hope than the therapeutic ones, whose objective is to prevent new infections. Various approaches have been examined, namely, recombinant live vector vaccines, protein and peptide vaccines, vaccines without DNA, and innocuous vaccines. The most advanced vaccines against HPV consist of particles that are similar to the virus called virus-like particles (VLP). These substances are created by L1 and L2 proteins. These particles do not contain DNA and are synthesised through self-assembly of the proteins of the upper antigen of the L1 capsid. VLPs, constructed by genetic engineering, are structures that are identical to the native virus but do not have an infectious capacity. The lower structural protein L2 can assemble with L1 and form an even more stable VLP. Their antigenic similarities with the genuine HPV virions explain why VLPs introduce a powerful humoral response with neutralising antibodies (Rodríguez-Cerdeira et al., 2009c, 2009d).

3.1 Do those vaccines activate the immune memory system?

The WHO explicitly stated that the induction of immune memory should be assessed by means of evaluating immune responses to additional doses of vaccine administered at planned intervals following the completion of the primary series. Subsequently, the immune-memory anamnestic response using an antigen challenge has been reported for the quadrivalent vaccine. Nevertheless, the questions in vaccinated women include the following: Does natural re-exposure to the same HPV type vaccine significantly boost antibody levels, which contributes to the long-term persistence of anti-HPV responses, and consequently, does it improve protection over the next few decades? Time is needed to suitably answer this question (WHO, 2006; Olsson et al., 2007)

Einstein *et al.* while comparing the immune response and reactogenicity of 2 vaccines by using the same pseudovirion-based neutralisation assay, stated that for any age strata, the positivity rates for the anti-HPV 16 and 18 neutralising antibodies in the cervicovaginal secretions and circulating HPV 16- and 18-specific memory B cell frequencies were higher after vaccination with the bivalent vaccine compared to the quadrivalent vaccine (Einstein et al., 2009). Regan *et al.* (24) considered transient infection in estimating the impact of an HPV

16 vaccine in Australia and showed that it has significant implications on patient immunity and overall vaccine effectiveness (Regan et al., 2007).

In our experience, the vaccines induced very high concentrations of neutralising antibodies, much higher than those for natural infection, and the seroconversion rates in the trials approached 100%. In a recent study, we evaluated whether women with naturally acquired HPV antibodies who were HPV DNA-negative at the baseline were less likely to develop new infection with the same HPV type than the HPV antibody-negative and DNA-negative women were. HPV infection rates were assessed over a year. New infections were detected by type-specific PCR according to the baseline HPV 6/11/16/18 serostatus. Our findings suggest that natural immunity does not reliably protect against new infections with HR-HPV types. Only a small proportion of women with naturally acquired antibodies had limited protection against incidental and persistent infection with 1 HPV type. Therefore, our results support vaccination of all women regardless of the naturally acquired-HPV antibody status (Rodríguez-Cerdeira C et al., 2009b). The medium-term objective of these vaccines is the prevention of precursory lesions of cervical cancer and cervical intraepithelial neoplasia (CIN), especially CIN 3. Furthermore, many studies have been published in favour of protection against vulvar and vaginal neoplasias by using the tetravalent vaccine (WHO, 2006). The final long-term objective of prophylactic vaccines for HPV is the prevention of invasive cervical carcinoma. Associated objectives include the prevention of other forms of HPV-related cancer, namely, those that target the vulva, vagina, anus, penis, and oropharynx (Olsson et al., 2007).

Some researchers are much more sceptical about the effectiveness of trying to establish vaccines and new models of transmission of HPV infection. They postulate that the future aim of globally eradicating HPV-associated pathologies will be achieved by the local production of antigens with cross-reactivity among the different HPV types. In addition, they state that while sensitive methods are available for the detection of viral genetic material (DNA and RNA), we do not have a definitive method for determining the infectious state of an individual, from the perspective of transmission of infections. Furthermore, currently, as we do not have any reliable correlates of immune protection against infection, we are unable to precisely report whether an individual has acquired immunity to infection, either through exposure to infection or vaccination; what level of protection has been conferred or how long it will last; or whether this protection will prevent further transmission (Olsson et al., 2007).

Clinical trials have shown that quadrivalent vaccine effective against anogenital warts but they have not ruled out the possibility that transient infection may lead to transmission. We have discussed several areas of uncertainty that are less important. The extent to which condoms and circumcision are protective against infections has not been firmly established. To date, modellers have assumed that transmission occurs via heterosexual penile-vaginal intercourse, because the greatest disease burden is cervical cancer and this mode of transmission is both the most studied and the best understood. However, other modes of transmission must be considered more closely if their role in other diseases such as anal and oropharyngeal cancers is to be studied. Unfortunately, for modellers, most studies of HPV natural history have not been designed to improve models but rather to answer broader questions. Studies of transmission in couples have not been carried out on a large enough scale or with sufficient sampling to clearly observe and measure transmission. It is our hope that as the demand for accurate quantitative modelling studies to evaluate the impact of vaccination programs increases, studies will increasingly be designed with model parameterisation in mind (WHO, 2006; Olsson et al., 2007; Regan et al., 2007). Other research regarding prevention indicates that oncogenic virus-mediated cell fusion induces chromosomal instability and tumours (Gao & Zheng , 2011).

An expanding body of work including tissue culture studies, mouse models, and human patients suggests that tetraploidy is a precursor of the chromosomal instability state and the diploid-tetraploid-aneuploid sequence. It has also been reported that tetraploid cells tend to activate a p53 response that leads to G1 arrest and ultimately senescence or apoptosis. Thus, deregulation of the cell cycle checkpoint and apoptosis will provide tetraploid cells an opportunity to undergo dysplasia and become oncogenic aneuploid cells, which has been verified by both *in vivo* and *in vitro* experiments. It is remarkable that all human oncogenic viruses can express proteins that have the ability to inhibit pRb and p53, two critical regulators of both the cell cycle and apoptosis (Storchova & Kuffer , 2008; Castedo et al., 2006).

Therefore, multicellular organisms need to be equipped with tools that allow them to detect and remove those cells. Multiple lines of evidence suggest that p53-dependent apoptosis is the major tool for eliminating accidental tetraploid cells, which cannot undergo normal mitosis and will trigger cell cycle checkpoints. Both p53 and pRb may function as tumour suppressors in this context. Nonetheless, tetraploid cells produced by oncogenic virus-mediated cell fusion can sometimes overcome this arrest and continuously proliferate as human oncogenic viruses, expressing oncoproteins and having the ability to perturb pRb, p53, and/or apoptotic proteins. For example, HR-HPV E6 and E7 can inhibit the functions of p53 and pRb, respectively (Castedo et al., 2006; Narisawa-Saito & Kiyono, 2007). Once the tetraploid cells resulting from oncogenic virus-mediated cell fusion survive and proliferate, they may undergo dysplasia, a hallmark of most malignant tumours (Holland & Cleveland, 2009).

Chromosome stability is related to mitosis. The oncoprotein HPV-16 E5 was recently determined to have fusogenic activity and to lead to increased incidence of CIN, particularly in the presence of p53 and pRb inhibitors HPV 16 E6 and E7, respectively. Moreover, it should be noted that HPV-16 E5 must be expressed on both cells for cell fusion to occur. In this model, 2 cervical cells both expressing E5 fuse at a high rate and the resulting tetraploid cell undergoes CIN with the help of E6 and E7 to ultimately become an aneuploid cervical cancer cell. Of course, accumulation of deleterious mutations in the fused cells may also lead to the extinction of pre-malignant lesions before they become cancerous (Hu & Ceresa, 2009).

However, this model is challenged by 2 facts. First, either HR-HPV E6 or E7 alone can also contribute to tetraploid cell formation by inducing cytokinesis failure (Incassati et al., 2006; Heilman et al., 2009; Duensing et al., 2001a). Second, it is widely accepted that increasingly deregulated expression of E6 and E7 has been identified as the major transforming factor in the pathogenesis of cervical dysplasia and derived cancers.

However, our model and these 2 facts are not mutually exclusive. First, *in vitro* and clinic studies have revealed that CIN and aneuploidisation seem to precede and favour HPV genome integration, prior to which the expression of E6 and E7 is low for tight restriction in host cells. Second, E5 is thought to play a role only in the early stage because E5 expression is inhibited by HPV genome integration, but E6 and E7 act throughout carcinogenesis, especially after integration. This model is also supported by a study showing that the formation of tetraploid cells is primarily attributed to E5 and E5-induced cell fusion rather than E6/E7 and cytokinesis failure. Therefore, cytokinesis failure induced by E6 or E7 in an over-expression system may only occur in the late stage, whereas E5-mediated cell fusion may play a key role in initial cell transformation (Duensing et al., 2001a, 2001b; Melsheimer et al., 2004).

According to the mechanisms discussed above, cell fusion is also a potential and necessary mechanism for cancer progression since tumour cells would degenerate and become extinct for fusion among cancer cells with distinct potency and may also accelerate cancer evolution. This conjecture has been confirmed in a study that showed that *in vitro* or *in vivo* spontaneous fusion between the bone- and lung-tropic sub lines of human breast cancer cell line MDA-MB-231 can produce hybrids with dual metastasis organotropism. Cell fusion with metastatic cancer cells can also endow primary cancer cells the ability to resist the cytolytic activity of cytotoxic T lymphocytes. Given these considerations, the development of fusion inhibitors would be beneficial for cancer prevention and treatment of virus-associated cancers, since they would inhibit the entry and spread of the virus and affect the oncogenic role (Lu & Kang, 2009; Lee et al., 2000).

4. Therapeutic vaccines

The investigation of therapeutic vaccines capable of providing specific cell-mediated immunity is justified. The possible indications for the therapeutic vaccine include: (1) post-exposure, (2) diagnosis of low-grade squamous intraepithelial lesion (L-SIL), and (3) diagnosis of high-grade squamous intraepithelial lesion (H-SIL) or invasive cancer (15,-17). Data from dog and rabbit models hint that vaccines with *E1* and *E2* genes as targets would be suitable for both post-exposed and L-SIL women. Nonetheless, in women affected by CIN 2/3 or cancer, continuous expression of *E6* and *E7* oncogenes is essential for progression and maintenance of the malignant phenotype. The experimental E6 and E7 vaccines have shown immunogenicity and effectiveness in transplantable tumour models in rodents. Nevertheless, human trials have demonstrated immunogenicity and safety but very limited effectiveness (Rodríguez-Cerdeira et al., 2009d; Fausch et al, 2002).

Therapeutic vaccines should be able to induce specific immunity mediated by the cells capable of preventing lesion development or eliminating existing lesions or even malignant tumours by using recombinant peptides derived from *E6* and *E7* oncogenes (minigenes) (Rodríguez-Cerdeira et al., 2009d). Various vaccine approaches based on the E7 protein or peptides representing the T cell epitopes have been developed and tested in preventive and therapeutic pre-clinical tumour models. Although effective in preventing the growth of transplantable E7-expressing tumours in mice, these vaccines have demonstrated only moderate efficacy in therapeutic settings. Although the exact mechanism of the vaccine failure is yet to be defined and is probably complex, the active immune evasion mechanisms employed by the tumour may play a critical role. The success of E7 TAA-based therapeutic vaccines against cervical cancer, therefore, may require vaccine formulations containing adjuvants that not only generate E7-specific potent immune responses but also overcome the tumour-mediated immune evasion mechanisms.

Co-stimulation plays a critical role for the generation of adaptive immune responses. We recently proposed that vaccine formulations containing co-stimulatory ligands may have efficacy in therapeutic cancer settings. We particularly focussed on the 4-1BBL, a co-stimulatory member of the tumour necrosis factor (TNF) family, because of the critical role played by 4-1BB signalling in the generation and maintenance of CD8+ T cell memory, which is critical for tumour eradication (Uno et al., 2006). Although 4-1BBL has no function as a soluble trimeric molecule, we generated a chimeric recombinant SA-4-1BBL in which the extracellular portion of this molecule was cloned at the C-terminus to the core streptavidin (SA). This chimeric molecule exists as tetramers and oligomers and has potent co-stimulatory activity on the CD4+ and CD8+ T cells in the soluble form. Vaccination with SA-4-1BBL and E7 peptide representing the dominant CD8+ T cell epitope resulted in effective eradication of the E7-expressing TC-1 tumours. The therapeutic efficacy of the vaccine was superior to other vaccine formulations containing an agonistic antibody (Ab) to the 4-1BB receptor or toll-like receptor agonists such as lipopolysaccharide, monophosphoryl lipid A, and CpG (Rabu et al., 2001; Elpek et al., 2007; Schabowsky et al., 2009).

Sharma *et al.* tested the efficacy of SA-4-1BBL as the immunomodulatory component of an E7 protein-based vaccine in the TC-1 tumour model as a prelude to phase I cancer. Use of whole E7 protein as the antigenic component of the vaccine alleviates the concerns related to the use of a single peptide representing a CD8+ T cell dominant epitope that includes the following: (i) saturation of immune response due to antigen exhaustion; (ii) lack of CD4+ T cell help, which can limit the vaccine's anti-tumour efficacy; (iii) lesser magnitude and duration of the immune response towards a single epitope compared to the collective responses to multiple epitopes; (iv) higher possibility of immune-edited escape variants; and (v) requirement for HLA compatibility that will limit the target patient populations (Sharma et al., 2010). .

We herein showed that single vaccination with SA-4-1BBL and a recombinant whole E7 protein resulted in the eradication of the established tumours in 70% of the test mice. The therapeutic efficacy of the vaccine was associated with robust primary and memory T cell responses, Th1 cytokines, enhanced intra-tumoural CD4+ and CD8+ T cell infiltration, and NK cell function. Taken together, these data corroborate the utility of SA-4-1BBL as a novel multifunctional immunomodulatory component of therapeutic vaccines and justify testing of the E7 protein-based vaccine formulation in human clinical trials. Sharma *et al.* in there studies concluded that the therapeutic efficacy of whole E7 protein and SA-4-1BBL vaccines in the TC-1 tumour model was comparable to the efficacy obtained using a synthetic peptide representing the dominant CD8+ T cell epitope for E7 protein as the antigenic component of the vaccine. The comparable therapeutic efficacies of the peptide and whole E7 protein-based vaccines may be due to both the vaccine formulation and the tumour model used in these studies. Both the vaccine formulations included equal amounts of antigen and therefore, more molar amounts of the peptide. The excess peptide amount and its faster kinetics of presentation by MHC class I molecules may allow robust generation of a CD8+ T cell response that curbs tumour growth (Sharma et al., 2010, Yan et al., 2009).

As much as the TC-1 tumour model uses transplantable tumours and has fast growth kinetics, antigen escape variants due to immunological pressure may not occur during the experiment. However, this may be different in a spontaneous tumour setting wherein immunological pressure may possibly give rise to antigen-loss variants. Therefore, use of either whole E7 protein-based vaccine or those with both and E7 proteins may have better efficacy in a spontaneous setting due to the availability of not only multiple CD8+ but also CD4+ T cell epitopes (44). Consistent with this notion, we demonstrated potent primary and memory CD4+ and CD8+ T cell responses in mice vaccinated with E7 protein and SA-4-1BBL. Although CD4+ T cells seem unnecessary for primary immune responses, it is critical for the generation and maintenance of long-term memory and recall responses (Gunn et al., 2001; Kumaraguru et al., 2005).

The development of non-toxic adjuvants that not only activate the effector arm of the immune system against tumours but also overcome various immune evasion mechanisms employed by the vaccines against cancer is important. Importantly, we previously reported the pleiotropic effects of SA-4-1BBL on the cells of innate, adaptive, and regulatory immunity (Alba et al., 2009), and treatment with SA-4-1BBL at therapeutic doses did not result in detectable signs of acute toxicity that were recently reported for agonistic antibodies to 4-1BB and were assessed by lymphadenopathy, lymphocyte proliferation, systemic cytokine response, and gross pathology (Fausch et al, 2002, 2003). Taken together, our findings support the notion that SA-4-1BBL is a potentially effective and safe adjuvant that can serve as a component of therapeutic vaccines. Testing its therapeutic efficacy in clinical trials will be important; if effective, this molecule may serve as a safe and effective platform for the development of therapeutic vaccines against cancer and chronic infections (Sharma et al., 2010).

In order to evaluate the therapeutic potential of the responses of L1-specific CD4+ and CD8+ T lymphocytes in cervical cancer patients, L1 VLP-loaded DCs were used to stimulate peripheral blood lymphocytes from the cervical cancer patients, and such responses were compared to those elicited by the E7 oncoprotein. We showed by reverse transcriptase (RT)-PCR that all the flash-frozen cervical biopsy samples collected from HPV 16-positive cervical cancer patients harboured L1 in addition to E6 and E7 RNA. The E7 RNA copy number (mean, 176.2) was significantly higher than those of E6 RNA (mean, 47.3) and L1 (mean, 58.3) in HPV 16-positive cervical cancers ($P < 0.0001$ and $P < 0.001$, respectively). However, no significant differences between the levels of expression of E6 and L1 were noted. Kinetic studies of E6, E7, and L1 RNA and protein expression levels in primary tumours showed sharp reductions in L1 expression versus E6 and E7 expression after multiple *in vitro* passages. Autologous DCs pulsed with HPV 16 VLPs or recombinant full-length E7 elicited strong type 1 L1- and E7-specific responses in CD4+ and CD8+ T cells from cervical cancer patients. Importantly, L1 VLP-specific CD8+ T lymphocytes expressed strong cytolytic activity against autologous tumour cells and were as effective as E7-specific cytotoxic T lymphocytes in lysing autologous tumour cells naturally infected by HPV 16. Taken together, these data demonstrate consistent expression of L1 in primary cervical tumours and the possibility of inducing effective L1/tumour-specific CD4+ and CD8+ T-lymphocyte responses in patients harbouring HPV-infected cervical cancer. These results may have important implications for the treatment of patients harbouring established HPV-infected lesions with L1 VLPs or combined E7/L1 DC-based vaccinations (Shedlock & Shen, 2003; Bellone et al, 2009).

One novel cancer therapy involves using the vascular disrupting agent 5,6-dimethylxanthenone-4-acetic acid (DMXAA). In the current study, we aimed to test the combination of DMXAA treatment and HPV-16 E7 DNA vaccination to enhance the anti-tumour effects and E7-specific CD8+ T cell immune responses in treated mice. We determined that DMXAA treatment generates significant therapeutic effects against TC-1 tumours but does not enhance antigen-specific immune responses in tumour-bearing mice. We then found that the combination of DMXAA treatment and E7 DNA vaccination generates potent anti-tumour effects and E7-specific CD8+ T cell immune responses in the splenocytes of the tumour-bearing mice. Furthermore, the DMXAA-mediated enhancement or suppression of E7-specific CD8+ T cell immune responses generated by CRT/E7 DNA vaccination depended on the time of DMXAA administration and was also applicable to other antigen-specific vaccines. DMXAA is a synthetic flavonoid that induces the production of local cytokines, including TNF-α. DMXAA has been shown to induce anti-tumour effects in animal models, especially in combination with established anti-cancer agents. It has also demonstrated a good safety profile and looks promising after phase I clinical trials (Peng et al., 2001 Shedlock & Shen, 2003; Silk & Finn, 2007).

Mice were immunised with 2 μg of various DNA vaccines and received boosters with the same regimen as indicated in the figure legends. For vaccinia encoding SigE7LAMP1 vaccination, 1×10^7 plaque-forming units (pfu) viruses were intraperitoneally injected in a volume of 100 μL. Splenocytes were harvested 1 week after the last vaccination. DMXAA treatment generates significant therapeutic effects against TC-1 tumours but does not enhance antigen-specific immune responses in tumour-bearing mice. To determine the anti-tumour effects of DMXAA treatment, we first challenged groups of C57BL/6 mice (5 per group) with TC-1 tumour cells and treated them with a single dose of DMXAA that was administered on day 13 after tumour challenge via intraperitoneal injection, and monitored the tumour size over time. Tumour-bearing mice treated with DMXAA showed significantly lower tumour volumes over time compared to tumour-bearing mice not treated with DMXAA. We also characterised the E7-specific CD8+ T cell immune responses in these mice. One week after DMXAA treatment, the splenocytes from tumour-bearing mice were harvested and characterised for E7-specific CD8+ T cells by using intracellular IFN-γ staining followed by flow cytometry analysis.

Combination of DMXAA treatment with E7 DNA vaccination generates potent anti-tumour effects and E7-specific CD8+ T cell immune responses in the splenocytes of tumour-bearing mice. In order to determine the therapeutic anti-tumour effects and E7-specific CD8+ T cell immune responses in TC-1 tumour-bearing mice treated with DMXAA and CRT/E7 DNA vaccination, we first challenged groups of C57BL/6 mice (5 per group) with TC-1 tumour cells and then treated them with CRT/E7 DNA vaccine with or without DMXAA. Seven days after the last vaccination, we harvested the splenocytes from the vaccinated mice and characterised them for the presence of E7-specific CD8+ T cells by using intracellular cytokine staining for IFN-γ followed by flow cytometry analysis. The tumour-bearing mice that were treated with CRT/E7 DNA vaccine in combination with DMXAA experienced better therapeutic anti-tumour effects than the mice treated with any other regimens. Furthermore, mice treated with the DNA vaccine in combination with DMXAA also generated the highest number of E7-specific CD8+ T cells compared to the mice treated with any of the other regimens.

In summary, the authors tried to show that the combination of DMXAA treatment and HPV-16 E7 DNA vaccination can enhance or suppress the anti-tumour effects and E7-

specific CD8+ T cell immune responses in treated mice depending on the time of DMXAA administration. These results may have potential implications for future clinical translation. Therefore, further work needs to be done to complete this study (Bellone et al, 2009; Peng et al., 2001; Shedlock & Shen, 2003; Silk & Finn, 2007).

5. Vaccines, prophylactics, and therapeutics

In the study by Petrone et al. (Petrone et al, 2011) that aimed to obtain a highly immunogenic E7 preparation, they did not focus on obtaining identical particles since particles of different sizes can be taken up by different types of antigen-presenting cells such as the DCs, macrophages, and polymorphonuclear leukocytes, sustaining a more potent immune response (Uno et al., 2006; Rabu et al., 2001). However, we standardised the different preparations by using semi-quantitative counting of the particles on EM micrographs (not shown). The immunogenicity of *Escherichia coli*-derived E7 fused through the N-terminus to either HPV16 E6 or GST was also investigated in mice. An antigen-specific immune response of Th2 polarity was obtained when the fusion proteins were administered to the mice without an adjuvant (data not shown). However, we were unable to observe the typical micro- and nanoparticles in these E7-fusion proteins prepared from *E. Coli.* Recently, the cytosolic accumulation of E7 oligomers shown in HPV 16 cervical cancer cell lines and in clinical samples by indirect methods supports a new hypothesis regarding the presence of E7 isoforms and their role in different cell compartments (Dantur et al., 2009; Knapp, et al. 2009). The presence of E7 in different aggregation forms and cell compartments could affect E7 processing and presentation by MHC I and II molecules, assessing both the strength as well as the quality of the host's anti-HPV immunity. More studies on recombinant *E. coli*-derived E7 assembled in different forms would contribute to explaining the stimulation of the different branches of the immune system in the HPV16 mouse tumour model (Knapp et al., 2009).

Significant differences exist between the HPV 16 mouse tumour model and human HPV 16-dependent diseases. However, studies on the immunoglobulin G (IgG) subclasses and their FcgR receptors between mice and humans are comparable. HPV 16 E7 immunogenicity studies in mouse will provide insights into the understanding of the protective immunity against human HPV 16 infections as well.

Commercial preventive HPV vaccines have high production costs, which has prevented the implementation of widespread vaccination programs. Recently combined preventive and therapeutic HPV vaccines produced in *E. coli* have been described (Knapp, et al. 2009; Schädlich et al., 2009; Bian et al., 2008), and the data presented here suggest a possible use of *E. coli*-derived E7 in the particle form in subunit vaccines. The *E. coli*-expressed proteins represent a well-studied and cost-effective means for vaccine production. These methods require reduced time, cost, and labour, and can be easily scaled up to industrial-scale production. Generation of new low-cost HPV vaccines could represent the only possibility for women living in developing countries to gain access to HPV vaccination programs in order to prevent or treat pre-cancerous lesions and cancer (Rubio I et al., 2009). In this paper, the author describes, for the first time, the use of recombinant HPV 16 E7 assembled *in vitro* into particulate form to induce protective immunity against an HPV 16-

related tumour in an HPV-16 mouse tumour model. Data show that E7 particles used without adjuvant are excellent stimulators of the immune system. In C57BL/6 mice, the E7 preparation induces anti-tumour immunity sustained by both humoral and cell-mediated immune responses. This E7 protein (derived from *E. coli*) that does not require an adjuvant could represent, along with the recently proposed *E. coli*-derived HPV antigens ((Knapp, et al. 2009; Yan et al., 2009), a low-cost constituent for the development of a new generation of HPV 16 vaccines that combines prophylactic and therapeutic activities.

Numerous methods have been developed to introduce foreign genes into mammalian cells, including chemical-based procedures, electroporation, gene gun, and mammalian viral vector-based systems. These methods have the following advantages: ease of use, gene capacity, cell specificity, cytotoxicity, efficiency, safety, and reproducibility. High cost of these methods can be the only limitation. To overcome this problem, recombinant baculoviruses have been widely developed using baculovirus/mammalian expression systems. These recombinant baculoviruses will be used extensively for gene therapy and vaccines, nevertheless, the authors did not observe substantial spot numbers in any of the mice treated with wild-type baculovirus. However, when we performed immunostaining for the splenocytes harvested from the mice intramuscularly injected with wild-type baculovirus, we observed non-specific IFN-γ production in 2 of the 6 mice. Several recent studies indicated that baculoviruses may induce innate immune responses (Strauss et al, 2007; Li et al., 2009; Abe et al, 2003, 2005; Huang et al.,2009). Although baculoviruses do not replicate in mammalian cells and thus can serve as safe DNA vaccine vectors, additional information is required on the pre-existing anti-vector immunity from the use of live baculoviruses for vaccine development.

In another study (Liao et al., 2008), a recombinant pseudotype baculovirus (BV-G-E) was generated by inserting the JEV E gene fragment into the pFastBac-VSV/G vector. The authors demonstrated that BV-G-E could elicit high protective immunity in mice. The amounts of BV-G-E injected into mice were 1×10^8, 1×10^9, and 1×10^{10} pfu. In yet another study, without the use of recombinant baculovirus, mice were inoculated intramuscularly with a single dose of 5×10^6 pfu of recombinant attenuated vesicular stomatitis virus (rVSV) expressing HPV16E7 protein. The authors suggested that rVSV-based vaccination should be explored as a therapeutic strategy for cervical carcinoma. Other recherche group (Lee et al., 2010) developed a novel DNA vaccine for HPV; a recombinant baculovirus-bearing human endogenous retrovirus (HERV) envelope protein, which cannot replicate in mammals, was used as a nano-carrier for the HPV-16L1 DNA vaccine (AcHERV-HP16L1). For the *in vivo* test, mice were injected intramuscularly with 107 particles of the constructs, with 2 boosters given at 2-week intervals. Compared to Gardasil® (25 µl/dose), the AcHERV-HP16L1-immunised mice showed similar high levels of humoral immunity in IgG/IgA and in HPV pseudovirion neutralisation. Combined immunisation (AcHERV-HP16L1 primer and Gardasil® booster) induced slightly higher neutralising activity. Compared to the group treated with Gardasil®, the mice immunised with AcHERV-HP16L1 showed 450- and 490-fold increases in IFN-γ at 5 and 20 weeks after the first priming, respectively. The safety levels were comparable. The combined immunisation conferred lower T cell immunity than AcHERV-HP16L1 treatment. The advantages of our novel AcHERVHP16L1 vaccine over Gardasil® include higher cellular immunogenicity and considerably lower production costs.

The recombinant baculovirus used for HPV16L1 gene delivery does not replicate in the host. Its advantages include safety, ease of processing, and most importantly, the ability to induce both humoral and cellular immunity. Therefore, we suggest that the AcHERV-HPV DNA vaccine be developed as an efficient prophylactic and therapeutic vaccine. On the basis of its advantages, we anticipate that the developed AcHERV- HP16L1 will contribute to global HPV prevention (Chen et al., 2000; Velders et al, 2001; Mahdavi & Monk, 2005).

Acceptance of the vaccine among adolescents and parents, protection against sexually transmitted infections (STIs), and adequate health support and recommendation are the keys to the success of HPV vaccines. Recent studies have shown that although some parents find the vaccine acceptable, others believed that their children are not at real risk of contracting an STI or expressed concern that vaccination may encourage the practice of risky sexual behaviours. In a recent survey, mothers of children aged between 8 and 14 years expressed a willingness to vaccinate their daughters (67%) or children (66%). Those who refused the vaccine cited the risk of unknown side effects, lack of sexual activity at the time, and the lack of a direct benefit in male children. In another parent survey, vaccination rates of 10–15-year-old children increased from 55% to 75% after the parents read a newsletter. Therefore, it is essential that accurate information about the disease and the vaccine be distributed by health professionals to ensure broad participation in the vaccination programs (Roberts et al., 2010; Tsakiroglou et al., 2011; Tan et al., 2010).

6. Future directions

In the development of therapeutic HPV vaccines, we have focused on identifying and targeting the most relevant antigens associated with cervical cancer, the E6 and E7 HPV oncoproteins, which represent tumor-specific antigens and potentially ideal targets for therapeutic HPV vaccines. It is important to consider using strategies such as prime-boost regimens and/or combinations strategies using molecules that are capable of blocking the negative regulators on T cells to further enhance the T cell immune responses. Furthermore, increasing understanding of the molecular mechanisms that hinder immune attack in the tumor microenvironment will lead to the identification of novel molecular targets that can be blocked in order to enhance the therapeutic effect of HPV vaccines. It is conceivable that effective therapy against HPV-associated malignancies will probably require a combination of therapeutic HPV vaccines with the employment of innovative agents that are capable of eliminating the suppressive factors present in the tumor microenvironment. With continued endeavor in the development of HPV therapeutic vaccines, it can foresee that HPV therapeutic vaccines will become an important approach that can be combined with existing forms of therapy such as chemotherapy and radiation therapy to generate better control of HPV-associated malignancies (Hung et al., 2008)

Neutralizing IL10 at the time of PV VLPs immunization increases cytotoxic T cell responses. PV VLPs incorporating PV early protein E2, 6 and 7, together with immune stimulator that promote strong type 1 responses, and at the same time blocking the effect of IL10 may have therapeutic effect against HPV infection related diseases and are worth further basic and clinical investigation (Chen et al., 2011).

After a long period of scepticism and disbelief, tumour viruses are today recognized as a significant cancer risk factor for humans. Much has been learned about the viral transforming mechanisms and prophylactic vaccines have been developed against tumour viruses' HPV. Yet, many important issues of tumour virology remain unresolved and exciting new ones are emerging from recent discoveries. They define future research directions for the field and include (Hoppe-Seyler et al., 2011):

- Novel strategies for tumour virus hunting.
- Tumour viruses as experimental tools to study human carcinogenesis.
- The interplay between viruses and the world of small non coding RNAs.
- Epigenetic interactions between tumour viruses and the host cell.
- The role of virus/virus interactions for viral carcinogenesis
- Novel strategies for prevention and therapy of virus-associated cancers.

Further study into the tumour microenvironment and molecular mechanisms impeding immune attack against HPV will lead to novel targets for therapeutic intervention in the future. Discovery of such targets, development of new adjuvants, and improved understanding of tumour biology will allow HPV vaccines to be used in combinational therapies in a synergistic manner in the future.

7. Conclusion

Doubts do remain unresolved, and therefore, the existence of cross-protection evidence in the bivalent vaccine against other subtypes of 16/18 capsular structure very similar protein suggested that the cause of this cross-immunity would be an extra-immune response induced by adjuvant use in the vaccine is unknown. Additional benefit that would represent this phenomenon in clinical practice, but how they behave subtypes prevalent highly uncertain risk to cause protection from the vaccine subtypes prevalent now? Will it be replaced? Because it has been reported that HPV 16/18-positive women are at 5–7-times greater risk of acquiring a subsequent infection with HPV 5/7 than the uninfected women, can infection be prevented using subtype vaccination?

We continue with the questions such as whether to vaccinate at-risk populations and what type of vaccine to use. We know that the vast majority of HPV infections are diagnosed in people at medium risk without appreciable risky behaviours. Protection of these people would be very effective because it would disrupt the chain of transmission. One option under discussion would be to vaccinate the gay population, which currently has relatively high rates of anal cancer linked to HPV and could greatly benefit from the preventive effects of the vaccine. Nonetheless, assuming that the vaccine does, in fact, prevent HPV-related anogenital and head and neck cancers in males and prevents male-to-female and male-to-male viral transmission, compelling arguments exist for a gender-neutral approach to vaccination. These arguments include the following: (1) female-only vaccination will not protect men who have sex with men from contracting HPV and HPV-related diseases and (2) the fastest way to achieve the greatest protection for females from cervical cancer and its precursors is to vaccinate both females and males.

Finally, the economic evaluation of any HPV vaccination strategy requires the measurement of clinical benefits and the economic benefits associated with an effective intervention. As newer vaccines targeting morbidity rather than mortality are being launched in the market, quantification of disease burden and modelling of the cost-effectiveness of intervention options are becoming more important when determining the best way to allocate scarce health care funds.

8. References

Abe T.; Takahashi H.; Hamazaki H.; Miyano-Kurosaki N.; Matsuura Y & Takaku H. (2003). Baculovirus induces an innate immune response and confers protection from lethal influenza virus infection in mice. *The Journal of Immunology*, Vol.171, No.3, (August 2003), pp. 1133–1139, ISSN 0022-1767

Abe T.; Hemmi H,; Miyamoto H,; Moriishi K.; Tamura S.; Takaku H. et al (2005). Involvement of the Toll-like receptor 9 signaling pathway in the induction of innate immunity by baculovirus. *Journal of Virology*, Vol.79, No.5, (March 2005), pp. 2847–2858, ISSN 0022-538X

Alba A.; Rodriguez-Cerdeira C. & Cararach M. (2009). The human papillomavirus (HPV) in human pathology: description, pathogenesis, oncogenic role, epidemiology and detection techniques. *The Open Dermatology Journal*, Vol.3, pp. 90- 6, ISSN 1874-3722

Bellone S.; El-Sahwi K.; Cocco E.; Casagrande F.; Cargnelutti M.; Palmieri M. et al (2009). Human papillomavirus type 16 (HPV-16) virus-like particle L1-specific CD8+ cytotoxic T lymphocytes (CTLs) are equally effective as E7-specific CD8+ CTLs in killing autologous HPV-16-positive tumor cells in cervical cancer patients: implications for L1 dendritic cell-based therapeutic vaccines. *Journal of Virology*, Vol.83, No.13, (July 2009), pp. 6779-6789, ISSN 0022-538X

Bian T.; Wang Y.; Lu Z.; Ye Z.; Zhao L.; Ren J.; Zhang H.; Ruan L. & Tian H. (2008). Human papillomavirus type 16 L1E7 chimeric capsomeres have prophylactic and therapeutic efficacy against papillomavirus in mice. *Molecular Cancer Therapeutics*, Vol.7, No.5, (May 2008), pp. 1329-1335, ISSN 1535-7163

Castedo M.; Coquelle A.; Vivet S.; Vitale I.; Kauffmann A.; Dessen P. et al (2006). Apoptosis regulation in tetraploid cancer cells. *The EMBO Journal*, Vol.25, No.11, (June 2006), pp. 2584–2595, ISSN 0261-4189

Chen CH.; Wang TL.; Hung CF.; Pardoll DM. & Wu TC. (2000). Boosting with recombinant vaccinia increases HPV-16 E7-specific T cell precursor frequencies of HPV-16 E7-expressing DNA vaccines. *Vaccine*, Vol.18, No.19, (April 2000), pp. 2015–2022, ISSN 0264-410X

Chen J.; Ni G. & Liu X. (2011). Papillomavirus virus like particle-based therapeutic vaccine against human papillomavirus infection related diseases: immunological problems and future directions. *Cell Immunol*, Vol. 269, No.1, (March 2011), pp. 5-9, ISSN 0818-9641

Dantur K.; Alonso L.; Castaño E.; Morelli L.; Centeno-Crowley JM.; Vighi S. & de Prat-Gay G. (2009). Cytosolic accumulation of HPV16 E7 oligomerssupports different transformation routes for the prototypic viral oncoprotein: the amyloid-cancer connection. *International Journal of Cancer*, Vol.125, No.8, (October 2009), pp. 1902-1911, ISSN 0020-7136

Duensing S.; Duensing A.; Crum CP. & Münger K. (2001). Human papillomavirus type 16 E7 oncoprotein-induced abnormal centrosome synthesis is an early event in the evolving malignant phenotype. *Cancer Research*, Vol.61, No.6, (March 2001), pp. 2356–2360, ISSN 0008-5472

Duensing S.; Duensing A.; Flores ER.; Do A.; Lambert PF. & Münger K. (2001). Centrosome abnormalities and genomic instability by episomal expression of human papillomavirus type 16 in raft cultures o human keratinocytes. *Journal of Virology*, Vol.75, No.16, (August 2001), pp. 7712–7716, ISSN 0022-538X

Einstein M.; Schiller JT.; Viscidi RP.; Strickler H.; Coursaget P.; Tan T.; Halsey N. & Jenkins D. (2009). Clinician's guide to human papillomavirus immunology: knowns and unknowns. *The Lancet infectious diseases*, Vol.9, No.6, (June 2009), pp 47–56, ISSN 1473-3099

Elpek KG.; Yolcu ES.; Franke DD.; Lacelle C.; Schabowsky RH. & Shirwan H. (2007). Ex vivo expansion of CD4 + CD25 + FoxP3+ T regulatory cells based on synergy between IL-2 and 4-1BB signaling. *Journal of Immunology*, Vol.179, No.11, (December 2007), pp. 7295–7304, ISSN 0022-1767

Fausch SC.; Da Silva DM.; Rudolf MP. & Kast WM. (2002). Human papillomavirus virus-like particles do not activate Langerhans cells: a possible immune escape mechanism used by human papillomaviruses. *The Journal of Immunology*, Vol.169, No.6, (September 2002), pp. 3242–9, ISSN 0022-1767

Fausch SC:, Da Silva DM. & Kast WM. (2003). Differential uptake and cross-presentation of human papillomavirus virus-like particles by dendritic cells and Langerhans cells. *Cancer Research*, Vol.63, No.13, (July 2003), pp. 3478–82, ISSN 0008-5472

Gao P. & Zheng J. (2011). Oncogenic virus-mediated cell fusion: New insights into initiation and progression of oncogenic viruses-related cancers. *Cancer Letters*, Vol.303, No.1, (April 2011), pp. 1–8, ISSN 0304-3835

González-Guerra E.; Guerra-Tapia A. & Rodríguez-Cerdeira C. (2009). Common clinical manifestations of HPV infection. *The Open Dermatology Journal*, Vol.3, pp. 97- 104, ISSN 1874-3722

Gunn GR.; Zubair A.; Peters C.; Pan ZK.; Wu TC. & Paterson Y. (2001). Two Listeria monocytogenes vaccine vectors that express different molecular forms of human papilloma virus-16 (HPV-16) E7 induce qualitatively different of established tumors immortalized by HPV-16. *Journal of Immunology*, Vol.167, No.11, (December 2001), pp. 6471–6479, ISSN 0022-1767

Heilman SA.; Nordberg JJ.; Liu Y.; Sluder G. & Chen JJ. (2009). Abrogation ofthe postmitotic checkpoint contributes to polyploidization in human papillomavirus E7-expressing cells. *Journal of Virology*, Vol.83, No.6, (March 2009), pp. 2756–2764, ISSN 0022-538X

Holland AJ. & Cleveland DW. (2009). Boveri revisited: chromosomal instability, aneuploidy and tumorigenesis. *Nature Reviews. Molecular Cell Biology*, Vol.10, No.7, (July 2009), pp. 478–7, ISSN 1471-0072

Hoppe-Seyler F. & Hoppe-Seyler K. (2011). Emerging topics in human tumor virology. *Int J Cancer*, Vol.129, No.6, (September 2011), pp. 1289-1299, ISSN 1097-0215

Hu L. & Ceresa BP. (2009). Characterization of the plasma membrana localization and orientation of HPV16 E5 for cell–cell fusion. *Virology*, Vol.393, No.1, (October 2009), pp. 135–143, ISSN 0042-6822

Hung C.; Ma B.; Monie A.; Tsen S. & Wu T. (2008). Therapeutic human papillomavirus vaccines: current clinical trials and future directions. *Expert Opin Biol Ther*, Vol.8, No.4, (April 2008), pp. 421-439, ISSN 1744-7682

Huang X.; Li Y. & Zheng CY. (2009). A novel single-cell quantitative real-time RT-PCRmethod for quantifying foot-and-mouth disease viral RNA. *Journal of Virologycal Methods*, Vol.155, No.2, (February 2009), pp. 150–156, ISSN 0166-0934

IARC Working Group on the evaluation of the evaluation of the carcinogenic risks to humans. Human Papillomavirus (1995*). Monographs of the Evaluation of Carcinogenic Risks to humans. Lyon: International Agency for Research on Cancer*, World Health Organisation, ISBN 92-4-156178-5, Lyon, France

Incassati A.; Patel ID. & McCance DJ. (2006). Induction of tetraploidy through loss of p53 and upregulation of Plk1 by human papillomavirus type-16 E6. *Oncogene*, Vol.25, No.17, (April 2006), pp. 2444–2451, ISSN 0950-9232

Kadish A.; Hagan RJ. & Ritter DB. (1992). Biologic Characteristics of Specific Human Papillomavirus. Types Predicted From Morphology of Cervical Lesions. *Human Pathology*, Vol.23, No.11, (November), pp. 1262-9, ISSN 0046-8177

Knapp AA.; McManus PM.; Bockstall K. & Moroianu J. (2009). Identification of thenuclear localization and export signals of high risk HPV16 E7 oncoprotein. *Virology*, Vol.383, No.1, (January 2009), pp. 60-68, ISSN 0042-6822

Kost TA. & Condreay JP. (2002). Recombinant baculoviruses as mammalian cell genedelivery vectors. *Trends in Biotechnology*, Vol.20, No.4, (April 2002), pp. 173–180, ISSN 0167-7799

Kumaraguru U.; Banerjee K. & Rouse BT. (2005). In vivo rescue of defective memory CD8+ T cells by cognate helper T cells. *Journal of Leukocyte Biology*, Vol.78, No.4, (October 2005), pp. 879–887, ISSN 0741-5400

Lee H-J.; Par N.; Cho H-J.; Yoon JK.; Dinh Van N.; Oh Y-K. & Kim YB. (2010). Development of a novel viral DNA vaccine against human papillomavirus: AcHERV-HP16L1. *Vaccine*, Vol.28, No.6, (February 2010), pp. 1613–1619, ISSN 0264-410X

Lee HM.; Timme TL. & Thompson TC. (2000). Resistance to lysis by cytotoxic T cells: a dominant effect in metastatic mouse prostate cancer cells. *Cancer Research*, Vol.60, No.7, (Apil 2000), pp. 1927- 1933, ISSN 0008-5472

Li Y.; Ye J.; Cao S.; Xiao S.; Zhao Q.; Liu X. et al (2009). Immunization with pseudotypebaculovirus expressing envelope protein of Japanese encephalitis virus elicits protective immunity in mice. *The Journal of Gene Medicine*, Vol.11, No.2, (February 2009), pp. 57–65, ISSN 1099-498X

Liao JB.; Publicover J.; Rose JK. & DiMaio D. (2008). Single-dose, therapeutic vaccination of mice with vesicular stomatitis virus expressing human papillomavirus type 16 E7 protein. *Clinical and vaccine immunology*, Vol.15, No.5, (May 2008), pp. 817-824, ISSN 1556-6811

Lu X.; & Kang Y. (2009). Efficient acquisition of dual metastasis organotropism to bone and lung through stable spontaneous fusion between MDA-MB-231 variants. *Proceedings of the National Academy of Sciences of the United States of America*, Vol.106, No.23, (Juny 2009), pp. 9385-9390, ISSN 0027-8424

Mahdavi A. & Monk BJ. (2005). Vaccines against human papillomavirus and cervical cancer: promises and challenges. *The Oncologist*, Vol.10, No.7, (August 2005), pp. 528-538, ISSN 1083-7159

Mariani L. & Venuti A. (2010). HPV vaccine: an overview of immune response, clinical protection, and new approaches for the future. *Journal of Translational Medicine*, Vol.8, pp. 105, ISSN 1479-5876

Melsheimer P.; Vinokurova S.; Wentzensen N.; Bastert G. & von Knebel DM. (2004). DNA aneuploidy and integration of human papillomavirus type 16 E6/E7 oncogenes in intraepithelial neoplasia and invasive squamous cell carcinoma of the cervix uteri. *Clinical Cancer Research*, Vol.10, No.9, (May 2004), pp. 3059-3063, ISSN 1078-0432

Mougin C.; Dalstein V. & Pretet JL. (2001). Epidemiology of cervical papillomavirus infections. Recent knowledge. *La Press Médicale*, Vol 30, No.20, (June 2001), pp. 1017-23, ISSN 0755-4982

Muñoz N.; Bosch FX.; de Sanjose S.; Herrero R.; Castellsague X.; Shah KV. et al (2003). Epidemiologic classification of human papillomavirus types associated with cervical cancer. *New Englan Journal of Medicine Med*, Vol.348, No.6, (February 2003), pp. 518-527, ISSN 0962-9351

Narisawa-Saito M. & Kiyono T. (2007). Basic mechanisms of high-risk human papillomavirus-induced carcinogenesis: roles of E6 and E7 proteins. *Cancer Science*, Vol 98, No.10, (October), pp. 1505-1511, ISSN 1347-9032

Nestle FO.; Di Meglio P.; Qin JZ. & Nickoloff BJ. (2009). Skin immune sentinels inhealth and disease. *Nature Reviews. Immunology*, Vol.8, No.10 (October 2009), pp. 679-691, ISSN 1474-1733

Olsson SE.; Kjaer SK.; Sigurdsson K.; Iversen OE.; Hernandez-Avila M.; Wheeler CM. et al (2009). Evaluation of quadrivalent HPV 6/11/16/18 vaccine efficacy against cervical and anogenital disease in subjects with serological evidence of prior vaccine type HPV infection. *Human Vaccines*, Vol 5, No 10, (October 2009), pp. 696-704, ISSN1554-8600

Olsson SE.; Villa LL.; Costa R.; Petta C.; Andrade R.; Malm C.; Iversen OE. et al (2007). Induction of immune memory following administration of a prophylactic quadrivalent human papillomavirus (HPV) types 6/11/16/18 L1 virus-like particle (VLP) vaccine. *Vaccine*, Vol.25, No.26, (June 2007), pp. 4931-4949, ISSN 0264-410X

Peng S.; Monie A.; Pang X.; Hung CF. & Wu TC. (2011). Vascular disrupting agent DMXAA enhances the antitumor effects generated by therapeutic HPV DNA vaccines. *Journal of Biomedical Science*, Vol.8, (March 2001), pp. 18-21, ISSN 1021-7770

Petrone L.; Ammendoli MG.; Cesolini A.; Caimi S.; Superti F.; Giorgi C. et al (2011). Recombinant HPV16 E7 assembled into particles induces an immune response and specific tumour protection administered without adjuvant in an animal model. *Journal of Translational Medicine*, Vol.9, (May 2011), pp. 69, ISSN 1479-5876

Rabu C.; Quemener A.; Jacques Y.; Echasserieau K.; Vusio P. & Lang F. (2005). Production of recombinant human trimeric CD137L (4-1BBL). Cross-linking is essential to its T cell co-stimulation activity. The *Journal of Biological Chemistry*, Vol.280, No.50, (December 2005), pp. 41472–41481, ISSN 0021-9258

Regan DG.; Philp DJ.; Hocking JS. & Law MG. (2007). Modelling the population-level impact of vaccination on the transmission of human papillomavirus type 16 in Australia. *Sex Health*, Vol.4, No.3, (September 2007), pp. 147–163, ISSN 1448-5028

Roberts ME.; Gerrard M.; Reimer R. & Gibbons FX. (2010). Mother-daughter communication and human papillomavirus vaccine uptake by college students. *Pediatrics*, Vol.125, No.5, (May 2010), pp. 982-989, ISSN 0031-4005

Rodríguez-Cerdeira C.; Menéndez A.; Bravo G. & Alcántara R. (2007). El virus del papiloma humano y su repercusión en la patología genital femenina. *Piel*, Vol.22, pp. 1171-1180, ISSN 1578-8830

Rodríguez-Cerdeira C. (2008). Tumores malignos. *Monografias Dermatologia*, Vol 21, pp. 393-401, ISSN 0214-4735

Rodríguez-Cerdeira C.; Gonzalez-Guerra E. & Guerra A (2008). Cáncer de vulva. *Mas Dermatología*, Vol.4, pp. 26-32, ISSN 1887-5181

Rodriguez-Cerdeira C. & Alba-Menéndez A. (2009). Vaccines for Papillomavirus (HPV) infection. *The Open Dermatology Journal*, Vol.3, pp. 123-6, ISSN 1874-3722

Rodríguez-Cerdeira C.; Alba Menéndez A. & Vilata Corell JJ. (2009). Desarrollo de nuevas vacunas contra el virus del papiloma humano. *Piel*, Vol.22, pp. 51-53, ISSN 1578-8830

Rodríguez-Cerdeira C.; Chillón R.; Díez-Moreno S. & Guerra-Tapia A. (2009). Prevalence and genotypic identification of human papillomavirus infection in a population from northwestern Spain. *The Open Dermatology Journal*, Vol.3, pp. 18-21, ISSN 1874-3722

Rodríguez-Cerdeira C.; Guerra-Tapia A.; Alcantara Caceres R. & Escalas J. (2009). Human Papilloma Virus (HPV) and genital cancer. *The Open Dermatology Journal*, Vol.3, pp. 111- 122, ISSN 1874-3722

Rodríguez Cerdeira C.; Cruces MJ. & Taboada JM. (2011). A quarter century of AIDS in North-western of Spain. *The Open AIDS Journal*, Vol 5, pp.1-8, ISSN: 1874-6136

Rubio I.; Bolchi A.; Moretto N.; Canali E.; Gissmann L. & Tommasino M. (2009). Potentanti-HPV immune responses induced by tandem repeats of the HPV16L2 (20-38) peptide displayed on bacterial thioredoxin. *Vaccine*, Vol.27, No.13, (March 2009), pp. 1949-1956, ISSN 0264-410X

Schabowsky RH.; Elpek KG.; Madireddi S.; Sharma RK.; Yolcu ES.; Bandura-Morgan L. et al (2009). A novel form of 4-1BBL has better immunomodulatory activity than an agonistic anti-4-1BB Ab without Ab-associated severe toxicity. *Vaccine*, Vol.28, No.2, (December 2009), pp. 512–522. ISSN 0264-410X

Schädlich L.; Senger T.; Kirschning CJ.; Müller M. & Gissmann L. (2009). Refining HPV 16 L1 purification from E. coli: reducing endotoxin contaminations and their impact on immunogenicity. *Vaccine*, Vol.27, No.10, (March 2009), pp. 1511-1522, ISSN 0264-410X

Sharma RK.; Srivastava AK.; Yolcu ES.; MacLeod KJ.; Schabowsky RH. & Madireddi S. (2010). SA-4-1BBL as the immunomodulatory component of a HPV-16 E7 protein based vaccine shows robust therapeutic efficacy in a mouse cervical cancer model. *Vaccine*, Vol.28, No.36, (August 2010), pp. 5794-5802, ISSN 0264-410X

Shedlock DJ. & Shen H. (2003). Requirement for CD4 T cell help in generating functional CD8 T cell memory. *Science*, Vol.300, No.5617, (April 2003), pp. 337-339, ISSN 0036-8075

Silk AW. & Finn OJ. (2007). Cancer vaccines: a promising cancer therapy against all odds. *Future Oncology*, Vol.3, No.3, (June 2007), pp. 299-306, ISSN 1479-6694

Storchova Z. & Kuffer C. (2008). The consequences of tetraploidy and aneuploidy. *Journal of Cell Science*, Vol.121, No.Pt 23, (December 2008), pp. 3859-66, ISSN 0021-9533

Strauss R.; Huser A.; Ni S.; Tuve S.; Kiviat N.; Sow PS. et al (2007). Baculovirus-based vaccination vectors allow for efficient induction of immune responses against plasmodium falciparum circumsporozoite protein. *Molecular therapy : the journal of the American Society of Gene Therapy*, Vol.15, No.1, (January 2007), pp. 193–202, ISSN 1525-0016

Tan J.; Farrell L. & Allen DG. (2010). The attitudes of Australian gynaecologists to HPV vaccination: an ASCCP survey. *Australian and New Zealand journal of obstetrics and gynaecology*, Vol.50, No.5, (October 2010), pp. 472-477, ISSN 0004-8666

Trottier H.; Mashmud S.; Costa MC.; Sobrinho JP.; Duarte-Franco E. & Rohan TE. (2006). Human papillomavirus infections with multiple types and risk of cervical neoplasia. *Cancer Epidemiol Biomarkers & Prevention*, Vol.15, No.7, (July 2006), pp. 1274-80, ISSN 1055-9965

Tsakiroglou M.; Bakalis M.; Valasoulis G.; Paschopoulos M.; Koliopoulos G. & Paraskevaidis E. (2011). Women's knowledge and utilization of gynecological cancer prevention services in the Northwest of Greece. *European Journal of Gynaecologycal Oncology*, Vol.32, No.2, pp. 178-181, ISSN 0392-2936

Uno T.; Takeda K.; Kojima Y.; Yoshizawa H.; Akiba H.; Mittler RS. et al (2006). Eradication of established tumors in mice by a combination antibody-based therapy. *Nature Medicine*, Vol.12, No.6, (Juny 2006), pp. 693–698, ISSN 1078-8956

Velders MP.; McElhiney S.; Cassetti MC.; Eiben GL.; Higgins T.; Kovacs GR. et al (2001). Eradication of established tumors by vaccination with Venezuelan equineencephalitis virus replicon particles delivering human papillomavirus 16 E7 RNA. *Cancer Research*, Vol.61, No.21, (November 2001), pp. 7861-7867, ISSN 0008-5472

Walboomers JM.; Jacobs MV.; Manos D.; Bosch FX.; Kummer JA.; Shah KV. et al (1999). Human papillomavirus is a necessary cause of invasive cancer worlwide. *The Journal of Pathology*, Vol.189, No.1, (September 1999), pp. 12-9, ISSN 1096-9896

World Health Organization (WHO) position paper, No. 15. 2009. pp. 118–132. (April 2009). In: *Weekly Epidemiological Record (WER),* 22.06.2010, Available from http://www.who.int/wer/2009/wer8415/en/index.html

World Health Organization (WHO). Guidelines to assure the quality, safety and efficacy of recombinant HPV virus-like particle vaccine. (October 2006). In: EXPERT COMMITTEE ON BIOLOGICAL STANDARDIZATION, 28.06.2010, Available from http://screening.iarc.fr/doc/WHO_vaccine_guidelines_2006.pdf

Yan J.; Reichenbach DK.; Corbitt N.; Hokey DA.; Ramanathan MP.; McKinney KA. et al (2009). Induction of antitumor immunity in vivo following delivery of a novelHPV-16 DNA vaccine encoding an E6/E7 fusion antigen. *Vaccine*, Vol.27, No.3, (January 2009), pp. 431–440, ISSN 0264-410X

6

Plant Production of Vaccine Against HPV: A New Perspectives

Markéta Šmídková[1,2], Marcela Holá[1], Jitka Brouzdová[1] and Karel J. Angelis[1]
[1]*Institute of Experimental Botany AS CR, Prague*
[2]*Institute of Organic Chemistry and Biochemistry, Prague*
Czech Republic

1. Introduction

Infection by human papilloma virus (HPV) attracted attention in connection with cervical cancer in humans (zur Hausen, 1996). HPV type 16 alone accounts for approximately 50% of all cases of cervical cancer. The virus icosahedral capsid is composed of the L1 major and the L2 minor proteins. L1 alone has the capacity to self-assemble into virus-like particles (VLPs) without participation of L2 or other proteins. Because of similar immunogenicity compared to infectious virions, VLPs can be produced and used as a safe prophylactic vaccine against viral transmission of cervical cancer. During recent years two highly efficient VLP-based HPV vaccines (e.g. Gardasil, *Merck MSD* and Cervarix, *GlaxoSmithKline*) become available. For commercial production of vaccines and recombinant therapeutics, plants are often considered as a cost-effective alternative with several benefits. Firstly, production in plants can be easily scaled up in the case of acute demand for production and secondly, produced proteins are unlikely to be contaminated by human or animal pathogens, toxins and oncogenic sequences. Moreover, plants provide a convenient environment for protein expression and storage including the possibility of direct administration as edible vaccine if expressed in the appropriate plant tissue. In this article, we report recent promising advances in the production of prophylactic and therapeutic vaccines against HPV by expression of the relevant antigens in plants, and discuss future prospects for the use of such vaccines.

2. HPV vaccines

2.1 Structure of HPV capsid and neutralizing epitopes on its surface

Papilloma viruses (PVs) are small tissue specific double-stranded DNA tumor viruses, classified in the taxonomic family of *Papillomaviridae*. The Human Papilloma Viruses (HPVs) are phylogenetically closely related with similar biological properties among each other and with animal papillomaviruses that are host-specific to other vertebrates including amphibians, reptiles, birds and a variety of land and sea mammals. Animal PVs have been studied either as disease carrier and transmitters in animals or as models of human PV infection (Brandsma et al.; 1994; Campo 1997). Due to etiological connection with the high-rate mortality cervical cancer, the main attention is concentrated on the genital high-risk HPV types 16, 18, 33 and 58 as the leading cause of cancer (Munoz et al., 2003). The low-risk types 6 and 11 are associated with benign epithelial papillomas or warts that occur in 5–12% of normal women (Heim et al,

1995), however, HPV6 and 11 are the most commonly diagnosed to coinfect and comorbid in immunosuppressed individuals with malignant HPVs (Jay & Moscicki, 2000).

Papillomavirus infection induces type-specific immune response, directed mainly against the major capsid protein L1, rather than L2 minor protein, which also participates in the formation of the shell of native HPV particles. The viral capsid is primarily composed of 360 copies of L1 protein organized into 72 L1-pentamers (capsomeres) and associated with 12 or more copies of the minor L2 protein. When expressed in various recombinant system, L1 readily self-assembles, even in the absence of L2, into noninfectious virus-like particles (VLPs). VLPs are also organized into 72 capsomeres of L1 protein (Fig. 1C) and are immunologically indistinguishable from the native virions (Fig. 1B). The 504-residue of the L1 protein chain contains 12 β-strands, 6 loops, and 5 α-helices that form "jelly roll" β-sandwich (Fig. 1D).

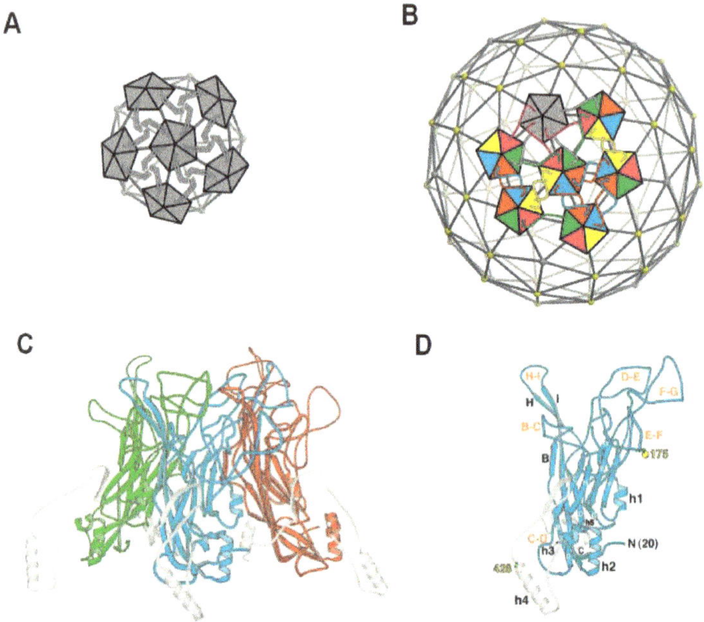

Fig. 1. Structure of the HPV capsid. (A) Small (T=1) VLPs derived from HPV-L1; (B) Full-size (T=7) Papillomavirus particles; (C) HPV16 capsomere (L1-pentamer) in the conformation found in small VLPs (Chen et al., 2000). Three subunits are shown in green, blue and red. The C'-terminal arms are in gray, to indicate that these portions of the subunit rearrange when L1-pentamers assemble into virions or into full-sized capsids; (D) The 3D structure of human papillomavirus 16 L1 monomer (HPV16L1). Secondary structural elements are labeled, with letters *B–J* for β-strands and h1–h5 for the 5 α-helices. Loops between strands are labeled *B–C, C–D*, etc. The first and the last residues are marked N (20) and C (474), respectively. The two cysteines that participate in the interpentamer disulphide bonding within the virion or in the virion-sized particles are shown in yellow, together with their residue numbers, 175 and 428. (Modis et al., 2002)

Some residues in the L1 protein, such as Asp202, Cys175, and Cys428 of HPV16 L1, are very important for VLP formation (Slupetzky et al., 2001), however some residues at the C'-

terminus can be truncated and replaced with heterologous epitopes or short polypeptides up to 60 amino acids without disrupting the assembly of VLPs (Paintsil et al., 1996; Müller et al., 1997; Paz De la Rosa et al., 2009). These chimeric VLPs (cVLPs) can induce strong immune responses against not only the inserted epitopes or polypeptides, but also the VLP shell (Freyschmidt et al., 2004; Varsani et al., 2003a; Xu et al., 2006). Experiments *in vitro* showed that a short N′-terminal segment of the L1 polypeptide chain acts as a switch between T=7 (72 L1-pentamer) and T=1 (12 L1-pentamer) VLP assembly (Fig. 1B) (Chen et al., 2000).

Structural analysis has revealed that BC, EF, FG, HI and DE hyper variable loops of L1 (Fig. 1D) are exposed on the outer surface of the L1-pentamer and form a broad pocket, which participate in receptor interaction. The rim of the pentamer pocket is extremely variable contrary to its floor. With a few exceptions, all HPV-neutralizing monoclonal antibodies analyzed so far are type-specific and recognize conformational epitopes within these surface-exposed hyper variable loops (Pastrana et al., 2004; Fleury et al., 2006). HPV16 and HPV11 VLPs epitopes recognized by neutralizing mAbs are shown on Fig. 2 (Roden et al., 1997a; Ludmerer et al., 1997).

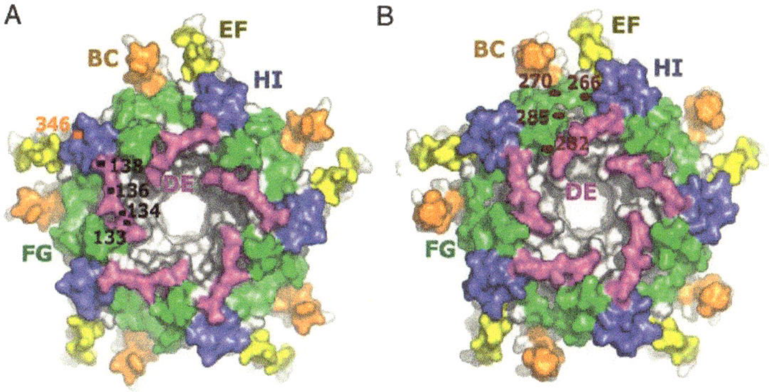

Fig. 2. Surface of the HPV 11 and 16 L1 pentamers. The surface loops are colored differently on the surface: BC (orange), DE (violet), EF (yellow), FG (green), and HI (slate). (A) HPV11; (B) HPV16. Neutralizing epitopes are schematically indicated on pentamers. Black squares, H11.F1 and H11.G5; orange square, H11.H3; red ellipse, H16.V5 and H16.E70. (Bishop et al., 2007)

2.2 HPV vaccines of the first generation. The need for second-generation vaccines

The first applied strategy for HPV prophylactic vaccination aimed on induction of neutralizing antibodies against L1 capsid proteins. Currently two vaccines composed of HPV-L1 self assembled into VLPs have been developed and are commercially available, a Glaxo-Smith Kline bivalent vaccine Cervarix and a Merck, Sharp and Dohme quadrivalent vaccine Gardasil (also marketed as Gardisil or Silgard). Bivalent vaccine Cervarix protects primarily against HPV 16 and 18 that are produced separately using a recombinant Baculovirus expression system. Purified VLPs of each HPV type are formulated with the AS04 adjuvant system composed of aluminium hydroxide and 3-*O*-desacyl-4.-monophosphoryl lipid A (MPL). Cervarix is stored as a sterile turbid liquid suspension for intramuscular injection at 2-8°C with a proposed shelf life 3 years. Gardasil is combination of *Saccharomyces cerevisce* produced HPV 16, 18, 6 and 11 VLPs and has amorphous aluminum hydroxy-phosphate sulfate (AAHS) as an adjuvant. Administrations of vaccine to HPV naive women have demonstrated almost complete protection against infection by the targeted HPV types. Number of medical trials confirmed the safety of currently used vaccines, their efficiency to induce immune response was equal or even higher than that observed during a natural infection and to maintain protection for 5 and 7.3 years in the case of Gardasil and Cervarix, respectively. (McCormack & Joura, 2010; Schwarz, 2009). The induction of HPV neutralizing antibody reaches maximum titers at month 7 after the first vaccination, i.e. 1 month after administration of the last, third dose. Then the titer decline until month 24 and remain stable thereafter (Dillner et al., 2007). Interestingly, the immune response to the Gardasil, the tetravalent vaccine, inversely correlates with the age. The induction of neutralizing antibody is higher in males and females aged 10 to 15 than in those of an age group 16 to 23 year (Villa et al., 2005). For sexually active women in the general population the efficiency of vaccination is expected to be much lower. Moreover, total period of protection afforded by vaccination is not yet known (Wright et al., 2006).

Along with the questions who should be vaccinated and at what age the vaccination is the most effective (Villa, 2011), issues related to vaccine formulation, production and administration have to be also adequately resolved (Schiller & Nardelli-Haefliger, 2006). Firstly, multispecific VLPs based vaccines are expensive to manufacture, since they are produced in eukaryotic cell culture and extensively purified. Both commercially available vaccines require 3 intramuscular injections over a 6 months course to achieve prophylaxis, and the direct vaccine cost excluding administration and medical visits is about USD 375 per recipient in the United States (Armstrong, 2010), reflecting also costly cold chain handling, distribution and storage of a vaccine. More to it, the protection with current vaccines is predominately type specific, and so they are not expected to protect against the almost 30% of cervical cancers that are HPV16 and 18 independent. Last, but not least, therapeutic activity against external genital lesions has not been reported (Villa, 2011).

Suitable vaccine formulations ensuring VLPs stability in liquid were established for both Gardasil (Shank-Retzlaff et al., 2006) and Cervarix (Le Tallec et al., 2009) vaccines. However during production fibrous aggregates of VLPs were occasionally observed. This is why marketed solutions of concentrated VLPs are protected against aggregation by high concentrations of salt. Many other factors including excipients maintaining pH, storage stability, temperature and time effectively influence VLPs. For example at high pH and low salt concentration, VLPs disassemble into capsomeres with weaker immune response than VLPs (Thönes et al., 2008) and denatured L1 protein does not induce any virus neutralizing antibody response (Shinje et al., 1991). Stabilization of protein antigens against aggregation and degradation in solution is important for antigen purification as well as vaccine formulation. Lyophilized VLPs might be an alternative to aqueous droplets for mucosal delivery in a powder formulation of a vaccine (Schiller & Nardelli-Haefliger, 2006; Gerber et al., 2001). Papillomavirus virions are resistant to desiccation and retain their native conformation after freeze-drying (Roden et. al, 1997b; Šmídková et al., 2010). However, both commercial vaccines contain an alum adjuvant, which during freeze-drying extensively coagulate into gel-like consistency, the state suspected to inhibit the release of antigen upon rehydration (Maa et al., 2006). The loss of efficient immune induction has been reported after freezing or freeze-drying of VLPs in aqueous solutions (Shinje et. al, 1991). The use of non-ionic stabilizers, such as methylcellulose (Corbett et al., 2010) or polysorbate PS80 (Shi et al., 2005) helps to avoid this effect. Another solution could be the use of another, physically and chemically more suitable adjuvant(s), but this strategy would further add to the cost of vaccine and principally could raise safety concerns. This is why convenient dry formulation, meaning at least longer shelf life at higher temperatures for marketing purposes is currently missing. The examples of the alternative adjuvants to alum are discussed in Section 3.

Several alternative methods of vaccine needle delivery have been developed. The tattoo delivery of DNA has been found as a cost-effective method that may be used in laboratory conditions when more rapid and more robust immune responses are required (Pokorná et al., 2009). The second method, a novel dry-coated densely packed Macroflux® microprojections array skin patch, was established as an alternate delivery system to intramuscular injection for delivering an alum adjuvanted vaccine Gardasil (Shi et al., 2005).

Besides the effort to improve the formulation, storing properties and methods of vaccine delivery, the first generation of HPV prophylactic vaccines based on IM delivery of HPV antigens of the recombinant VLPs reached its limits with two vaccines produced in baculovirus and yeast cell culture on the market. In parallel with development of these vaccines there were successful attempts to produce recombinant VLPs also in various plant expression systems (see Section 2.4). Plant expression of HPV vaccines pursues several objectives as the cost efficiency, production of uncontaminated safe product, scale up and potential edible vaccine format. Currently HPV VLPs are readily produced in several plant systems with newly developed technologies for industrial large-scale transient production that can successfully compete with current production of L1 based VLPs vaccines. Nevertheless the cost of clinical trials, of approval and implementation of new technologies is so inhibitory high that there will be hardly any HPV vaccine of the first generation produced in plants that will reach the market. More realistic expectation is that developed plant technologies will compete with established procedures for production of new, improved generation of vaccines, when their advantages will surplus currently marketed vaccines and expected market success will justify the cost of clinical trials and production.

2.3 Vaccines of the second generation

2.3.1 L2 based vaccines

The limitation of current vaccines is that neutralizing antibodies induced by immune response to L1 based VLPs are type-restricted (Wakabayashi et al., 2002). Addition of other HPV types VLPs to the existing vaccines would be viable approach only in the case of a small increase in the overall cost of the vaccination scheme. In contrast to L1, Pastrana et al. (2005) showed in *in vitro* assays that antigen determinant present on the N'-end of L2 coat protein can induce broad range of cross neutralizing antibodies in mouse and rabbit sera. These results raise the possibility that a monovalent vaccine could protect against a broad range of genital HPV types. Unfortunately, neutralizing antibody titers against the papillomavirus type from which the L2 vaccine was derived were generally higher than the titers against heterologous types and lower than those induced by L1 VLPs (Pastrana et al., 2005; Roden et al., 2000). This can be avoided by construction of concatenated multiple L2 fusion proteins derived from known cross-protective epitopes of several divergent HPV types. These fusion proteins, consisting of L2 epitopes of 3-22 HPV types, were able to induce high neutralizing antibody titers against all heterologous HPVs tested at a level comparable to that induced by L1 VLPs. In addition, L2 polypeptides have the advantage that they could be produced in *E. coli,* and therefore manufacturing would be easier and cheaper in comparison to production of VLPs. The most promising approach of the non-VLPs second generation of HPV vaccines includes L1 capsomeres and L2 protein (Stanley, 2010).

2.3.2 Therapeutical vaccines

The therapeutic vaccines reduce or eradicate existing disease or infections by targeting cells expressing tumor-associated or tumor-specific antigens on their surface (Ma et al., 2010). There are many different types of therapeutic vaccine candidates based on viral gene peptides and proteins (Xie et al., 2011; Kenter et al., 2008; Melief et al., 2007; Fiander et al., 2006), DNA (Alvarez-Salas et al.; 2008, Sheets et al., 2003) and various viral and bacterial vectors (Brandsma et al, 2009, Davison et al, 2003). They all aim to induce specific cell-mediated immunity and in most cases the targets are the E6 and E7 proteins. Whereas L1 and L2 are expressed only in terminally differentiated keratinocytes, E6 and E7 are constitutively expressed at all layers of epithelium-infected cells (Fig. 3).

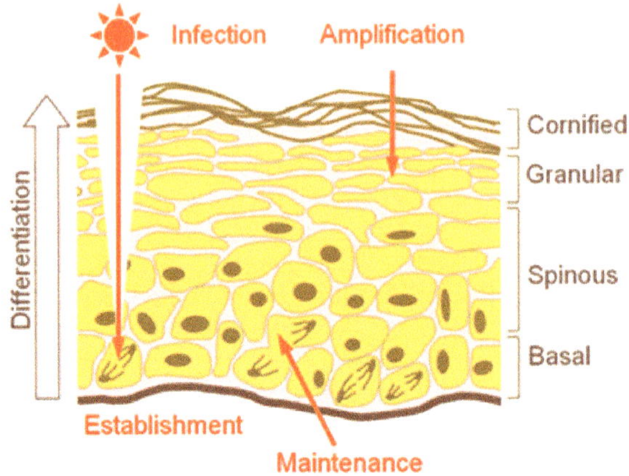

Fig. 3. Cervical stratified squamous epithelial cell architecture and the expression of HPV proteins after infection. Daughter cells of epithelial stem cells divide along the basement membrane and then mature vertically through the epithelium without further division. After introduction of HPV into stem cells in the basal layer of the epithelium, expression of viral non-structural proteins E1-E7 occurs. Under the regulation of these proteins, the dividing-cell population expands vertically and epithelial cell differentiation is delayed and is less complete. Viral proteins are expressed sequentially with differentiation as shown, and mature virions are produced only in the most superficial layers of the epithelium. Intraepithelial antigen-presenting cells (APCs) are depleted in the HPV-infected epithelium. (http://www.ircm.qc.ca/LARECHERCHE/axes/Biologie/Virologie/Pages/Projets.aspx)

E6 and E7 bind p53 and pRB human tumor suppressor genes (Duensing et al., 2000). These oncoproteins are involved in the malignant transformation of HPV-infected cells and are thought to be required for continued tumor growth. They are the primary targets of therapeutic vaccines, most of which have been designed to treat later stages of the disease. The E1 and E2 proteins are necessary for HPV replication within the cell before the virus is integrated into the host DNA (Doorbar et al., 1991). Because E1 and E2 are expressed already early in the progress of at HPV infection and at higher levels than E6 and E7, they may be the best targets for a therapeutic vaccine designed to treat early stages of the disease, such as low-grade dysplasia (Carvajal et al., 2007). Many candidate vaccines with therapeutic potential are currently tested in ongoing trials; however, there is low expectation that any of the current therapeutic vaccines will have a substantial public health impact in the near future (Ma et al., 2010).

2.4 Vaccine production in plants

2.4.1 Posttranslational modification of the therapeutic proteins in plants

Therapeutic recombinant proteins are produced in many hosts from prokaryotes to human cells. When the protein of interest is of eukaryotic origin, one of the production objectives besides yield, solubility and stability is a posttranslational modifications (PTM) required for structural integrity and biological activity of the protein. Microbial expression systems are generally used for expression of simple proteins, because, PTM, including signal peptide cleavage, propeptide processing, protein folding, disulfide bond formation and glycosylation, might not be achieved in prokaryotes. Contrary to prokaryotes, plants are capable of PTM as other higher eukaryotes for safe and low cost production biologically active proteins (Dieryck et al., 1997; Ma et al., 1995). The correct folding and assembly of plant-produced antibody molecules, which requires interactions with several chaperones and with processing and glycosylation enzymes, illustrates that most co- and posttranslational events are similar in plants and mammals (Table 1).

Protein glycosylation is assumed as the most important PTM with significant effects on protein folding, conformation, distribution, stability and activity. In plant cells, as in other eukaryotic cells, N-glycosylation starts during co-translation in ER, when an oligosaccharide precursor is added to Asn residues that is constituent of the N-glycosylation-specific sequences Asn-X-Ser/Thr. The differences in the maturation of plant and mammalian N-glycans appear during the late processing in Golgi apparatus, when core alpha(1,6)-linked fucose residues and terminal sialic acid are attached in mammals, whereas beta(1,2)-xylose and core alpha(1,3)-fucose residues in plants (Fig.4).

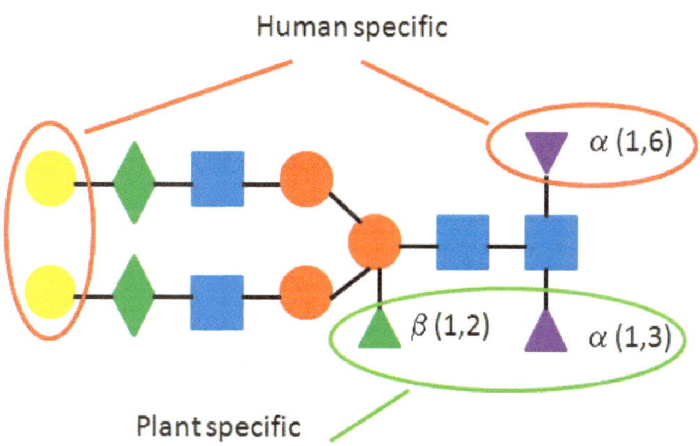

Fig. 4. N-glycan structures in human and plant. N-glycosylation patterns processed in plant cells differ from those of mammal

Posttranslational modification	Location of the reaction in animal cell	Identification in plants and location
Glycosylation		
O-glycosylation	Secretory pathway, nucleus and cytosol	Yes. Sugar addition on Hyp, Ser, Thr
N-glycosylation	Secretory pathway	Yes. Minor differences in modification
Glycation		Yes
Proteoglycan	Secretory pathway	Yes
Attachment of fatty acids		
S-acylation	Cytosol	Yes
N-myristoylation	Cytosol	Yes
Prenylation	Cytosol	Yes
Glypiation	Cytosol	Yes
Cholesterol link	Cytosol	Not identified.
Attachment of ions		
Phosphorylation	Cytosol, secretory pathway	Yes. No mannose-6-phosphate in plant N-glycans
Sulfatation	Secretory pathway	Not identified in secretory pathway
Gamma-carboxylation	ER	Not identified.
Proteolysis		
Cleavage of signal peptide	ER	Yes. ER
Cleavage of propeptide	ER/Golgi	Yes. ER, Golgi, vacuole
Other posttranslational modifications		
Hydroxylation	ER	Yes. ER, Golgi
Cross-linking modifications	ER	Yes. ER, cytosol
Acetylation	Secretory pathway and cytosol	Yes. Function not yet understood in plants
Oligomerization	ER	Yes. ER
Selenoprotein	Cytosol	Not identified in higher plants, described in *C. reinhardtii*
Deamidation	Intra- and extracellular	Yes
Oxidation	Intra- and extracellular	Yes

Table 1. Protein modifications in plant and animal cells. (Gomord & Faye, 2004, modified)

Plant specific residues were described to be constituents of the glycol-epitopes of some plant allergens, showing IgE binding and causing mediator release by human basofils (van Ree et al., 2000). Moreover, the injection of a plant glycoproteins or plant-made antibodies containing plant-specific N-glycans was found to elicit production of antibodies specific for beta(1,2)-xylose and alpha(1,3)-fucose-containing glyco-epitopes in most laboratory mammals and non-allergic human blood donors. Their presence may induce a rapid immune clearance of plant-glycosylated therapeutics from the blood steam (Bardor et al., 2003). One strategy to prevent the addition of immunogenic glycans is to store therapeutic proteins carrying KDEL signal within ER (Ko et al., 2003). Second strategy is based on the inhibition of Golgi glycosyltransferases of plants. The moss *Physcomitrella patens* is the only known plant with high frequency of homologous recombination, thus allowing relatively easy knockouting of target genes. The knockout of alpha(1,3)-fucosyltransferase and beta(1,2)-xylosyltransferase genes in the moss *Physcomitrella patens* prevents the production of plant-specific glyco-epitopes without effecting the secretion of the protein (Koprivova et al., 2004). Third attractive strategy to "humanize" plant N-glycans is expressing of mammalian glycosyltransferases in plants. Like N-glycosylation, O-glycosylation is important for protein function. Surprisingly, little attention is paid so far to O-glycosylation status of plant produced therapeutic proteins.

2.4.2 L1 based prophylactic vaccines and the yields of L1 produced in different plant systems

L1 when expressed in plants readily assemble into VLPs indistinguishable in size from baculovirus expressed VLPs in insect cells (Fig. 5). Sucrose sedimentation analysis also showed that there is a large amount of not, or only partially assembled molecules, presumably capsomeres (fractions 18–24), as well as other larger aggregates (fractions 1–8) when compared to the insect cell-produced protein (Maclean et al., 2007). L1VLPs can be produced either in transgenic plants stably transformed with an expression cassette or transiently using one of several available plant-virus derived expression systems. Initially published yields of L1 expression was low, in a range of 1% of the total soluble protein, which is far lower than industrial demand of more than 5% (Rybicky, 2010). For example, Warzecha et al. (2003) obtained approximately 20 ng HPV-11 L1 per g in transgenic potato tubers; Varsani et al., 2003b, 2006 obtained 4 ng HPV-16 L1 per g of leaf tissue in transgenic tobacco and approximately 40 ng per g of *Nicotiana benthamiana* leaves transiently transformed with a tobacco mosaic virus vector and Kohl et al. (2006) and Liu et al. (2005) achieved approximate yield of L1 at the range 0.05% TSP in transgenic tobacco.

Nevertheless, during passed years, necessary steps to improve *L1* gene expression were recognized and applied. Firstly it was removal of the carboxy-terminal nuclear localization signal sequence (NLS) of L1 that has been shown to enhance expression in transgenic plants. Moreover, the results indicated that full-length L1 is localized essentially entirely within the nucleus (Fig. 6A), whereas cells that express truncated form of L1 in a diffuse pattern within entire cell (Fig. 6B.) (Warzecha et al., 2003). Transient expression of full-length L1 protein in cytoplasm of tobacco leaf cells after agroinfection was described by Šmídková et al. (2010) (Fig. 6C).

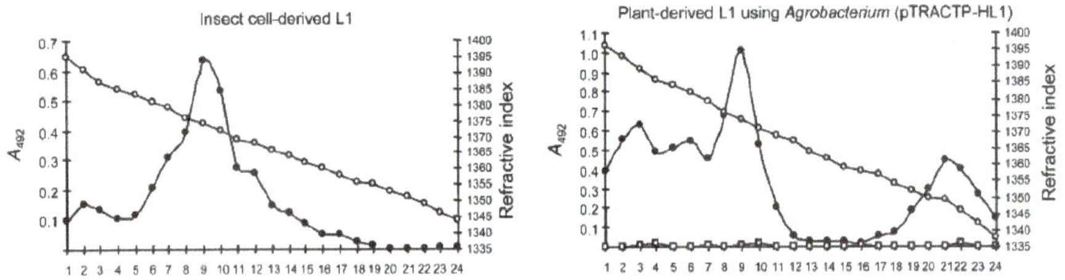

Fig. 5. Sedimentation analysis of transiently expressed HPV-16 L1 protein isolated from *Nicotiana benthamiana* plants (left panel) and insect cells (right panel) in sucrose gradient. The concentration of L1 in fractions was estimated by capture ELISA (closed circles); open squares - ELISA analysis of control, no expressing plants; open circles and right axis - refractive index. Fraction 1 corresponds to the bottom of the centrifuge tube (Maclean et al., 2007).

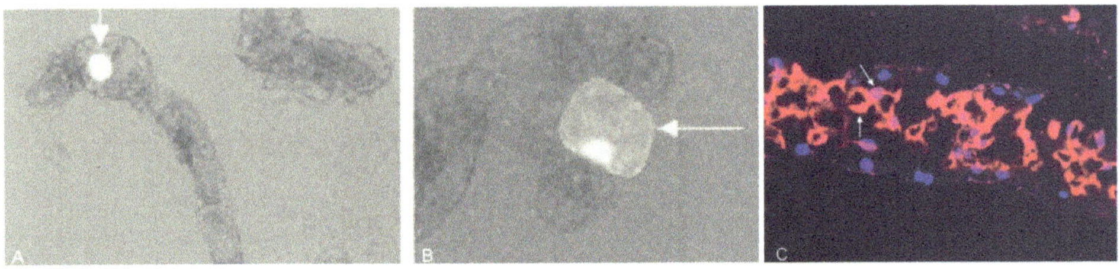

Fig. 6. Expression of HPV L1 proteins in tobacco cells. Transgenic tobacco expressing either full-length (A) or truncated (B) L1 coding sequence fused in frame at the carboxy terminus of GFP. Fluorescence appears as bright areas (Warzecha et al., 2003) (C) Localization of L1 in cryosections of *Nicotiana benthamiana* leaves agroinfected with plant TRV viral vector expressing optimized *L1h* gene (pTVL1h). The protein was detected by immunofluorescence microscopy at 400X magnification. Nuclei were counterstained with DAPI (Šmídková et al., 2010).

Biemelt et al. (2003) after failure to express L1 in transgenic potatos, changed amino-acid codon usage of *L1* gene to that of potato (*L1p*) and of canonic human cells (*L1h*). Despite the presence of codons rarely used by plant cells and for plant genes atypical high GC content, expression of *L1h* led to high accumulation of L1 protein in transgenic plants, even higher than expression of *L1p*. The effect of increased GC content on expression efficiency of *L1* in plants has been confirmed by several groups (Maclean et al., 2007; Šmídková et al., 2010), nevertheless the published yields of L1 differ significantly one from each other, depending on the plant expression system used. For example the change of tobacco cultivar used for transgenic expression from *Nicotiana tabacum* cv. Xanthi to cv. SR1 allowed a 100-fold increase in expression of the native *L1* from viral isolate (Rybicky, 2010). The transient expression of the same *L1* using TMV plant viral expression vector resulted in further, one order of magnitude, increase of L1 over the expression in transgenic tobacco (Varsani et al., 2006). A strategy of optimization procedure for L1 transient expression described recently Šmídková et al. (2010). The results are summarized on Fig. 7, depicting A) The course of L1 expression from original virus isolate sequence (41% GC) and *L1p* sequences optimized for

Solanace plants expression (39% GC) and from canonic human cell optimized sequence *L1h* (61% GC); B) In three plants: tomato and *Nicotiana benhamiana* and *Nicotiana tabacum* tobaccos; C) In two plant viral expression vectors: PVX and TRV and by D) Two transformation methods: agroinfection (method in which a virus infects a host as a part of T-DNA of Ti plasmid carried by *Agrobacterium tumefaciens*) and *Agrobacterium* mediated transfer of expression cassette into cells after infiltration of leaves. The optimization of L1h transient expressed from pTRV vector after *Agrobacterium* infiltration of tomato host plants yielded 45 mg of VLPs per kilo of fresh leaves, the yield that is close to industrial acceptable level.

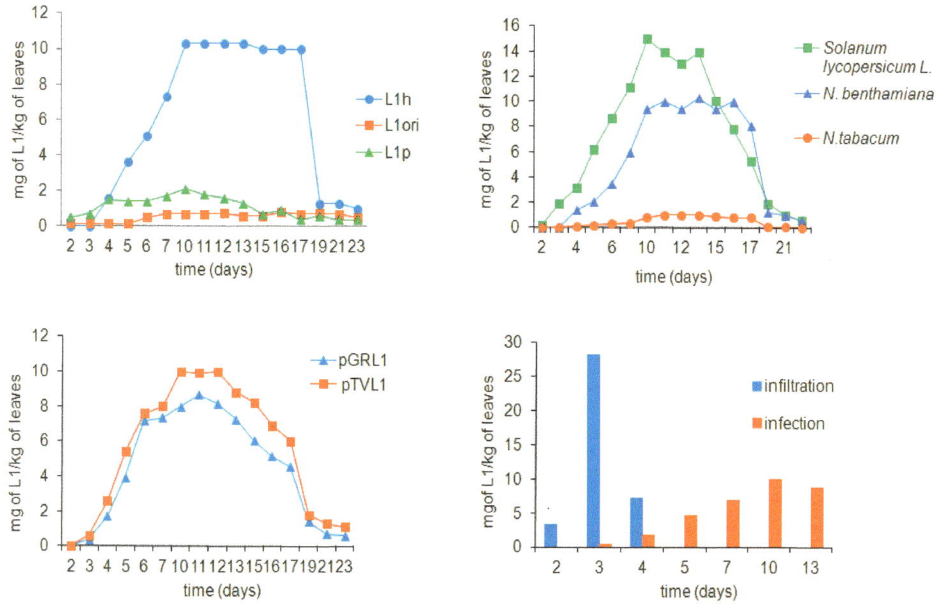

Fig. 7. Time course of the L1 transient expression. (A) Expression of original native HPV *L1* gene sequence *L1ori* and sequences optimized for expression either in plants *L1p* or in mammalian cells *L1h* from plant TRV-based vector pTV00; (B) Expression of *L1h* from pTV00 vector in leaves of *Nicotiana benthamiana, Nicotiana tabacum* and *Solanum lycopersicum L.* (tomato); (C) Comparison of the expression of *L1h* gene from plant tobamo virus (TRV) based expression vector pTV00 and from potato virus X (PVX) based vector pGR106; (D) The yield of L1protein reached by viral agroinfection or by *Agrobacterium* mediated transfer of expression cassette into leaf cells of *Nicotiana bentamiana* (Šmídková et al., 2010).

Nevertheless the highest yield (3 g/ kg fresh leaves; 24% TSP) of plant-produced L1 ever was achieved by Fernández-San Millán et al. (2008) when expressing unmodified *L1* sequence of primary HPV16 virus isolate from expression cassette stably integrated in tobacco chloroplasts genome. Expression in plant chloroplasts is an emerging system when compared to nuclear transformation. Plastid genome engineering offers many advantages over nuclear genome, including targeted recombination based integration, high levels of transgene expression due to high copy number, absence of epigenetic effects, transgene containment via maternal inheritance and multi-gene expression in a single transformation event (Chebolu and Daniell, 2009). Recently the expressions of transgenes in plastids as high as 70% and 72% of total leaf protein was reported by Oey et al. (2009) and Ruhlman et al. (2010), respectively.

Results of L1 expression in various plant systems up to date are summarized in Table2.

Antigen	Production system and yield	Efficacy data
HPV-16 L1	*Agrobacterium*-transformed *Nicotiana tabacum* cv. Xanthi plants Assembled in VLPs 4 µg/kg ww	Weakly immunogenic in rabbit
HPV-11 L1	Transgenic potato tubers Assembled in VLPs 20 µg/kg	Weakly immunogenic in orally vaccinated mice
HPV-16 L1	Transgenic potato tubers Assembled in VLPs 12 mg/kg	Weakly immunogenic in orally vaccinated mice
HPV-16 L1	Transgenic tobacco plants Assembled in VLPs 20 mg/kg ww	Highly immunogenic in mice injected with purified product
HPV-16 L1	Protein expressed in *Nicotiana benthamiana* by TMV-derived vector 40 µg/kg wet leaves	ND
HPV-11 L1	Transgenic *N. tabacum* 2 mg/kg ww Transgenic *Arabidopsis thaliana* 12 mg/kg ww *N. benthamiana* via rTMV 10 mg/kg ww	ND
HPV-16 L1	Agroinfiltrated *N. benthamiana*, human codon usage-optimized gene; protein targeted to chloroplasts, assembled in VLPs 500 mg/kg ww	Antibodies elicited in mice by injection of crudely purified extracts neutralized HPV-16 pseudovirion transfection of HEK293TT cells
HPV-16 L1-Rubisco/ ATPase peptide fusion	Protein produced in chloroplasts of transplantomic tobacco plants from native or chloroplast-optimized genes 60 mg/kg ww	ND
HPV-16 L1	Protein produced from unmodified genes in chloroplasts of transplantomic tobacco plants 3 g/kg ww	Mice injected intraperitoneally with partially purified VLPs with Freund's or aluminium hydroxide adjuvants produced neutralizing antibodies

Table 2. Plant-derived HPV antigens for the development of prophylactic vaccines. HPV: Human papillomavirus; ND: No data; PVA: Potato virus A; PVX: Potato virus X; rTMV: Recombinant tobacco mosaic virus; TMV: Tobacco mosaic virus; VLP: Virus-like particle; ww: Wet weight. (Giorgi et al., 2010)

2.4.3 The structure and stability of plant derived L1

The assembly of VLPs in plants after transient (Fig. 8 A, C) or stable (Fig. 8D) L1 expression was confirmed by electron microscopy of leaf crude extracts.

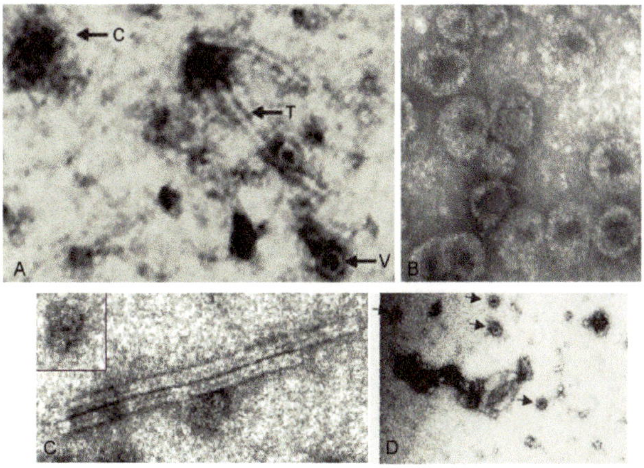

Fig. 8. Electron microscope images of uranyl acetate negatively stained HPV VLPs expressed in various systems: (A) Extracts prepared from freeze-dried leaves of *Nicotiana benthamiana* transiently expressing L1. V - HPV16L1 55-nm VLPs particles, C - HPV16 L1 capsomeres, T - flexible rods of plant TRV virus (Šmídková et al., 2010); (B) CsCl-purified baculovirus expressed VLPs in insect cells; (C) Crude extracts from top leaves of *Nicotiana benthamiana* expressing HPV VLPs from plant TMV virus. Two rods of TMV are shown together with VLPs (Varsani et al., 2006); (D) CsCl-purified VLPs from transgenic potato plants. VLPs have band density 1.32g/ml (Biemelt et al., 2003).

The structure of VLPs is not stable upon freezing and thawing, but plant expressed VLPs retain their structure during freeze-drying in both, the plant extracts and the plant tissue Fig. 8 and 9 (Maclean et al, 2007).

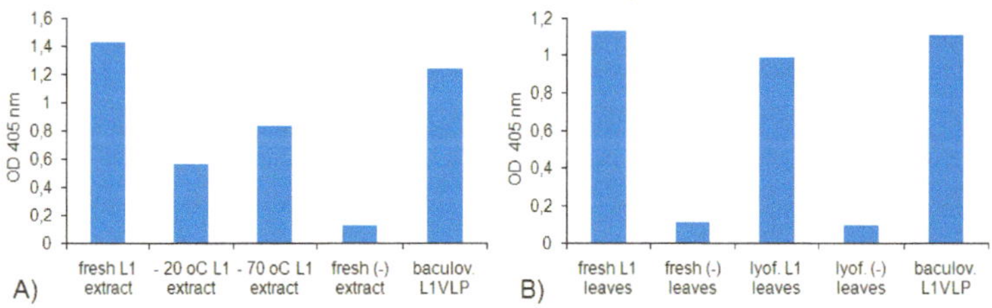

Fig. 9. Stability of L1 VLPs transiently expressed from pTV00 vector in *Nicotiana benthamiana* leaves: (A) after freezing and thawing extract from fresh leaves. Approximately 50% of VLPs loses 3D structure when extract is stored at -20°C or –70°C, respectively; (B) Upon freeze-drying of leaves and extraction cycle. More than 90 % of L1 retains conformation in extracts from freeze-dried leaves (*third column*) in comparison to extract prepared from fresh leaves (first column). Controls are extracts from leaves prepared the same way, but from plants inoculated with an empty pTV00 vector.

2.4.4 Immunogenicity of plant derived L1

The first report on production of HPV VLPs in plants and testing of their immunogenicity appeared in literature in 2003. Varsani et al. (2003b) was the first to express full-length native *HPV-16 L1* gene in transgenic *Nicotiana tabacum* cv. Xanthi. This plant-produced protein assembled into recognizable VLPs and was immunogenic, when injected into rabbits with Freund's incomplete adjuvant. Since then, several groups has observed induction of specific antibodies after subcutaneous injection of either purified plant-derived HPV16 L1 VLPs (Biemelt et al., 2003) or of the crude extract from the tobacco leaves expressing HPV16 L1 protein (Fig. 11A) (Maclean et al., 2007; Šmídková et al., 2010). Despite the fact that in plant extracts majority of expressed L1 protein was present as capsomeres besides VLPs Fig. 8A, the extracts were highly immunogenic without any additional adjuvant (Maclean et al., 2007, Šmídková et al., 2010). The antibodies induced by immunization with plant extract depicted on Fig. 8A preferentially recognized fully assembled L1 VLPs (Fig. 12A) and neutralized in vitro HPV16 virions (Fig. 12B). Plant expressed L1 in crude extract also induces CTL (Fig. 11B).

These findings suggests that principal antigenic determinant is either entire VLP or 3D structure specific for fully assembled VLPs and these antigens are present in crude extracts from plants transiently expressing L1 in enough quantity to elicit immune response equal or higher than purified VLPs from insect cells. Moreover immunization with plant L1 crude extracts induce cellular responses characteristic for active vaccine (Šmídková et al., 2010).

Mucosal delivery has several advantages over needle administration. Immune response is best achieved by direct application of a vaccine to mucosal surfaces and in addition mucosal application of a vaccine can also induce humoral, cell-mediated and systemic immune responses (Rigano & Walmsley, 2005). HPV VLPs are immunogenic when administered orally and stable in the environment of the gastrointestinal tract. Rose et al (1999) and Gerber et al. (2001) reported that as little as 1-10 micrograms are sufficient to induce high titers of L1 specific antibodies after oral application when administered with LT or CpG DNA adjuvants. Besides VLPs also capsomeres (L1-pentamers) and T=1 particles (12 L1-pentamers) depicted on Fig. 10 were investigated for oral immunogenicity in mice. Mutated L1 gene (L1_2xCysM) with two cysteines replaced by serines was used to generate capsomeres and T=1 particles. Compared to capsomeres, VLPs induced higher titers of neutralizing and IgA secreted antibodies, while cytotoxic T cell responses was comparable. The induction of secreted IgA antibodies was observed after oral but not after subcutaneous immunization (Thönes & Müller, 2007).

The concept of using tissue of plants expressing vaccine antigens as an edible vaccines attracted already a lot of attention and is still of special interest. A number of clinical studies demonstrated the induction of specific antibodies after oral immunization using crude plant material containing, for example, hepatitis B or Norwalk virus antigens (Lal et al., 2007). Likewise, oral immunization using crude potato tubers expressing L1 protein can induce specific antibody (Warzecha et al., 2003, Biemelt et al., 2003). Moreover, HPV L1-E6/E7 based chimeric VLPs have been successfully expressed in tomato fruits, which were able to elicit humoral and cytotoxic T-cell activity in mice (Paz De la Rosa et al., 2009).

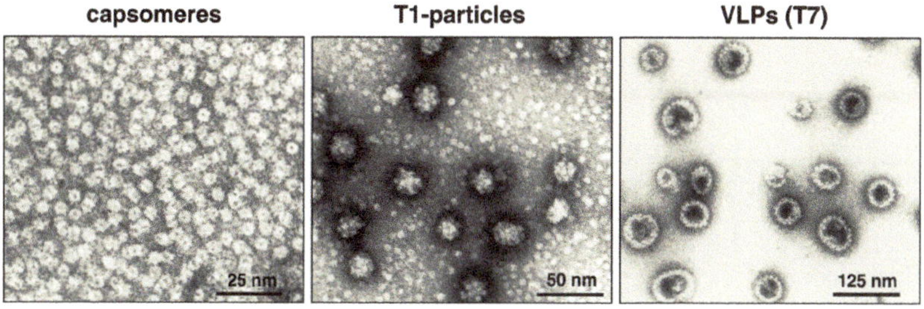

Fig. 10. Analysis of different L1 assembly forms by electron microscopy. Capsomeres (L1-pentamers), T1-particles (12 L1-pentamers) and VLPs (T7 particles of 71 L1-pentamers) purified from infected insect cells expressing the wild-type HPV 16 L1 gene (L1wt) or mutated L1 (L1_2xCysM) were analyzed by electron microscopy after uranyl acetate negative staining (Thönes & Müller, 2007).

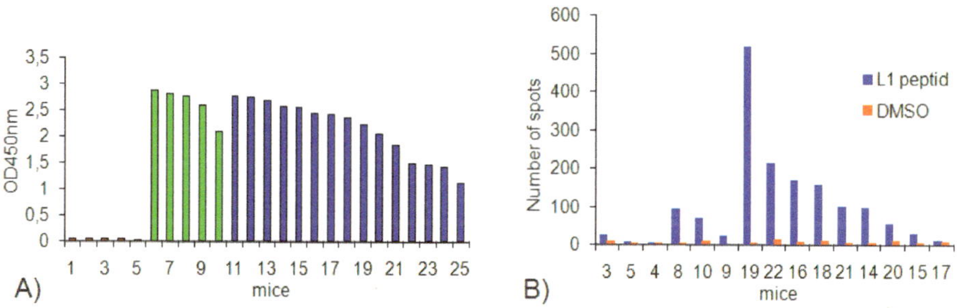

Fig. 11. Antibody (A) and cytotoxic T-lymphocytes (B) induction by L1-VPLs. Response elicited by control plant extracts (mice 1 - 5), control plant extract from *Nicotiana benthamiana* containing purified VLPs from insect cells (mice 6 - 10) and crude plant extracts from leaves expressing L1 (mice 11 - 25) in C57BL/6 mice. Collected sera from individual mice were tested by ELISA for induction of specific antibody (y-axis in OD 450 units). CTLs induction was measured by ELISPOT analysis of splenocytes recovered from scarified animals. The number of CTLs spots was recorded by an ELISPOT reader and expressed as a mean per 10^6 splenocytes

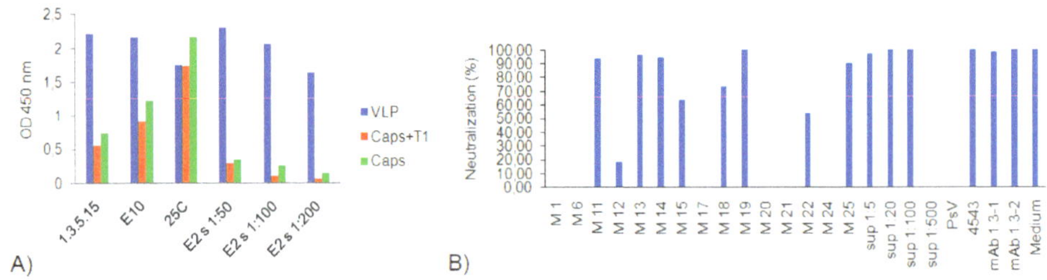

Fig. 12. (A) The specificity of mAb E2 toward various L1 assembly structures. VLPs, T1-particles (12 L1-pentamers) and capsomeres produced in insect cells were absorbed on the microtiter plates and analyzed by ELISA. Interactions of hybridoma E2 supernatant is compared to antibodies obtained after immunization with insect cell-derived VLPs (1.3.5.15, E10 and 25C). (B) Neutralization assay. Sera of mice and of E2 hybridoma supernatant were tested for neutralization of infection of 293T cells by HPV pseudovirions (Psv). Percent of neutralization obtained by incubation with mice sera diluted 1:50 and that of E2 hybridoma supernatant diluted 1:5, 1:20, 1:100, 1:500. Neutralization activity of mice sera was compared to a high titer rabbit polyclonal anti-L1 antiserum 4543 (100 %) and to the mAb's 1.3.1 and 1.3.2 as additional positive controls.

2.4.5 Plant based therapeutic and second-generation vaccines

Capsomeres can be used as a potential cost-saving substitute of VLPs, as L1-pentameric capsomeres are considered thermo-stable, the advantageous feature for the use in developing countries where cold chain administration and delivery of vaccine is difficult to maintain (Stanley et al., 2008). A promising step towards a capsomeres-based vaccine was described by Yuan et al. (2001) when dogs were completely protected against canine oral papillomavirus (COPV) infection by capsomeres vaccination. Capsomeres have been also reported to induce neutralizing antibodies and L1-specific cytotoxic T-lymphocytes (CTLs) upon oral, intranasal and subcutaneous immunization (Dell et al., 2006; Thönes & Müller, 2007; Schadlich et al., 2009). To increase immunogenicity, L1_2xCys mutant version of HPV16 L1 protein was fused with LTB as an adjuvant and expressed in chloroplasts (Waheed et al, 2011a, 2011b).

Plant expressed HPV antigens to be used as therapeutic vaccine to date are summarized in Table 3:

Antigen	Production system and yield	Efficacy data
HPV-16 E7	*N. benthamiana* tobacco leaves infected with PVX-E7 3-4 µg/g fresh leaves	40% of mice immunized with E7-containing crude leaf extract were protected from growth of cancer induced by E7-expressing C3 cells
HPV-16 E7	*N. benthamiana* tobacco leaves infected with PVX-E7; protein targeted to secretory pathway 15-20 µg/g fresh leaves	80% of mice immunized with E7-containing crude leaf extract were protected from growth of cancer induced by E7-expressing C3 cells
HPV-16 E7	*N. benthamiana* tobacco leaves infected with PVX-E7; protein targeted to secretory pathway	Mice vaccinated orally with freeze-dried E7-containing leaf extract mixed with feed produced high titer of anti-E7 antibodies
HPV-16 E7	*N. benthamiana* tobacco leaves infected with PVX-E7	Dendritic cells pulsed with E7-containing leaf extract were able to prime naive lymphocytes to induce E7-specific CTLs
LicKM-E7GGG	*N. benthamiana* tobacco leaves infected with LicKM-E7GGG, using a launch vector expression system 400 µg purified protein per gram of fresh leaves	Purified protein injected into mice induced IgG and CTL response and protected them against challenge with E7-expressing tumor cells in both prophylactic and therapeutic vaccination regimen
11-kDa Zera zein-derived peptide-E7 mut	*N. benthamiana* via agroinfiltration	Mice vaccinated with the protein were protected against tumor cells expressing E7
PVX CP-HPV-16 E7GGG	DNA vaccine	DNA vaccine was able to protect vaccinated mice from the growth of tumors induced by E7-expressing TC-1 cells
PVX CP-HPV-16 E7	Tobacco chloroplast	ND
SAP-KQ-E7GGG	a) DNA vaccine b) Expressed in N. benthamiana	a) DNA vaccine tested in therapeutic setting was able to block tumor growth in the 40% of challenged mice b) Not performed
HPV-16 L2-PVA CP-E7 epitope fused protein	Expressed by PVX in Nicotiana tabacum, N. benthamiana using Agrobacterium tumefaciens-mediated inoculation	ND
HPV-16 VLPs carrying L1 fused to a string of epitopes from E6 and E7	Tomato seedling cotyledons HPV-16 VLPs carrying L1 fused to string of epitopes from E6 and E7 using A. tumefaciens-mediated inoculation	Mice injected with chimeric VLPs were able to develop neutralizing antibodies and specific CTLs

Table 3. Plant-derived HPV antigens for the development of therapeutic vaccines. CP: Coat protein; CTL: Cytotoxic T lymphocyte; HPV: Human papillomavirus; ND: No data; PVA: Potato virus A; PVX: Potato virus X; SAP-KQ: Mutagenized type I ribosome inhibiting proteins from *Saponaria officinalis;* VLP: Virus-like particle. (Giorgi et al., 2010)

The important proof of the L2 plant-produced nonhuman papillomavirus vaccine efficiency was published in connection with the purified rTMV particles displaying cottontail rabbit papillomavirus (CRPV) or rabbit oral papillomavirus (ROPV) L2 protein peptides on their surface (Palmer et al., 2006). This pseudovirion system was also used to express entire native *L1* gene of CRPV. Intramuscular injection with of CRPV L1-containing concentrated plant extract derived from transgenic tobacco protected rabbits against CRPV challenge (Kohl et al., 2006).

Since VLPs based vaccines are not effective in the therapy of diseases, an important goal is development of anti-HPV vaccines with either therapeutic or both prophylactic and therapeutic properties. Few studies were performed with viral oncoproteins expressed in plants. HPV-16 E7 was transiently expressed using a viral vector based on potato virus X (PVX) in the *Nicotiana benthamiana, Nicotiana rustica, Nicotiana tabacum, Chenopodium quinoa* and the tomato *Solanum lycopersicum L.* cv. Micro-Tom. The highest expression of HPV-16 E7 3–4 µg/g of fresh leaves was achieved in *Nicotiana benthamiana* and the expressed E7 induced specific humoral and cell-mediated immune responses in mice (Franconi et al., 2002, 2006). The efficiency of chimeric constructs when E7 is fused to other proteins and expressed in plants was also reported. The expression of HPV-16 E7 fused with the PVX CP in tobacco chloroplasts has been recently reported. The expression of the fusion protein in this system was higher than E7 alone (Morgenfeld et al., 2009). Mutated E7, E7GGG, which lacks the retinoblastoma binding site, and thus the native transformation potential, was fused to the *Clostridium thermocellum* b-1,3–1,4-glucanase (LicKM) as a carrier molecule for expression in plants. The expression of fusion protein in *Nicotiana benthamiana* yielded 400 µg of purified protein per gram of leaf (Musiychuk et al., 2007). Injection of the purified LicKM-E7GGG fusion protein into mice induced both E7-specific IgG and cytotoxic T-cell responses, and protected mice against challenge with E7-expressing tumor cells (Massa et al., 2007). The successful expression of chimeric HPV-16 L1 protein fused to a string of three E7 and one E6 epitopes in transgenic tomatoes demonstrates that a combination prophylactic / therapeutic HPV vaccine could be produced in plants (Paz de la Rosa et al., 2009; Monroy-García et. al, 2011). Unfortunately, while the produced VLPs stimulated both antibody and T-cell responses, yields were low in the range 0.05 - 0.1% of total soluble protein. Similarly, combined vaccine based on minor capsid protein L2 and an epitope of E7 oncoprotein was successfully expressed in plants, when an epitope of the L2 protein and an epitope of E7 oncoprotein were fused to the N′- and C′-end of PVA CP, respectively. The construct was cloned into a PVX-based vector and transiently expressed in plants using *Agrobacterium*-mediated inoculation (Čeřovská et al., 2008).

3. Vaccine formulation

3.1 Parenteral administration

3.1.1 Adjuvants

The goal of vaccination is to generate a strong immune response to the administered antigen. Papillomavirus VLPs themselves are good "inducers" of immune response and antigen determinants present on their surface are able to activate dendritic cells (DCs) for triggering T-cell activation (Bontkes et al., 2005; Yang et al., 2005). Nevertheless, for efficient clinical use additional adjuvants are needed not only to enhance the immune response, but also assuring achievement of appropriate type of protective immunity in each situation.

The aluminum (alum) salts or gel-based adjuvant formulations used e.g. in HPV Gardasil vaccine are currently approved in vaccines licensed for human use in the US. Nevertheless a significant number of compounds tested for adjuvant effect are clearly more effective than alum, albeit usually accompanied with a higher toxicity as e.g. Freund's complete adjuvant. This is the main reason preventing their use as adjuvants in human vaccine formulations. As adjuvants were successfully tested low toxic mutants of the cholera toxin (CT) (Yamamoto et al., 1997) and *E.coli* heat-labile enterotoxin (LT) (Chong et al., 1998). The inactive B-subunits of these toxins proved to be a strong mucosal (oral, nasal, vaginal, etc.) adjuvants (e.g. Salmonella toxin B subunit is used in commercial Cervarix vaccine) for a wide variety of antigens in mice and other animal species so far tested, however their use in humans is limited (Chong et al., 1998). This is why there is a growing interest to develop new adjuvants eliciting high mucosal, humoral and cellular immune response accompanied by negligible or low toxicity.

Antigen delivery systems	**Immunopotentiators**
Insoluble aluminum compounds	MPL and synthetic derivates
Calcium phosphate	MDP and derivatives
Liposomes	Oligonucleotides (CpG, etc.)
Virosomes™	Double-stranded RNA (dsRNA)
ISCOMS®	Alternative pathogen-associated Molecular patterns (PAMPs) (*E. coli* heat Labile enterotoxin (LTB); flagellin)
Microparticles (e.g., PLG)	Saponins (Quils, QS-21)
Emulsions (e.g., MF59, Montanides)	Small-molecule immune potentiators (SMIPs) (e.g., resiquimod [R848])
Virus-like particles & viral vectors	Cytokines & chemokines

Table 4. Examples of adjuvant classes (O'Hagan & Rappuoli, 2004)

3.1.2 Adjuvant effect of plant extracts

Plant extracts are known to contain various compounds, which supposedly have immunostimulatory and immunosuppressive effects (Wagner & Proksh, 1985). Plant crude extracts and their components were tested for their adjuvant capacity. The extract from leaves of *Nicotiana bethamiana* co-administrated subcutaneously with HPV16E7 (Franconi et al., 2002) or HPV16L1 VLP´s (Maclean et. al, 2007; Šmídková et al., 2010) enhanced specific humoral and cellular immune response in tested mice. Freund's adjuvant added to the plant extract did not increased noticeably humoral response elicited by HPV16L1 VLP´s in subcutaneously immunized mice and results indicate that the addition of Freund's adjuvant to plant extract might be even deleterious (Maclean et. al, 2007). The study of Isfar et al. (2004) compares adjuvant effect of CT and of aqueous extract of *Solanum torvum* (STE). STE was shown to evoke an increase in IgA titer comparable to that of CT when co-administrated with ovalbumin intraperitoneally. No acute toxic effects were evident with the used dose range. Plant extract has been shown to induce DC maturation of dendritic cells. This effect was not caused by lipopolysaccharide (LPS) but rather by presence of heat-resistant products mimicking the effect of LPS in foliar extract (Di Bonito et al, 2009).

Probably the most studied plant compound with adjuvant effect is the saponin fractions isolated from *Quillaja saponaria* (Newman et al., 1992). The mechanism of saponin effect is complex and, apart from direct cellular stimulation, there is also evidence that saponins may enhance oral immunization by protection of antigen from degradation by digestive enzymes and by increasing permeability of the intestine to macromolecules (Campbell, 1995).

All these findings are promising for development of needle-free administration route of immunization as an alternative to intramuscular vaccine application. For this purposes intranasal, intravaginal, transdermal, sublingual and intramuscular administration routes were tested for systemic immune responses against HPV16L1 using (Cho et al., 2010). The sublingual route provided the most effective mucosal secretory IgA (sIgA) and serum IgG responses, cholera toxin subunit B (CTB) showed the most promising adjuvant activity.

3.2 HPV L1 antigens as an edible vaccine?

The majority of currently licensed vaccines are administered parenterally, even though they have the disadvantages of patient reluctance to tolerate needle sticks and lack of mucosal immune induction (Velasquez et al 2010). Edible vaccine represents further approach to self-administrated nonparenteral vaccine that could solve the problem of high cost and need for appropriate storage of currently available preventive HPV vaccines.

Thönes & Müller (2007) investigated the oral immunogenicity of different assembly forms of HPV 16 L1: T7-VLPs, T1 particles and capsomeres produced from Baculovirus expression vector in insect cells and showed that all three assembly forms induce humoral and cellular immune responses after oral vaccination of mice. The anti-L1 antibodies were conformation-specific and showed neutralizing activity in a pseudovirion-based assay. They also investigated whether adjuvants have an effect on oral immunogenicity when co-administrated with different L1 forms. Besides saponins, which were significantly toxic if applied orally, co-administration of either CpG DNA or *Escherichia coli* heat-labile enterotoxin LT(R192G) had no apparent enhancing effect on the production of anti-L1 antibodies. Compared to capsomeres, VLPs induced stronger humoral immune responses while the CTL responses were induced at comparable levels.

To establish an edible HPV16 vaccine Sasagawa et al., (2005) constructed a recombinant HPV16 L1-expressing *Schizosaccharomyces pombe* yeast strain to be administrated as freeze-dried yeast powder orally as an edible vaccine, with or without the mucosal adjuvant heat-labile toxin LT (R192G), to mice. After the third immunization, none of the mice that received the edible HPV16 vaccine showed specific antibody responses, whereas all of the positive controls that were administered intranasally with 5 µg of HPV16-virus-like particles (VLP) had serum IgG, and genital IgA and IgG that reacted with HPV16-VLP in enzyme-linked immunosorbent assays (ELISAs).

HPV L1 antigens that proof to be highly immunogenic when administrated parenterally induce only mild or none response when administrated orally. In light of these experiments it seems unlikely that current design of L1 based HPV vaccines will reach the market as an edible replacement of existing vaccines. More research is needed to establish vaccine concentration and formulation to boost its effect. It is also obvious that the highly phrased concept of edible vaccine administrated as plants or fruits for direct consumption in the less developed countries is rather romantic dream than reality and have to be corrected. It is now clear that if there will be an edible vaccine, it will have complex formulation that will be strictly controlled.

A good nonparenteral alternative for vaccine delivery could be nasal immunization, which already proved to be effective in tests with animals. The obstacles imposed by the normal process of mucociliary clearance limiting residence time of applied antigens could be circumvent by presence of an inert *in situ* gelling polysaccharide (GelSite) extracted from Aloe vera for nasal delivery of NV VLP antigen (Hefferon, 2010). The nasal cavity is a promising site for vaccine delivery because it is easy to access, is highly vascularized, has a relatively large surface area, has low proteolytic activity, and is able to induce systemic immunity as well as both local and distal mucosal immunity via the Common Mucosal Immune System (CMIS)

4. Conclusions

The major reason for the vaccine production in plants is that the vaccine antigen production is safe and could be potentially cheap and both transient and transgenic productions are scalable. Biologically active proteins can be produced more easily in plants than in other eukaryotic systems; and that the use of food plants could eventually allow edible and/or oral vaccines to be produced cheaper. The recent reports indicate very high yields of human vaccine candidates to be obtained via plastid transformation or large scale transient expression what could enable to meet the expected requirement of antigen for oral route as is required parenterally for the same immune response. A recent review on human trials of plant-based oral vaccines summarizing human studies of oral transgenic plant derived vaccines against enterotoxigenic *E. coli* infection, norovirus and HBV adds weight to the growing body of evidence that plant-made oral vaccines to these viruses are not only feasible, but could effective (Rybicki, 2010). Nevertheless there is still long way to go from improvement of antigen yields, to formulation of the vaccine including auxiliary factors improving efficacy and stability, to translation of the proposed vaccines into clinical trials and, not least, governmental and/or regulatory body approvals.

5. Acknowledgements

This work was supported by the Grant Agency of the Czech Republic contract 521/01/1418 and 521/04/0971, Grant Agency of the Czech Academy of Sciences A6038201 and S5038304 and by Ministry of Education, Youth and Sports of the Czech Republic projects 1M0505.

6. References

Alvarez-Salas, L.M. (2008). Amolimogene bepiplasmid, a DNA-based therapeutic encoding the E6 and E7 epitopes from HPV, for cervical and anal dysplasia. *Current opinion in molecular therapeutics*, Vol.10, No.6, (December 2008), pp. 622-6288, ISSN 1464-8431

Armstrong, E. P. (2010). Prophylaxis of cervical cancer and related cervical disease: a review of the cost-effectiveness of vaccination against oncogenic HPV types. *Journal of managed care pharmacy*, Vol.16, No.3, (April 2010), pp. 217-230, ISSN 1083-4087

Bardor, M.; Faveeuw, C.; Fitchette, A.C.; Gilbert, D.; Galas, L.; Trottein, F.; Faye, L. & Lerouge, P. (2003). Immunoreactivity in mammals of two typical plant glyco-epitopes, core alpha(1,3)-fucose and core xylose. *Glycobiology*, Vol.13, No.6, (June 2003), pp.427-434, ISSN 0959-6658

Biemelt, S.; Sonnewald, U.; Gaimbacher, P.; Willmitzer, L. & Müller, M. (2003). Production of human papillomavirus type 16 virus-like particlesin transgenic plants. *Journal of virology*, Vol.77, No. 17, (September 2003), pp.9211-9220, ISSN 0022-538X

Bishop, B.; Dasgupta, J.; Klein, M.; Garcea, R.L.; Christensen, N.D.; Zhao, R. & Chen , X.S. (2007). Crystal structures of four types of human papillomavirus L1 capsid proteins: Understanding the specificity of neutralizing monoclonal antibodies. *The Journal of Biological Chemistry*, Vol.282, No.43, (October 2007), pp. 31803–31811, ISSN 0021-9258

Bontkes, H.J.; Ruizendaal, J.J.; Kramer, D.; Meijer, C.J. & Hooijberg, E. (2005). Plasmacytoid dendritic cells are present in cervical carcinoma and become activated by human papillomavirus type 16 virus-like particles. *Gynecologic Oncology*, Vol.96, No.3, (March 2005), pp. 897–901, ISSN 0090-8258

Brandsma, J. L. (1994). Animal models of human-papillomavirus-associated oncogenesis. *Intervirology*, Vol.37, No.3-4, (March 1994), pp. 189–200, ISSN 0300-5526

Brandsma, J.L.; Shlyankevich, M.; Su, Y.; Zelterman, D.; Rose, J.K. & Buonocore, L. (2010). Reversal of papilloma growth in rabbits therapeutically vaccinated against E6 with naked DNA and/or vesicular stomatitis virus vectors. *Vaccine*, Vol.29, No.52, (December 2010), pp. 8345-8351, ISSN 1873-2518

Campbell, J.B. (1995). Saponins. In: *The theory and practical application of adjuvants*, Stewart-Tull, D.E.S. (Ed.), pp. 95–127, John Wiley & Sons, New York

Campo, M.S. (1997). Vaccination against papillomavirus in cattle. *Clinics in dermatology*, Vol.15, No.2, (July 1997), pp. 275-83, ISSN 0738-081X

Carvajal, A. A.; de la Garza, A.; Quiroz, B. J.; Zea, E. V.; Estrada, I. D.; Fuentez, E. M.; Contreras, M. L.; Andrade-Manzano, A.; Padilla, S. & Varela, A. R. (2007). MVA E2 recombinant vaccine in the treatment of human papillomavirus infection in men presenting intraurethral flat condyloma: a phase I/II study. *Biodrugs* , Vol. 21, No.1, (January 2007), pp. 47-59, ISSN 1173-8804

Čeřovská, N.; Hoffmeisterová, H.; Pečenková, T.; Moravec, T.; Synková, H.; Plchová, H. & Velemínský J. (2008). Transient expression of HPV16 E7 peptide (aa 44–60) and HPV16 L2 peptide (aa 108–120) on chimeric potyvirus-like particles using potato virus X-based vector. *Protein Expression and Purification*, Vol.58, No.1, (August 2008), pp. 154–161, ISSN 1046-5928

Chebolu, S. & Daniell, H. (2009). Chloroplast-derived vaccine antigens and biopharmaceuticals: expression, folding, assembly and functionality. *Current topics in microbiology and immunology*, Vol.332, (July 2009), 33-54, ISSN 0070-217X

Chen, X. S.; Garcea, R. L.; Goldberg, I.; Casini, G. & Harrison, S. C. (2000). Structure of small virus-like particles assembled from the L1 protein of human papillomavirus 16. *Molecular Cell*, Vol. 5, No.3, (March 2000), pp. 557-567, ISSN 1097-2765

Cho, H.J.; Kim, J.Y.; Lee Y., Kim, J.M.; Kim, Y.B.; Chun, T. & Oh, Y.K. (2010). Enhanced humoral and cellular immune responses after sublingual immunization against human papillomavirus 16 L1 protein with adjuvants. *Vaccine*, Vol. 28, No.14, (March 2010), pp. 2598-2606, ISSN 1873-2518

Chong, C.; Friberg, M. & Clements, J.D. (1998). LT (R192G), a non-toxic mtant of the heat-labile enterotoxin of Escherichia coli,elicits enhanced humoral and cellular immune responses associated with protection against lethal oral challenge with Salmonella spp. *Vaccine*, Vol.16, No.7, (April 1998), pp.732–740, ISSN 0264-410X

Davidson, E.J.; Boswell, C.M.; Sehr, P.; Pawlita, M.; Tomlinson, A.E.; McVey, R.J.; Dobson, J.; Roberts, J.S.; Hickling, J.; Kitchener, H.C. & Stern, P.L. (2003). Immunological and clinical responses in women with vulval intraepithelial neoplasia vaccinated with a vaccinia virus encoding human papillomavirus 16/18 oncoproteins. *Cancer research*, Vol.63, No.18, (September 2003), pp. 6032-6041, ISSN 0008-5472

Dell, K.; Koesters, R.; Linnebacher, M.; Klein, C. & Gissmann, L. (2006). Intranasal immunization with human papillomavirus type 16 capsomeres in the presence of non-toxic cholera toxin-based adjuvants elicits increased vaginal immunoglobulin levels. *Vaccine*, Vol.24, No.13, (March 2006), pp. 2238–2247, ISSN 0264-410X

Di Bonito, P.; Grasso, F.; Mangino, G.; Massa ,S.; Illiano, E.; Franconi, R.; Fanales-Belasio, E.; Falchi, M.; Affabris, E. & Giorgi, C. (2009). Immunomodulatory activity of a plant extract containing human papillomavirus 16-E7 protein in human monocyte-derived dendritic cells. *International journal of immunopathology and pharmacology*, Vol.22. No. 4, (October-December 2009), pp. 967-978, ISSN 0394-6320

Dieryck, W.; Pagnier, J.; Poyart, C.; Marden, M.C.; Gruber, V.; Bournat, P.; Baudino, S. & Merot, B. (1997). Human haemoglobin from transgenic tobacco. *Nature*, Vol.386, No.6620, (March 1997), pp. 29-30, ISSN 0028-0836

Dillner, J.; Arbyn, M. & Dillner, L. (2007). Translational mini-review series on vaccines: Monitoring of human papillomavirus vaccination. *Clinical and experimental immunology*, Vol.148, No.2, (May 2007), pp. 199-207, ISSN 0009-9104

Doorbar, J.; Ely, S.; Sterling, J.; McLean, C. & Crawford, L. (1991). Specific interaction between HPV-16 E1-E4 and cytokeratins results in collapse of the epithelial cell intermediate filament network. *Nature*, Vol. 352, No.6338, (August 1991), pp. 824-827, ISSN 0028-0836

Duensing, S.; Lee, L. Y.; Duensing, A.; Basile, J.; Piboonniyom, S.; Gonzalez, S.; Crum, C.P. & Munger, K. (2000). The human papillomavirus type 16 E6 and E7 oncoproteins cooperate to induce mitotic defects and genomic instability by uncoupling centrosome duplication from the cell division cycle. *Proceedings of the National Academy of Sciences of the United States of America*, Vol.97, No. 18, (August 2000), pp. 10002-10007, ISSN 0027-8424

Fiander, A.N.; Tristram, A.J.; Davidson, E.J.; Tomlinson, A.E.; Man, S.; Baldwin, P.J.; Sterling, J.C. & Kitchener HC. (2006). Prime-boost vaccination strategy in women with high-grade, noncervical anogenital intraepithelial neoplasia: clinical results from a multicenter phase II trial. *International journal of gynecological cancer*,Vol.16, No.3, (May-June 2006), pp. 1075-1081, ISSN 1048-891X

Fernández-San Millán, A.; Ortigosa, S.M.; Hervás-Stubbs, S.; Corral-Martínez, P.; Seguí-Simarro, J.M., Gaétan, J., Coursaget, P. & Veramendi, J. (2008). Human papillomavirus L1 protein expressed in tobacco chloroplasts self-assembles into virus-like particles that are highly immunogenic. *Plant biotechnology journal*, Vol.6, No.5, (Jun 2008), pp. 427–44, ISSN 1467-7652

Fleury, M.J.; Touzé, A.; Alvarez, E.; Carpentier, G.; Clavel, C.; Vautherot, J.F. & Coursaget, P. (2006). Identification of type-specific and cross-reactive neutralizing conformational epitopes on the major capsid protein of human papillomavirus type 31. *Archive sof virology*, Vol.151, No.8, (August 2006), pp. 1511-1523, ISSN 0304-8608

Franconi, R.; Di Bonito, P.; Dibello, F; Accardi, L.; Müller, A.; Cirilli, A.; Simeone, P.; Donà, G.; Venuti, A. & Giorgi, C. (2002). Plant-derived human papillomavirus 16 E7 oncoprotein induces immune response and specific tumor protection. *Cancer Research*, Vol.62, No.13, (July 2002), pp. 3654-3658, ISSN 0008-5472

Franconi, R.; Massa, S.; Illiano, E.; Mullar, A.; Cirilli, A.; Accardi, L.; Di Bonito, P.; Giorgi, C. & Venuti, A. (2006). Exploiting the plant secretory pathway to improve the anticancer activity of a plant-derived HPV16 E7 vaccine. *International journal of immunopathology and pharmacology*, Vol. 19, No.1, (January-March 2006), pp. 187-197, ISSN 0394-6320

Freyschmidt, E.J.; Alonso, A.; Hartmann, G. & Gissmann, L. (2004). Activation of dendritic cells and induction of T cell responses by HPV 16 L1/E7 chimeric virus-like particles are enhanced by CpG ODN or sorbitol. *Antiviral Therapy*, Vol.9, No.4, (August 2004), pp. 479–489, ISSN 1359-6535

Gerber, S.; Lane, C.; Brown, D.M.; Lord, E.; DiLorenzo, M.; Clements, J.D.; Rybicki, E., Williamson, A.L. & Rose, R.C. (2001). Human papillomavirus virus-like particles are efficient oral immunogens when coadministered with Escherichia coli heat-labile enterotoxin mutant R192G or CpG DNA. *Journal of Virology*, Vol.75, No.10, (May 2001), pp. 4752–60, ISSN 0022-538X

Giorgi, C.; Franconi, R. & Rybicki, E.P. (2010). Human papillomavirus vaccines in plants. *Expert Review of Vaccines*, Vol. 9, No.8, (August 2010), pp. 913–924, ISSN 1744-8395

Gomorod, V. & Faye L. (2004). Posttranslational modification of therapeutic proteins in plants. *Current opinion in plant biology*, Vol.7, No.2, (April 2004), pp. 171-181, ISSN 1369-5266

Hefferon, K.L. (2010). The mucosal immune response to plant-derived vaccines. *Pharmaceutical research*, Vol.27, No.10, (October 2010), pp. 2040–2042, ISSN 0724-8741

Heim, K.; Christensen, N.D.; Hoepfl, R.; Wartusch, B.; Pinzger, G.; Zeimet, A.; Baumgartner, P.; Kreider, J.W. & Dapunt, O. (1995). Serum IgG, IgM, and IgA reactivity to human papillomavirus types 11 and 6 viruslike particles in different gynecologic patient groups. *The Journal of Infectious Diseases*, Vol.172, No.2, (August 1995), pp. 395-402, ISSN 0022-1899

Corbett H.J.; Fernando, G.J.P.; Chen, X.; Frazer, I.H. & Kendall, M.A.F. (2010). Skin vaccination against cervical cancer associated human papillomavirus with a novel micro-projection array. *PLoS One*, Vol.5, No.10, (October 2010), pp. e13460, ISSN 1932-6203

Israf, D.A.; Lajis, N.H.; Somchit, M.N. & Sulaiman, M.R. (2004). Enhancement of ovalbumin-specific IgA responses via oral boosting with antigen coadministered with an aqueous *Solanum torvum* extract. *Life Science*, Vol.75, No.4, (January 2004), pp. 397–406, ISSN 0024-3205

Jay, N. & Moscicki, A.B. (2000). Human papillomavirus infections in women with HIV disease: prevalence, risk, and management. *The AIDS Reader*, Vol.10, No.11, (November 2000), pp. 659-668, ISSN 1053-0894

Kenter, G.G.; Welters, M.J.; Valentijn, A.R.; Lowik, M.J.; Berends-van der Meer, D.M.; Vloon, A.P.; Drijfhout, J.W.; Wafelman, A.R.; Oostendorp, J.; Fleuren, G.J.; Offringa, R.; van der Burg, S.H. & Melief, C.J. (2008). Phase I immunotherapeutic trial with long peptides spanning the E6 and E7 sequences of high-risk human papillomavirus 16 in end-stage cervical cancer patients shows low toxicity and robust immunogenicity. *Clinical cancer research,* Vol.14, No.1, (January 2008), pp. 169-177, ISSN 1078-0432

Ko, K.; Tekoah, Y.; Rudd, P.M.; Harvey, D.J.; Dwek, R.A.; Spitsin, S.; Hanlon, C.A.; Rupprecht, C.; Dietzschold, B.; Golovkin, M. & Koprowski, H. (2003). Function and glycosylation of plant-derived antiviral monoclonal antibody. *Proceedings of the National Academy of Sciences of the United States of America,* Vol.100, No.13, (June 2003), p.p. 8013-8018, ISSN 0027-8424

Kohl, T.; Hitzeroth, I.I.; Stewart, D.; Varsani, A.; Govan, V. A.; Christensen, N. D.; Williamson, A.L. & Rybicki E. P. (2006). Plant-produced cottontail rabbit papillomavirus L1 protein protects against tumor challenge: a proof-of-concept study. *Clinical and vaccine immunology,* Vol.13, No.8, (January 2006), pp. 845–853, ISSN 1556-6811

Koprivova, A.; Stemmer, C.; Altmann, F.; Hoffmann, A.; Kopriva, S.; Gorr, G.; Reski, R. & Decker, E.L. (2004). Targeted knockouts of Physcomitrella lacking plant-specific immunogenic N-glycans. *Plant biotechnology journal,* Vol.2, No.6, (November 2004), p.p. 517-523, ISSN 1467-7644

Le Tallec, D.; Doucet, D.; Elouahabi, A.; Harvengt, P.; Deschuyteneer, M. & Deschamps, M. (2009). Cervarix, the GSK HPV-16/HPV-18 AS04-adjuvanted cervical cancer vaccine, demonstrates stability upon long-term storage and under simulated cold chain break conditions. *Human vaccines,* Vol.5, No.7, (July 2009), pp. 467–474, ISSN 1554-8619

Lal, P.; Ramachandran, V.G.; Goyal, R. & Sharma, R. (2007). Edible vaccines: current status and future. *Indian journal of medical microbiology,* Vol.25, No.2, (April 2007), pp. 93-102, ISSN 0255-0857

Liu, H.L.; Li, W.S.; Lei, T.; Zheng, J.; Zhang, Z.; Yan, X.F.; Wang, Z.Z.; Wang, Y.L. & Si, L.S. (2005). Expression of human papillomavirus type 16 L1 protein in transgenic tobacco plants. Acta Biochim. Biophys. Sin. (Shanghai) 37, 153–158. *Acta biochimica et biophysica Sinica (Shanghai),* Vol.37, No.3, (March 2005), pp. 153–158, ISSN 1672-9145

Ludmerer, S.W.; Benincasa, D.; Mark, G.E. 3rd & Christensen, N.D. (1997). A neutralizing epitope of human papillomavirus type 11 is principally described by a continuous set of residues which overlap a distinct linear, surface-exposed epitope. *Journal of virology,* Vol.71, No.5, (May 1997), pp. 467–474, ISSN 0022-538X

Ma, B.; Xu, Y.; Hung, C.F. & Wu T.C. (2010). HPV and Therapeutic Vaccines: Where are We in 2010? *Current cancer therapy reviews,* Vol.6, No.2, (May 2010), pp. 81-103, ISSN 1573-3947

Ma, J.K.; Hiatt, A.; Hein, M.; Vine, N.D.; Wang, F.; Stabila, P.; van Dolleweerd, C.; Mostov, K. & Lehner, T. (1995). Generation and assembly of secretory antibodies in plants. *Science,* Vol.268, No.5211, (May 1995), p.p. 716-719, ISSN 0036-8075

Maa, Y.F.; Shu, C.; Ameri, M.; Zuleger, C.; Che, J.; Osorio, J.E.; Payne, L.G. & Chen, D. (2003). Optimization of an alum-adsorbed vaccine powder formulation for epidermal powder immunization. *Pharmaceutical Research,* Vol.20, No.7, (July 2003), pp. 969–977, ISSN 0724-8741

MacLean, J.; Koekemoer, M.; Olivier, A.J.; Stewart, D.; Hitzeroth I.I.; Rademacher, T.; Fischer, R.; Williamson, A.L. & Rybicki, E.P. (2007). Optimization of human papillomavirus type 16 (HPV-16) L1 expression in plants: comparison of the suitability of different

HPV-16 L1 gene variants and different cell-compartment localization. Journal of General Virology, Vol.88, No.Pt 5, (May 2007), pp. 1460-1469, ISSN 0022-1317

Massa, S.; Franconi, R.; Brandi, R.; Müller, A.; Mett, V.; Yusibov, V. & Venuti, A. (2007). Anti-cancer activity of plant-produced HPV16 E7 vaccine. *Vaccine,* Vol.25, No.16, (April 2007), pp. 3018–3021, ISSN 0264-410X

McCormack, P.L. & Joura, E.A. (2010). Quadrivalent human papillomavirus (types 6, 11, 16, 18) recombinant vaccine (Gardasil®): a review of its use in the prevention of premalignant genital lesions, genital cancer and genital warts in women. *Drugs,* Vol.70, No.18, (December 2010), pp. 2449-2474, ISSN 0264-410X

Melief, C.J.; Welters, M.J.; Lowik, M.J.; Vloon, A.P. & Kenter, G.G. (2007). Long peptide vaccine-induced migration of HPV16-specific type 1 and 2 T cells into the lesions of VIN III patients associated with complete clinical responses. *Cancer Immunity,* Vol.7, Suppl.1, (May 2007), pp. 20, ISSN 1424-9634

Modis, Y.; Trus, B.L. & Harrison, S.C. (2002). Atomic model of the papillomavirus capsid. *The EMBO Journal,* Vol. 21,No.18, (September 2002), pp. 4754-4762, ISSN 0261-4189

Monroy-García, A.; Gómez-Lim, M.A.; Weiss-Steider, B.; la Rosa, G. V & Hernández-Montes, J. (2011). A novel HPV 16 L1-based chimeric virus-like particle containing E6 and E7 seroreactive epitopes permits highly specific detection of antibodies in patients with CIN 1 and HPV-16 infection.*Virology Journal,* Vol. 8, (February 2002), pp. 59, ISSN 1743-422X

Morgenfeld, M., Segretin, M.E. & Wirth, S. (2009). Potato virus X coat protein fusion to human papillomavirus 16 E7 oncoprotein enhance antigen stability and accumulation in tobacco chloroplast. *Molecular Biotechnology,* Vol.43, No.3, (July 2009), pp. 243–249, ISSN 1073-6085.

Müller, M.; Zhou, J.; Reed, T.D.; Rittmüller, C.; Burger, A.; Gabelsberger, J.; Braspenning, J. & Gissmann, L. (1997). Chimeric papillomavirus-like particles. *Virology,* Vol.234, No.1, (July 1997), pp. 93–111, ISSN 0042-6822

Munoz, N.; Bosch, F.X.; de Sanjose, S.; Herrero, R.; Castellsague, X.; Shah, K.V.; Snijders, P.J. & Meijer, C.J. (2003). Epidemiologic classification of human papillomavirus types associated with cervical cancer. *The new england journal of medicine,* Vol.348, No.6, (February 2003) pp. 518-527, ISSN 0028-4793

Musiychuk, K.; Stephenson, N.; Bi, H.; Farrance, C.E.; Orozovic, G.; Brodelius, M.; Brodelius, P.; Horsey, A.; Ugulava, N.; Shamloul, A.M.; Mett, V.; Rabindran, S.; Streatfield, S.J. & Yusibov V. (2007). A launch vector for the production of vaccine antigens in plants. *Influenza and Other Respiratory Viruses,*Vol.1, No.1, (January 2007) pp. 19–25, ISSN 1750-2640

Newman, M.J.; Wu, J.; Gardner, B.H.; Munroe, K.J.; Leombruno, D.; Recchia, J.; Kensil, C.R. & Coughlin, R.T. (1992). Saponin adjuvant induction of ovalbumin-specific CD8+ cytotoxic T lymphocyte responses. *Journal of Immunology,* Vol.148, No.8, (April 1992), pp. 2357–2362, ISSN 0022-1767

Oey, M.; Lohse, M.; Kreikemeyer, B. & Bock, R. (2009). Exhaustion of the chloroplast protein synthesis capacity by massive expression of a highly stable protein antibiotic. *The Plant Journal,.* Vol.57, No.3, (February 2009), pp. 436–445., ISSN 1365-313X

O'Hagan, D.T. & Rappuoli R. (2004). Novel approaches to vaccine delivery. *Pharmaceutical Research,* Vol.21, No.4, pp. 1519-1530, ISSN 0724-8741

Paintsil, J.; Müller, M.; Picken, M.; Gissmann, L. & Zhou, J. (1996). Carboxyl terminus of bovine papillomavirus type-1 L1 protein is not required for capsid formation. *Virology*, Vol.223, No.1, (September 1996), pp. 238–244, ISSN 0042-6822

Palmer, K.E.; Benko, A.; Doucette, S.A.; Cameron, T.I.; Foster, T.; Hanley, K.M., McCormick, A.A.; McCulloch, M.; Pogue G.P.; Smith, M.L. & Christensen, N.D. (2006). Protection of rabbits against cutaneous papillomavirus infection using recombinant tobacco mosaic virus containing L2 capsid epitopes. *Vaccine*, Vol.24, No. 26, (May 2006), pp. 5516–5525, ISSN 0264-410X

Pastrana, D.V.; Buck, C.B.; Pang, Y.Y.; Thompson, C.D.; Castle, P.E.; FitzGerald, P.C.; Kruger Kjaer, S.; Lowy, D.R. & Schiller, J.T.(2004). Reactivity of human sera in a sensitive, high-throughput pseudovirus-based papillomavirus neutralization assay for HPV16 and HPV18. *Virology*, Vol.321, No.2, (April 2004), pp. 205-216, ISSN 0042-6822

Pastrana, D.V.; Gambhira, R.; Buck, C.B.; Pang, Y.Y.; Thompson, C.D.; Culp, T.D.; Christensen, N.D.; Lowy, D.R.; Schiller, J.T. & Roden R.B. (2005). Cross-neutralization of cutaneous and mucosal Papillomavirus types with anti-sera to the amino terminus of L2. *Virology*, Vol.337, No.2, (July 2005), pp. 365–372, ISSN 0042-6822

Paz De la Rosa, G.; Monroy-García, A.; Mora-García, M.L.; Reynaga Peña, C.G.; Hernández-Montes, J.; Weiss-Steider B. & Gómez Lim, M.A. (2009). An HPV 16 L1-based chimeric human papillomavirus-like particles containing a string of epitopes produced in plants is able to elicit humoral and cytotoxic T-cell activity in mice. *Virology Journal*, Vol. 6, (January 2009), pp. 2 ISSN 1743-422X

Pokorná, D., Poláková, I., Kindlová, M., Dušková, M., Ludviková, V., Gabriel, P., Kutinová, L., Müller, M. & Šmahel M. (2009). Vaccination with human papillomavirus type 16-derived peptides using a tattoo device. *Vaccine*, Vol.27, No.27, (April 2009), pp. 3519-3529, ISSN ISSN 0264-410X

Rigano, M.M. & Walmsley, A.M. (2005). Expression systems and developments in plant-made vaccines. *Immunology and cell biology*, Vol.83, No.3, pp. 271-277, ISNN 0818-9641

Roden, R.B.; Armstrong, A.; Haderer, P.; Christensen, N.D.; Hubbert, N.L.; Lowy, D.R.; Schiller, J.T. & Kirnbauer, R. (1997a). Characterization of a humanpapillomavirus type 16 variant-dependent neutralizing epitope. *Journal of Virology*, Vol.71, No.8, (August 1997), pp. 6247-6252, ISSN 0022-538X

Roden, R.B.; Lowy, D.R. & Schiller, J.T. (1997b). Papillomavirus is resistant to desiccation. *The Journal of infectious diseases*, Vol.176, No.4, (October 1997), pp. 1076–1079, ISSN 0022-1899

Roden, R.B.; Yutzy, W.I.; Fallon, R.; Inglis, S; Lowy, D.R. & Schiller, J.T. (2000). Minor capsid protein of human genital papillomaviruses contains subdominant, cross-neutralizing epitope. *Virology*, Vol.270, No. 2, (May 2000), pp. 254 - 257, ISSN 0042-6822

Rose, R. C.; Lane, C.; Wilson, S.; Suzich J. A., Rybicki, E.P. & A. L. Williamson A. L. (1999). Oral vaccination of mice with human papillomavirus virus-like particles induces systemic virus-neutralizing antibodies. *Vaccine*, Vol.17, No.17, (April 1999), pp. 2129- 2135, ISSN 0264-410X

Ruhlman, T.; Verma, D.; Samson, N. & Daniell, H. (2010) The role of heterologous chloroplast sequence elements in transgene integration and expression. *Plant Physiology*, Vol.152, No.4., (April 2010) ,pp. 2088–2104, ISSN 1532-2548

Rybicki E.P. (2010). Plant-made vaccines for humans and animals. *Plant Biotechnology Journal,* Vol.8, No.5, (June 2010) ,pp. 620–637, ISSN 1467-7644

Sasagawa, T.; Tani, M.; Basha, W.; Rose, R.C.; Tohda, H.; Giga-Hama, Y.; Azar, K.K.; Yasuda, H.; Sakai, A. & Inoue, M. (2005). A human papillomavirus type 16 vaccine by oral delivery of L1 protein. *Virus Research*, Vol.110, No.1-2, (June 2005), pp. 81–90, ISSN 0168-1702

Schadlich, L.; Senger, T.; Gerlach, B.; Mucke, N.; Klein, C.; Bravo, I.G.; Müller, M. & Gissmann, L. (2009). Analysis of modified human papillomavirus type 16 L1 capsomeres: the ability to assemble into larger particles correlates with higher immunogenicity. *Journal of Virology*, Vol.83, No.15, (August 2009), pp. 7690–7705, ISSN 0022-538X

Shank-Retzlaff, M.L.; Zhao, Q.; Anderson, C; Hamm, M.; High, K.; Nguyen, M.; Wang, F.; Wang, N.; Wang, B.; Wang, Y.; Washabaugh, M.; Sitrin, R. & Shi, L. (2006). Evaluation of the thermal stability of Gardasil. *Human Vaccines*, Vol.2, No.4, (July-August 2006), pp. 147–154, ISSN 1554-8600

Sheets, E.E.; Urban, R.G.; Crum, C.P.; Hedley, M.L.; Politch, J.A.; Gold, M.A.; Muderspach, L.I.; Cole, G.A. & Crowley-Nowick, P.A. (2003). Immunotherapy of human cervical high-grade cervical intraepithelial neoplasia with microparticle-delivered human papillomavirus 16 E7 plasmid DNA. *American journal of obstetrics and gynecology*, Vol.188, No.4, (April 2003), pp. 916-926, ISSN 0002-9378

Shi, L.; Sanyal, G.; Ni, A.; Luo, Z.; Doshna, S.; Wang, B.; Graham, T. L.; Wang, N. & Volkin, D. B. (2005). Stabilization of human papillomavirus virus-like particles by non-ionic surfactants. *Journal of pharmaceutical sciences,* Vol.94, No.7, (July 2005), pp. 1538-1551, ISSN 0022-3549

Schiller, J.T. & Nardelli-Haefliger, D. (2006). Chapter 17: Second generation HPV vaccines to prevent cervical cancer. *Vaccine*, Vol. 24, Suppl 3, (August 2006), pp. S3/147-153, ISSN 0264-410X

Schwarz, T.F. (2009). Clinical update of the AS04-adjuvanted human papillomavirus-16/18 cervical cancer vaccine, Cervarix. *Advances in therapy.* Vol.26, No.11, (November 2009), pp.983-998, ISSN 0741-238X

Shinje, G.; Neil, D.C.; John, W.K. & Jenson, A.B. (1991). Comparison of neutralization of BPV-1 infection of C127 cells and bovine fetal skin xenografts. *International journal of cancer,* Vol.49, No.2, (September 1991), pp. 285–289, ISSN 0020-7136

Slupetzky, K..; Shafti-Keramat, S.; Lenz, P.; Brandt, S.; Grassauer, A.; Sara, M. & Kirnbauer, R. (2001). Chimeric papillomavirus-like particles expressing a foreign epitope on capsid surface loops. *The Journal of general virology*. 82, No.Pt 11, (November 2001), pp. 2799-2804, ISSN 0022-1317

Šmídková, M.; Müller, M.; Thönes, N.; Puiko, K.; Angelisová, P.; Velemínský J. & Angelis K.J. (2010). Transient expression of human papillomavirus type 16 virus-like particles in tobacco and tomato using a tobacco rattle virus expression vector. *Biologia Plantarum,*Vol. 54, No.3, (September 2009), pp. 451-460, ISSN 0006-3134

Stanley, M. (2010). Prospects for new human papillomavirus vaccines. *Current opinion in infectious diseases,* Vol.23, No.1, (February 2010), pp. 70-75, ISSN 0951-7375

Thönes, N. & Müller, M. (2007). Oral immunization with different assembly forms of the HPV 16 major capsid protein L1 induces neutralizing antibodies and cytotoxic T-lymphocytes. *Virology*, Vol.369, No.2, (September 2007), pp. 375–388, ISSN 0042-6822

Thönes, N.; Herreiner, A.; Schadlich, L.; Piuko, K. & Müller, M. (2008). A Direct Comparison of Human Papillomavirus Type 16 L1 Particles Reveals a Lower Immunogenicity of Capsomeres than Viruslike Particles with Respect to the Induced Antibody Response. *Journal of Virology*, Vol.82, No.11, (Jun 2008), pp. 5472–5485, ISSN 0022-538X

van Ree, R.; Cabanes-Macheteau, M.; Akkerdaas, J.; Milazzo, J.P.; Loutelier-Bourhis, C.; Rayon, C.; Villalba, M.; Koppelman, S.; Aalberse, R.; Rodriguez, R.; Faye, L. & Lerouge P. (2000). Beta(1,2)-xylose and alpha(1,3)-fucose residues have a strong contribution in IgE binding to plant glycoallergens. *The Journal of biological chemistry*, Vol.275, No.15, (April 2000), pp.114751-11458, ISSN 0021-9258

Varsani, A.; Williamson, A.L.; deVilliers, D., Becker, I., Christensen, N.D. & Rybicki E.P. (2003a). Chimeric human papillomavirus type 16 (HPV-16) L1 particles presenting the common neutralizing epitope for the L2 minor capsid protein of HPV-6 and HPV-16. *Journal of Virology*, Vol.77, No.15, (August 2003), pp. 8386–8393, ISSN 0022-538X

Varsani, A.; Williamson, A.L.; Rose, R.C.; Jaffer, M. & Rybicki, E.P. (2003b). Expression of Human papillomavirus type 16 major capsid protein in transgenic Nicotiana tabacum cv. Xanthi. *Archives of virology*, Vol.148, No., (9), (September 2003), pp. 1771–1786, ISSN 0304-8608

Varsani, A.; Williamson, A.L.; Stewart, D. & Rybicki, E.P. (2006). Transient expression of Human papillomavirus type 16 L1 protein in Nicotiana benthamiana using an infectious tobamovirus vector. *Virus research*, Vol.120, No. 1-2, (March 2006), pp. 91-96, ISSN 0168-1702

Velasquez, L.S.; Shira, S.; Berta, A.N.; Kilbourne, J.; Medi, B.M.; Tizard, I.; Ni, Y.; Arntzen, C.J. & Herbst-Kralovetz, M.M. (2011). Intranasal delivery of Norwalk virus-like particles formulated in an in situ gelling, dry powder vaccine. Vaccine, Vol.29, No. 32., (June 2011), pp. 5221– 5231, ISSN 0264-410X

Villa, L.L.; Costa, R.L.; Petta, C.A.; Andrade, R.P.; Ault, K.A.; Giuliano, A.R.; Wheeler, C.M.; Koutsky, L.A.; Malm, C.; Lehtinen, M.; Skjeldestad, F.E.; Olsson, S.E.; Steinwall, M.; Brown, D.R.; Kurman, R.J.; Ronnett, B.M.; Stoler, M.H.; Ferenczy, A.; Harper, D.M.; Tamms, G.M.; Yu, J.; Lupinacci, L.; Railkar, R.; Taddeo, F. J.; Jansen, K. U.; Esser, M.T.; Sings, H.L.; Saah, A. J. & Barr, E. (2005). Prophylactic quadrivalent human papillomavirus (types 6, 11, 16, and 18) L1 virus-like particle vaccine in young women: a randomised double-blind placebo-controlled multicentre phase II efficacy trial. *The lancet oncology*, Vol.6, No.5, (May 2005), pp. 271-278, ISSN 1470-2045

Villa, L. (2011). HPV prophylactic vaccination: The first years and what to expect from now. *Cancer Letters*, Vol.305, No.2, (Jun 2011), pp. 106–112, ISSN 0304-3835

Wagner, H. & Proksh, A. (1985). Immunostimulatory drugs of fungi and higher plants. In: Wagner H, editor. Economic and medicinal plant research, pp. 113-153, Academic Press, New York

Waheed, M.T.; Thönes, N.; Müller, M.; Hassan, S.W.; Razavi, M.; Lössl, E.; Kaul, H.P. & Lössl, A.G. (2011a). Transplastomic expression of a modified human papillomavirus L1 protein leading to the assembly of capsomeres in tobacco: a step towards cost-effective second-generation vaccines. *Transgenic research,* Vol.20, No.2, (Jun 2011), pp. 271–282, ISSN 0962-8819

Waheed, M.T.; Thönes, N.; Müller, M.; Hassan, S.W.; Gottschamel, J.; Lössl, E., Kaul H.P. & Lössl A.G. (2011b). Plastid expression of a double-pentameric vaccine candidate containing human papillomavirus-16 L1 antigen fused with LTB as adjuvant: transplastomic plants show pleiotropic phenotypes. *Plant Biotechnology Journal* , Vol.9, No.6, (March 2011), pp. 651-660, ISSN 1467-7652

Wakabayashi, M.T.; Da Silva, D.M.; Potkul, R.K. & Kast, W.M. (2002). Comparison of human papillomavirus type 16 L1 chimeric virus-like particles versus L1/L2 chimeric virus-like particles in tumor prevention. *Intervirology*, Vol.45, No.4-6 , (April 2002) ,pp. 300–307, ISSN 0300-5526

Warzecha, H.; Mason, H.S.; Lane, C.; Tryggvesson, A.; Rybicki, E.; Williamson, A.L.; Clements, J.D. & Rose, R.C. (2003). Oral immunogenicity of human papillomavirus-like particles expressed in potato. *Journal of Viroogy*, Vol.77, No. 16, (August 2003) pp. 8702-8711, ISSN 0022-538X

Wright, T.C.; Bosch, F.X.; Franco, E.L.; Cuzick, J.; Schiller, J.T.; Garnett, G.P. & Meheus, A. (2006). Chapter 30: HPV vaccines and screening in the prevention of cervical cancer; conclusions from a 2006 workshop of international experts. *Vaccine,* Vol. 24, Suppl 3, (August 2006) pp. S3251-261, ISSN 0264-410X

Xie Q.; Zhou Z.X.; Li Z.L. & Zeng Y. (2011). Transforming activity of a novel mutant of HPV16 E6E7 fusion gene. *Virologica Sinica*, Vol.26, No.3, (Jun 2011), pp. 206-213, ISSN 1995-820X

Xu, Y.F.; Zhang, Y.Q.; Xu, X.M. & Song, G.X. (2006). Papillomavirus virus like particles as vehicles for the delivery of epitopes or genes. *Archives of virology,* Vol.151, No.11, (November 2006) pp. 2133-2148, ISSN 0304-8608

Yamamoto, S.; Kiyono, H.; Yamamoto, M.; Imaoka, K.; Fujihashi, K.; Van Ginkel, F.W.; Noda, M.; Takeda, Y. & McGhee, J.R. (1997). A nontoxic mutant of cholera toxin elicits Th2-type responses for enhanced mucosal immunity. *Proceedings of the National Academy of Science USA*, Vol. 94, No.10, (May 1997), pp. 5267–5272, ISSN 0027-8424

Yang, R.; Murillo, F.M.; Cui, H.; Blosser, R.; Uematsu, S.; Takeda, K.; Akira, S.; Viscidi, R.P. & Roden, R.B. (2004). Papillomavirus-like particles stimulate murine bone marrow-derived dendritic cells to produce alpha interferon and Th1 immune responses via MyD88. *Journal of Virology,* Vol.78, No.20, (October 2004), pp. 11152–11160, ISSN 0022-538X

Yuan, H.; Estes, P.A.; Chen, Y.; Newsome, J.; Olcese, V.A.; Garcea, R.L. & Schlegel, R. (2001). Immunization with a pentameric L1 fusion protein protects against papillomavirus infection. *Journal of vorology*, Vol.75, No.17, (September 2001), pp. 7848–7853, ISSN 0022-538X

zur Hausen, H. (1996). Papillomavirus infections - a major cause of human cancers. *Biochimica et biophysica acta*, Vol.1288, No.2, (October 1996), pp. F55-F78, ISSN 0006-3002

http://www.ircm.qc.ca/LARECHERCHE/axes/Biologie/Virologie/Pages/Projets.aspx

Development of Vaccines and Gene Therapy Against HPV Infection and Cervical Cancer

Zoraya De Guglielmo Cróquer[1]
and Armando Rodríguez Bermúdez[2]
[1]*Instituto de Oncología y Hematología, Laboratorio de Genética Molecular, Ciudad Universitaria, Calle Minerva, Los Chaguaramos, Caracas*
[2]*Universidad Central de Venezuela, Instituto de Investigaciones Económicas y Sociales, Ciudad Universitaria, Los Chaguaramos, Caracas*
Venezuela

1. Introduction

From the establishment of etiologic relationship between HPV and cervical cancer, researchers have emphasized the importance of prevention by education of people, especially teenagers. This virus is associated with diseases of the cutaneous and mucosal human epithelia, including benign warts and invasive cancer that affect different anatomical regions as skin, cervix, vagina, vulva, anus, penis, head and neck. Controversial evidence suggests a relationship between HPV infection and breast cancer (de Villiers et al., 2005; Khan et al., 2005; Heng et al., 2009) (Table 1).

Clinical manifestation	HPV types often detectable
Verrucae vulgares, verrucae palmares et plantares	1, 2, 4
Verrucae planare	3, 10
Butcher´s warts	7
Squamous cell carcinoma of the finger, Bowen´s disease	16
Epidermodysplasia verruciformis (EV)	3, 5, 8
EV- squamous cell carcinoma	5, 8
Condylomata acuminata	6, 11
High grade-squamous intraepithelial neoplasias and invasive carcinomas of the anogenital tract	16
Bowenoid papulosis, erythroplasia of Queyrat	16
Buschke-Lowenstein tumor	6, 11
Respiratory Papillomatosis	6, 11
Heck´s disease	13, 32
Head and neck cancers (larynx, tonsils, tongue, sinuse, lung)	16, 18, 6, 11
Breast cancer?	16, 18

Table 1. Clinical manifestations and associated HPV types (taken and modified of Handisurya et al., 2009).

Noted that a variety of diseases caused by HPV is largely due to viral tropism, i.e., the preference of a certain type of HPV by a tissue or cell group in particular, depending on factors of virus and host, mainly receptors, transcriptional activators, enhancers, and tissue-specific promoters (Graham, 2010). Based on the tropism, HPV has been classified into two main phylogenetic genera, the α-HPV and the β-HPV, which correspond to the mucosal and cutaneous infective HPV, respectively (de Villiers et al., 2004). The temporal organization of the virus replication cycle is also different between different HPV types perhaps reflecting differences in sites of infection and transmission modes.

Traditionally, cancer and associated lesions have been treated with surgery, radiotherapy and chemotherapy, these treatments produced widely known adverse effects (American Cancer Society, 2007; Instituto Nacional del Cáncer, 2008). However, many efforts have been done in order to find effective preventive and curative options less invasive and with minimal or no side effects. These options are mainly based on molecular biology techniques to develop vaccines and the use of molecules that stimulate the immune and cytotoxic response against HPV infection and cervical cancer. The development of these vaccines and therapeutic procedures is based on *in vitro* culture and knowledge of the life cycle, genome and regulation of viral transcription, which has allowed the identification of potential targets to control genes expression in infectious and / or neoplastic processes (Table 2).

Genome region	Gen/ protein	Expression site	Function
Early	E1	Basal, parabasal and intermediate cells of the host	ATP- dependent DNA helicase; unique enzyme expressed by the virus, which is essential for viral replication
	E2		Helps E1 to locate the origin of replication in LCR, cell cycle and apoptosis regulation
	E4		Cell Cycle arrest, virion assembly, remodels cytokeratin network
	E5		Control of cell growth and differentiation, immune modulation
	E6		Inhibits apoptosis and differentiation
	E7		Cell cycle control, controls centrosome duplication
Late	L1	Superficial cells	Major capsid protein
	L2		Minor capsid protein, recruits L1, virus assembly
Long control region (LCR)			Binds many cellular transcription activators, confers keratinocyte specificity to transcription

Table 2. Role of HPV genome regions

2. Prophylactic vaccines to prevent HPV infection

Prophylactic vaccines currently exist to prevent the spread of HPV infections; these vaccines have the objective to create antigens capable to induce neutralizing antibodies that prevent the entry of virus into host cells. They are based on preventing infection of HPV types most prevalent around the world: types 6 and 11, of low oncogenic risk, associated with the formation of warts and benign condylomata, and types 16 and 18 of high cancer risk, associated with cancerous and precancerous lesions, which are responsible for approximately 70% of all cervical cancers worldwide (Muñoz et al., 2004).Initially it was suggested to produce a vaccine based on attenuated virus, but its implementation and evaluation in humans was a very high risk due to the presence of oncogenic viral DNA; in addition the growth of virus in *in vitro* culture had been limited until recently when a researchers group managed to establish a reproducible and highly efficient production of HPV type 18 in human keratinocytes, which has a potential value for establishing research models of *ex vivo* viral expression (Castellsagué et al., 2006; Wang et al., 2009).

Moreover, although the studies on the immunology of HPV have shown antibodies against many different viral products, the best characterized and most type-specific antibodies are those directed against conformational epitopes of the L1 capsid protein. In the 90's it was possible to produce *in vitro*, genetically engineered virus-like particles or VLPs, which consist of L1 or L1 + L2 recombinant protein, obtained by introducing one or both genes, respectively, in cultures of eukaryotic cells (yeast, insect or bacteria). These recombinant proteins have the ability to self-assemble to form three-dimensional structures that are morphological and antigenically identical to the original HPV virions, but not containing the viral genome, so these structures can not replicate or cause infection or cancer (Muñoz et al., 2008).

There have been studies in experimental animal models and humans, where there was a good tolerance to systemic vaccination with L1- VLPs, and induction of serum antibody titers of at least 40 times higher than the titles produced in an natural infection (Lowy & Frazer, 2003). The first large multicenter, double-blind study, with phase III results, was published in 2002, on a monovalent vaccine developed by Merck Laboratories HPV type 16 (Brull & Carrera, 2005). This company created another quadrivalent vaccine called Gardasil, synthesized in the yeast *Saccharomyces cerevisiae*, based on L1- VLPs of oncogenic types most commonly found in cervical dysplasia (HPV types 16 and 18) and non-oncogenic types responsible for approximately 90% of warts genitals and recurrent respiratory papillomatosis (types 6 and 11), which is considered to act on two different hyperproliferative diseases (Schiller & Lowy, 2006). It was approved by the U.S. Food and Drug Administration (FDA) in 2006 and is administered in 3 doses, spread over 6 months (0, 2 and 6 months). Follow-up studies for 3 ½ years after vaccination showed an effectiveness of 94% in persistent infection with HPV types 16, as well as 100% in preventing high-grade intraepithelial lesions associated with types 16 and 18, and prevention of genital lesions related to HPV types 6 and 11 (Mao et al., 2006; Villa et al., 2005). The efficacy against vulvar and vaginal neoplasia grade II and III was 72-100% (Joura et al., 2007). In well designed clinical trials in young women aged 15-25 years who were HPV 16/18 seronegative and DNA negative to 14 HPV high-risk types, high levels of immunogenicity and protection were sustained for follow-up periods of up to 8.4 years (McKeage & Romanowski, 2011).

Each 0.5-mL dose contains 20 μg HPV 6 L1 protein, 40 μg HPV 11 L1 protein, 40 μg HPV 16 L1 protein, and 20 μg HPV 18 L1 protein. VLPs are adsorbed on an aluminum-containing adjuvant. Each 0.5-mL dose contains 225 μg amorphous aluminum hydroxyphosphate sulfate. The formulation also includes sodium chloride, L-histidine, polysorbate 80, sodium borate, and water for injection. The quadrivalent HPV vaccine contains no thimerosal or antibiotics. The vaccine should be stored at 2°C--8°C (36°F--46°F) and not frozen.

GlaxoSmithKline laboratories developed a bivalent vaccine called Cervarix for HPV types 16 and 18, produced in insect cells with baculovirus as expression system, which is also administered in three doses (0, 1 and 6 months). Studies reported 100% efficacy in preventing infections with involved HPV types, with an almost absolute immunogenicity for 4 ½ years after vaccination and the detection of antibody titers from 16 to 26 times higher than detected after natural infection (McKeage & Romanowski, 2011; Bhatla et al., 2010; Muñoz et al., 2008; Harper et al., 2004; Kahn, 2005).

Both vaccines (Gardasil and Cervarix) use aluminum-based adjuvants, which reduces the dose required to induce antibodies peak titer and helps to stabilize the vaccine during storage (Schiller & Lowy, 2006). Overall adverse effects reported in vaccination protocols are limited and include reactions at the injection site (erythema, pain and swelling) and systemic adverse effects (headache, fever and nausea) which were of middle nature, transitory and common for individuals receiving the vaccine or placebo (Paavonen et al., 2007).

Whereas the onset of sexual activity during adolescence, the FDA approved the vaccine Gardasil for girls and women aged between 9 to 26 years, while the Advisory Committee on Immunization Practices of the USA Center for Disease Control and Prevention (ACIP) recommended vaccination in females aged between 11 to 26 years and added males to the population who can benefit from Gardasil vaccination (FDA, 2010).

There has been controversy regarding the vaccination of women alone or the inclusion of men. In this regard, it has been noted that vaccinating girls aged 12 years old, can reduce cases of cervical cancer associated with types 16 and HPV 18 in about 95% and the introduction of vaccination in children would increase this figure three points (Taira et al., 2004). We must also take into account the potential role of vector that man can exert on the transmission of HPV infection, so the inclusion of the male population in vaccination programs could contribute to optimal control of transmission (Tirado-Gómez et al., 2005).

Currently the vaccine is not recommended for pregnant women. The long-term effects of the vaccine on fertility are not known, but no effects are anticipated. Although studies on the toxicity to the fetus are inconclusive, FDA has classified the HPV vaccine as a pregnancy Category B medication, meaning that the medication does not appear to cause harm to the fetus in animal studies. Initially, the trials for Gardasil and Cervarix excluded pregnant women. Pregnancy was determined by a sensitive human chorionic gonadotropin (HCG) test on the day of expected vaccination. However, some women became pregnant during the few weeks or months following the receipt of a vaccine or placebo injection. Overall, the proportions of pregnancies with an adverse outcome were comparable in subjects who received Gardasil and subjects who received placebo. However, the clinical trials had a relatively small sample size. Though receiving the HPV vaccine while pregnant is generally considered safe, it is still recommended to wait until after pregnancy to get the vaccine (American Cancer Society, 2008).

Vaccination at early age has led to concerns of parents, researchers and health specialists because of the need to talk with children about sexuality and sexually transmitted diseases, the vaccination charges received by children, the possibility that immunization may lead to the adoption of risky sexual behaviors and concerns about the safety of vaccines (Kahn,

2005). Some researchers have pointed out as risk of vaccination the possible selection of not included HPV types in vaccines or the increase in the prevalence of rare oncogenic HPV types, which can only be known over time, after the mass vaccination had been effective.

Other weaknesses of the prophylactic vaccine against HPV is that it only protects against specific HPV types, leaving out a wide range of viral types, although rare, are also present, and have also been reported conflicting results regarding the existence of cross protection. In addition, the vaccine is preventive (not cure existing infections or injuries) and there is a low percentage of cervical cancer and precursor lesions in which no association has been established with HPV, existing other factors associated with the development of this malignancy, as exposure to mutagens, genetic susceptibility, hormonal status and immune status (Tirado-Gómez et al., 2005; del Amo et al., 2005); unknown the duration of protection provided by the vaccine, it may be necessary to administer a booster dose (Brull & Carrera, 2005; Diestro Tejeda et al., 2007). In this regard, an evaluation showed that the quadrivalent vaccine provides strong and sustained protection against condiloma and vulvovaginal and cervical low grade neoplasia, related to types 6, 11, 16 and 18, for more than four years. The same study suggests that the effectiveness of the vaccine might be less in cases where coinfection with HPV types absent in the vaccine is present (Dillner, 2010).

It is important to take into account the high cost of the vaccines listed, however, this is not comparable to the loss of life or money spending for the treatments of lesions associated with HPV infection. Since vaccines are prophylactic and only provide preventive (no therapeutic) effect, most benefits are gained by vaccinating before infection occurs, ideally before the onset of sexual intercourse. In this sense, the ACIP has recommended the introduction of HPV vaccine in national immunization programs of governments worldwide. It is therefore essential to determine the HPV types circulating in each region and assess the potential impact of preventive vaccination in the respective populations.

Various researchers have emphasized that even with the globalization of preventive vaccination, screening schemes should continue due to multifactorial nature of cervical cancer, only 2 of 15 oncogenic HPV types are included in the vaccine and vaccination programs initially cover women into a limited range of ages, anticipating that at least during 2-3 decades unvaccinated sexually active women remain at risk for the disease (Giuliano, 2007; Stanley, 2008; Hutchinson & Klein, 2008).

The efficacy of L2 vaccination has been proved in pre-clinical and clinical studies. Natural infection does not induce anti-L2 antibodies and many L2 epitopes are not on the virus surface, but during the infection cellular protease furin removes an L2 N-terminal sequence rendering L2 accessible on the capsid surface and displaying the L2-neutralizing epitopes. The L2-neutralizing epitope was inserted on the surfaces of VLPs increasing the titers of neutralizing antibodies approximately 10-fold. A synthetic L2 lipopeptide with concatenated multitype L2 fusion proteins from different papillomavirus types have already been utilized in inducing cross-neutralizing antibodies against several clinically relevant HPV types. This polymeric L2 approach gives rise to antisera, that neutralize at higher titers, not only the types included in the multimeric immunogen but also other types. So, immunization against L2 could be a candidate prophylactic pan-human papillomaviruses vaccine (Alphs et al., 2008; Jagu et al., 2009).

3. Therapeutic vaccines and gene therapy for treatment of cervical cancer

Another line in the study of cervical cancer treatment has pursued in the implementation of therapeutic vaccines and / or gene therapy to cure existing cases, through the transfer of DNA, inserting the normal gene or gene expression regulation.

Therapeutic vaccines are composed of peptides homologous to the viral proteins, as indicated in the treatment of dysplasia and invasive cervical cancer or as adjuvant therapy for locally recurrent or metastatic (Diestro Tejada et al., 2007). DNA vaccines have also been developed, which are considered as stable, safe, can be prepared in large quantities and repeatedly administered without significant adverse effects. In addition, the DNA tends to be preserved in the receptor cells, ensuring long-term expression of the encoded antigen and reinforcing the maintenance of immunological memory.

Generally, the immune response generated from DNA alone is weak, so it has been tested the adjuvant effect of several molecules, and the combination of specific genes (Kim et al., 2004). However, vaccines have been developed based on naked DNA, viral or bacterial vector, tumor cells and dendritic modified cells.

Other molecules in use for gene therapy of cervical cancer are cytokines which has immunoregulatory effect that promotes maturation, activation and migration of effector cells of the immune response to the tumor site. Of particular interest are interferons, interleukin 2 or IL-2 (which activates T cells, NK cells, macrophages and the release of other cytokines) and the aforementioned IL-12 (whose anti-tumor effect individually or in combination with *E6* and *E7* is dependent on the activation of CD8 + cytotoxic T lymphocytes and NK cells at the site of immunization). Intratumoral administration of these molecules significantly reduced the progression of HPV-associated tumors and inhibited recurrent tumor formation after being removed by surgery (Frechtel, 2005; Bubenik et al., 2003).

In 1999, a group of researchers developed and tested the vaccine TA-GW based on the L2 and E7 fusion proteins of HPV type 6, with Alhydrogel as adjuvant, for the treatment of condilomas, reporting immunogenicity and cure in approximately 62% of lesions 8 weeks after vaccination, without considerables adverse effects (Lacey et al., 1999).

In 2002, Kaufmann et al. performed one of the first multicenter and multinational studies with a recombinant vaccine, TA-HPV, consisting of attenuated vaccinia virus genetically engineered to express the E6 and E7 proteins of HPV types 16 and 18. The protocol included two doses of the vaccine in patients with early-stage cervical cancer, and the induction of humoral and cell-mediated response with low side and/or toxic effects was observed.

In 2004, Gutierrez et al. evaluated the effect of the recombinant vaccine MVAE2, consisting of attenuated vaccinia virus and the E2 gene of HPV, in squamous intraepithelial lesions of high and low grade. Treatment consisted in the administration of six doses, one every week, injected directly into the cervix. During the observation of treatment results, the reduction of injuries was monitored by colposcopy and histological analysis. The immune response was determined by measuring of antibodies againts MVAE2 and analysis of cytotoxic lymphocyte activity against cancer cells with oncogenic human papillomavirus. The presence of viral DNA and viral load were determined using the Hybrid Capture method (Digene).

After treatment it was possible the elimination of pre-cancerous lesions and even cancer (cancer *in situ*), with an efficiency of 95% in the first and 40% in the latter. All patients developed antibodies to the vaccine and a specific cytotoxic response against HPV-transformed cells. These results were compared with those obtained in a similar group of patients treated with cryosurgery, a technique that is able to eliminate low-grade lesions in all patients; but there was not observed cytotoxic activity against cancer cells.

As for of the virus detection, there was no evidence in 50% of the treated sample after treatment and in the remaining 50% was only detected 10% of the original viral load. Assessments of MVAE2 vaccine in women with cervical cancer are in Phase III, consisting of a multicenter study in 250 patients with cancer *in situ* in the Juarez Hospital of the Ministry of Health of Mexico.

This vaccine was also tested in men for the treatment of urethral condilomas, showing the stimulation of the immune response against HPV and regression of lesions in 93% of cases, 4 weeks after therapy. These assessments are in phase II. The results are promising and show that local therapeutic vaccination with MVAE2 is an effective tool for stimulating the immune response to HPV infection and the presence of virus-transformed cells, as well as regression of high and low grade cancer lesions (Albarran y Carvajal et al., 2007).

On the other hand, researchers have highlighted the potential utility of gene gun used in the administration of DNA-based vaccines as part of the antigenic systems strategy for the control of cancer and infectious diseases, projecting itself as an important tool in antigen-specific immunotherapy (Kim et al., 2008a).

In the particular case of uterine cancer, Kim et al. (2008b), in a mouse model, used a Helio gun to dispense gold microparticles coated with E6 DNA of HPV type 16 attached to an expression regulator of major histocompatibility complex class I molecules (human calreticulin). They observed an increased cellular and humoral immune response and antitumor effect, from the increased processing and presentation of antigens to T cells, together with the regression of tumors, enhanced antigen-specific memory and prolonged survival of vaccinated mice. The authors highlight the potential clinical benefits of this therapeutic strategy in humans, which may include co-administration of molecules with other properties, e.g. DNA encoding anti-apoptotic or angiogenic proteins (Kim et al., 2004; Kim et al., 2008b).

This vaccine was combined with E7 and L2 proteins of HPV, also observed significant therapeutic effects against E6/E7 expressing tumor cells, and generate a potent L2-antigen specific response, thereby protecting against pseudovirion infection. These results highlight the potential clinical benefits of this vaccine (Kim et al., 2008b).

Ahn et al. (2004) performed in mice, direct intratumoral injection of an adenoviral vaccine carrier *E7* sequence of HPV type 16 and interleukin 12 (IL-12) as adjuvant, which induces cellular immune responses for protection against tumor formation. They observed partial or complete regression of the tumors and long-term immunity against recurrence of the malignancy, and this effect was much greater with the vaccine formed with the all components, compared with the injection of any of the separate components. The IL-12 is one of the most widely used cytokine on gene therapy against cervical cancer, due to its effect in inhibiting tumor growth and experimental metastasis, dependent on the activation of NK cells.

However, Sin (2009) reported that IL-12 and *E7* HPV type 16 cDNA-based vaccine lost its antitumor and immunoprotective effect when it was combined with nitric oxide (used and known for its adjuvant effect in routine protocols for vaccination), which demonstrates an immunosuppressive effect of the compound (nitric oxide) in the system used.

Peng et al. (2010) in a preclinical model about recurrent respiratory papillomatosis (RRP), generated a DNA vaccine that encodes the HPV-11 *E6* and *E7* genes in a pcDNA3 backbone plasmid. Vaccinated mice generated strong CD8+ T cell response against the $E6_{aa44-51}$ peptide, which is presented by the major histocompatibility complex class I molecule. Results revealed that the $E6_{aa44-51}$ peptide contains the most immunogenic region for HPV-11 viral type, making it a candidate for the development and evaluation of novel vaccine strategies targeting the RRP patient population.

On the other hand, it has been established that an L1 molecule of various HPV types contains several cysteine residues at markedly similar relative positions, strongly suggesting that these cysteine residues play important roles in the structure and function of the HPV capsids, especially in the viral capsid assembly. Ishii et al. (2007) , in an *in vitro* model (HeLa cells), observed that HPV type 16-pseudovirions lost their infectivity after incubation with thiol-reactive reagents that bound to the free thiol of pseudovirions major capsid protein L1, due to conformational changes that result in the inhibition of the entry and trafficking of this molecules. Therefore, the authors suggest that these reagents might function as practical inhibitors of HPV infection. These reagents could be used in drug design or in combination with preventive and/or therapeutic strategies. It would be necessary further evaluation on this topic.

3.1 Antisense molecules and RNA interference in cervical cancer treatment

Another line of investigation for the treatment of cervical cancer by gene therapy has been successful in testing antisense molecules as the ribozyme R434 (which, through its catalytic activity, specifically destroys the HPV types 16 *E6* and *E7* mRNA and prevents the growth of immortalized cells in the presence of virus), antisense oligonucleotides (AS-ODN) that hybridize with viral messenger blocking viral translation, and interference RNA (RNAi) (Álvarez Salas, 2006; Hamada et al., 1996; Hall & Alexander, 2003) (table 3).

Both technologies, antisense and RNAi, consist of gene silencing (interruption or suppression of the expression of a gene at transcriptional or translational levels).

Agent	Mechanism	Result
Most drugs	Bind to target protein	Protein inhibition
RNase H-independent ODNs	Hybridize to target mRNA	Inhibition of translation of the target protein
RNase H-dependent ODNs	Hybridize to target mRNA	Degradation of the mRNA by RNase H
Ribozymes and DNA enzymes	Catalyze cleavage of target mRNA	Degradation of the mRNA
siRNA	Hybridize to target mRNA by its antisense strand and guide it into endoribonuclease enzyme complex RISC	Degradation of the mRNA

Table 3. Comparison of different gene silencing strategies.

The second, based on double-stranded RNA has proven to be more powerful than the first, based on single-stranded RNA (Mao et al., 2007).

The antisense oligonucleotides have shown effectiveness in inhibiting the expression of *E6* and *E7* oncogenes, and also produced the release and / or activation of molecules involved in defense mechanisms (such as cytochrome c and procaspases 3 and 9), the induction of apoptosis and inhibition of telomerase activity. However, it has been reported that these molecules are unstable and design and management are very expensive (Choo et al., 2000).

RNA interference (RNAi) is a process of RNA-based gene silencing, which relies on nucleotide sequence complementarity and is involved in the mobilization of transposable genetic elements, in defense mechanisms and in different cellular events (such as differentiation, metabolism , stress response, propagation and apoptosis). This natural RNA-dependent gene silencing process is controlled by the RNA-induced silencing complex (RISC) and is initiated by short double-RNA molecules in a cell´s cytoplasm, where they interact with the catalytic RISC component, protein argonauta, and the enzyme Dicer (Humayun et al., 2008) (figure 1).

This process occurs through effector molecules identified in many eukaryotes, called microRNAs (miRNAs), highly conserved in orthologous species, indicating their importance in basic cellular processes. miRNAs are endogenous short RNA molecules with space-time independents expression patterns that determine inhibition of translation or degradation of target mRNAs when complementarity is incomplete or perfect, respectively (Raia & Calin, 2011). Hence, this methodology has a potential therapeutic for various diseases, additionally it can be used in the evaluation of molecular and metabolic pathways. MiRNAs originate from populations of non-coding small RNAs (they are one of several small non-coding RNAs, including ribosomal RNA, transfer RNA and small nuclear RNA) resulting from transcription of DNA sequences by RNA polymerase II and form secondary structures hairpin loop type. Several investigators have found alterations of these molecules (particularly single nucleotide polymorphism or SNP) in all cancers studied to date and have indicated that miRNAs are expressed abnormally in these patologies and are involved in predisposition, development and progression of cancer, so they can be used for diagnostic and prognostic purposes. In this regard, miRNAs have been detected in body fluids, which favors its use as biomarkers, because their assessment would be less invasive compared with other conventional markers, such as Pap smears and biopsies. Also, they can become as tumor suppressor, inhibiting cancer development, and as oncogenes, stimulate their development, depending on its expression pattern (Patel & Sauter 2011, Vitale et al. 2011).

In the biogenesis of mature miRNAs, act two type III Rnases, Drosha and Dicer, which cut precursor RNAs in double-stranded RNA (dsRNA) molecules with a length of 21 to 25 nucleotides, which will separated to generate single strand molecules (Ketting et al., 2001). In addition to miRNAs, in the RNAi mechanism have also identified other endogenous small RNAs called short interfering RNAs (siRNA) which, like miRNAs, originate from endogenous complementary dsRNA transcripts, but have an exact length of 21 nucleotides and most interesting is that they can derive from mRNA-coding sequences, transposons and heterochromatin (Ghildiyal et al., 2008).

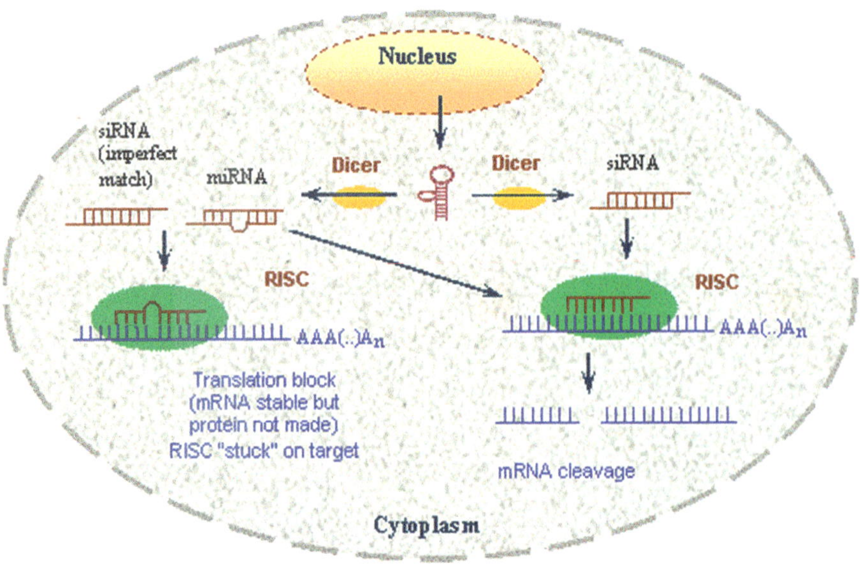

Fig. 1. A simplified model for the RNAi pathway.
The model has two steps, each involving ribonuclease enzyme. In the first step, the trigger RNA (either dsRNA or miRNA primary transcript) is processed into an short, interfering RNA (siRNA) by the RNase II enzymes Dicer and Drosha. In the second step, siRNAs are loaded into the effector complex RNA-induced silencing complex (RISC). The siRNA is unwound during RISC assembly and the single-stranded RNA hybridizes with mRNA target. Gene silencing is a result of nucleolytic degradation of the targeted mRNA by the RNase H enzyme Argonaute (Slicer). If the siRNA/mRNA duplex contains mismatches the mRNA is not cleaved. Moreover, gene silencing is a result of translational inhibition.
Source: National Center for Biotechnology Information
(http://www.ncbi.nlm.nih.gov/projects/genome/probe/doc/TechRnai.shtml)

siRNAs can be designed and artificially synthesized by chemical methods or by molecular cloning vectors and have been used to induce gene silencing *in vitro* and *in vivo* models, showing that perform the same biological functions as the natural miRNAs. The synthetic siRNAs can be transfected into mammalian cells by cationic lipofection, where they bind to liposomes as transport vehicle. In general, although it has achieved the efficient silencing of target genes, this strategy has a high cost and initially required the administration of multiple dose in mice, because a considerable percentage of the siRNAs is degraded by the action of endogenous endonucleases. Recently, the application of liposomes contained in Biogels, has overcome this limitation. The main disadvantage is that synthetic siRNAs have a short half-life after application (Sioud & Sorensen, 2003; Jiang et al., 2004).

It has been suggested that the efficiency of silencing by RNAi not only depends on the activity of RISC by itself, but also other factors such as accessibility of RISC to the target sequence (which is affected by RNA secondary structure and interaction of target mRNA with other molecules) and cleavage and release of cleaved RNA. Moreover, recent studies have shown that siRNA has nonspecific effects, ie in addition to its complementary target sequence (Schubert et al., 2005); studies of cervical cancer reported the silencing of the gene of interest and the production of inflammatory cytokines and interferon, simultaneously. This was particularly evident when using high concentrations of siRNA. That is the reason because the researchers recommend dose-response studies on a given system in order to select the lowest concentration of siRNA to observe the desired result, eliminating or reducing non-specific responses (Yamato et al., 2008). These nonspecific responses may also be caused by mismatches present in a siRNA in a tolerable level with its mRNA target (Haley et al., 2004). All these elements must be taken into account to design siRNA sequences and protocols in order to obtain the greatest effectiveness and specificity. Currently there is software that facilitates the design of these molecules.

The DNA sequence to silence can also be introduced into a vector that allows the transcription of siRNA. These vectors include siRNA expression plasmids, in which the DNA insert is placed under the control of the promoter of RNA Pol III (H1 gene or U6 gene) and form hairpin secondary structures that are processed by RISC and hybridize to target mRNA for its degradation (Brummelkamp et al., 2002).

Another type of widely used vectors are viruses, because they have a wide capacity of cell infection, especially retroviruses and adenoviruses. The former have the ability to integrate into the genome of replicating cells and therefore are useful for stable transfection of cancer cells. However, it has been reported that the transfection rate is low (de Felipe & Izquierdo, 2000). Adenoviruses have the ability to infect quiescent cells and dividing cells and produce a higher transfection rate than the retroviruses, but are more difficult to handle because of the size of its genome (Carette et al., 2004).

Noted that the use of this technology in the treatment of cervical cancer is possible because while *E6* and *E7* sequester the activities of p53 and pRb proteins in HPV-induced malignancies, copies of *p53* and *pRb* wild genes are usually conserved, which confers a reversible character of the malignancy, whereas reducing the expression of *E6* and *E7* in HPV-transformed cells could restore the activity of endogenous tumor suppressor and thus prevent the proliferation of these cells (Webster et al., 2000).

It has also been shown that RNAi technology against *E6* and *E7* genes induces senescence, apoptosis or inhibition of cancer cell growth in cell models (Webster et al., 2000; Butz et al., 2003; Niu et al., 2006) and destroys or suppresses the growth of tumors in mice injected directly with short molecules of RNAi (siRNA) against E6/E7 (Niu et al., 2006; Fujii et al., 2006). The first work on gene silencing by RNAi in uterine cancer was conducted by Jiang and Millner (2002). The researchers, in an *in vitro* model, administered synthetic siRNAs against *E6* and *E7* oncogenes of HPV 16. They observed the degradation of the *E6* and *E7* mRNA, with consequent expression of *p53*, decreased cell proliferation and induction of cell death by apoptosis. In particular, the induction of apoptosis or senescence in tumor cells has been effective since the introduction of the transcriptional regulator *E2* and the reduction or inhibition of *E6* and *E7* genes expression (Butz et al., 2003).

At the molecular level, it was observed that *E6* silencing induced accumulation of p53 cellular protein and transactivation of *p21* cell cycle control gene (Jiang & Milner, 2005). On the other hand, has been demonstrated the specificity of the technique since it was found that *E6* RNAi of HPV type 16 was less efficient in silencing *E6* gene in cells infected with other HPV types (Niu et al., 2006). These findings support the usefulness of this technique as a tool for investigating the mechanisms involved in the establishment and development of malignancy, as for the creation of therapies for treatment and healing.

It is noteworthy that there are studies that report the simultaneous silencing of *E6* and *E7*, while in others there was particular silencing of only one of these oncogenes, when using the mechanism of siRNA. It was explained that this is due to the existence of the bicistronic E6/E7, and simultaneous or individual silencing will depend largely on the particulars sequences of siRNA used and their positions of complementarity with the target mRNA (they may hybridize at a point where affect the expression of both genes or only one). In this sense, it has been suggested that alternative splicing events of *E6* and *E7* oncogenes of HPV preced events of silencing by siRNA (Lea et al., 2007).

Another target in the treatment of cervical cancer with RNAi is the telomerase *hTERT* gene, which has been cloned in several siRNA expression plasmids. This enzyme helps in maintaining the genomic stability by synthesizing the telomeres of eukaryotic chromosomes to protect them from degradation events, fusion and recombination. Overexpression of this enzyme void aging and cell death, as in most somatic cells telomerase activity is very low or absent, whereas in undifferentiated or immortal cells is considerable. Using siRNA plasmids for *hTERT in vivo* and *in vitro* models, it has been observed the target gene silencing, with the consequent decrease of telomerase activity, inhibition of cell proliferation, increased activity of caspase 3 and death of tumor cells by apoptosis (Wang et al., 2007).

It has also been observed that the application of siRNA technology increases the sensitivity of malignant cells to chemotherapy and radiotherapy. This has been demonstrated with cisplatin (study where *E6* and *E7* oncogenes were silenced), which can then be used in lower concentrations with the consequent reduction of its negative effects (Putral et al., 2005). The sensitivity of HeLa cells to radiotherapy increased with the *hTERT* gene silencing by siRNA, which allowed the establishment of a relationship between sensitivity to radiotherapy and telomerase activity in this type of cancer (Wang et al., 2007). This observation can be taken into account when designing treatment protocols for a given patient. Thus, the combination of siRNA with chemotherapy or radiotherapy may be synergistic in reducing cancer resistance to conventional therapies, which may promote recovery and / or survival with these therapies.

4. Conclusions

While it has been estimated the impact that preventive vaccination may have on the transmission of HPV infection and the development of cervical cancer and precursor lesions, is important to note the existence of other factors that may affect or influence the development of this pathology as well as existing cases prior to vaccination, so the effect of a preventive vaccine in the prevalence of cervical cancer may involve several decades. Moreover, prophylactic vaccines do not protect against infection (or malignancy) caused by other HPV types not contained in them, so cases of disease will still arise and require treatment.

Faced with these limitations of preventive vaccines, therapeutic vaccines based primarily on molecular resources and gene therapy are currently being evaluated and could become as an effective tool for the treatment of cervical cancer and low or high grade lesions, contributing together to preventive vaccines for a better control of this disease.

In this regard, studies carried out until to date about the effect of gene therapy on cervical cancer, project this technology as an useful and specific tool for the activation of the short and long term immune response, reducing metastasis and regression and even producing the elimination of tumors when applied alone or in combination with routine therapies (chemotherapy and radiotherapy) and surgery.

5. References

Ahn WS, Bae SM, Kim TY, Kim TG, Lee JM, Nam Koong S et al. (2004). A therapy modality using recombinant IL-12 Adenovirus plus E7 protein in a Human Papillomavirus 16 E6/E7-associated cervical cancer animal model. *Human Gene Therapy,* Vol. 14, No.15, (October 2003), pp.1389-1399, ISSN: 1043-0342 .

Alphs H, Gambhira R, Karanam B, Roberts J, Jagu S et al. (2008). Protection against heterologous human papillomavirus challenge by a synthetic lipopeptide vaccine containing a broadly cross-neutralizing epitope of L2. *Proceedings of the National Academy of Sciences,* Vol. 105, No. 15 (April 2008), pp. 5850-5855, ISSN 1091-6490.

Albarran y Carvajal A, de la Garza A, Cruz Quiroz B, Vazquez E, Diaz I, Mendez E et al. (2007). MVA E2 Recombinant Vaccine in the Treatment of Human Papillomavirus Infection in Men Presenting Intraurethral Flat Condyloma: A Phase I/II Study. *BioDrugs,* Vol. 21, No. 1, pp. 47-59, ISSN: 1173-8804.

Álvarez Salas L (2006). Ácidos nucleicos terapeúticos contra cáncer cervical: una alternativa viable. Cinvestav Publicaciones, oct-dec 2006, pp .44-48.

American Cancer Society. Chemotherapy: What it is, how it helps, 10. 09. 2007, Online ISSN: 1542-4863, Available from http: //www.cancer.org/docroot/ETO/content/ETO_1_2X_Chemotherapy_What_It_Is _How_It_Helps.asp

American Cancer Society. CA: A Cancer Journal for Clinicians, 20.02.2008, Online ISSN: 1542-4863, Available from http: //caonline.amcancersoc.org/cgi/content/full/57/1/7

Bhatla N, Suri V, Basu P, Shastri S, Datta S, Bi D et al. (2010). Immunogenicity and safety of human papillomavirus-16/18 AS04-adyuvant cervical cancer vaccine in healthy Indian women. *Journal of Obstetrics and Gynaecology Research,* Vol. 36, No. 1 (February 2010), pp 123-132, eISSN 1447-0756.

Brull P, Carrera R (2005). Vacunas VPH para la prevención del cáncer de cérvix. *Ginecología y Obstetricia Clínica,* Vol. 6, No.3, pp. 129-133, ISSN: 1695-3827.

Brummelkamp TR, Bernards R & Agami R (2002). A system for stable expression of short interfering RNAs in mammalian cells. *Science,* Vol. 296, No. 5567, pp. 550-553, ISSN 0036-8075.

Bubenik J, Miky R, Vonka V, Mendoza L, Imova J, Smahel M & Indrova M (2003). Interleukin-2 and dendritic cells as adjuvants for surgical therapy of tumours associated with human papillomavirus type 16. *Vaccine,* Vol.21, No. 9-10 (June 2002), pp. 891-896, ISSN 0264-410X.

Butz K ,Ristriani T, Hengstermann A, Denk C,Scheffner M, Hoppe-Seyler F (2003). siRNA targeting of the viral E6 oncogene efficiently kills human papillomavirus-positive cancer cells. *Oncogene,* Vol. 22 (Junio 2003), pp. 5938–5945, ISSN 0950-9232.

Carette JE, Overmeer RM, Schagen FH, Alemany R, Barski OA, Gerritsen WR, van Beusechem VW (2004). Conditionally replicating adenoviruses expressing short hairpin RNAs silence the expression of a target gene in cancer cells. *Cancer Research,* Vol. 64 (Abril 2004), pp. 2663-2667, ISSN: 0008-5472.

Castellsagué X, Albero G, Martí D, Plà Farnós M, Ortega P, Belloví C (2006). Prevención primaria: vacunas frente al VPH para la prevención del cáncer de cuello uterino, In: *4ta Monografía de la Sociedad Española de Epidemiología. Virus de papiloma Humano y Cáncer: epidemiología y prevención*, De Sanjosé S & García A (Eds), pp. 107-130, EMISA, ISBN: 690-0811-0, ISBN 690-0811-0, Madrid, España.Choo CK, Ling MT, Suen CK, Chan KW, Kwong YL (2000). Retrovirus- mediated delivery of HPV 16 antisense RNA inhibited tumorigenicity of CaSKi cells. *Gynecologic Oncology*, Vol. 78, No.3 (September 2000), pp. 293-301, ISSN: 0090-8258.

de Felipe P, Izquierdo M (2000). Tricistronic and tetracistronic retroviral vectors for gene transfer. *Human Gene Therapy* , Vol. 11, No. 13 (September 2000), pp. 1921-1931, ISSN:1043-0342 .

De Villiers E, Fauquet C, Broker T, Bernard H, zur Hausen H (2004). Classification of papillomavirus. *Virology*, Vol. 324, No.1 (March 2004), pp. 17-24, ISSN: 1743-422X.

De Villiers E, Sandstrom R, zur Hausen H, Buck C (2005). Presence of papillomavirus sequences in condylomatous lesions of the mamillae and invasive carcinoma of the breast. *Breast Cancer Research*, Vol. 7, No.1 (October 2004), pp. R1-R11, ISSN: 1465-5411.

del Amo J, González C, Losana J, Clavo P, Muñoz L, Ballesteros J et al. (2005). Influence of age and geographical origin in the prevalence of high risk human papillomavirus in migrant female sex workers in Spain. *Sexually Transmitted Infections*, Vol. 81, No. 1 (February 2004), pp. 79-84, ISSN 1472-3263.

Diestro Tejeda M, Serrano Velasco M, Gómez Pastrana F (2007). Cáncer de cuello uterino. Estado actual de las vacunas frente al VPH. *Oncología*, Vol. 30, No.2 (February 2007), pp. 42-59, ISSN 0378-4835.

Dillner J (The Future I/II Study Group)(2010). Four year efficacy of prophylactic human papillomavirus quadrivalent vaccine against low grade cervical, vulvar and vaginal intraepithelial neoplasia and anogenital warts: randomized controlled trial. *British Medical Journal*, Vol. 340 (July 2010), pp.340-349, ISSN 1468-5833.

Food and Drug Administration (2010). Clinical Review for male indication for Gardasil, In: *FDA News*, 05.09.2011, Online ISSN 15-324648, Available from http: //www.fda.gov/downloads/BiologicsBloodVaccines/Vaccines/ApprovedProducts/UCM190977.pdf

Frechtel G (2005). El ARN de interferencia. *Bioquimia*, Vol. 30, No.4(October 2005), pp. 99-100, ISSN 0185-5751.

Fujii T, Saito M, Iwasaki E, Ochiya T, Takei Y, Hayashi S (2006). Intratumor injection of small interfering RNA-targeting human papillomavirus 18 E6 and E7 successfully inhibits the growth of cervical cancer. *International Journal of Oncology*, Vol. 29, No. 3(April 2006), pp. 541-548, ISSN 1791-2423.

Ghildiyal M, Seitz H, Horwich M, Li C, Du T, Lee S et al. (2008). Endogenous siRNAs derived from transposons and mRNAs in Drosophila somatic cells. *Science Express*, Vol. 320, No. 5879, pp. 1077-1081, ISSN 1095-9203.

Giuliano A (2007). Human papillomavirus vaccination in males. *Gynecologic Oncology*, Vol. 107, No. 1, pp. S24- S26, ISSN 1095-6859.

Gutierrez C, Tinoco A, Navarro T, López M, Risco R, Calzado P et al. (2004). Therapeutic vaccination with MVA E2 can eliminate precancerous lesions (CIN 1, CIN 2, and

CIN 3) associated with infection by oncogenic human papillomavirus. *Human Gene Therapy*, Vol. 15, No. 5 (May 2004), pp. 421-431, ISSN 1557-7422.

Haley B, Zamore P (2004). Kinetic analysis of the RNAi enzyme complex. *Nature Structural and Molecular Biology*, Vol. 11, No. 7 (July 2004), pp. 599-606, ISSN 1545-9985 .

Hall A, Alexander K (2003). RNA interference of human papillomavirus type 18 E6 and E7 induces senescence in hela cells. *Journal of Virology*, Vol. 77, No. 10 (May 2003), pp. 6066-6069, ISSN: 1098-5514.

Hamada K, Sakaue M, Alemany R, Zhang W, Horio Y, Roth J (1996). Adenovirus-mediated transfer of HPV 16 E6/E7antisense RNA to human cervical cancer cells. *Gynecologic Oncology*, Vol. 63, No. 2 (March 1996), pp. 219-227, ISSN: 0090-8258.

Handisurya A, Schellenbacher Ch, Kirnbawer R (2009). Diseases caused by human papillomaviruses (HPV). *Journal of German Society of Dermatology* ,Vol. 7, No. 5 (November 2008), pp. 453-466, ISSN 1610-0387.

Harper D, Franco E, Wheeler C, Ferris D, Jenkins D, Schuind A et al. (2004). Efficacy of a bivalent L1 virus-like particle vaccine in prevention of infection with human papillomavirus types 16 and 18 in young women: a randomised controlled trial. *Lancet*, 2004; Vol. 364, No. 9447, pp. 1757-1765, ISSN 1474-547X.

Heng B, Glenn W, Ye Y, Tran B, Delprado W, Lutze-Mann L, Whitaker N, Lawson J (2009). Human papillomavirus is associated with breast cancer. *British Journal of Cancer*, Vol. 101, No. 8 (October 2009), pp. 1345-1350, ISSN: 0007-0920.

Humayun M, Abdul S, Hassan S, Ahn J, Wang MH (2008). RNAi: An emerging field of molecular research. *African Journal of Biotechnology*, Vol. 7, No. 25 (December 2008), pp. 4784-4788, ISSN 1684-5315.

Hutchinson D, Klein K (2008). Human papillomavirus disease and vaccines. *American Journal of Health-System Pharmacy*, Vol.65, No. 22 (November 2008), pp. 2105-2112, ISSN: 1535-2900.

Instituto Nacional del Cáncer (2008) . Efectos de la quimioterapia, In: *La quimioterapia y usted: Apoyo para las personas con cáncer*, 26.02.2008, Available from: http://www.cancer.gov/espanol/cancer/quimioterapia-y-usted/page5

Ishii Y, Kondo K, Matsumoto T, Tanaka K, Shinkai-Ouchi F et al. (2007). Thiol-reactive reagents inhibits intracellular trafficking of human papillomavirus type 16 pseudovirions by binding to cysteine residues of major capsid protein L1. *Virology Journal*, Vol. 4, No. 110 (October 2007), ISSN: 1743-422X.

Jagu S, Karanam B, Gambhira R, Chivukula S, Chaganti R et al. (2009). Concatenated multitype L2 fusion proteins as candidate prophylactic pan-human papillomavirus vaccines. *Journal of the National Cancer Institute*, Vol. 101, No. 11 (January 2009), pp.782-792, ISSN 1460-2105.

Jiang M, Milner J (2005). Selective silencing of viral gene E6 and E7 expression in HPV-positive human cells using small interfering RNAs. *Methods in Molecular Biology*, 292 (July 2005), pp. 401-420, ISSN 1940-6029.

Jiang M, Milner J (2002). Selective silencing of viral gene expression in HPV-positive human cervical carcinoma cells treated with siRNA, a primer of RNA interference. *Oncogene*, Vol. 21 (July 2002), pp. 6041-6048, ISSN: 1476-5594.

Jiang M, Rubbi C, Milner J (2004). Gel-based application of siRNA to human epithelial cancer cells induces RNAi-dependent apoptosis. *Oligonucleotides*, Vol. 14 (August 2004), pp. 239-248, ISSN: 2159-3345.

Joura E, Leodoter S, Hernández-Ávila M, Wheeler C, Pérez G, Koustsky L et al. (2007). Efficacy of a quadrivalent prophylactic human papillomavirus (types 6, 11, 16 and 18) L1 virus-like particle vaccine against high grade vulval and vaginal lesions: a combined analysis of three clinical trials. *Lancet*, Vol. 369, No. 9574 (May 2007), pp. 1693-1702, ISSN: 0140-6736.

Kahn J (2005). Vaccination as a prevention strategy for human papillomavirus-related diseases. *Journal of Adolescent Health*, Vol. 37, No. 6 (August 2005), pp. S10 - S16, ISSN: 1054-139X.

Kaufmann A, Stern P, Rankin E, Sommer H, Nuessler V, Schneider A et al. (2002). Safety and Immunogenicity of TA-HPV, a recombinant vaccinia virus expressing modified human papillomavirus (HPV)-16 and HPV 18 *E6* and *E7* genes, in women with progressive cervical cancer. *Clinical Cancer Research*, Vol. 8 (December 2002), pp. 3676-3685, ISSN 1557-3265.

Ketting RF, Fisher SE, Bernstein E, Sijen T, Hannon G, Plasterk R (2001). Dicer functions in RNA interference and in synthesis of small RNA involved in developmental timing in *C. elegans*. *Genes & Development*, Vol. 15 (September 2001), pp. 2654-2659, ISSN 0890-9369.

Khan CY, Iacopetta B, Lawson J, Whitaker N (2005). Identification of human papillomavirus DNA gene sequences in human breast cancer. *British Journal of Cancer*, Vol. 93 (August 2005), pp. 946-948, ISSN 1532-1827.

Kim D, Gambhira R, Karanam B, Monie A, Hung CF, Roden R, Wu TC (2008). Generation and characterization of a preventive and therapeutic HPV DNA vaccine. *Vaccine*, Vol. 26, No. 3 (January 2008), pp. 351-360, ISSN 1873-2518.

Kim D, Hoory T, Monie A, Ting J, Hung CF, Wu T (2008). Enhancement of DNA vaccine potency through coadministration of CIITA DNA with DNA vaccines via gene gun. *The Journal of Immunology*, Vol. 180 (March 2008), pp. 7019-7027, ISSN: 1550-6606.

Kim JW, Hung CF, Juang J, Woo T, Armstrong DK, Pai SI et al. (2004). Comparison of HPV DNA vaccines employing intracellular targeting strategies. *Gene Therapy*, Vol. 11 (February 2004), pp. 1011-1018, ISSN 1476-5462.

Lacey C, Thompson H, Monteiro E, O´Neill T, Davies M, Holding F (1999). Phase IIa safety and Immunogenicity of a therapeutic vaccine, TA-GW, in persons with genital warts. *The Journal of Infectious Diseases*, Vol. 179, No. 3 (March 1999), pp. 612-618, ISSN 1537-6613.

Lea JS, Sunaga N, Sato M, Kalahasti G, Miller DS, Minna JD, Muller CY (2007). Silencing of HPV 18 oncoproteins with RNA interference causes growth inhibition of cervical cancer cells. *Reproductive Sciences*, Vol. 14, No. 1 (January 2007), pp. 20-28, ISSN 1933-7205.

Lowy D, Frazer I (2003). Prophylactic human papillomavirus vaccines. *Journal of the National Cancer Institute Monographs*, Vol. 2003, No. 31 (June 2003), pp. 111-116, ISSN 1745-6614.

McKeage K, Romanowski B (2011). AS04-Adjuvanted Human Papillomavirus (HPV) Types 16 and 18 vaccine (Cervarix): a review of its use in the prevention of premalignant cervical lesions and cervical cancer causally related to certain oncogenic HPV types. *Drugs*, Vol. 71, No. 4 (March 2011), pp. 465-488, ISSN 0012-6667.

Mao C, Koutsky L, Ault K, Wheeler C, Brown D, Wiley D et al. (2006). Efficacy of Human Papillomavirus-16 Vaccine to Prevent Cervical Intraepithelial Neoplasia . A Randomized Controlled Trial. *Obstetrics and Gynecology*, Vol. 107, No.1 (January 2006), pp. 18-27, ISSN 1873-233X .

Mao Ch P, Hung Ch F, Wu T C (2007). Immunotherapeutic strategies employing RNA interference technology for the control of cancers. *Journal of Biomedical Science*, Vol. 14 (October 2006), pp. 15-29, ISSN 1423-0127 .

Muñoz N, Bosch F, Castellsague X, Díaz M, de Sanjose S, Hammouda D, Shah KV, Meijer CJ (2004). Against which human papillomaviruses types shall we vaccinate and screen? The international perspective. *International Journal of Cancer,* Vol. 111, No. 2 (August 2004), pp. 278-285, ISSN 1097-0215.

Muñoz N, Reina J, Sánchez G (2008). La vacuna contra el virus del papiloma humano (VPH): una gran arma para la prevención primaria del cáncer de cuello uterino. *Colombia Médica*, Vol.39, No. 2 (April 2008), pp. 196-204, ISSN 1657-9534.

Niu X, Peng Z, Duan W, Wang H, Wang P(2006). Inhibition of HPV 16 E6 oncogen expression by RNA interference *in vitro* and *in vivo*. *International Journal of Gynecological Cancer*, Vol.16, No. 2 (April 2006), pp. 743-751, ISSN 1525-1438.

Paavonen J, Jenkins D, Bosh F, Naud P, Salmerón J, Wheeler C et al. (2007). Efficacy of a prophylactic adyuvant bivalent L1 virus-like particle vaccine against human papillomavirus types 16 and 18 in young women: an interim analysis of a phase III double-blind, randomized controlled trial. *Lancet,* Vol. 369, No. 9580 (June 2007), pp. 2161-2170, ISSN 0140-6736.

Patel N, Sauter E (2011). Body fluid micro (mi)RNAs as biomarkers for human cancer. *Journal of Nucleic Acids Investigations*, Vol.2, No. 1 (January 2011), pp. 1-4, eISSN: 2035-6005.

Peng S, Best S, Hung C, Loyo M, Lyford-Pike S, Flint P et al. (2010). Characterization of Human Papillomavirus Type 11-Specific Immune Responses in a Preclinical Model. *Laryngoscope*, Vol. 120, No. 3 (March 2010), pp 504-510, ISSN: 1531-4995.

Putral L, Bywater M, Gu W, Saunders N, Gabrielli B, Leggatt G, McMillan N (2005) . RNA Interference against Human Papillomavirus oncogenes in cervical cancer cells results in increased sensitivity to Cisplatin. *Molecular Pharmacology* , Vol. 68, No. 5 (August 2005), pp. 1311-1319, ISSN 1521-0111.

Raia R, Calin G. Non-coding RNAs and cancer: microRNAs and beyond (2011). *Journal of Nucleic Acid Investigation*, Vol. 2, No. 1 (March 2011), pp. 27-30, eISSN: 2035-6005.

Schiller J, Lowy D (2006). Prospects for cervical cancer prevention by human papillomavirus vaccination. *Çancer Research*, Vol. 66, No. 21 (November 2006), pp. 10229-10233, eISSN 1538-7445.

Schubert S, Grunweller A, Erdmann V, Kurreck J (2005). Local RNA target structure influences siRNA efficacy: systematic analysis of intentionally designed binding regions. *Journal of Molecular Biology*, Vol. 348, No. 4 (May 2005), pp. 883-893, eISSN 1089-8638.

Sin JI (2009). Supression of antitumour protective cytotoxic T lymphocyte responses to a human papillomavirus 16 E7 DNA vaccine by coinfection of IL-12 complementary DNA: involvement of nitric oxide in immune suppression. *Immunology*, Vol. 128, No. 1 (January 2009), pp. 707-717, eISSN 1365-2567.

Sioud M, Sorensen DR (2003). Cationic liposome-mediated delivery of siRNAs in adult mice. *Biochemical and Biophysical Research Communications*, Vol. 312, No.4 (December 2003), pp. 1220-1225, eISSN 1090-2104.

Stanley M (2008). Human papillomavirus vaccines versus cervical cancer screening. *Clinical Oncology*, Vol. 20, No. 6, (August 2008), pp. 388-394, ISSN 1433-2981.

Taira AV, Neukermans CP, Sanders GD (2004). Evaluating human papillomavirus vaccination programs. *Emerging Infectious Diseases*, Vol. 10, No. 11 (November 2004), pp. 1915-1923, eISSN 1080-6059.

Tirado-Gómez L, Mohar-Betancourt A, López-Cervantes M, García-Carrancá A, Franco-Marina F, Borges G (2005). Factores de riesgo de cáncer cervicouterino invasor en mujeres mexicanas. *Salud Pública de México*, Vol. 47, No. 5 (October 2005): 342-350, eISSN 1606-7916.

Villa L, Costa R, Petta C, Andrade R, Ault K, Giuliano A et al.. (2005). Prophylactic quadrivalent human papillomavirus (types 6, 11, 16, and 18) L1 virus-like particle vaccine in young women: a randomised double-blind placebo controlled multicentre phase II efficacy trial. *The Lancet Oncology*, Vol. 6, No. 5 (May 2005), pp. 271–278, eISSN 1474-5488.

Vitale A, Tan H, Jin P (2011). MicroRNAs, SNPs and cancer. *Journal of Nucleic Acids Investigations,* Vol. 2, No. 6 (March 2011), pp. 32-38, eISSN: 2035-6005.

Wang HK, Duffy A, Broker T, Chow L (2009). Robust production and passaging of infectious HPV in squamous epithelium of primary human keratinocytes. *Genes & Development*, Vol. 23, No. 2 (November 2008), pp. 181-194, ISSN 0890-9369/09.

Wang R, Lin F, Wang X, Gao P, Dong K, Wei SH et al. (2007). The therapeutic potential of surviving promoter-driven siRNA on suppressing tumor growth and enhancing radiosensitivity of human cervical carcinoma cells via down regulating *hTERT* gene expression. *Cancer Biology & Therapy*, Vol. 6, No. 8(August 2008), pp. 1295-1301, eISSN 1555-8576.

Webster K, Parish J, Pandya M, Stern P, Clarke A, Gaston K. The HPV 16 E2 protein induces apoptosis in the absence of other HPV proteins and via a p53-dependent pathway. *The Journal of Biological Chemistry*, Vol. 275, No. 1 (January 2000), pp. 87-94, eISSN 1083-351X.

Yamato K, Yamada T, Kisaki M, Ui-Tei K, Natori Y, Fujino M, Nishihara T, Ikeda Y et al. (2008). New highly potent and specific E6 and E7 siRNAs for treatment of HPV 16 positive cervical cancer. *Cancer Gene Therapy*, Vol. 15, No, 3 (March 2008), pp. 140-153, eISSN 1476-5500.

8

Current Insight into Anti-HPV Immune Responses and Lessons for Prophylactic and Therapeutic Vaccines

Isabelle Bourgault-Villada[1,2] and Simon Jacobelli[2]
[1]*AP-HP, Hôpital Ambroise Paré, Boulogne Billancourt, UVSQ, Versailles,*
[2]*Institut Cochin, Paris, Université Paris Descartes*
France

1. Introduction

Human Papillomavirus (HPV) are epitheliotropic for stratified malpighian epithelia such as those of the cervix, vulva or anal canal. Mucosal papillomaviruses are responsible for several clinical lesions and can be classified as non oncogenic and oncogenic viruses. The first ones are responsible for benign lesions such as external genital warts (EGW) or condyloma due to HPV 6 and 11. The second ones include oncogenic viruses such as HPV 16 and 18, the most common ones, and HPV 45, 31, 33, 52 etc which are involved in invasive cancers preceded by cervical, vulvar, penile or anal intraepithelial neoplasia. Oncogenic HPV are detectable in 99.7% of cervical cancers (Bosch et al, 1995). Cellular immunity plays a key role in controlling and killing infected or transformed keratinocytes. Nevertheless, around 10% of women having infected cervical mucosa are not able to control oncogenic HPV and develop cervical intraepithelial neoplasia (CIN). High grade CIN (CIN3) require surgical treatment before their progression to invasive cancers in 30% of cases (McCredie et al, 2008; Ostor et al, 1993). A great priority is then to develop a preventive vaccine to protect against HPV infection. In women with CIN, therapeutic vaccine could be used to eliminate previously infected or transformed keratinocytes and avoid surgical treatment.

2. Virology

Following a breach in the malpighian pluristratified epithelium, HPVs infect basal stem cells of keratinocytes. The virus initially remains in episomal form with synthesis of E2 protein. This protein is a major regulator of viral vegetative cycle and is required for transcriptional regulation as well as viral DNA replication together with the E1 helicase (Desaintes et al, 1996). In contrast, E2 is generally undetectable in cancers due to a preferential integration of the viral genome in the cell genome and disruption of the E2 open reading frame (Berumen et al, 1994; Collins et al, 2009). Therefore E2 is a marker of viral infection and is specific for the early stages of the viral gene expression in infected cells. This was formally demonstrated in a recent work that showed a strong staining of the E2 protein in the intermediate differentiated layers of HPV16-infected tissues and low grade CIN (Xue et al,

2010). The high expression of HPV16 E2 in low grade lesions therefore represents a marker for HPV infection even before any clinical manifestation.

After integration of the genome of oncogenic HPVs into the host genome, viral oncogenic E6 and E7 proteins are synthesized in large quantities in the inner third of the epithelium. During maturation of keratinocytes from the basal layer to the epithelial surface, viral capside proteins L1 and L2 are synthesized and expressed at the surface of mature keratinocytes in order to form a new viral particle which is able to infect adjacent healthy epithelium and to contaminate sexual partners.

3. Epidemiology of oncogenic HPV and related diseases

HPV infections occur preferentially in young women under 25 years of age (Boulanger et al, 2004). Several stages of lesions can be observed following oncogenic HPV infection. The first stage is a simple infection of keratinocytes that become koilocytes and develop into condyloma. The following stages are related to the transformation of infected keratinocytes into malignant cells. The depth at which malignant cells are found defines the disease stage: low (as CIN1) or high grade squamous intraepithelial lesions as CIN2/3. The latter is diagnosed on the basis of Pap smears, followed by colposcopy and biopsies and can evolve towards invasive cancer. HPV16 is found in more than 50% of cervical cancer cases and HPV18 in 17%. The incidence of cervical cancer remains very high with 500 000 new cases per year in the world, essentially in developing countries where the level of screening by Pap smear is very low. It annually leads to 230 000 deaths.

The premalignant lesions of HPV-related grade 3 usual vulvar intraepithelial neoplasia (usual VIN or VIN3) involve the mucosal and/or cutaneous epithelium of the vulva, perineal and perianal region. Usual VIN occurs in adult women and commonly resembles persistent anogenital warts that are often multifocal pigmented papular lesions disseminated on the vulva and/or the perianal skin. Usual VIN is characterized by the presence of poorly differentiated or undifferentiated basal cells and highly atypical squamous epithelial cells (McClugagge et al, 2009). The oncogenic HPV most frequently found in usual VIN is HPV16 that plays a direct role in up to 91% of the cases (Srodon et al, 2006).

The overall incidence rates of anal cancer has recently increased, particularly among men who have sex with men (MSM) and HIV-infected patients (Piketty et al, 2008) Combination antiretroviral therapy does not prevent nor revert anal cancer in the latter patients (Piketty et al, 2010). Despite several HPV coinfections in particular in HIV-infected patients, HPV16 is the most common one in anal cancer (Abramowitz et al, 2011).

4. Humoral immune response after HPV infection

Serum antibodies against HPV are directed against viral capside antigens and in particular against L1 protein. Their synthesis is late (6 to 12 months after infection) and antibody concentration remains limited because of the absence of HPV viremia (Carter et al, 2000). However, these antibodies persist in many women for at least 10 years (af Geijersstam et al, 1998). Only 70% of women having persistent HPV16 DNA in the genital mucosa have detectable antibodies (Ho et al, 2004; Kirnbauer et al, 1994). These antibodies do not play any neutralizing role against HPV after virus entry in basal stem cells of keratinocytes (de Gruijl et al, 1999) because L1 protein is not expressed at the surface of these cells.

5. Antibodies detected after HPV infection do not protect against a new infection

Antibodies synthesized after HPV infection do not protect against a new infection with the same HPV genotype, as observed in a cohort study of women with and without such antibodies (Viscidi et al, 2004, 2005). There was no difference over time between the two groups with respect to HPV16 DNA detection in the genital mucosa. This is not surprising since the level of the anti-HPV antibodies found in mucosal secretions is lower than in the serum where the level of antibodies is already very low (Lowe et al, 1997; Nardelli-Haefliger et al, 2003). Local secretory IgA could not stop the spread of HPV infection (Bard et al, 2004).

6. Cellular immune response after HPV infection

Cellular immune responses play a critical role in HPV infections by controlling or eliminating the virus. The incidence of HPV-induced diseases is increased in T-cell immunodeficient individuals, such as HIV-infected (Sun et al, 1997), transplanted patients (Arends et al, 1997), patients treated by immunosuppressive drugs (Ulrich et al, 2008) or in primary immunodeficiencies (Lawrence et al, 2005). In patients with high-grade CIN 2/3 or invasive cervical carcinoma, blood cytotoxic T lymphocytes (CTL) directed against HPV-16 E6 or E7 proteins are barely detectable (Nakagawa et al, 1997, 2000). Proliferative responses of CD4-lymphocytes against these two proteins seem to correlate with the infection stage. Indeed, high frequency specific interleukin-2 (IL2)–producing CD4 lymphocytes have been observed in asymptomatic HPV-16–infected women (de Jong et al, 2002) whereas they decrease during disease progression toward high-grade CIN or invasive cancer (Tsukui et al, 1996).

In a woman who completely cleared usual vulvar intraepithelial neoplasia (VIN) lesions eight months after disease onset (Figure 1), an immunohistochemical study showed a marked dermal infiltrate containing a majority of CD4+ T lymphocytes and an epidermal infiltrate made up of both $CD4^+$ and $CD8^+$ T cells (Figure 2) (Bourgault Villada et al, 2004). Before clinical regression, high frequency anti-E6 and anti-E7 effector blood T-cells by *ex vivo* IFNγ ELISPOT assay was evidenced (Figure 3). This appears to be the first evidence of an association between spontaneous regression of usual VIN lesions and HPV-specific T cell responses detectable in the blood. Hence, an increase of HPV-specific effector T lymphocyte responses by vaccine-based therapeutic strategies might be useful to clear the lesions in usual VIN disease.

On the contrary, in chronic nonregressive CIN3, lymphocyte infiltrates in the epidermis mainly contain CD8+ lymphocytes and no CD4+ cells. It is likely that CD8+ lymphocytes play a major role in the defense against HPV infections by killing infected keratinocytes. However, CD4+ lymphocytes that synthesize IFNγ and IL2 are required for an optimal induction of high affinity tumor-specific memory CD8+ effector T-cells.

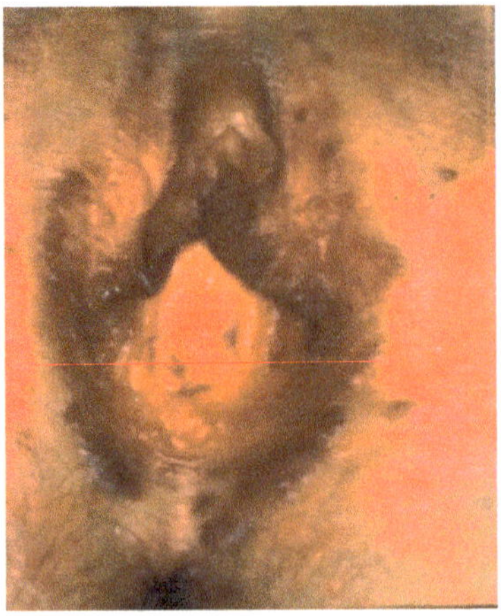

Fig. 1. Clinical lesions of multifocal pigmented usual VIN before spontaneous clinical regression

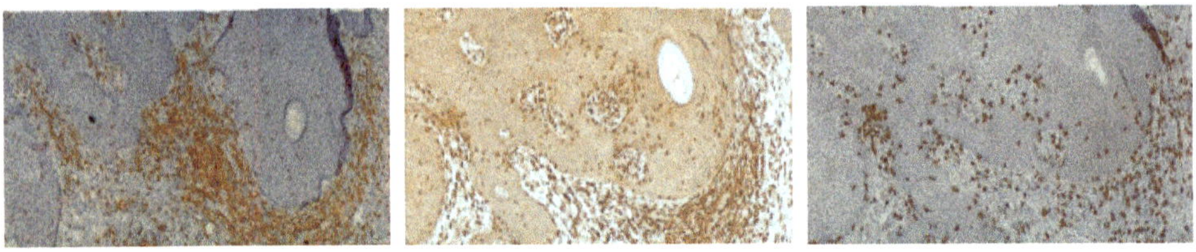

CD3 lymphocytes CD4 lymphocytes CD8 lymphocytes

Fig. 2. Immunohistochemical study of the vulvar biopsy just before spontaneous regression

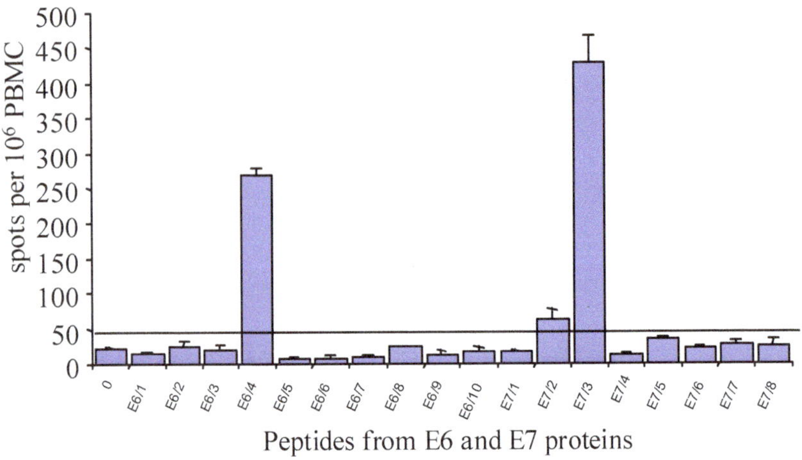

Fig. 3. IFNγ ELISPOT assay performed just before clinical regression

7. Presentation of HPV antigens to T and B lymphocytes after HPV infection

During infection, viral particles enter through epithelium up to basal basal stem cells of keratinocytes and sometimes can penetrate into the chorion. In the epithelium, they can be captured by Langerhans cells and they are quickly internalized (Bousarghin et al, 2005; Fausch et al, 2005; Malejczyk et al, 1997) and degraded into short and large peptides (Combadière et al, 2008; Herbst et al, 1996; Offringa et al, 2003; Yan et al, 2004). The classical view of the role of Langerhans cells is one of antigen uptake in the epidermis, and migration through the dermal lymphatics to the lymphoid organs, where they present antigen to lymphocytes that then home back to the tissue to carry out their effector function. Matthews et al (2003) have previously reported that Langerhans cells number is significantly reduced in HPV16 lesions without Langerhans cells depletion in the surrounding uninfected tissue. During HPV infection, the migration of Langerhans cells towards mucosal follicle is followed by presentation of short and large viral peptides by HLA class I and HLA class II molecules to CD4+ and CD8+ T lymphocytes, respectively. After stimulation, CD4+ and CD8+ T lymphocytes can circulate and migrate within the HPV-infected epithelium by using their surface molecules such as cutaneous lymphocyte antigen (Grover et al, 2006). The presentation of whole viral particles to B lymphocytes requires that HPV binds to dermal dendritic cells that are able to carry the whole virus to follicular dendritic cells present in mucosal follicle (Palucka et al, 2010).

8. Does a T-cell marker of viral control exist?

We recently tested by proliferative assays, intracellular cytokines synthesis and IFNγ ELISPOT the cellular immune responses against the HPV16 E2 protein that is early synthesized after HPV infection when the virus is episomal in eight women presenting with HPV16-related usual VIN and their healthy male partners (Jacobelli et al, 2011, unpublished data). We showed that anti-E2 polyfunctional CD4 T-cell responses (proliferative responses and synthesis of IFNγ and/or IL2) appear when the clinical lesions heal or when the HPV infection remains silent. Blood proliferative T-cell responses against HPV16 E2 peptides have been also observed in 50% of healthy women, who presumably previously cleared HPV16 infection (de Jong et al, 2004) and in 9 out of 22 regressive CIN3 cases (Dillon et al, 2007). In another studies, the lack of anti-E2 proliferative responses was reported in 16 of 18 patients (89%) affected with usual VIN lesions (Davidson et al, 2003) and in 7 of 8 and 9 of 12 women affected with CIN3 (Dillon et al, 2007; de Jong et al, 2004). These observations reinforce the strong role of T-cells in the control of HPV replication.

9. Why the male partners of women having CIN3 or usual VIN do not have any lesion?

Men are vectors of oncogenic HPV infection (Buckley et al, 1981). However, while HPV infection was found in 71 to 90% of the partners of HPV-infected women (Hippelainen et al, 1994; Nicolau et al, 2005), only 52% harbored the same HPV subtypes (Reiter et al, 2010). Moreover, penile intra-epithelial neoplasia is rare and detected in less than 2% of the men in contact with oncogenic HPV (Giraldo et al, 2008). We thus analyzed HPV infection and anti-HPV16 E2 blood T-cell responses in asymptomatic male partners chronically exposed to HPV16 during sexual intercourses with their wives affected with usual VIN (Jacobelli et al,

2011, , unpublished data). We had hypothesized that male partners exposed to replicative HPV16 could develop immunologic responses against the early E2 viral protein and thus clear infection. We indeed observed HPV16-E2-specific proliferative responses and intracellular synthesis of single IFNγ, dual IFNγ/IL2 and single IL2. These T-cell responses indicate a striking link between the absence of HPV-related lesions and the presence of spontaneous anti-E2 specific polyfunctional T-cell response in male partners. It is tempting to speculate that E2-specific responses prevent HPV16-related lesions. Since E2 protein is not encapsidated in the viral particle, the strong E2-specific T cells responses measured in partners of women with usual VIN demonstrates that the virus effectively replicates in males. Our results suggest that male are an important reservoir of genital HPVs and provide a strong argument in favor of prophylactic HPV vaccination of young men with Virus Like Particles to decrease HPV16 infection in men, and thus fight against the spread of mucosal HPV diseases in the population.

10. Balance between cellular immunity and infected / tumoral cells: Mechanisms of tumor escape

The impairment of HPV-16–specific CD4 lymphocytes and CTL responses can occur many years after infection / transformation of keratinocytes. It could be related to the tumor or to T-cell responses. The tumor cells can down-regulate their MHC class I molecules, synthesize TGFβ or decrease the number of viral peptides on their surface. Mechanisms of T-cell tolerance to HPV includes presence of regulatory T-cells (Treg) at proximity of the tumor cells (van der Burg et al, 2007) and sometimes in the blood (Molling et al, 2007; Visser et al, 2007), engagement of PD1 or CTLA4 in the immune synapse and inhibition of CD3 zeta expression on infiltrating tumor T-cells (Patel et al, 2009; Zehbe et al, 2006).

11. Prophylactic vaccines can prevent infection

The vaccination against HPV can have two different purposes. The first one is a preventive strategy aiming at blocking primary infection by preventing the entry of the virus into their target cells i.e. the basal basal stem cells of keratinocytes. In this aim, a vaccination able to induce transudated serum antibodies at the epithelial surface is a good strategy and is obtained by using viral L1 particles as vaccine. Large quantities of L1 are produced in vitro by splicing the L1 gene into plasmids (for expression in yeast) or recombinant baculoviruses (for expression in insect cells). The Virus Like Particle is formed by self aggregation of 72 L1 capsomers into a sphere. This spherical structure is similar to the viral capside, but it is empty without DNA or RNA and non infectious. After systemic immunization, it is able to induce the synthesis of neutralizing antibodies that can recognize the conformational structure of the real viral capside. Inversely, after HPV infection, antibodies are ineffective and only therapeutic vaccines can be considered to induce T lymphocytes able to kill HPV infected keratinocytes. These therapeutic vaccines must target oncogenic E6 and E7 viral proteins early expressed in the basal epithelial cells.

Merck has developed Gardasil®, a vaccine directed against four HPV types. It contains Virus Like Particles (L1) from HPV-6, 11, 16, and 18, with aluminum hydroxyphosphate as an adjuvant. Cervarix® is a bivalent vaccine developed by GSK. It targets HPV-16/18 VLP (L1) and contains a novel adjuvant named ASO4 co-formulated with aluminum. ASO4 contains phospholipids from *Salmonella minnesota* membrane and binds to TLR4 at the surface of dendritic cells. Activated dendritic cells synthesize type I IFN, IL6, IL12, TNFα that allows recruitment and stimulation of Th follicular cells that increase antibodies production by B lymphocytes. Both vaccines must be administrated by intramuscular route. Three injections should be performed, at M0, M2 and M6 for Gardasil® and M0, M1 and M6 for Cervarix®. Gardasil® and Cervarix® have been commercialized worldwide and each country should define their own recommendations.

Phase I trials of Gardasil® were performed with only HPV16 L1 VLP in 300 16 to 23 years old women, who had less than 5 sexual partners and had never been exposed to HPV16 (Harro et al, 2001). The immunogenicity of the vaccine was excellent with the induction of very high levels of blood anti-L1 antibodies, 50 to 100 times those observed after natural HPV infection. The tolerance of the vaccine was good with only a slight pain, swelling and erythema at the injection sites. Phase II trials included about 2 000 subjects, they showed preliminary proof of efficacy using also HPV16 VLP versus a placebo (Koutsky et al, 2002). Subsequent phase III trial were carried out on more than 25 000 subjects, using the quadrivalent vaccine containing VLP from HPV 6, 11, 16 and 18. 98 to 100% protection was obtained against HPV -6, 11, 16, and 18 related diseases such as CIN2/3, vulvar and vaginal condyloma, usual VIN and VaIN3 (Garland et al, 2007; Joura et al, 2007; Munoz et al, 2010). Protection against persistent infection (for 6 months) by HPV16 or 18 was obtained in 99% of cases. Gardasil® obtained an FDA approval for the vaccination of girls and women aged 9 to 26 years to prevent cervical cancer, precancerous genital lesions and genital warts. Recently, 90% protection was obtained against extragenital warts in males (Giuliano et al, 2011). Efficacy of Gardasil® obtained against HPV31-induced CIN2/3 is around 55%. Finally, 43% protection was obtained against CIN2/3 induced by 14 oncogenic and non oncogenic genotypes of HPV (HPV 6, 11, 16, 18, 31, 33, 35, 39, 45, 51, 52, 56, 58, 59) 3.7 years after vaccination.

As for Cervarix®, phases I and II (Harper et al, 2004, 2006) studies showed 98 to 100% protection against CIN 2/3 similar to that of Gardasil®. The phase III trial involved more than 20 000 subjects (Paavonen et al, 2007) and was approved by the FDA and European Medical Agency. 70% protection was obtained against CIN2/3 related to 14 oncogenic HPV genotypes (HPV 16, 18, 31, 33, 35, 39, 45, 51, 52, 56, 58, 59, 66, 68) 3 years following vaccination (Paavonen et al, 2009). The efficacy of Cervarix® against HPV31-induced CIN2/3 is around 92%. Protection against persistent infection (for 6 months) by HPV33 and 45 was obtained in 76 and 77% of cases respectively.

Nevertheless, many questions remain unanswered. How long will the protection last ? Does thresholds of antibodies exist to allow the protection ? What will be the impact of the vaccination on the ecology of other HPVs, HPV screening by Pap smears and on adolescent sexual behavior and their use of condoms for HIV protection ? Will parents, preteens, physicians and the public at large, accept vaccination of young girls ? Will it be interesting to vaccinate young men to decrease HPV16 infection in men, viral transmission from men to women and more importantly spread of mucosal HPV diseases in the population ? Are MSM the future candidates for vaccination against anal cancer ?

12. Protection by the quadrivalent prophylactic vaccine against cutaneous external genital warts

A paradox exits between the protection by prophylactic vaccines against cutaneous EGW (related to HPV6 and 11 replicative viruses) and the absence of detectable antibodies on the keratinized skin surface. Following a breach in the epithelium, HPVs bind via L1 first to the basement membrane and then to the cellular receptor on the basal stem keratinocytes (Kines et al, 2009). Anti-L1 antibodies induced by prophylactic vaccines could block both of these interactions (Day et al, 2007). Indeed, this process of virus entry is slow, between 12 to 14 hours (Sapp et al, 2009) and, since the breach is accompanied by a serum exudate, exposure to serum antibodies is rapid. Another explanation for protection could be a stronger stimulation of anti-HPV CD4+ and CD8+ T-cells after infection. Indeed, in the presence of memory anti-L1 CD4+ T-cell, the CD8+ cytotoxic T-lymphocytes could be more strongly stimulated, with multiple specificities and higher affinity (Sauzet et al, 1995). The killing of infected keratinocytes could be then more effective.

13. Prevention of infection by other oncogenic HPVs by divalent prophylactic vaccine

Recently, it has been demonstrated that Cervarix® is able to prevent CIN2/3 induced by HPV 16 and 18 and also by HPV 31, 33 and 45 (http://www.ema.europa.eu/, cervarix®, summary of product characteristics). An efficacy of 70% and 43% was obtained against CIN2/3 related to 14 oncogenic HPVs (16, 18, 31, 33, 35, 39, 45, 51, 52, 56, 58, 59, 66, 68) with Cervarix® and 12 oncogenic HPVs (16, 18, 31, 33, 35, 39, 45, 51, 52, 56, 58, 59) with Gardasil®, respectively (http://www.ema.europa.eu/, gardasil®, summary of product characteristics). A high level of anti-HPV antibodies usually correlates with a broad recognition of B-cell epitopes. Such epitopes can be shared by several other closely related HPVs. In Cervarix®, the use of ASO4 adjuvant allows to obtain high anti-HPV16 and 18 antibodies levels, that are able to prevent infection by numerous other oncogenic HPVs (McKeage et al, 2011).

14. Alternative to L1 VLP vaccines

A particularly attractive strategy is to vaccinate with a linear N-terminal highly conserved sequence of the viral capsid L2 protein. In a properly immunogenic context, neutralizing antibodies to this B cell epitope-containing region are elicited and they have broadly neutralizing capacities against a wide range of HPVs (Conway et al, 2011). Immunization with adjuvanted chimeric HPV16L1-HPV16L2 VLP have also induced neutralization or cross-neutralization of HPV16, -18, -31, -45, -52, and -58; HPV6 and -11; and HPV5 (Schellenbacher et al, 2009). These new types of vaccine are very promising.

15. How to cure infection / tumorigenesis? Therapeutic vaccines

Preventive vaccines do not address the current need for better treatment for women previously infected by HPV 16 or 18. Other types of vaccines must be used to increase or induce new specific anti-HPV cellular immunity (CD4+ and CD8+ T lymphocytes) in order to kill transformed epithelial cells. Several approaches can be used in this aim. To stimulate cytotoxic or antiviral CD8+ T lymphocytes, the vaccines must target the cytoplasm of dendritic cells. The degradation of vaccine antigens by proteasomes results in short peptides that can bind to HLA class I molecules and migrate at the surface of dendritic cells. To stimulate CD4+ T lymphocytes, endocytosis of vaccinal antigens is essential, followed by degradation of antigens by lysosome/endosome in large peptides that associate with HLA class II molecules before migrating at the surface of dendritic cells. All these therapeutic vaccines must target E6 and E7 viral proteins and contain recombinant viruses (vaccinia viruses for example), DNA or peptides.

Peptidic or lipopeptidic vaccines were tested within phases I-II for treatment of women having CIN3 or metastatic cervical cancer. The chosen peptides were E7 11-20 and E7 86-93, two peptides able to bind HLA-A2 molecules in association with a CD4+ epitope (PADRE) able to bind numerous HLA-DR molecules (Ressing et al, 2000; Steller et al, 1998; van Driel et al, 1999). In women with invasive cervical cancer, 25 to 30% of cellular immune responses were observed without any clinical improvement. Another trial in 18 women with CIN3 has shown a clinical improvement in 50% of them (Muderspach et al, 2000). Recently, an open clinical trial was performed by the Melief's group (Kenter et al, 2009) in twenty women presenting with usual VIN using 13 large peptides spanning the whole E6 and E7 proteins. Forty five percent of complete (9/20 women) and 25 % (5/20) of partial remission were observed 12 months after immunization. These important results would be even more interesting if the investigators had included a placebo group (Bourgault Villada, 2010a). A new trial with a placebo group is currently under way.

Vaccinia virus was used in a recombinant vaccine containing E6 and E7 genes from HPV16 and HPV18 (TA-HPV) to vaccinate usual VIN patients. A clinical complete or partial response was observed in 8/18 treated women (Davidson et al, 2003). More recently, vaccination against usual VIN was also performed with another recombinant vaccinia virus, TA-L2E6E7 from HPV16 (Daayana et al, 2010). Two months before vaccination, 19 women were treated by topical imiquimod and then vaccinated by intramuscular route with 3 doses of recombinant vaccinia virus. Imiquimod is an immunomodulator that increases the synthesis of type I IFN by dendritic cells after its fixation to the TLR7 in human dendritic cells. Complete remission was obtained in 58% of vaccinated women.

Vaccination against CIN 2/3 was also performed by Transgene using a recombinant vaccinia virus, MVA, associated with the genes coding for E6 and E7 proteins and IL2 cytokine in 18 women. The disappearance of the lesions was observed by colposcopy 6 months later in 10 patients, without any CIN at biopsy in 9 cases. The important conclusion of this trial was that the vaccine was clinically effective, thus avoiding conization for 50% of the women with HPV16-related CIN2/3. A phase II trial including a placebo group is presently undertaken.

A phase II clinical trial has also been performed to evaluate the potential use of the MVA-E2 in treating CIN 2/3 (Garcia-Hernandez et al, 2006). Thirty-four women received the therapeutic vaccine injected directly into the cervix once every week over a 6-week period. Nineteen patients (59%) showed no lesion nine weeks later and histological analysis showed total elimination of high-grade lesions in 20 patients. All patients developed Ab against the MVA-E2 vaccine and showed a specific cytotoxic response against papilloma-transformed cells.

DNA containing E6 and E7 genes from HPV 16 and 18 (ZYC101a) was administered on 86 women having CIN2/3 (Garcia et al, 2004). Conization was performed 6 months later. Resolution of CIN was observed in 73% of the younger (less than 25 years old) women with a significant difference compared to a control group. This therapeutic vaccine is also very promising as CIN 2/3 treatment. New phase II trial is currently under way, testing DNA from E6 and E7 genes versus placebo.

All these results are very important and encouraging for the development of therapeutic vaccines for HPV induced cancers. Nevertheless the proof of efficacy in CIN 2/3 should be carefully demonstrated because therapeutic vaccine should be more efficient that surgery. It is important to note that these therapeutic vaccines should avoid relapse of HPV infection after treatment by increasing HPV-specific cellular immunity.

Other vaccines were tested to fight high grade anal intraepithelial neoplasia (AIN3) in HIV+ patients. HSPE7 including Mycobacterium bovis BCG heat-shock protein 65 (Hsp65) and HPV16 E7 protein was tested. Clinical complete and partial responses were observed in 5 vaccinated patients out of 15 (33% of efficacy) (Palefski et al, 2006). A better vaccine with adjuvant is presently developed.

The safety and immunogenicity of the human papillomavirus type 16 (HPV16) or HPV18 (HPV16/18) E7 protein-pulsed mature dendritic cell vaccination (phase I) were evaluated as adjuvant therapy for 10 patients with stage IB cervical cancer treated by radical hysterectomy (Santin et al, 2008). All patients developed CD4+ T-cell and Ab responses to DC vaccination and 8 of them E7-specific CD8+ T-cells. DC vaccination was well tolerated and no significant toxicity was recorded. New trials (phase II) in cervical cancer patients harboring a limited tumor burden or who are at significant risk of tumor recurrence are warranted to show an efficacy of this immunotherapy.

Condyloma have been also treated by immunotherapy. Two trials were performed using the VLP of HPV6 (Zhang et al, 2000) or the fusion protein L2E7 fron HPV6 (Lacey et al, 1999; Thompson et al, 1999; Vandepapeliere et al, 2005) with a clearance of condyloma obtained in 75 and 20% of cases, respectively. In the absence of control group in these trials, it is too early to make conclusions about the efficacy of these vaccines. In a phase I/II trial, thirty males presenting with intraurethral flat condyloma were treated with either a recombinant vaccinia viral vaccine MVA-E2 (expressing the E2 gene of bovine papillomavirus) (Albarran et al, 2007). 28/30 patients treated with MVAE2 vaccine were free of clinical or histological lesion or HPV at 4 weeks.

16. How to determine the epitopic regions for a therapeutic vaccine?

In a study including 16 women presenting with usual VIN, we have determined the strongly immunogenic regions from HPV16 E6 and E7 proteins for CD4+ and/or CD8+ T lymphocytes (Bourgault Villada et al, 2010b). Among 18 large peptides of the proteins E6 and E7, two were recognized in proliferative assays as immunodominant by T cells from 10 out of 16 women (62%) at the entry in the study, namely E6/2 (aa 14-34) and E6/4 (aa 45-68) peptides. Four other peptides, E6/7 (aa 91-110), E7/2 (aa 7-27), E7/3 (aa 21-40) and E7/7 (aa 65-87) were recognized by only 12% of the women in proliferative or IFNγ ELISPOT tests. The regions of E6 and E7 proteins implicated in T cell recognition during HPV infection were not yet well defined because of the usually low frequency of anti-HPV blood T cell responses and of the difficulties of their study.

In protein E6, some peptides included in, including or overlapping our peptides E6/2 (aa 14-34) and E6/4 (aa 45-68) have already been described as preferentially recognized by

CD4+ T cells. Among them, peptide E6 42-57 that is restricted by HLA-DR7 has already been identified (Strang et al, 1990). Regions E6 1-31, 22-51 and 24-45 can be also immunogenic for CD4+ T cells as shown in CIN or sexually active healthy women (Kadish et al, 1997). The region E6 42-71, which includes peptide E6/4 (aa 45-68), has also been described as a target of proliferative responses in CIN patients (Kadish et al, 1997). Another E6 111-158 region was previously described as inducing proliferative responses in infected asymptomatic subjects or in patients with CIN3 (Kadish et al, 1997; Strang et al, 1990) as well as E6 127-141 peptide in healthy young women (Gallagher et al, 2007). Similarly, peptides E7 43-77, E7 50-62 and E7 58-68 which are restricted by DR3, DR15 and DR17, respectively, were defined as epitopic peptides for CD4 + T cells (Strang et al, 1990; van der Burg et al, 2001; Wang et al, 2009). E7 region 51-98, including our E7/7 (aa 65-87) peptide, is also very immunogenic for proliferating T lymphocytes (de Gruijl et al, 1998; Luxton et al, 1996; Nakagawa et al, 1996).

The characterization of E6 and E7 HPV-16 epitopes and the HLA restriction of their recognition by CD8+ T lymphocytes are more precise: E6 29-38, E7 11-20, E7 82-90 and E7 86-93 epitopes are presented by HLA-A2 (Evans et al, 2001; Ressing et al, 1995, 1996), E6 80-88 and E7 44-52 by HLA-B18 (Bourgault Villada et al, 2000) and E6 49-57 by HLA-A24 (Morishima et al, 2007). In women who cleared HPV 16 infection, cytotoxic T lymphocytes (CTL) responses are directed against epitopes preferentially located in the N-terminal half of the E6 protein (region 16-40) (Nakagawa et al, 2005). In this fragment, the dominant epitope E6 29-37 is restricted by HLA-B48, E6 31-38 by HLA-B4002 and the subdominant epitope E6 52-61 by HLA-B35 (Nakagawa et al, 2007). The same group had also shown that the peptide E6 33-42 61 is recognized by CD8+ T lymphocytes in association with HLA-A68, peptide E6 52-61 in association with HLA-B57 and -B35, peptide E6 75-83 in association with HLA-B62, peptide E7 7-15 in association with HLA-B48 and peptide E7 79-87 in association with HLA-B60 (Nakagawa et al, 2004, 2007; Wang et al, 2008). In addition, E7 7-15 is also able to bind HLA-A2 and -B8 to be recognized by CTL (Oerke et al, 2005; Ressing et al, 1995). From the latter results, two hot spots of CD8+ T-cell epitopes in protein E6 may be located in the regions E6 29-38 and 52-61 and another one in protein E7 (E7 7-15) (Nakagawa et al, 2007). Nevertheless, a poor immunogenicity of E7 protein was observed in many studies during both HPV 16 infection and after peptidic vaccination using long peptides spanning both E6 and E7 (Kenter et al, 2008; Welters et al, 2008) such as those used in our study.

The epitopes E6/2 (aa 14-34) and E6/4 (aa 45-68) hence could be strongly recognized by CD4+ and / or CD8+ T lymphocytes and could be particularly relevant in the design of a peptide vaccination. We may hypothesize that the T cell responses that we observed were able to contain the tumor cells into the epithelium. Therefore, E6/2 (aa 14-34) and E6/4 (aa 45-68) peptides could play a major role in the protection against invasive cancer by stimulating T lymphocytes.

17. Conclusion

HPV infections are very frequent. Eighty percent of women more than 25 years old have been infected. Two third of them have been infected by a oncogenic HPV and 10% of them will develop an intraepithelial neoplasia, mainly CIN. Preventive vaccines are very effective means of avoiding CIN and cervical cancer with an efficacy of 70% against CIN 2/3 related to 14 oncogenic HPVs. Some questions persist about this preventive vaccine: How long will the protection last ? Boosts will be necessary ? Young boys should be also vaccinated ? What is the best age to perform the vaccine with the highest immunogenicity ?

Women previously infected by HPV 16 or 18 and presenting with intraepithelial neoplasia are not good candidate for prophylactic vaccines. Therapeutic vaccines should be good alternatives to surgery for CIN2/3, VIN3 and AIN3 and they are being continuously improved.

18. References

Abramowitz, L., Jacquard, A. C., Jaroud, F., Haesebaert, J., Siproudhis, L., Pradat, P., Aynaud, O., Leocmach, Y., Soubeyrand, B., Dachez, R., Riethmuller, D., Mougin, C., Pretet, J. L., & Denis, F. (2011). Human papillomavirus genotype distribution in anal cancer in France: The EDiTH V study. *Int J Cancer* 129:433-9.

Af Geijersstam, V., Kibur, M., Wang, Z., Koskela, P., Pukkala, E., Schiller, J., Lehtinen, M., & Dillner, J. (1998). Stability over time of serum antibody levels to human papillomavirus type 16. *J Infect Dis* 177:1710-4.

Albarran, Y. C. A., De La Garza, A., Cruz Quiroz, B. J., Vazquez Zea, E., Diaz Estrada, I., Mendez Fuentez, E., Lopez Contreras, M., Andrade-Manzano, A., Padilla, S., Varela, A. R., & Rosales, R. (2007). MVA E2 recombinant vaccine in the treatment of human papillomavirus infection in men presenting intraurethral flat condyloma: a phase I/II study. *BioDrugs* 21:47-59.

Arends, M. J., Benton, E. C., Mclaren, K. M., Stark, L. A., Hunter, J. A., & Bird, C. C. (1997). Renal allograft recipients with high susceptibility to cutaneous malignancy have an increased prevalence of human papillomavirus DNA in skin tumours and a greater risk of anogenital malignancy. *Br J Cancer* 75:722-8.

Bard, E., Riethmuller, D., Meillet, D., Pretet, J.L., Schaal, J.P., Mougin, C., & Seilles, E. (2004); High-risk papillomavirus infection is associated with altered antibody responses in genital tract: non-specific responses in HPV infection. *Viral Immunol* 17:381-9.

Berumen, J., Casas, L., Segura, E., Amezcua, J. L., & Garcia-Carranca, A. (1994). Genome amplification of human papillomavirus types 16 and 18 in cervical carcinomas is related to the retention of E1/E2 genes. *Int J Cancer* 56:640-5.

Bosch, F. X., Manos, M. M., Munoz, N., Sherman, M., Jansen, A. M., Peto, J., Schiffman, M. H., Moreno, V., Kurman, R., & Shah, K. V. (1995). Prevalence of human papillomavirus in cervical cancer: a worldwide perspective. International biological study on cervical cancer (IBSCC) Study Group. *J Natl Cancer Inst* 87:796-802.

Boulanger, J. C., Sevestre, H., Bauville, E., Ghighi, C., Harlicot, J. P., & Gondry, J. (2004). [Epidemiology of HPV infection]. *Gynecol Obstet Fertil* 32:218-23.

Bourgault Villada, I., Beneton, N., Bony, C., Connan, F., Monsonego, J., Bianchi, A., Saiag, P., Levy, J. P., Guillet, J. G., & Choppin, J. (2000). Identification in humans of HPV-16 E6 and E7 protein epitopes recognized by cytolytic T lymphocytes in association with HLA-B18 and determination of the HLA-B18-specific binding motif. *Eur J Immunol* 30:2281-9.

Bourgault Villada, I., Moyal Barracco, M., Ziol, M., Chaboissier, A., Barget, N., Berville, S., Paniel, B., Jullian, E., Clerici, T., Maillere, B., & Guillet, J. G. (2004). Spontaneous regression of grade 3 vulvar intraepithelial neoplasia associated with human papillomavirus-16-specific CD4(+) and CD8(+) T-cell responses. *Cancer Res* 64:8761-6.

Bourgault Villada, I. (2010a). Vaccination against HPV-16 for vulvar intraepithelial neoplasia. *N Engl J Med* 362:655-6.

Bourgault Villada, I., Moyal Barracco, M., Berville, S., Bafounta, M. L., Longvert, C., Premel, V., Villefroy, P., Jullian, E., Clerici, T., Paniel, B., Maillere, B., Choppin, J., & Guillet, J. G. (2010b). Human papillomavirus 16-specific T cell responses in classic HPV-related vulvar intra-epithelial neoplasia. Determination of strongly immunogenic regions from E6 and E7 proteins. *Clin Exp Immunol* 159:45-56.

Bousarghin, L., Hubert, P., Franzen, E., Jacobs, N., Boniver, J., & Delvenne, P. (2005). Human papillomavirus 16 virus-like particles use heparan sulfates to bind dendritic cells and colocalize with langerin in Langerhans cells. *J Gen Virol* 86:1297-305.

Buckley, J. D., Harris, R. W., Doll, R., Vessey, M. P., & Williams, P. T. (1981). Case-control study of the husbands of women with dysplasia or carcinoma of the cervix uteri. *Lancet* 2:1010-5.

Carter, J. J., Koutsky, L. A., Hughes, J. P., Lee, S. K., Kuypers, J., Kiviat, N., & Galloway, D. A. (2000). Comparison of human papillomavirus types 16, 18, and 6 capsid antibody responses following incident infection. *J Infect Dis* 181:1911-9.

Collins, S. I., Constandinou-Williams, C., Wen, K., Young, L. S., Roberts, S., Murray, P. G., & Woodman, C. B. (2009). Disruption of the E2 gene is a common and early event in the natural history of cervical human papillomavirus infection: a longitudinal cohort study. *Cancer Res* 69:3828-32.

Combadiere, B., & Mahe, B. (2008). Particle-based vaccines for transcutaneous vaccination. *Comp Immunol Microbiol Infect Dis* 31:293-315.

Conway, M. J., Cruz, L., Alam, S., Christensen, N. D., & Meyers, C. (2011). Cross-neutralization potential of native human papillomavirus N-terminal L2 epitopes. *PLoS One* 6:e16405.

Daayana, S., Elkord, E., Winters, U., Pawlita, M., Roden, R., Stern, P. L., & Kitchener, H. C. (2010). Phase II trial of imiquimod and HPV therapeutic vaccination in patients with vulval intraepithelial neoplasia. *Br J Cancer* 102:1129-36.

Davidson, E. J., Boswell, C. M., Sehr, P., Pawlita, M., Tomlinson, A. E., Mcvey, R. J., Dobson, J., Roberts, J. S., Hickling, J., Kitchener, H. C., & Stern, P. L. (2003). Immunological and clinical responses in women with vulval intraepithelial neoplasia vaccinated with a vaccinia virus encoding human papillomavirus 16/18 oncoproteins. *Cancer Res* 63:6032-41.

Day, P. M., Thompson, C. D., Buck, C. B., Pang, Y. Y., Lowy, D. R., & Schiller, J. T. (2007). Neutralization of human papillomavirus with monoclonal antibodies reveals different mechanisms of inhibition. *J Virol* 81:8784-92.

De Gruijl, T. D., Bontkes, H. J., Walboomers, J. M., Stukart, M. J., Doekhie, F. S., Remmink, A. J., Helmerhorst, T. J., Verheijen, R. H., Duggan-Keen, M. F., Stern, P. L., Meijer, C. J., & Scheper, R. J. (1998). Differential T helper cell responses to human papillomavirus type 16 E7 related to viral clearance or persistence in patients with cervical neoplasia: a longitudinal study. *Cancer Res* 58:1700-6.

De Gruijl, T. D., Bontkes, H. J., Walboomers, J. M., Coursaget, P., Stukart, M. J., Dupuy, C., Kueter, E., Verheijen, R. H., Helmerhorst, T. J., Duggan-Keen, M. F., Stern, P. L., Meijer, C. J., & Scheper, R. J. (1999). Immune responses against human papillomavirus (HPV) type 16 virus-like particles in a cohort study of women with cervical intraepithelial neoplasia. I. Differential T-helper and IgG responses in relation to HPV infection and disease outcome. *J Gen Virol* 80 (Pt 2):399-408.

De Jong, A., Van Der Burg, S. H., Kwappenberg, K. M., Van Der Hulst, J. M., Franken, K. L., Geluk, A., Van Meijgaarden, K. E., Drijfhout, J. W., Kenter, G., Vermeij, P., Melief, C. J., & Offringa, R. (2002). Frequent detection of human papillomavirus 16 E2-specific T-helper immunity in healthy subjects. *Cancer Res* 62:472-9.

De Jong, A., Van Poelgeest, M. I., Van Der Hulst, J. M., Drijfhout, J. W., Fleuren, G. J., Melief, C. J., Kenter, G., Offringa, R., & Van Der Burg, S. H. (2004). Human papillomavirus type 16-positive cervical cancer is associated with impaired CD4+ T-cell immunity against early antigens E2 and E6. *Cancer Res* 64:5449-55.

Desaintes, C., & Demeret, C. (1996). Control of papillomavirus DNA replication and transcription. *Semin Cancer Biol* 7:339-47.

Dillon, S., Sasagawa, T., Crawford, A., Prestidge, J., Inder, M. K., Jerram, J., Mercer, A. A., & Hibma, M. (2007). Resolution of cervical dysplasia is associated with T-cell proliferative responses to human papillomavirus type 16 E2. *J Gen Virol* 88:803-13.

Evans, M., Borysiewicz, L. K., Evans, A. S., Rowe, M., Jones, M., Gileadi, U., Cerundolo, V., & Man, S. (2001). Antigen processing defects in cervical carcinomas limit the presentation of a CTL epitope from human papillomavirus 16 E6. *J Immunol* 167:5420-8.

Fausch, S. C., Da Silva, D. M., & Kast, W. M. (2005). Heterologous papillomavirus virus-like particles and human papillomavirus virus-like particle immune complexes activate human Langerhans cells. *Vaccine* 23:1720-9.

Gallagher, K. M., & Man, S. (2007). Identification of HLA-DR1- and HLA-DR15-restricted human papillomavirus type 16 (HPV16) and HPV18 E6 epitopes recognized by CD4+ T cells from healthy young women. *J Gen Virol* 88:1470-8.

Garcia, F., Petry, K. U., Muderspach, L., Gold, M. A., Braly, P., Crum, C. P., Magill, M., Silverman, M., Urban, R. G., Hedley, M. L., & Beach, K. J. (2004). ZYC101a for treatment of high-grade cervical intraepithelial neoplasia: a randomized controlled trial. *Obstet Gynecol* 103:317-26.

Garcia-Hernandez, E., Gonzalez-Sanchez, J. L., Andrade-Manzano, A., Contreras, M. L., Padilla, S., Guzman, C. C., Jimenez, R., Reyes, L., Morosoli, G., Verde, M. L., & Rosales, R. (2006). Regression of papilloma high-grade lesions (CIN 2 and CIN 3) is stimulated by therapeutic vaccination with MVA E2 recombinant vaccine. *Cancer Gene Ther* 13:592-7.

Garland, S. M., Hernandez-Avila, M., Wheeler, C. M., Perez, G., Harper, D. M., Leodolter, S., Tang, G. W., Ferris, D. G., Steben, M., Bryan, J., Taddeo, F. J., Railkar, R., Esser, M. T., Sings, H. L., Nelson, M., Boslego, J., Sattler, C., Barr, E., & Koutsky, L. A. (2007). Quadrivalent vaccine against human papillomavirus to prevent anogenital diseases. *N Engl J Med* 356:1928-43.

Giraldo, P. C., Eleuterio, J., Jr., Cavalcante, D. I., Goncalves, A. K., Romao, J. A., & Eleuterio, R. M. (2008). The role of high-risk HPV-DNA testing in the male sexual partners of women with HPV-induced lesions. *Eur J Obstet Gynecol Reprod Biol* 137:88-91.

Giuliano, A. R., Palefsky, J. M., Goldstone, S., Moreira, E. D., Jr., Penny, M. E., Aranda, C., Vardas, E., Moi, H., Jessen, H., Hillman, R., Chang, Y. H., Ferris, D., Rouleau, D., Bryan, J., Marshall, J. B., Vuocolo, S., Barr, E., Radley, D., Haupt, R. M., & Guris, D. (2011). Efficacy of quadrivalent HPV vaccine against HPV Infection and disease in males. *N Engl J Med* 364:401-11.

Grover, A., Kim, G. J., Lizee, G., Tschoi, M., Wang, G., Wunderlich, J. R., Rosenberg, S. A., Hwang, S. T., & Hwu, P. (2006). Intralymphatic dendritic cell vaccination induces tumor antigen-specific, skin-homing T lymphocytes. *Clin Cancer Res* 12:5801-8.

Harper, D. M., Franco, E. L., Wheeler, C., Ferris, D. G., Jenkins, D., Schuind, A., Zahaf, T., Innis, B., Naud, P., De Carvalho, N. S., Roteli-Martins, C. M., Teixeira, J., Blatter, M. M., Korn, A. P., Quint, W., & Dubin, G. (2004). Efficacy of a bivalent L1 virus-like particle vaccine in prevention of infection with human papillomavirus types 16 and 18 in young women: a randomised controlled trial. *Lancet* 364:1757-65.

Harper, D. M., Franco, E. L., Wheeler, C. M., Moscicki, A. B., Romanowski, B., Roteli-Martins, C. M., Jenkins, D., Schuind, A., Costa Clemens, S. A., & Dubin, G. (2006). Sustained efficacy up to 4.5 years of a bivalent L1 virus-like particle vaccine against human papillomavirus types 16 and 18: follow-up from a randomised control trial. *Lancet* 367:1247-55.

Harro, C. D., Pang, Y. Y., Roden, R. B., Hildesheim, A., Wang, Z., Reynolds, M. J., Mast, T. C., Robinson, R., Murphy, B. R., Karron, R. A., Dillner, J., Schiller, J. T., & Lowy, D. R. (2001). Safety and immunogenicity trial in adult volunteers of a human papillomavirus 16 L1 virus-like particle vaccine. *J Natl Cancer Inst* 93:284-92.

Herbst, B., Kohler, G., Mackensen, A., Veelken, H., Kulmburg, P., Rosenthal, F. M., Schaefer, H. E., Mertelsmann, R., Fisch, P., & Lindemann, A. (1996). In vitro differentiation of CD34+ hematopoietic progenitor cells toward distinct dendritic cell subsets of the birbeck granule and MIIC-positive Langerhans cell and the interdigitating dendritic cell type. *Blood* 88:2541-8.

Hippelainen, M. I., Yliskoski, M., Syrjanen, S., Saastamoinen, J., Hippelainen, M., Saarikoski, S., & Syrjanen, K. (1994). Low concordance of genital human papillomavirus (HPV) lesions and viral types in HPV-infected women and their male sexual partners. *Sex Transm Dis* 21:76-82.

Ho, G. Y., Studentsov, Y. Y., Bierman, R., & Burk, R. D. (2004). Natural history of human papillomavirus type 16 virus-like particle antibodies in young women. *Cancer Epidemiol Biomarkers Prev* 13:110-6.

Jacobelli S., Sanaa. F.., Moyal Barracco M., Pelisse M., Berville S., Villefroy P., North M.O., Figueiredo S., Charmeteau B., Clerici T., Plantier F., Dupin N., Avril M.F., Guillet J.G., & Bourgault Villada I. (2011). Anti-HPV16 E2 protein T-cell responses and viral control in women with usual vulvar intraepithelial neoplasia and their healthy partners. *Submitted.*

Joura, E. A., Leodolter, S., Hernandez-Avila, M., Wheeler, C. M., Perez, G., Koutsky, L. A., Garland, S. M., Harper, D. M., Tang, G. W., Ferris, D. G., Steben, M., Jones, R. W., Bryan, J., Taddeo, F. J., Bautista, O. M., Esser, M. T., Sings, H. L., Nelson, M.,

Boslego, J. W., Sattler, C., Barr, E., & Paavonen, J. (2007). Efficacy of a quadrivalent prophylactic human papillomavirus (types 6, 11, 16, and 18) L1 virus-like-particle vaccine against high-grade vulval and vaginal lesions: a combined analysis of three randomised clinical trials. *Lancet* 369:1693-702.

Kadish, A. S., Ho, G. Y., Burk, R. D., Wang, Y., Romney, S. L., Ledwidge, R., & Angeletti, R. H. (1997). Lymphoproliferative responses to human papillomavirus (HPV) type 16 proteins E6 and E7: outcome of HPV infection and associated neoplasia. *J Natl Cancer Inst* 89:1285-93.

Kenter, G. G., Welters, M. J., Valentijn, A. R., Lowik, M. J., Berends-Van Der Meer, D. M., Vloon, A. P., Drijfhout, J. W., Wafelman, A. R., Oostendorp, J., Fleuren, G. J., Offringa, R., Van Der Burg, S. H., & Melief, C. J. (2008). Phase I immunotherapeutic trial with long peptides spanning the E6 and E7 sequences of high-risk human papillomavirus 16 in end-stage cervical cancer patients shows low toxicity and robust immunogenicity. *Clin Cancer Res* 14:169-77.

Kenter, G. G., Welters, M. J., Valentijn, A. R., Lowik, M. J., Berends-Van Der Meer, D. M., Vloon, A. P., Essahsah, F., Fathers, L. M., Offringa, R., Drijfhout, J. W., Wafelman, A. R., Oostendorp, J., Fleuren, G. J., Van Der Burg, S. H., & Melief, C. J. (2009). Vaccination against HPV-16 oncoproteins for vulvar intraepithelial neoplasia. *N Engl J Med* 361:1838-47.

Kines, R. C., Thompson, C. D., Lowy, D. R., Schiller, J. T., & Day, P. M. (2009). The initial steps leading to papillomavirus infection occur on the basement membrane prior to cell surface binding. *Proc Natl Acad Sci U S A* 106:20458-63.

Kirnbauer, R., Hubbert, N. L., Wheeler, C. M., Becker, T. M., Lowy, D. R., & Schiller, J. T. (1994). A virus-like particle enzyme-linked immunosorbent assay detects serum antibodies in a majority of women infected with human papillomavirus type 16. *J Natl Cancer Inst* 86:494-9.

Koutsky, L. A., Ault, K. A., Wheeler, C. M., Brown, D. R., Barr, E., Alvarez, F. B., Chiacchierini, L. M., & Jansen, K. U. (2002). A controlled trial of a human papillomavirus type 16 vaccine. *N Engl J Med* 347:1645-51.

Lacey, C. J., Thompson, H. S., Monteiro, E. F., O'neill, T., Davies, M. L., Holding, F. P., Fallon, R. E., & Roberts, J. S. (1999). Phase IIa safety and immunogenicity of a therapeutic vaccine, TA-GW, in persons with genital warts. *J Infect Dis* 179:612-8.

Lawrence, T., Puel, A., Reichenbach, J., Ku, C. L., Chapgier, A., Renner, E., Minard-Colin, V., Ouachee, M., & Casanova, J. L. (2005). Autosomal-dominant primary immunodeficiencies. *Curr Opin Hematol* 12:22-30.

Lowe, R. S., Brown, D. R., Bryan, J. T., Cook, J. C., George, H. A., Hofmann, K. J., Hurni, W. M., Joyce, J. G., Lehman, E. D., Markus, H. Z., Neeper, M. P., Schultz, L. D., Shaw, A. R., & Jansen, K. U. (1997). Human papillomavirus type 11 (HPV-11) neutralizing antibodies in the serum and genital mucosal secretions of African green monkeys immunized with HPV-11 virus-like particles expressed in yeast. *J Infect Dis* 176:1141-5.

Luxton, J. C., Rowe, A. J., Cridland, J. C., Coletart, T., Wilson, P., & Shepherd, P. S. (1996). Proliferative T cell responses to the human papillomavirus type 16 E7 protein in women with cervical dysplasia and cervical carcinoma and in healthy individuals. *J Gen Virol* 77 (Pt 7):1585-93.

Malejczyk, J., Majewski, S., & Jablonska, S. (1997). Cellular immunity in cutaneous and genital HPV infections. *Clin Dermatol* 15:261-74.

Matthews, K., Leong, C. M., Baxter, L., Inglis, E., Yun, K., Backstrom, B. T., Doorbar, J., & Hibma, M. (2003). Depletion of Langerhans cells in human papillomavirus type 16-infected skin is associated with E6-mediated down regulation of E-cadherin. *J Virol* 77:8378-85.

McCluggage, W. G. (2009). Recent developments in vulvovaginal pathology. *Histopathology* 54:156-73.

McCredie, M. R., Sharples, K. J., Paul, C., Baranyai, J., Medley, G., Jones, R. W., & Skegg, D. C. (2008). Natural history of cervical neoplasia and risk of invasive cancer in women with cervical intraepithelial neoplasia 3: a retrospective cohort study. *Lancet Oncol* 9:425-34.

McKeage, K., & Romanowski, B. (2011). AS04-adjuvanted human papillomavirus (HPV) types 16 and 18 vaccine (Cervarix(R)): a review of its use in the prevention of premalignant cervical lesions and cervical cancer causally related to certain oncogenic HPV types. *Drugs* 71:465-88.

Molling, J. W., De Gruijl, T. D., Glim, J., Moreno, M., Rozendaal, L., Meijer, C. J., Van Den Eertwegh, A. J., Scheper, R. J., Von Blomberg, M. E., & Bontkes, H. J. (2007). CD4(+)CD25hi regulatory T-cell frequency correlates with persistence of human papillomavirus type 16 and T helper cell responses in patients with cervical intraepithelial neoplasia. *Int J Cancer* 121:1749-55.

Morishima, S., Akatsuka, Y., Nawa, A., Kondo, E., Kiyono, T., Torikai, H., Nakanishi, T., Ito, Y., Tsujimura, K., Iwata, K., Ito, K., Kodera, Y., Morishima, Y., Kuzushima, K., & Takahashi, T. (2007). Identification of an HLA-A24-restricted cytotoxic T lymphocyte epitope from human papillomavirus type-16 E6: the combined effects of bortezomib and interferon-gamma on the presentation of a cryptic epitope. *Int J Cancer* 120:594-604.

Muderspach, L., Wilczynski, S., Roman, L., Bade, L., Felix, J., Small, L. A., Kast, W. M., Fascio, G., Marty, V., & Weber, J. (2000). A phase I trial of a human papillomavirus (HPV) peptide vaccine for women with high-grade cervical and vulvar intraepithelial neoplasia who are HPV 16 positive. *Clin Cancer Res* 6:3406-16.

Munoz, N., Kjaer, S. K., Sigurdsson, K., Iversen, O. E., Hernandez-Avila, M., Wheeler, C. M., Perez, G., Brown, D. R., Koutsky, L. A., Tay, E. H., Garcia, P. J., Ault, K. A., Garland, S. M., Leodolter, S., Olsson, S. E., Tang, G. W., Ferris, D. G., Paavonen, J., Steben, M., Bosch, F. X., Dillner, J., Huh, W. K., Joura, E. A., Kurman, R. J., Majewski, S., Myers, E. R., Villa, L. L., Taddeo, F. J., Roberts, C., Tadesse, A., Bryan, J. T., Lupinacci, L. C., Giacoletti, K. E., Sings, H. L., James, M. K., Hesley, T. M., Barr, E., & Haupt, R. M. (2010). Impact of human papillomavirus (HPV)-6/11/16/18 vaccine on all HPV-associated genital diseases in young women. *J Natl Cancer Inst* 102:325-39.

Nakagawa, M., Stites, D. P., Farhat, S., Judd, A., Moscicki, A. B., Canchola, A. J., Hilton, J. F., & Palefsky, J. M. (1996). T-cell proliferative response to human papillomavirus type 16 peptides: relationship to cervical intraepithelial neoplasia. *Clin Diagn Lab Immunol* 3:205-10.

Nakagawa, M., Stites, D. P., Farhat, S., Sisler, J. R., Moss, B., Kong, F., Moscicki, A. B., & Palefsky, J. M. (1997). Cytotoxic T lymphocyte responses to E6 and E7 proteins of human papillomavirus type 16: relationship to cervical intraepithelial neoplasia. *J Infect Dis* 175:927-31.

Nakagawa, M., Stites, D. P., Patel, S., Farhat, S., Scott, M., Hills, N. K., Palefsky, J. M., & Moscicki, A. B. (2000). Persistence of human papillomavirus type 16 infection is associated with lack of cytotoxic T lymphocyte response to the E6 antigens. *J Infect Dis* 182:595-8.

Nakagawa, M., Kim, K. H., & Moscicki, A. B. (2004). Different methods of identifying new antigenic epitopes of human papillomavirus type 16 E6 and E7 proteins. *Clin Diagn Lab Immunol* 11:889-96.

Nakagawa, M., Kim, K. H., & Moscicki, A. B. (2005). Patterns of CD8 T-cell epitopes within the human papillomavirus type 16 (HPV 16) E6 protein among young women whose HPV 16 infection has become undetectable. *Clin Diagn Lab Immunol* 12:1003-5.

Nakagawa, M., Kim, K. H., Gillam, T. M., & Moscicki, A. B. (2007). HLA class I binding promiscuity of the CD8 T-cell epitopes of human papillomavirus type 16 E6 protein. *J Virol* 81:1412-23.

Nardelli-Haefliger, D., Wirthner, D., Schiller, J. T., Lowy, D. R., Hildesheim, A., Ponci, F., & De Grandi, P. (2003). Specific antibody levels at the cervix during the menstrual cycle of women vaccinated with human papillomavirus 16 virus-like particles. *J Natl Cancer Inst* 95:1128-37.

Nicolau, S. M., Camargo, C. G., Stavale, J. N., Castelo, A., Dores, G. B., Lorincz, A., & De Lima, G. R. (2005). Human papillomavirus DNA detection in male sexual partners of women with genital human papillomavirus infection. *Urology* 65:251-5.

Oerke, S., Hohn, H., Zehbe, I., Pilch, H., Schicketanz, K. H., Hitzler, W. E., Neukirch, C., Freitag, K., & Maeurer, M. J. (2005). Naturally processed and HLA-B8-presented HPV16 E7 epitope recognized by T cells from patients with cervical cancer. *Int J Cancer* 114:766-78.

Offringa, R., De Jong, A., Toes, R. E., Van Der Burg, S. H., & Melief, C. J. (2003). Interplay between human papillomaviruses and dendritic cells. *Curr Top Microbiol Immunol* 276:215-40.

Ostor, A. G. (1993). Natural history of cervical intraepithelial neoplasia: a critical review. *Int J Gynecol Pathol* 12:186-92.

Paavonen, J., Jenkins, D., Bosch, F. X., Naud, P., Salmeron, J., Wheeler, C. M., Chow, S. N., Apter, D. L., Kitchener, H. C., Castellsague, X., De Carvalho, N. S., Skinner, S. R., Harper, D. M., Hedrick, J. A., Jaisamrarn, U., Limson, G. A., Dionne, M., Quint, W., Spiessens, B., Peeters, P., Struyf, F., Wieting, S. L., Lehtinen, M. O., & Dubin, G. (2007). Efficacy of a prophylactic adjuvanted bivalent L1 virus-like-particle vaccine against infection with human papillomavirus types 16 and 18 in young women: an interim analysis of a phase III double-blind, randomised controlled trial. *Lancet* 369:2161-70.

Paavonen, J., Naud, P., Salmeron, J., Wheeler, C. M., Chow, S. N., Apter, D., Kitchener, H., Castellsague, X., Teixeira, J. C., Skinner, S. R., Hedrick, J., Jaisamrarn, U., Limson, G., Garland, S., Szarewski, A., Romanowski, B., Aoki, F. Y., Schwarz, T. F., Poppe,

W. A., Bosch, F. X., Jenkins, D., Hardt, K., Zahaf, T., Descamps, D., Struyf, F., Lehtinen, M., Dubin, G., & Greenacre, M. (2009). Efficacy of human papillomavirus (HPV)-16/18 AS04-adjuvanted vaccine against cervical infection and precancer caused by oncogenic HPV types (PATRICIA): final analysis of a double-blind, randomised study in young women. *Lancet* 374:301-14.

Palefsky, J. M., Berry, J. M., Jay, N., Krogstad, M., Da Costa, M., Darragh, T. M., & Lee, J. Y. (2006). A trial of SGN-00101 (HspE7) to treat high-grade anal intraepithelial neoplasia in HIV-positive individuals. *Aids* 20:1151-5.

Palucka, K., Ueno, H., Roberts, L., Fay, J., & Banchereau, J. (2010). Dendritic cell subsets as vectors and targets for improved cancer therapy. *Curr Top Microbiol Immunol* 344:173-92.

Patel, S., & Chiplunkar, S. (2009). Host immune responses to cervical cancer. *Curr Opin Obstet Gynecol* 21:54-9.

Piketty, C., Selinger-Leneman, H., Grabar, S., Duvivier, C., Bonmarchand, M., Abramowitz, L., Costagliola, D., & Mary-Krause, M. (2008). Marked increase in the incidence of invasive anal cancer among HIV-infected patients despite treatment with combination antiretroviral therapy. *Aids* 22:1203-11.

Piketty C, A. S.-M., E. Lanoy, B. Cochand-Priollet, S. Trabelsi, P-M. Girard, R. Tubiana, L. Abramowitz, E. Tartour, L. Weiss, D. Costagliola, & the Valparaiso Study Group. (2010). Lack of regression of anal squamous intraepithelial lesions and anal HPV infection despite immune restoration under cART. *18th International AIDS Conference*.

Reiter, P. L., Pendergraft, W. F., 3rd, & Brewer, N. T. (2010). Meta-analysis of human papillomavirus infection concordance. *Cancer Epidemiol Biomarkers Prev* 19:2916-31.

Ressing, M. E., Sette, A., Brandt, R. M., Ruppert, J., Wentworth, P. A., Hartman, M., Oseroff, C., Grey, H. M., Melief, C. J., & Kast, W. M. (1995). Human CTL epitopes encoded by human papillomavirus type 16 E6 and E7 identified through in vivo and in vitro immunogenicity studies of HLA-A*0201-binding peptides. *J Immunol* 154:5934-43.

Ressing, M. E., Van Driel, W. J., Celis, E., Sette, A., Brandt, M. P., Hartman, M., Anholts, J. D., Schreuder, G. M., Ter Harmsel, W. B., Fleuren, G. J., Trimbos, B. J., Kast, W. M., & Melief, C. J. (1996). Occasional memory cytotoxic T-cell responses of patients with human papillomavirus type 16-positive cervical lesions against a human leukocyte antigen-A *0201-restricted E7-encoded epitope. *Cancer Res* 56:582-8.

Ressing, M. E., Van Driel, W. J., Brandt, R. M., Kenter, G. G., De Jong, J. H., Bauknecht, T., Fleuren, G. J., Hoogerhout, P., Offringa, R., Sette, A., Celis, E., Grey, H., Trimbos, B. J., Kast, W. M., & Melief, C. J. (2000). Detection of T helper responses, but not of human papillomavirus-specific cytotoxic T lymphocyte responses, after peptide vaccination of patients with cervical carcinoma. *J Immunother* 23:255-66.

Santin, A. D., Bellone, S., Palmieri, M., Zanolini, A., Ravaggi, A., Siegel, E. R., Roman, J. J., Pecorelli, S., & Cannon, M. J. (2008). Human papillomavirus type 16 and 18 E7-pulsed dendritic cell vaccination of stage IB or IIA cervical cancer patients: a phase I escalating-dose trial. *J Virol* 82:1968-79.

Sapp, M., & Bienkowska-Haba, M. (2009). Viral entry mechanisms: human papillomavirus and a long journey from extracellular matrix to the nucleus. *Febs J* 276:7206-16.

Sauzet, J. P., Deprez, B., Martinon, F., Guillet, J. G., Gras-Masse, H., & Gomard, E. (1995). Long-lasting anti-viral cytotoxic T lymphocytes induced in vivo with chimeric-multirestricted lipopeptides. *Vaccine* 13:1339-45.

Schellenbacher, C., Roden, R., & Kirnbauer, R. (2009). Chimeric L1-L2 virus-like particles as potential broad-spectrum human papillomavirus vaccines. *J Virol* 83:10085-95.

Srodon, M., Stoler, M. H., Baber, G. B., & Kurman, R. J. (2006). The distribution of low and high-risk HPV types in vulvar and vaginal intraepithelial neoplasia (VIN and VaIN). *Am J Surg Pathol* 30:1513-8.

Steller, M. A., Gurski, K. J., Murakami, M., Daniel, R. W., Shah, K. V., Celis, E., Sette, A., Trimble, E. L., Park, R. C., & Marincola, F. M. (1998). Cell-mediated immunological responses in cervical and vaginal cancer patients immunized with a lipidated epitope of human papillomavirus type 16 E7. *Clin Cancer Res* 4:2103-9.

Strang, G., Hickling, J. K., Mcindoe, G. A., Howland, K., Wilkinson, D., Ikeda, H., & Rothbard, J. B. (1990). Human T cell responses to human papillomavirus type 16 L1 and E6 synthetic peptides: identification of T cell determinants, HLA-DR restriction and virus type specificity. *J Gen Virol* 71 (Pt 2):423-31.

Sun, X. W., Kuhn, L., Ellerbrock, T. V., Chiasson, M. A., Bush, T. J., & Wright, T. C., Jr. (1997). Human papillomavirus infection in women infected with the human immunodeficiency virus. *N Engl J Med* 337:1343-9.

Thompson, H. S., Davies, M. L., Holding, F. P., Fallon, R. E., Mann, A. E., O'neill, T., & Roberts, J. S. (1999). Phase I safety and antigenicity of TA-GW: a recombinant HPV6 L2E7 vaccine for the treatment of genital warts. *Vaccine* 17:40-9.

Tsukui, T., Hildesheim, A., Schiffman, M. H., Lucci, J., 3rd, Contois, D., Lawler, P., Rush, B. B., Lorincz, A. T., Corrigan, A., Burk, R. D., Qu, W., Marshall, M. A., Mann, D., Carrington, M., Clerici, M., Shearer, G. M., Carbone, D. P., Scott, D. R., Houghten, R. A., & Berzofsky, J. A. (1996). Interleukin 2 production in vitro by peripheral lymphocytes in response to human papillomavirus-derived peptides: correlation with cervical pathology. *Cancer Res* 56:3967-74.

Ulrich, C., Hackethal, M., Meyer, T., Geusau, A., Nindl, I., Ulrich, M., Forschner, T., Sterry, W., & Stockfleth, E. (2008). Skin infections in organ transplant recipients. *J Dtsch Dermatol Ges* 6:98-105.

Van Der Burg, S. H., Ressing, M. E., Kwappenberg, K. M., De Jong, A., Straathof, K., De Jong, J., Geluk, A., Van Meijgaarden, K. E., Franken, K. L., Ottenhoff, T. H., Fleuren, G. J., Kenter, G., Melief, C. J., & Offringa, R. (2001). Natural T-helper immunity against human papillomavirus type 16 (HPV16) E7-derived peptide epitopes in patients with HPV16-positive cervical lesions: identification of 3 human leukocyte antigen class II-restricted epitopes. *Int J Cancer* 91:612-8.

Van Der Burg, S. H., Piersma, S. J., De Jong, A., Van Der Hulst, J. M., Kwappenberg, K. M., Van Den Hende, M., Welters, M. J., Van Rood, J. J., Fleuren, G. J., Melief, C. J., Kenter, G. G., & Offringa, R. (2007). Association of cervical cancer with the presence of CD4+ regulatory T cells specific for human papillomavirus antigens. *Proc Natl Acad Sci U S A* 104:12087-92.

Van Driel, W. J., Ressing, M. E., Kenter, G. G., Brandt, R. M., Krul, E. J., Van Rossum, A. B., Schuuring, E., Offringa, R., Bauknecht, T., Tamm-Hermelink, A., Van Dam, P. A., Fleuren, G. J., Kast, W. M., Melief, C. J., & Trimbos, J. B. (1999). Vaccination with

HPV16 peptides of patients with advanced cervical carcinoma: clinical evaluation of a phase I-II trial. *Eur J Cancer* 35:946-52.

Vandepapeliere, P., Barrasso, R., Meijer, C. J., Walboomers, J. M., Wettendorff, M., Stanberry, L. R., & Lacey, C. J. (2005). Randomized controlled trial of an adjuvanted human papillomavirus (HPV) type 6 L2E7 vaccine: infection of external anogenital warts with multiple HPV types and failure of therapeutic vaccination. *J Infect Dis* 192:2099-107.

Viscidi, R. P., Schiffman, M., Hildesheim, A., Herrero, R., Castle, P. E., Bratti, M. C., Rodriguez, A. C., Sherman, M. E., Wang, S., Clayman, B., & Burk, R. D. (2004). Seroreactivity to human papillomavirus (HPV) types 16, 18, or 31 and risk of subsequent HPV infection: results from a population-based study in Costa Rica. *Cancer Epidemiol Biomarkers Prev* 13:324-7.

Viscidi, R. P., Snyder, B., Cu-Uvin, S., Hogan, J. W., Clayman, B., Klein, R. S., Sobel, J., & Shah, K. V. (2005). Human papillomavirus capsid antibody response to natural infection and risk of subsequent HPV infection in HIV-positive and HIV-negative women. *Cancer Epidemiol Biomarkers Prev* 14:283-8.

Visser, J., Nijman, H. W., Hoogenboom, B. N., Jager, P., Van Baarle, D., Schuuring, E., Abdulahad, W., Miedema, F., Van Der Zee, A. G., & Daemen, T. (2007). Frequencies and role of regulatory T cells in patients with (pre)malignant cervical neoplasia. *Clin Exp Immunol* 150:199-209.

Wang, X., Moscicki, A. B., Tsang, L., Brockman, A., & Nakagawa, M. (2008). Memory T cells specific for novel human papillomavirus type 16 (HPV16) E6 epitopes in women whose HPV16 infection has become undetectable. *Clin Vaccine Immunol* 15:937-45.

Wang, X., Santin, A. D., Bellone, S., Gupta, S., & Nakagawa, M. (2009). A novel CD4 T-cell epitope described from one of the cervical cancer patients vaccinated with HPV 16 or 18 E7-pulsed dendritic cells. *Cancer Immunol Immunother* 58:301-8.

Welters, M. J., Kenter, G. G., Piersma, S. J., Vloon, A. P., Lowik, M. J., Berends-Van Der Meer, D. M., Drijfhout, J. W., Valentijn, A. R., Wafelman, A. R., Oostendorp, J., Fleuren, G. J., Offringa, R., Melief, C. J., & Van Der Burg, S. H. (2008). Induction of tumor-specific CD4+ and CD8+ T-cell immunity in cervical cancer patients by a human papillomavirus type 16 E6 and E7 long peptides vaccine. *Clin Cancer Res* 14:178-87.

Xue, Y., Bellanger, S., Zhang, W., Lim, D., Low, J., Lunny, D., & Thierry, F. (2010). HPV16 E2 is an immediate early marker of viral infection, preceding E7 expression in precursor structures of cervical carcinoma. *Cancer Res* 70:5316-25.

Yan, M., Peng, J., Jabbar, I. A., Liu, X., Filgueira, L., Frazer, I. H., & Thomas, R. (2004). Despite differences between dendritic cells and Langerhans cells in the mechanism of papillomavirus-like particle antigen uptake, both cells cross-prime T cells. *Virology* 324:297-310.Zehbe, I., Schmidt, M., Maeurer, M., Leo, C., Hockel, M., & Pilch, H. (2006). Different T-cell receptor (TCR) zeta chain expression in cervical cancer and its precursor lesions. *Zentralbl Gynakol* 128:266-70.

Zehbe I., Schmidt M., Maeurer M., Leo C., Höckel M., & Pilch H. (2006). Different T-cell receptor (TCR) zeta chain expression in cervical cancer and its precursor lesions. *Zentralbl Gynakol* 128:266-70.

Zhang, L. F., Zhou, J., Chen, S., Cai, L. L., Bao, Q. Y., Zheng, F. Y., Lu, J. Q., Padmanabha, J., Hengst, K., Malcolm, K., & Frazer, I. H. (2000). HPV6b virus like particles are potent immunogens without adjuvant in man. *Vaccine* 18:1051-8.

Part 3

Human Papillomavirus in Non-Uterine Disease

9

Epidemiology of HPV in Head and Neck Cancer

Márcio Campos Oliveira, Maria da Conceição Andrade
and Fabrício dos Santos Menezes
*State University of Feira de Santana - Bahia/State
University of Southwest Bahia
Brazil*

1. Introduction

The Human papillomavirus (HPV) is etiologically related to the development of uterine cervical and other genital cancers (Bosch et al., 1995; Frisch et al., 1999; Melbye & Frisch, 1998), and may be involved also in the etiology of cancers of the upper aerodigestive tract comprising the head and neck (HN) tumors (Franceschi et al., 1996). Some molecular and epidemiological studies support such possibility, once that an increased risk of cancer of the oral cavity, pharynx and larynx subsequent to the occurrence of cancer of the cervix has been found. Moreover, the incidence of some head and neck tumors has been increasing around the world and this high prevalence was attributed to the influence of risk factors, being the human papillomavirus important in this role.

The present chapter aims at investigating epidemiologic features of HPV in head and neck cancer worldwide in order to determine the prevalence and the type distribution of HPV by means of a literature review of published studies.

2. Epidemiology of head and neck cancer

The head and neck cancer comprises malignancies arising in the upper respiratory and digestive tracts and is a relatively frequent type of cancer (Parkin et al., 2002). Thus, the term "head and neck cancer" includes lesions at several anatomic sites, such as the lip, oral cavity, nose and paranasal sinuses, naso-pharynx, oro-pharynx, hypo-pharynx, larynx, oesophagus, salivary glands, as well the soft tissues of the neck and ear. Unfortunately, many papers lack the exact location of the head and neck lesions, making the material poorly characterised. The human papillomavirus (HPV) detection rates reported in the so-called head and neck cancer do not give us a detailed view of the association of HPV in distinct entities, unless detailed anatomic locations are given (Syrjänen, 2005).

The malignant tumors of the head and neck consist of a rather heterogeneous group of neoplasias arising in the epithelium of the upper aerodigestive tract. The most common histologic type is squamous cell carcinomas (SCC), occurring in the oral cavity, pharynx (nasopharynx, oropharynx and hypopharynx) and larynx (Lassen, 2010).

Worldwide annually, over 650,000 patients are diagnosed with HNSCC and some 350,000 die from this disease every year (Ferlay et al., 2010; Syrjänen, 2010). Head and neck cancer is the sixth most common cancer worldwide (Parkin et al., 2002), and the table 1 summarizes the global incidence and mortality of head and neck cancer per anatomic site.

CANCER	INCIDENCE	MORTALITY
Oral cavity and lip		
Male	170,496	83,109
Female	92,524	44,545
Total	263,020	127,654
Nasopharynx		
Male	57,852	35,984
Female	26,589	15,625
Total	84,441	51,609
Other pharynx		
Male	108,588	76,458
Female	28,034	19,092
Total	136,622	95,550
Larynx		
Male	129,651	70,336
Female	21,026	11,556
Total	150,677	81,892

Table 1. Global incidence and mortality of head and neck cancer per anatomic site (Ferlay et al., 2010). GLOBOCAN (IARC).

The rates of incidence and mortality around the world of head and neck squamous cell carcinomas have been broadly varying, with notably high rates in Southeast Asia and Eastern Europe (Franceschi et al., 1996). In addition, there is a considerable global variation in the incidence of the disease due to geographic differences in ethnicity, culture and socio-economics (Lassen, 2010). Figure 1, obtained through the Globocan project (Ferlay et al., 2010) illustrates the global incidence of head and neck cancer.

Incidence and survival trends have recently been reported in various types of cancer based on 1994–2003 data from cancer registries in a large number of European countries. Oral cavity and pharyngeal cancer were analysed as a group and divergent incidence trends were observed when different countries were compared. For some countries, there was an increase in incidence (England, Wales and Czech Republic), whereas for other countries there was no change (a.o. Switzerland and Denmark) or a decrease (a.o. Finland, France and Germany) (Karim et al., 2008).

Jemal et al. (2008) estimated that 47,500 people were diagnosed with head and neck cancer in the United States, representing approximately 3% of new cancer diagnoses, and an estimated 11,260 people died from this disease, with squamous cell carcinomas in the majority of these cases.

Shiboski et al. (2005) showed, with an analysis of the National Cancer Institute's Surveillance, Epidemiology and End Results (SEER) data from 1973-2001, an annual increase in the incidence of oral tongue, palatine tonsil, and base-of-tongue cancers, by 2.1%, 3.9%, and 1.7%, respectively, in 20- to 44-year-old white patients, while the incidence of HNSCC at other sites declined.

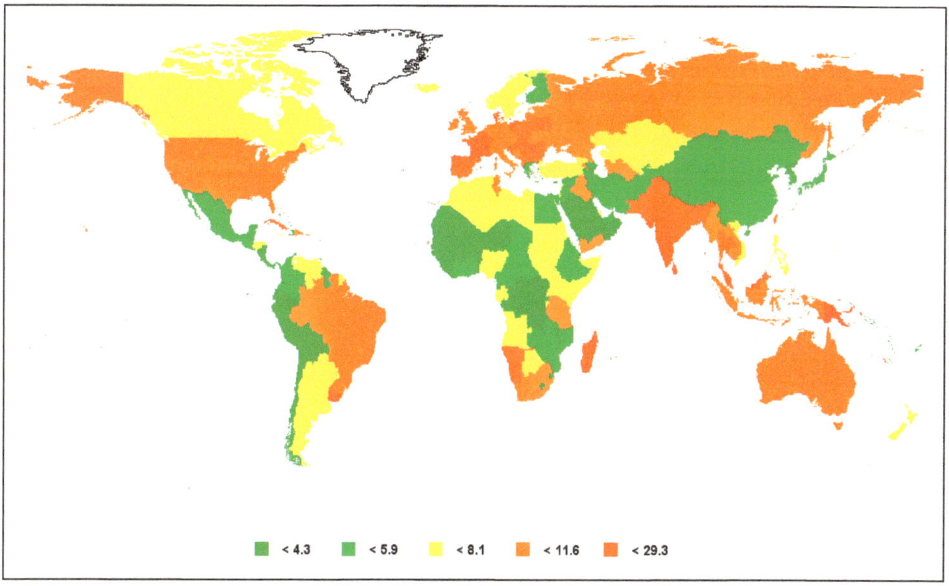

Fig. 1. Global incidence of head and neck tumors (oral cavity and lip, larynx, nasopharynx and other pharynx). Estimated age-standardized incidence rate per 100,000, both sexes, all ages (Ferlay et al., 2010). GLOBOCAN (IARC).

3. Head and neck cancer and HPV

Since the first description of a potential link between HPV infection and head and neck cancer (Syrjänen, 1984), several studies have strongly supported an etiologic role for HPV in cancers arising from specific mucosal sites within the head and neck (D'Souza et al., 2007; Gillison et al., 2000; Herrero et al., 2003). Thus, the detection of HPV genomic deoxyribonucleic acid (DNA) has been found in approximately 25.9% of 5,046 HNSCC cancer specimens from 60 studies using sensitive polymerase chain reaction-based methods (Kreimer et al., 2005).

Head and neck squamous cell carcinoma (HNSCC) typically affects male smokers older than 55 years. Recently, an increase in the incidence of HNSCC in young adults has been recognized, many of them nonsmokers and females. Functional inactivation of p16 is known to be a common event in HNSCC, mainly by either deletion or epigenetic changes. A previous study by this group has shown that p16 deletions in HNSCC are significantly associated with age. The primary objective of this study was to evaluate additional molecular alterations of p16 in HNSCC, specifically in relation to age, site, and human papillomavirus (HPV) status. Patients ranging in age from 22 to 76 years with HNSCC were prospectively identified (n = 24). Methylation-specific polymerase chain reaction and immunohistochemistry were used to evaluate p16 gene inactivation and p16 protein expression, respectively. HPV 16 status was determined for each case. Overall, p16 inactivation was a frequent event detected in 46% of cases. Methylation of p16 was more often detected in females than males (P = .05). All cases showing p16 methylation were from the anterior tongue, and 75% of them were young patients. The results indicate that p16 methylation is a more common event in those younger than 40 years in contrast to p16 deletions, which are more common in those older than 40 years. Consequently, it appears that specific modes of inactivation of p16 in HNSCC are related to specific patient risk profiles. Interestingly, HPV 16 messenger RNA was detected exclusively in HNSCC from the base of tongue lesions and was only found in males. This differs from the patient profile of HNSCC in the young, which affects the anterior tongue and commonly females, thus, making it highly unlikely that this virus is a primary causative agent of HNSCC in these young adults (O'Regan et al., 2008).

Despite successful efforts to control tobacco and alcohol consumption in the western world, several developed countries report rising oropharyngeal squamous cell carcinoma (OPSCC) incidence figures, specifically in young individuals. Similar to anogenital cancers, a significant proportion of OPSCC (up to 60%) is caused by sexually acquired HPV infection and the rise in OPSCC has been attributed to changing sexual behaviours in the Western World. Accordingly, patients with HPV-positive OPSCC report divergent sexual histories and absence of classical risk factors as tobacco and alcohol exposure compared to patients with HPV-negative OPSCC. The profile of HPV-positive OPSCC differs from HPV-negative OPSCC in several other significant aspects, including a unique molecular biologic tumor characteristics and improved clinical behaviour. Thus, a further increase in HPV-positive OPSCC will impact significantly upon clinical management of OPSCC, unless it is halted by adequate preventive measures aimed at reduction of HPV-associated disease. HPV vaccination has been recently offered to young females in an attempt to reduce HPV-induced cervical cancer and may ultimately result in a decline of OPSCC incidence as well. Until then, close collaboration between otolaryngologists/head and neck surgeons and anogenital/genitourinary specialists is warranted to optimize clinical management of HPV-induced malignancy and improve detection of second primary tumor development (Monsj et al., 2010).

In addition, some researches revealed differences between positive and negative tumors for human papillomavirus being the HPV-positive HNSCC patients approximately 5 years younger than HPV-negative HNSCC patients with equal distribution between the sexes (Haraf et al., 1996; Cruz et al., 1996; Sisk et al., 2002; Strome et al., 2002). For a better understanding, although the epidemiology of HPV in head and neck cancer is the aim in this chapter, a brief explanation on the risk factors in HPV infection is necessary before beginning this approach.

3.1 Risk factors

Over the last two decades, biological agents have been implicated in the etiology of this tumor. Among these agents, human papillomavirus (HPV) is particularly important (Badaracco et al.,2000; Cortezzi et al., 2004; Lo Muzio et al., 2004; Smith et al., 2004; Ibieta et al., 2005). HPV is a DNA virus which encodes two oncoproteins that play an important role in carcinogenesis, i.e., E6 which binds, sequesters and degrades p53, and E7 which binds and degrades pRb; thus facilitating the development of tumors (Badaracco et al.,2000; Cortezzi et al., 2004; Lo Muzio et al., 2004; Remmerbach et al., 2004). Although the relationship between this virus and malignant uterine cervix tumors has been well established in the literature, with more than 90% of these tumors being positive for the virus, the same does not apply to oral carcinogenesis (Miller et al., 2001; Sugiyama et al., 2003). The HPV detection rates at this anatomical site is very variable, probably due to differences in sample size, in the population studied and in the sensitivity of the techniques used.

The presence of HPV in oral cancers suggests that HPV may play a similar role in transforming the oral epithelia. Persistent infection with high-risk types of HPV plays a critical role in the pathogenesis of cervical cancer, as well as OSCC. HPVs are 8-kb circular DNA viruses that specifically target the basal cells of the epithelial muscosa. The HPV family is comprised of more than 100 genotypes, classified in accordance with the type of epithelial cells infected and the ability to effect cellular transformation. The ability of HPV to transform epithelial cells is divided into high-risk and low-risk types. Low-risk types are associated with benign lesions such as warts, while infections with high-risk types progress to malignant lesions. The HPV genome is comprised of several early (E1 to E7) and late (L1 and L2) genes, as well as a non-coding region, all of which play roles in viral replication, transcription, and carcinogenesis (Ragin et al., 2007).

The primary risk factors for the majority of head and neck cancer worldwide are tobacco and alcohol consumption (Hennessey et al., 2009). In spite of these traditional risk factors, the HPV-positive HNSCC, in particular high-risk HPV type 16, appears more frequently than HPV-negative HNSCC in non-smokers and non-drinkers (Gillison et al., 2000; Hafkamp et al., 2003; Ritchie et al., 2003; Haraf et al., 1996). In case-control researches, the association between tobacco or alcohol use and the development of HPV-positive HNSCC was not found (D'Souza et al., 2007; Gillison et al., 2008). Furthermore, human papillomaviruses have recognized influence in the development of HNSCC in such sites as oropharynx, being considered as an independent risk factor (Schwartz et al., 1998; Gillison et al., 2000; Mork et al., 2001; Wiest et al., 2002; Herrero et al., 2003; Hobbs et al., 2006; Ernster et al., 2007; Andrews et al., 2008). Nevertheless, there is controversy in the literature as to the combination of HPV infection with tobacco and/or alcohol increasing the risk of cancer. Schwartz et al. (1998) and Smith et al. (2004) showed an additive effect between oral HPV infection, tobacco or alcohol use, and oral cancer, but more researches are necessary to evaluate possible interactions among these exposures (Vidal & Gillison, 2008).

The two most prevalent HPV types in oral carcinomas are HPV 16 and 18, far exceeding the detection rate of all the other types (Snijders et al., 1996, 1997, Badaracco et al., 2000; Syrjänen and Syrjänen, 2000; Miller and Johnstone, 2001; Ringströmet al., 2002). Interestingly, the low-risk HPV types 6 and 11 can also be identified in some oral carcinomas, similar to laryngeal carcinomas (Yamaguchi et al., 1991; Fife et al., 1996; Chang et al., 2002). A study by Sisk et al. (2000) showed that the incidence of HPV in younger patients is not significantly different from older patients, suggesting a similar role for HPV in all age groups.

Sexual contact has been associated to cervical cancer through high-risk mucosatropic HPVs (IACR, 1995), but the means by which HPV is transmitted to the upper airways are still unclear (Mannarini et al., 2009). Studies showed a rare oral HPV infection in newborn babies of infected mothers (Watts et al. 1998) and children prior to sexual activity (Koch et al., 1997) being the infections rate increased from the first sexual intercourse (Kellokoski et al., 1992).

Sexual behavior has an association with HPV-positive cancer in head and neck cancer, as observed by D'Souza et al. (2007) in a case-control study of 100 individuals with oropharyngeal cancer and 200 control persons, which found that the development of oropharyngeal cancer is linked with a high lifetime number of vaginal sex partners (≥ 26) and with a high lifetime number of oral sex partners (≥ 6). Gillison et al. (2008) found with a case-control study of 240 individuals with oropharyngeal cancer that the risk of developing an HPV-16-positive HNSCC increased with increasing numbers of oral sex partners. In addition, oral-anal contacts are very strongly associated with the risk of HPV-positive tumor (Rosenquist et al., 2005; Rajkumar et al., 2003).

In a research, Rintala et al. (2006) observed the natural history of oral and genital HPV infection. The results showed that oral sex had no association to oral HPV infection; however, a persistent oral HPV infection of the spouse increased the risk of persistent oral HPV infection 10-fold in the other spouse.

Although the relation of *cannabis sativa* with HPV infections of head and neck sites is unclear (Mannarini et al., 2009), such behavior has been proposed as a reason for increasing numbers of young patients with head and neck cancer (Báez, 2008). Gillison et al. (2008) observed a strong association between *cannabis sativa* use and HPV-16 - positive HNSCC, with a relation of increasing intensity and duration of use.

Among the risk factors for HPV infection in head and neck tumors, there is the immunosuppression, as observed in human immunodeficiency virus (HIV)-positive cases (Adamopoulou et al., 2008). The genetic susceptibility is also an important risk factor to increase the risk of HPV infection, as noted in Fanconi anemia (Park et al., 2010).

3.2 Epidemiology of head and neck cancer with HPV involvement

3.2.1 Premalignant lesions

According to Axell et al. (1996), premalignant lesions, or pre-cancer lesions, of the oral mucosa are epithelial changes more likely to undergo malignant transformation than normal tissue at other mucosal sites. There are two types of clinical premalignant lesions: white lesions (leukoplakia) and reddish lesions (erythroplakia) (Axell et al., 1996). These two terms are purely clinical, and have no association with the underlying histopathology (Syrjänen, 2005).

3.2.1.1 Erythroplakia

Erythroplakia lesions are defined as a bright red patches that cannot be diagnosed as any other lesions (Axell et al., 1996). There are few researches about erythroplakia lesions involving human papillomavirus in head and neck. Nielsen et al. (1996), in a case-control study with 49 patients with oral premalignant lesions, observed 10 cases of oral erythroplakia (1 man and 9 women). The presence of HPV was examined immunohistochemically, through DNA-DNA *in situ* hybridization and through PCR. The investigations revealed that HPV was found in 50.0% of the erythroplakias and 33.3% of erythroleucoplakias. The authors concluded that HPV may be an etiologic co-factor, because 100% of patients who developed oral cancer within 4-12 years were all positive for HPV, with one being HPV-16-positive. This sample had few cases and a critical analysis of these results is necessary. Further confirmatory data are needed before any conclusions can be drawn on the possible causal role of HPV in this disease (Syrjänen, 2005).

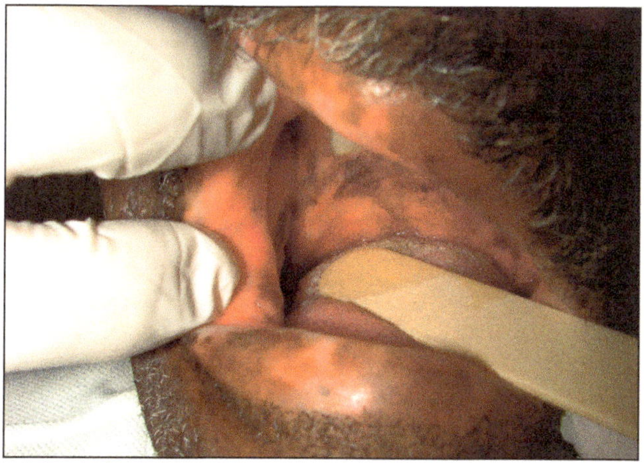

Fig. 2. Erythroplakia in soft palate

3.2.1.2 Leukoplakia

Oral leukoplakia is considered as a premalignant lesion for the development of oral squamous cell carcinoma (OSCC) and several risk factors have been reported to contribute to this step-wise carcinogenesis, including human papillomavirus (HPV) (Yang et al., 2009).

Syrjänen (2005) observed in the literature 964 leukoplakia biopsies, of which 31.1% contained HPV DNA. The HPV types 6/11 were the most prevalent (55.8%), followed by HPV types 16/18 evidenced in 28.2% of the cases (Miller & Johnstone, 2001).

However, Yang et al. (2009) analyzed, using PCR in paraffin sections, 167 patients with oral leukoplakia, including 12 who had malignant transformation from the pre-existing oral leukoplakia. The HPV prevalence in patients with oral leukoplakia was approximately 22.8%, and the most prevalent viral strain was HPV-18 (78.9%). This research also suggested that HPV in oral leukoplakia is not a prognostic indicator of malignant transformation.

Ostwald et al. (2003) examined 72 oral leukoplakia for the presence of HPV 6/11, 16 and 18 DNA through PCR/Southern blot hybridization. The HPV DNA was found in 16/72 (22.2%) leukoplakias, and HPV 16 and 18 DNA were present in 12/72 (16.7%) leukoplakias, being 11.1% the detection rate of HPV 6/11.

In a case-control study, the HPV presence was found in 62.5% of the verrucous leukoplakias, 45.5% of the homogeneous leukoplakias and in 12.5% of the nodular leukoplakias (Nielsen et al., 1996).

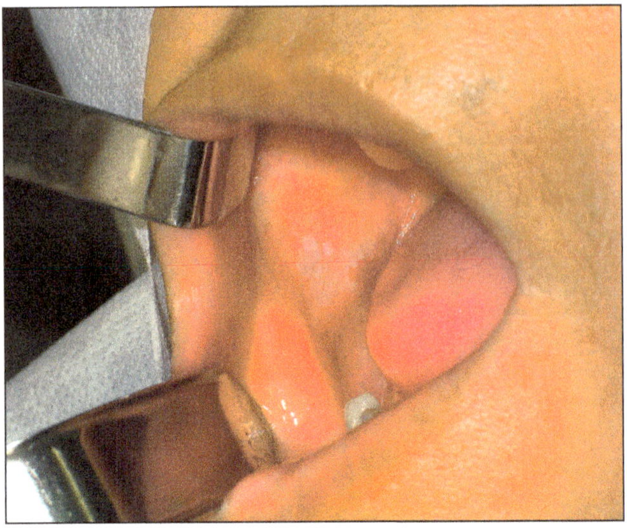

Fig. 3. Leukoplakia in buccal.

3.2.2 Oral cavity and lips

Clinical presentation of oral cancer is highly variable. On clinical examination, oral SCC lesions may be preceded by mucosal alterations with histologically detectable dysplastic changes. However, a malignancy involving a complex genetic process may also occur directly "de novo" without any pre-existing clinically detectable mucosal changes. All head and neck carcinomas tend to be diagnosed late because there is no pain until the late stages. Thus, the overall survival is only 40-50% (Johnson et al., 1991; Berrino et al., 1999; Franceschi et al., 2000).

Studies that support a causal relationship between HPV and OSCC include: a consistent detection of HPV DNA in tumor specimens (Hansson et al., 2005); E6/E7 viral oncogene expression in oral lesions (Braakhuis et al., 2004); the requirement of oral carcinoma cell lines to express E6/E7, to maintain a malignant phenotype; and epidemiological data highlighting HPV infection as a risk factor for the development of OSCC (Ragin et al., 2007). At least three proteins (E5, E6, E7) coded by the high-risk HPVs, which are expressed throughout the viral life cycle, are considered oncogenic, due to their transforming and growth-stimulating properties. These proteins have the ability to deregulate tumor suppressor function by binding to and abrogating the functions of p21 (Tsai & Chen., 2003), p53 (Camus, 2007), and pRb (Huh et al.,2007) proteins, resulting in defects in apoptosis, DNA repair, cell cycle control, and eventually leading to cellular immortalization.

Oliveira et al. (2009) showed that the presence of HPV DNA by PCR was detected in only 29.5% of OSCC cases, 80.8% of which were identified for HPV 18. Although this investigation have detected only 29.5% of HR-HPV DNA in OSCC, it is possible that this virus contribute to the development of some case of this tumor. Furthermore, it seems that the immunohistochemical expression of p53 and bcl-2 and the presence of HPV DNA are independent events in OSCC.

Cancers involving the oral cavity account for 2-3% of all malignancies and the tongue is the subsite with the highest incidence of cancer in the oral cavity (Silverman Jr, 2001). The tongue may be the first site of exposure to viral microorganisms in the aerodigestive tract and oral tongue cancer could be susceptible to HPV exposure, directly or indirectly. The prevalence of HPV in oral tongue cancer is extremely diverse, ranging from 0% to 100% in the literature, and the prevalence of HPV in HNSCC is not uncommon (Bouda et al., 2000, Gillison et al., 2001, Matzow , 1998, Ringström , 2002). The markedly different reports of prevalence of HPV in oral tongue cancer may be due to: mixed samples with the oropharynx; methodological differences for detecting HPV, including less accurate methods; various tumour stages and racial and geographical differences between the studies.

In a study made in the Republic of Korea for Lee et al. (2010), HPV prevalence in early oral tongue cancer was 36% (13/36). In the HPV-positive tumours, 11 cases (84.8%) were infected with HPV-16 and the others were infected with non-16 highrisk type and low-risk type HPV each and multiple infections were not found in these cases.

Sugiyama et al. (2007) examined 66 oral squamous cell carcinomas (OSCCs) for human papillomavirus-16 (HPV-16) infection to evaluate its prognostic significance. Cox regression analysis of 5-year survival demonstrated that patients without nodal metastasis or with intratumoural HPV-16 showed better prognoses compared with each counterpart. In Kaplan-Meier survival analysis, nodal status but not HPV-16 status was statistically significant. The 5-year survival rate of HPV-16 positive patients without nodal metastasis (94%) was extremely high, compared with that of HPV-16 negative patients with nodal metastasis (25%). These results suggest that HPV-16 status as well as nodal status may provide prognostic significance in patients with OSCC.

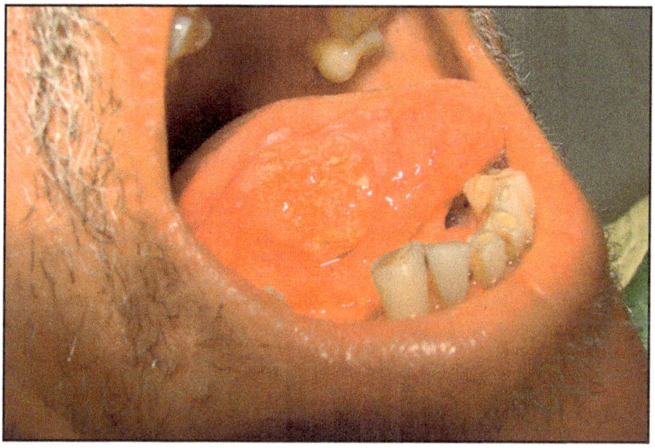

Fig. 4. Oral cancer in tongue.

3.2.3 Pharynx

3.2.3.1 Oropharynx

The oropharynx is the predominant site where HPV-induced squamous cell carcinomas develop (Braakhuis et al., 2009). This region of interest for HPV infection comprises predominantly the vallecula, walls of the oropharynx, and in particular the tonsils (Kreimer et al., 2005).

In some countries, such as the United States and the Netherlands, the incidence of oropharyngeal cancer is increasing (Braakhuis et al., 2009; Ernster et al., 2007), and it represents an emerging public health problem (St Guily et al., 2011). One potential way to explain this increase would be to demonstrate an increasing prevalence of oncogenic HPV in palatine or lingual tonsil tissue over time (Ernster et al., 2009).

Studies found a strong association between oropharynx cancers and HPV infection, with detection rates of 50% or more (Hammarstead et al., 2006; Klussmann et al., 2001; Venuti et al., 2004; Paz et al., 1997). The biological explanation for why the prevalence of HPV is higher in tumors from the oropharynx compared with other sites in the head and neck remains unclear (Kreimer et al., 2005). However, it is possibly explained because of "specific virus-tissue interactions" (Kreimer et al., 2005) that allow a facilitated viral access to basal mucosal cells in the tonsillar crypts and an apparent predilection for this anatomic site for transformation by HPVs, analogous to the cervical transformation zone (Vidal & Gillison, 2008).

In a systematic review of HNSCC biopsies that employed PCR-based methods to detect and genotype HPV, Kreimer et al. (2005) observed a HPV prevalence significantly higher in oropharyngeal squamous cell carcinomas (35.6% of 969) than in oral squamous cell carcinomas (23.5% of 2,642) or laryngeal squamous cell carcinomas (24.0% of 1,435). Furthermore, the human papillomavirus type 16 was found in a larger majority of HPV-positive oropharyngeal squamous cell carcinomas (86.7%). However, the HPV18 infection was rare in HPV-positive oropharyngeal SCCs (2.8%) compared with other head and neck sites. Aside from HPV16 and HPV18, other oncogenic HPVs were rarely detected in oropharynx. This research also found geographic differences in HPV-positivity of oropharyngeal carcinomas possibly linked to differences in HPV exposure or variation in host susceptibility factors among countries.

From a literature review worldwide, Syrjänen (2004) identified 422 tonsillar SCCs and 51% of these tumors contained HPV DNA. The HPV 16 was the most frequent type, identified in 84% of the 216 HPV DNA-positive tumors, but also the low-risk HPV types 6/11 DNA have been detected in 3% of the HPV-positive carcinomas, and the following HPV types have been detected in occasional tonsillar carcinomas: HPV 5, 12, 31, 35, and 59.

In a research developed in France, the overall HPV prevalence was 57% in tonsil cancers, and was significantly higher in female than in male cases (28/35 versus 78/150 in tonsil cases). Among HPV positive samples, HPV 16 was found in 89% of tonsil cases, and all other HPV types had prevalence below 5% (St Guily et al., 2011).

In Norway, a study with 137 patients about the prevalence of HPV with tonsillar carcinomas observed HPV infection in 52% of the tumors being the HPV-16 the most frequent subtype (87%). Furthermore, the study showed that the survival of the HPV-positive group was significantly better in males (Hannisdal et al., 2010).

In Stockholm, 98 pretreatment biopsies of tonsillar squamous cell carcinoma were analyzed. The HPV DNA was present in 83 cases (85%) of the tonsillar SCC biopsies and 77 of these were HPV-16 positive. HPV-16 E6 and E7 RNA were found in 98% of 52 HPV-16 positive cases analyzed. In addition, the incidence rate of HPV-positive tumors almost doubled each decade between 1970 and 2007, in parallel with a decline of HPV-negative tumors. The study suggested that the incidence of HPV-positive cancers is still increasing in Stockholm, and also an epidemic of a virus-induced carcinoma, with soon practically all tonsillar SCC being HPV positive, as in cervical cancer (Nasman et al., 2009).

A study developed in the United States in the state of Colorado through PCR observed an increase of oropharyngeal cancer in males from 2.54 per 100,000 to 3.47 or 36.6%. Of the 72 cases, 50 (69%) were positive for HPV subtype 16. The ratio of HPV-positive to HPV-negative cases prior to 1995 was 0.72 (8:11), but it was 3.81 (42:11) afterwards. The survival was positively affected by HPV status, being 83% in the HPV-positive patients and 15% in the HPV-negative group (Ernster et al., 2007).

A research in Puerto Rico evaluated through PCR 118 head and neck squamous cell carcinoma, and 16 cases were found in the oropharynx. Furthermore, in 52 patients, HPV16 was detected, being 19% or 10 cases in oropharynx that had a slightly higher incidence of HPV16 DNA (Báez et al., 2004).

In Australia, a study involving 86 tonsil cancers analyzed the HPV status through PCR and immunohistochemistry. The HPV status could be established in 67 of the tumors, and 31 (46%) of these were HPV-positive, predominantly (28/31) for HPV16 (Li et al., 2003).

Overall, the percentage of HPV-positive oropharyngeal carcinomas varies among different reports, which is not only explained by the varying inclusion of tumors from different anatomic sublocations among studies (van Monsjou et al., 2010). Therefore, further standardized seroepidemiologic studies are important to answer some questions.

3.2.3.2 Nasopharynx

Nasopharyngeal carcinoma (NPC) is a tumor that arises in the epithelium surface of the posterior nasopharynx and shows a peculiar geographic and ethnic distribution (Parkin et al., 1997). Despite the strong association with Epstein-Barr virus (EBV), the human papillomavirus (HPV) has also been linked as a cofactor for the development of nasopharyngeal carcinoma (Punwaney et al., 1999).

Although NPC is rare in most populations, it is a leading form of cancer in a few well-defined populations, including natives of southern China, Southeast Asia, the Arctic, and the Middle East/North Africa. Thus, the distinctive racial/ethnic and geographic distribution of NPC worldwide suggests that both environmental factors and genetic traits contribute to its development (Chang & Adami, 2006).

In North Africa, 70 Moroccan patients with NPC were screened for EBV and HPV. The EBV was detected in all NPC tumors, whereas HPV DNA was revealed in 34% of cases (24/70). Molecular analysis showed that 20.8% (5/24) were infected with HPV31, and the remaining were infected with other oncogenic types (i.e., HPV59, 16, 18, 33, 35 and 45). The mean age of HPV-positive patients was 37.3, whereas the mean age of HPV-negative cases was 43.0 years old. Nonetheless, the statistical analysis showed that there's no association between sex or age and HPV infection. The study revealed that EBV is commonly associated with NPC in Moroccan patients and that NPC tumors from Moroccan patients harbor high-risk HPV genotypes (Laantri et al., 2011).

In Iran, a retrospective study analyzed the prevalence of EBV and HPV infection subtypes 6/11 and 16/18 in 20 patients with NPC. Thus, 16 cases were classified as undifferentiated carcinoma (WHO type III) and 4 as non-keratinizing SCC (WHO type II). About the HPV infection, two of 20 NPC (10%) contained HPV 6/11 sequences and two of 20 NPC (10%) contained HPV 16/18 sequences, and combined EBV and HPV infection was detected in 3 of the 20 (15%) patients (Mirzamani et al., 2006).

A research involving North Americans with NPC showed that five (5.6%) of 89 cases had nasopharyngeal carcinoma, all with non-keratinizing histology. Of the 5 patients with NPC, 4 (80%) were HPV-positive for subtypes 16 (1 patient), 18 (2 patients), and 59 (1 patient). All 4 cases were white North Americans with age ranging between 58-76 years old. Therefore, it suggests that HPV may be the etiologic factor in some EBV-negative, nonkeratinizing NPCs among whites (Maxwell et al., 2010).

An investigation developed by Punwaney et al. (1999) with 30 patients (6 Caucasian Americans, 1 Chinese American, 14 and 9 patients from Korea and China, respectively) found in 7 (23%) HPV sequences. The human papillomavirus appears to be uncommonly (17%) associated with NPC in patients from the Far East and was detected more often (50%) in NPC from American Caucasian patients. There appears to be a broad profile in the relationship between HPV, EBV, and NPC histologic subtype. However, strong conclusions are not possible because of a low number of American Caucasian cases studied.

In Hong Kong Chinese people, 16 of nasopharyngeal were examined for the presence of HPV 16 and 18 using PCR on paraffin-wax-embedded biopsy specimens. However, no DNA of either human papillomavirus subtype was detected. The number of cases in this series was small, and further studies are warranted using fresh biopsy material and including other viral subtypes (Dickens et al., 1992).

Singhi et al. (2011) analyzed 45 carcinomas of the nasopharynx through immunohistochemistry and *in situ* hybridization for EBV and HPV. In this series, only 4 cases (9%) were HPV-positive being all these specimens EBV-negative. The HPV was more likely to be detected in carcinomas from white patients than non-white patients (16% vs 0%), and in 3 HPV-positive patients, there was the finding of an extension into the oropharynx.

Further studies are still required to associate the coexistence of EBV and HPV in the development of nasopharyngeal carcinomas (Mirzamani et al., 2006; Tyan et al., 1993). Moreover, epidemiology studies would also be of interest to determine whether the incidence of HPV-positive NPC is increasing in concert with the increased frequency of HPV-positive oropharyngeal cancers (Maxwell et al., 2010).

3.2.3.3 Larynx and hypopharynx

The larynx is among the most significant anatomic sites in terms of HPV involvement, exceeded in clinical importance perhaps only by the genital tract and skin infections (Syrjänen, 2005). However, the HPV role in anatomic sites in the upper aerodigestive tract such as the larynx is less clear (Herrero, 2003), and data on HPV involvement in preneoplastic and neoplastic lesions of the larynx and other locations are limited and conflicting (Gorgoulis et al., 1999).

The hypopharynx comprises the postcricoid region, hypopharyngeal region of the aryepiglottic fold, and posterior wall of the hypopharynx (Kreimer et al., 2005). Unfortunately, there are few researches involving only hypopharynx in association with HPV presence in the literature. In this chapter, the hypopharynx and larynx were combined because of few reports observed in hypopharynx with HPV involvement and for the reason that some manuscripts aggregated these anatomical sites. Therefore, this group of diseases was called "larynx cancers" or laryngeal squamous cell carcinomas (SCCs) in accordance to Kreimer et al. (2005).

3.2.3.4 Larynx cancers

Most malignancies in the larynx are squamous cell carcinomas (>90%). Similar to oral and pharyngeal cancers, multiple case series have reported prevalences of HPV DNA in laryngeal cancer (Herrero, 2003). Although the association and clinical significance of human papillomavirus (HPV) infections with a subset of head and neck cancers, particularly for oropharyngeal carcinoma, has recently been well documented, the involvement of HPV in laryngeal cancer has been inadequately evaluated (Torrente et al., 2011).

In a systematic review worldwide comprising 1,435 cases (1,222 of larynx and 213 of hypopharynx cancers), the overall HPV prevalence was of 24% in laryngeal SCCs. The HPV was detected in 21.3%, 13.8%, and 38.2% of SCCs of the larynx from Europe, North America, and Asia, respectively. In addition, the HPV16 was the most common type detected in samples accounted for 69.2% of all HPV-positive laryngeal SCCs, followed by HPV18 detected in 3.9% of cases (Kreimer et al., 2005).

A study of Syrjänen & Syrjänen (2000) involving 1,252 cases had a detection rate of 25% for HPV DNA in 313 samples. Furthermore, the HPV 16 was the single most common HPV type detected in these lesions, with other high-risk types being occasionally reported.

In the United States, 21 hypopharynx cases and 86 larynx cases were evaluated through PCR, Southern blot hybridization and *in situ* hybridization. Thus, the HPV positivity was identified in 10% of hypopharynx samples and 19% of larynx samples (Gillison et al., 2000).

In Poland, the HPV 16 DNA presence was analyzed using PCR technique in 72 samples of laryngeal carcinoma. The human papillomavirus was detected in 26 (36.1%) of the 72 patients. However, there was no statistically significant correlation HPV positivity and clinical-pathological features of the group analyzed (Morshed et al., 2005).

In France, the human papillomavirus was detected in 5% in larynx squamous cell carcinoma, and no patient analyzed had p53 gene mutations in cancer cells (Fouret et al., 1997).

In Belgium, the laryngeal squamous cell carcinomas were evaluated for the presence of HPV DNA through E6/E7 type-specific PCR, and 75% of patients (44 out of 59) presented high-risk HPV types with a high prevalence of HPV-16 (Duray et al., 2011).

In the Puerto Rican population, of 118 head and neck squamous cell carcinoma evaluated through PCR, the larynx was the most common site affected (52 out of 118). Separately, the HPV 16 detected in larynx was 85.7% and 55.6% in hypopharynx. When aggregated, the hypopharynx and larynx showed 56% (29 cases) of all HPV16 DNA detected in the study (Báez et al., 2004).

In Northeast China, 102 patients with laryngeal squamous cell carcinomas were examined for HPV DNA. The HPV DNA was found in 60 cases (58.8%), being the HPV-16, -18, -6, -11, and -33 DNA detected in 30 cases, 22 cases, 25 cases, 2 cases and 1 case, respectively. Moreover, co-infection either with HPV-6 and -16 or with HPV-6 and -18 was detected in 20 cases (33.3% of HPV DNA-positive cases) (Ma et al., 1998).

A retrospective study examining early larynx malignancies from 38 patients detected a rate of 16% in HPV DNA, and the HPV types 16, 26, 31, 39, and 52 were identified. Although the

HPV-26 is related to uterine cervical cancer, the research found the first evidence of this subtype in a laryngeal carcinoma (Baumann et al., 2009).

Although several researches support the HPV presence in hypopharynx/larynx cancer with prevalences ranging of 13.8% to 38.2% (Kreimer et al., 2005), Ribeiro et al. (2011) observed in 78 fresh tissue biopsies a low prevalence of 3.8% in cases from Central Europe and Latin America. These wide variations in HPV prevalence which are reported may depend on the HPV diagnostic methodologies, especially in earlier studies (St Guily et al., 2010). Researches for the development of accurate, specific, and confirmatory methods for the detections of HPV in laryngeal squamous cell carcinoma are necessary, being standardized seroepidemiologic studies important to answer some questions.

Table 2. summarizes some researches of head and neck lesions with HPV involvement.

	AUTHORS (YEAR)	GEOGRAPHIC LOCATION	METHOD*	HPV TYPE**	POSITIVE/ CASES	%
ORAL CAVITY AND LIP	Kreimer et al. (2005)	Australia, Canada, China, Cuba, Finland, France, Germany, India, Ireland, Italy, Japan, Korea, Netherlands, Norway, Poland, Spain, Slovenia, Sudan, Sweden, Switzerland, Taiwan, United Kingdom, United States, Venezuela	PCR-based HPV testing methods	HPV-16	423/ 2,642	16%
	Oliveira et al. (2009)	Brazil	PCR	HPV-18	21/88	23,9%
	Lee et al. (2010)	Republic of Korea	HPV genotyping chip and RT-PCR	HPV-16	11/36	30,6%
OROPHARYNX	Kreimer et al. (2005)	Australia, Canada, Cuba, Finland, France, Germany, India, Ireland, Italy, Japan, Netherlands, Norway, Poland, Spain, Slovenia, Sudan, Sweden, Switzerland, United States	PCR-based HPV testing methods	HPV-16	299/969	30,9%
	St Guily et al. (2011)	France	INNO-LiPA HPV Genotypingextra test	HPV-16	94/185	50,8%
	Nasman et al. (2009)	Stockholm	PCR	HPV-16	77/98	78,6%
	Ernster et al. (2007)	United States	PCR	HPV-16	50/72	69,4%
	Li et al. (2003)	Australia	PCR and IHC	HPV-16	28/67	41,8%

	AUTHORS (YEAR)	GEOGRAPHIC LOCATION	METHOD*	HPV TYPE**	POSITIVE/ CASES	%
	Báez et al. (2004)	Puerto Rico	PCR	HPV-16	10/16	62,5%
NASOPHARYNX	Laantri et al. (2011)	Morocco	PCR	HPV-31	5/70	7,1%
	Mirzamani et al. (2006)	Iran	ISH	HPV-6/11; HPV-16/18	2/20; 2/20	10%; 10%
	Dickens et al. (1992)	Hong Kong	PCR	none	0/16	0%
LARYNX AND HYPOPHARYNX	Kreimer et al. (2005)	Canada, Cuba, Denmark, Finland, France, Germany, Greece, India, Italy, Japan, Netherlands, Norway, Spain, Slovenia, Sweden, Switzerland, United Kingdom, United States	PCR-based HPV testing methods	HPV-16	238/1,435	16,6%
	Morshed et al. (2005)	Poland	PCR	HPV-16	26/72	36.1%
	Ma et al. (1998)	Northeast China	PCR, SB, and IHC	HPV-16	30/102	29,4%
ERYTHROPLAKIA	D'Costa et al. (1998), Giovannelli et al. (2002), Syrjänen & Syrjänen (2000)	India, Italy, ???	PCR, ???	HPV-16	9/32	28,1%
LEUKOPLAKIA	Ostwald et al. (2003)	Germany	PCR, SB	HPV-16/18	12/72	16.7%

*Abbreviations: PCR = Polymerase chain reaction, RT-PCR = Real Time PCR, IHC = Immunohistochemistry, SB = Southern Blotting, ISH = *In situ* hybridization.
**Most common HPV types found in studies.

Table 2. Prevalence of HPV in lesions of the head and neck.

4. Conclusion

The present review showed heterogeneous prevalence between different anatomical sites in HNSCC with HPV involvement around the world. These results must be interpreted with caution because most researches conducted for data on HPV and HNSCC have been, with rare exception, small (<100 cases). The methods employed for case identification have often been unclear, and it is difficult to differentiate studies that enrolled consecutive patients from studies that used alternative inclusion criteria. Moreover, poor quality of some biopsy specimens may also have affected the prevalence estimates with some false-negative findings (Kreimer et al., 2005).

Further standardized seroepidemiologic studies are important to answer some questions, among them the impact of HPV vaccination on HNSCC. Thus, epidemiology studies are interesting to determine whether the incidence of HPV-positive is increasing, mainly in sites frequently affected such as oropharynx, in particular the tonsils.

In conclusion, with a clear understanding of the prevalence of oncogenic HPV in specific populations, an estimate of the progression rate from HPV infection to HPV-positive carcinoma may be derived. This effort could help guide screening and prevention strategies in the future (Ernster et al., 2009), such as the development of screening programs, new therapeutic approaches and specific methods of prevention, especially in high incidence areas (Laantri et al., 2011).

5. Acknowledgements

The authors are grateful to Mr. Abílio Borghi for the critical reading of the chapter.

6. References

Adamopoulou M, Vairaktaris E, Panis V, Nkenke E, Neukam FW & Yapijakis C (2008). HPV detection rate in saliva may depend on the immune system efficiency. *In Vivo,* Vol. 22, pp. 599-602

Andrews E, Seaman WT & Webster-Cyriaque J (2009). Oropharyngeal carcinoma in non-smokers and non-drinkers: a role for HPV. *Oral Oncol,* Vol. 45, pp. 486-491

Badaracco G, Venuti A, Bartolazzi A, Morillo R, Marzetti F, Marcante ML. (2000), Overexpression of p53 and bcl-2 proteins and the presence of HPV infection are independent events in head and neck cancer. *J Oral Pathol Med.* Vol. 29, pp. 173–179

Báez A, Almodovar JI, Cantor A, Celestin F, Cruz-Cruz L, Fonseca S et al (2004). High frequency of HPV16-associated head and neck squamous cell carcinoma in the Puerto Rican population. *Head Neck,* Vol. 26, pp. 778-784

Báez A (2008). Genetic and environmental factors in head and neck cancer genesis. *J Environ Sci Health C Environ Carcinog Ecotoxicol Rev,*Vol. 26, pp. 174-200

Baumann JL, Cohen S, Evjen AN, Law JH, Vadivelu S, Attia A et al (2009). Human papillomavirus in early laryngeal carcinoma. *Laryngoscope,* Vol. 119, pp. 1531-1537

Berrino F, Capocaccia R, Esteve J, et al., Survival of cancer patients in Europe: the EUROCARE-2 study. IARC Scientific Publication No. 151. Lyon, France; 1999

Bosch FX, Manos MM, Munoz N, Sherman M, Jansen AM, Peto J, et al (1995). Prevalence of human papillomavirus in cervical cancer: a worldwide perspective. International biological study on cervical cancer (IBSCC) Study Group. *J Natl Cancer Inst,* Vol. 87, pp. 796–802

Bouda M, Gorgoulis VG, Kastrinakis NG, Giannoudis A, Tsoli E, Danassi-Afentaki D, et al. (2000)''High risk'' HPV types are frequently detected in potentially malignant and malignant oral lesion, but not in normal oral mucosa. *ModPathol.* Vol. 13, pp.644–653

Braakhuis BJ, Snijders PJ, Keune WJ. (2004). Genetic patterns in head and neck cancers that contain or lack transcriptionally active human papillomavirus. J Natl Cancer Inst . Vol. 96, pp. 998–1006

Braakhuis BJ, Visser O & Leemans CR (2009). Oral and oropharyngeal cancer in The Netherlands between 1989 and 2006: Increasing incidence, but not in young adults. *Oral Oncol,* Vol. 45, pp. e85-89

Camus S, Menendez S, Cheok CF, Stevenson LF (2007). Ubiquitinindependent degradationof p53 mediated by high-risk human papillomavirus protein E6. Oncogene.Vol. 26, pp. 4059–470

Chang ET & Adami HO (2006). The enigmatic epidemiology of nasopharyngeal carcinoma. *Cancer Epidemiol Biomarkers Prev,* Vol. 15, pp. 1765-1777

Chung CH & Gillison ML (2009). Human papillomavirus in head and neck cancer: its role in pathogenesis and clinical implications. *Clin Cancer Res. [Review],* Vol. 15, No. 22, pp. 6758-62

Cortezzi SS, Provazzi PJ, Sobrinho JS, Mann-Prado JC, Reis PMP, Freitas SEN, et al. (2004), Analysis of human papillomavirus prevalence and TP53 polymorphism in head and neck squamous cell carcinomas. *Cancer Genet Cytogenet.* Vol.150, pp:44–49

Cruz IB, Snijders PJ, Steenbergen RD, Meijer CJ, Snow GB, Walboomers JM, et al (1996). Age-dependence of human papillomavirus DNA presence in oral squamous cell carcinomas. *Eur J Cancer B Oral Oncol,* Vol. 32, No. 1, pp. 55–62

D'Costa J, Saranath D, Dedhia P, Sanghvi V, Mehta AR (1998). Detection of HPV-16 genome in human oral cancers and potentially malignant lesions from India. *Oral Onco, Vol.* 34, pp. 413-420

D'Souza G, Kreimer AR, Viscidi R, et al (2007). Case-control study of human papillomavirus and oropharyngeal cancer. *N Engl J Med,* Vol. 356 , pp. 1944–56

Dickens P, Srivastava G & Liu YT (1992). Human papillomavirus 16/18 and nasopharyngeal carcinoma. *J Clin Pathol,* Vol. 45, pp. 81-82

Duray A, Descamps G, Arafa M, Decaestecker C, Remmelink M, Sirtaine N et al (2011). High incidence of high-risk HPV in benign and malignant lesions of the larynx. *Int J Oncol,* Vol. 39, pp. 51-59

Ernster JA, Sciotto CG, O'Brien MM, Finch JL, Robinson LJ, Willson T, et al. (2007). Rising incidence of oropharyngeal cancer and the role of oncogenic human papilloma virus. *Laryngoscope,* Vol. 117, pp. 2115-2128

Ernster JA, Sciotto CG, O'Brien MM, Robinson LJ & Willson T (2009). Prevalence of oncogenic human papillomavirus 16 and 18 in the palatine tonsils of the general adult population. *Arch Otolaryngol Head Neck Surg,* Vol. 135, pp. 554-557

Ferlay J, Shin HR, Bray F, Forman D, Mathers C & Parkin DM. (2010). Cancer Incidence and Mortality Worldwide: IARC CancerBase No. 10 [Internet], In: *GLOBOCAN 2008 v1.2*, 16/07/2011, Available from: < http://globocan.iarc.fr >

Fouret P, Monceaux G, Temam S, Lacourreye L & St Guily JL (1997). Human papillomavirus in head and neck squamous cell carcinomas in nonsmokers. *Arch Otolaryngol Head Neck Surg*, Vol. 123, pp. 513-516

Franceschi S, Bidoli E, Herrero R. (2000). Comparison of cancers of the oral cavity and pharynx worlwide: etiological clues. *Oral Oncol.* Vol. 36, pp.106-15

Franceschi S, Munoz N, Bosch XF, Snijders PJ & Walboomers JM (1996). Human papillomavirus and cancers of the upper aerodigestive tract: a review of epidemiological and experimental evidence. *Cancer Epidemiol Biomarkers Prev*, Vol. 5, pp. 567 - 75

Frisch M, Fenger C, van den Brule AJC, Sørensen P, Meijer CJLM, Walboomers JMM, et al (1999). Variants of squamous cell carcinoma of the anal canal and perianal skin and their relation to human papillomaviruses. *Cancer Res*, Vol. 59, pp. 753–7

Frisch M, Goodman MT. (2000). Human papillomavirus-associated carcinomas in Hawaii and the mainland. Cancer. Vol. 88, pp. 1464–1469

Gillison ML, D'Souza G, Westra W, Sugar E, Xiao W, Begum S et al (2008). Distinct risk factor profiles for human papillomavirus type 16-positive and human papillomavirus type 16-negative head and neck cancers. *J Natl Cancer Inst*, Vol. 100, pp. 407-420

Gillison ML, Koch WM, Capone RB, Spafford M, Westra WH, Wu L et al (2000). Evidence for a causal association between human papillomavirus and a subset of head and neck cancers. *J Natl Cancer Inst*, Vol. 92, pp. 709-720

Gillison ML, Shah KV (2001). Human papillomavirus-associated head and necksquamous cell carcinoma: mounting evidence for an etiologic role for human papillomavirus in a subset of head and neck cancers. *Curr Opin Oncol*. Vol. 13, pp.183–188

Giovannelli L, Campisi G, Lama A, Giambalvo O, Osborn J, Margiotta V, et al. (2002), Human papillomavirus DNA in oral mucosal lesions. *J Infect Dis*. Vol. 185, pp. 833–836

Gorgoulis VG, Zacharatos P, Kotsinas A, Kyroudi A, Rassidakis AN, Ikonomopoulos JA et al (1999). Human papilloma virus (HPV) is possibly involved in laryngeal but not in lung carcinogenesis. *Hum Pathol*, Vol. 30, pp. 274-283

Hafkamp HC, Speel EJ, Haesevoets A, Bot FJ, Dinjens WN, Ramaekers FC, et al (2003). A subset of head and neck squamous cell carcinomas exhibits integration of HPV 16/18 DNA and overexpression of p16INK4A and p53 in the absence of mutations in p53 exons 5–8. *Int J Cancer*, Vol. 107, No. 3, pp. 394–400

Hammarstedt L, Lindquist D, Dahlstrand H, Romanitan M, Dahlgren LO, Joneberg J et al (2006). Human papillomavirus as a risk factor for the increase in incidence of tonsillar cancer. *Int J Cancer*, Vol. 119, pp. 2620-2623

Hannisdal K, Schjolberg A, De Angelis PM, Boysen M & Clausen OP (2010). Human papillomavirus (HPV)-positive tonsillar carcinomas are frequent and have a favourable prognosis in males in Norway. *Acta Otolaryngol*, Vol. 130, pp. 293-299

Hansson BG, Rosenquist K, Antonsson A, Wennerberg J. (2005). Strong association between infection with human papillomavirus and oral and oropharyngeal squamous cell carcinoma: a population-based case-control study in southern Sweden. Acta Otolaryngol. Vol. 25, pp. 1337–1344

Haraf DJ, Nodzenski E, Brachman D, Mick R, Montag A, Graves D, et al (1996). Human papilloma virus and p53 in head and neck cancer: clinical correlates and survival. *Clin Cancer Res,* Vol. 2, No. 4, pp. 755–62

Hennessey PT, Westra WH & Califano JA (2009). Human papillomavirus and head and neck squamous cell carcinoma: recent evidence and clinical implications. *J Dent Res. [Research Support, N.I.H., Extramural Review],* Vol. 88, No. 4, pp. 300-6

Herrero R, Castellsague X, Pawlita M, Lissowska J, Kee F, Balaram P et al (2003). Human papillomavirus and oral cancer: the International Agency for Research on cancer multicenter study. *J Natl Cancer Inst,* Vol. 95, pp. 1772–83

Herrero R (2003). Chapter 7: Human papillomavirus and cancer of the upper aerodigestive tract. *J Natl Cancer Inst Monogr,* pp. 47-51

Hobbs CG, Sterne JA, Bailey M, Heyderman RS, Birchall MA & Thomas SJ (2006). Human papillomavirus and head and neck cancer: a systematic review and meta-analysis. *Clin Otolaryngol,* Vol. 31, pp. 259-266

Huh K, Zhou X, Hayakawa H, Cho JY, Libermann TA. (2007). The Human Papillomavirus type 16 E7 oncoprotein associates with the cullin 2 ubiquitin ligase complex, which contributes to degradation of the retinoblastoma tumor suppressor. *J Virol,* Vol. 81, pp. 9737-47

IARC Working Group on the Evaluation of Carcinogenic Risks to Humans (1995). Human papillomaviruses. *IARC Monogr Eval Carcinog Risks Hum,* Vol. 64, pp. 1-378

Ibieta BR, Lizano M, Frıas-Mendivil M, Barrera JL, Carrillo A, Ruíz-Godoy LM, et al. Human papilloma virus in oral squamous cell carcinoma in a Mexican population (2005). *Oral Surg Oral Med Oral Pathol Oral Radiol Endod.,* Vol.99, pp. 311–5

Jemal A, Siegel R, Ward E, Murray T, Xu J & Thun MJ (2007). Cancer statistics. *CA Cancer J Clin,* Vol. 57, No. 1, pp. 43–66

Jemal A, Siegel R, Ward E, Hao Y, Xu J, Murray T, et al. (2008). Cancer statistics, 2008. *CA Cancer J Clin,* Vol. 58, pp. 71-96

Johnson NW, et al. (1991). Orofacial neoplasms: global epidemiology, risk factors and recommendations for research. *Int Dent J.* Vol. 41, pp. 365–375

Karim-Kos HE, de Vries E, Soerjomataram I, Lemmens V, Siesling S & Coebergh JW (2008). Recent trends of cancer in Europe: a combined approach of incidence, survival and mortality for 17 cancer sites since the 1990s. *Eur J Cancer,* Vol. 44, No. 10 , pp. 1345–89

Kellokoski JK, Syrjänen SM, Chang F, Yliskoski M & Syrjänen KJ (1992). Southern blot hybridization and PCR detection of oral human papillomavirus (HPV) infections in women with genital HPV infections. *J Oral Pathol Med,* Vol. 21, pp. 459-64

Kim SH, Koo BS, Kang S, Park K, Kim H, Lee KR, Lee MJ, Kim JM, Choi EC, Cho NH. (2007), HPV. Integration begins in the tonsillar crypt and leads to the alteration of p16, EGFR and c-myc during tumor formation. *Int J Cancer.* Vol. 120, pp. 1418–1425

Klussmann JP, Weissenborn SJ, Wieland U, Dries V, Kolligs J, Jungehuelsing M et al (2001). Prevalence, distribution, and viral load of human papillomavirus 16 DNA in tonsillar carcinomas. *Cancer,* Vol. 92, pp. 2875-2884

Koch A, Hansen SV, Nielsen NM, Palefsky J & Melbye M (1997). HPV detection in children prior to sexual debut. *Int J Cancer,* Vol. 73, pp. 621-4

Kreimer AR, Clifford GM, Boyle P, et al (2005). Human papillomavirus types in head and neck squamous cell carcinomas worldwide: a systematic review. *Cancer Epidemiol Biomarkers Prev,* Vol. 14, pp. 467–75

Laantri N, Attaleb M, Kandil M, Naji F, Mouttaki T, Dardari R et al (2011). Human papillomavirus detection in moroccan patients with nasopharyngeal carcinoma. *Infect Agent Cancer,* Vol. 6, pp. 3

Lassen P (2010). The role of Human papillomavirus in head and neck cancer and the impact on radiotherapy outcome. *Radiother Oncol. [Research Support, Non-U.S. Gov't Review],* Vol. 95, No. 3, pp. 371-80

Lee S Y, Cho N H, Choi E C, Baek S J, Kim W S, Shin D. H. et al. (2010). Relevance of human papilloma virus (HPV) infection to carcinogenesis of oral tongue cancer. *Int. J. Oral Maxillofac. Surg.,* Vol. 39, pp. 678–683

Li W, Thompson CH, O'Brien CJ, McNeil EB, Scolyer RA, Cossart YE et al (2003). Human papillomavirus positivity predicts favourable outcome for squamous carcinoma of the tonsil. *Int J Cancer,*Vol. 106, pp. 553-558

Lo Muzio L, Campisi G, Giovannelli L, Ammatuna P, Greco I, Staibano S, et al. HPV DNA and surviving expression in epithelial oral carcinogenesis: a relationship? (2004), *Oral Oncol;* Vol. 40, pp. 736–741

Ma XL, Ueno K, Pan ZM, Hi SZ, Ohyama M & Eizuru Y (1998). Human papillomavirus DNA sequences and p53 over-expression in laryngeal squamous cell carcinomas in Northeast China. *J Med Virol,* Vol. 54, pp. 186-191

Mannarini L, Kratochvil V, Calabrese L, Gomes Silva L, Morbini P, Betka J, et al (2009). Human Papilloma Virus (HPV) in head and neck region: review of literature. *Acta Otorhinolaryngol Ital. [Review],* Vol. 29, No. 3, pp. 119-26

Matzow T, Boysen M, Kalantari M, Johansson B, Hagmar B. (1998). Low detection rate of HPV in oral and laryngeal carcinomas. *Acta Oncol.* Vol. 37, pp. 73–76

Maxwell JH, Kumar B, Feng FY, McHugh JB, Cordell KG, Eisbruch A et al (2010). HPV-positive/p16-positive/EBV-negative nasopharyngeal carcinoma in white North Americans. *Head Neck,* Vol. 32, pp. 562-567

McKing RG, Baric RS, Olhsan AF. (1998). Human papillomavirus and head and neck cancer: epidemiology and molecular biology. *Head Neck.* Vol. 20, pp. 250–265

Melbye M, Frisch M (1998). The role of human papillomaviruses in anogenital cancers. *Semin Cancer Biol,* Vol. 8, pp. 307-313

Mellin H, Friesland S, Lewensohn R, Dalianis T & Munck-Wikland E (2000). Human papillomavirus (HPV) DNA in tonsillar cancer: clinical correlates, risk of relapse, and survival. *Int J Cancer,* Vol. 89, No. 3, pp. 300–4

Miller CS & Johnstone BM. (2001). Human papillomavirus as a risk factor for oral squamous cell carcinoma: a meta-analysis, 1982–1997. Oral *Surg Oral Med Oral Pathol Oral Radiol Endod.* Vol. 91, pp.622–635

Mirzamani N, Salehian P, Farhadi M & Tehran EA (2006). Detection of EBV and HPV in nasopharyngeal carcinoma by in situ hybridization. *Exp Mol Pathol,* Vol. 81, pp. 231-234

Mork J, Lie AK, Glattre E, Clark S, Hallmans G, Jellum E, et al. (2001). Human papillomavirus infection as a risk factor for squamous-cell carcinoma of the head and neck. *N Engl J Med,* Vol. 344, pp. 1125-1131

Morshed K, Polz-Dacewicz M, Rajtar B, Szymanski M, Ziaja-Soltys M & Golabek W (2005). [The prevalence of E6/E7 HPV type 16 in laryngeal cancer and in normal mucosa]. *Pol Merkur Lekarski,* Vol. 19, pp. 291-293

Nasman A, Attner P, Hammarstedt L, Du J, Eriksson M, Giraud G et al. (2009). Incidence of human papillomavirus (HPV) positive tonsillar carcinoma in Stockholm, Sweden: an epidemic of viral-induced carcinoma? *Int J Cancer,* Vol. 125, pp. 362-366

Nielsen H, Norrild B, Vedtofte P, Praetorius F, Reibel J & Holmstrup P (1996). Human papillomavirus in oral premalignant lesions. *Eur J Cancer B Oral Oncol. [Research Support, Non-U.S. Gov't],* Vol. 32B, No. 4, pp. 264-70

Oliveira MC, Soares RC, Pinto LP, Souza LB, Medeiros SRB & Costa ALL (2009). High-risk human papillomavirus (HPV) is not associated with p53 and bcl-2 expression in oral squamous cell carcinomas. *Auris Nasus Larynx,* Vol. 36, pp. 450–456

O'Regan E M, Toner M E, Finn S P, Fan C Y, Ring M, Hagmar B. et al. (2008). p16INK4A genetic and epigenetic profiles differ in relation to age and site in head and neck squamous cell carcinomas. Human Pathology Vol., 39, pp.452–458

Ostwald C, Rutsatz K, Schweder J, Schmidt W, Gundlach K & Barten M (2003). Human papillomavirus 6/11, 16 and 18 in oral carcinomas and benign oral lesions. *Med Microbiol Immunol,* Vol. 192, pp. 145-148

Pan HY, Zhang ZY, Zhou XJ, Li J. (2006). The establishment of a carcinogenesis model of oral squamous cell carcinoma in vitro. Zhonghua Kou Qiang Yi Xue Za Zhi. Vol. 41, pp.: 20–24

Park JW, Pitot HC, Strati K, Spardy N, Duensing S, Grompe M, et al. (2010). Deficiencies in the Fanconi anemia DNA damage response pathway increase sensitivity to HPV-associated head and neck cancer. *Cancer Res. [Research Support, N.I.H., Extramural],* Vol. 70, No. 23, pp. 9959-68

Parkin DM, Whelan SL, Ferlay J, Raymond L & Young J. (1997). In: *Scientific publications Cancer incidence in five continents,* IARC, Lyon

Parkin DM, Bray F, Ferlay J & Pisani P (2005). Global cancer statistics, 2002. *CA Cancer J Clin,* Vol. 55, No. 2, pp. 74–108

Paz IB, Cook N, Odom-Maryon T, Xie Y & Wilczynski SP (1997). Human papillomavirus (HPV) in head and neck cancer. An association of HPV 16 with squamous cell carcinoma of Waldeyer's tonsillar ring. *Cancer,* Vol. 79, pp. 595-604

Punwaney R, Brandwein MS, Zhang DY, Urken ML, Cheng R, Park CS et al. (1999). Human papillomavirus may be common within nasopharyngeal carcinoma of Caucasian Americans: investigation of Epstein-Barr virus and human papillomavirus in eastern and western nasopharyngeal carcinoma using ligation-dependent polymerase chain reaction. *Head Neck,* Vol. 21, pp. 21-29

Ragin CCR, Modugno F, Gollin SM. (2007). The epidemiology and risk factors of head and neck cancer: a focus on human papillomavirus. J Dent Res. Vol. 86, pp. 104–14

Rajkumar T, Sridhar H, Balaram P, Vaccarella S, Gajalakshmi V, Nandakumar A et al. (2003). Oral cancer in Southern India: the influence of body size, diet, infections and sexual practices. *Eur J Cancer Prev,* Vol. 12, pp. 135-143

Remmerbach TW, Brinckmann UG, Hemprich A, Chekol M, Ku¨hndel K, Liebert UG. (2004). PCR detection of human papillomavirus of the mucosa: comparison between MY09/11 and GP5+/GP6+ primer sets, *J Clin Virol* . Vol. 30, pp. 302–308

Ribeiro KB, Levi JE, Pawlita M, Koifman S, Matos E, Eluf-Neto J et al. (2011). Low human papillomavirus prevalence in head and neck cancer: results from two large case-control studies in high-incidence regions. *Int J Epidemiol,* Vol. 40, pp. 489-502

Ringström E, Peters E, Hasegawa M, Posner M, Liu M, Kelsey KT. (2002). Human papillomavirus type 16 and squamous cell carcinoma of the head and neck. *Clin Cancer Res.* Vol. 8, pp.3187–3192

Rintala M., Grénmana S., Puranen M., Syrjänen S. (2006). Natural history of oral papillomavirus infections in spouses: A prospective Finnish HPV Family Study. *Journal of Clinical Virology,* Vol. 35, pp. 89–94

Ritchie JM, Smith EM, Summersgill KF, Hoffman HT, Wang D, Klussmann JP, et al. (2003). Human papillomavirus infection as a prognostic factor in carcinomas of the oral cavity and oropharynx. *Int J Cancer,* Vol. 104, No. 3, pp. 336–44

Rosenquist K, Wennerberg J & Schildt EB (2005). Oral status, oral infections and some lifestyle factors as risk factors for oral and oropharyngeal squamous cell carcinoma. A populationbased case-control study in southern Sweden. *Acta Otolaryngol,* Vol. 125, pp. 1327-36

Schwartz SM, Daling JR, Doody DR, Wipf GC, Carter JJ, Madeleine MM, et al. (1998). Oral cancer risk in relation to sexual history and evidence of human papillomavirus infection. *J Natl Cancer Inst,* Vol. 90, pp. 1626-1636

Shiboski CH, Schmidt BL, Jordan RC (2005). Tongue and tonsil carcinoma: increasing trends in the U.S. population ages 20-44 years. *Cancer,* Vol. 103, pp. 1843-1849

Silverman Jr S. (2001). Demographics and occurrence of oral and pharyngeal cancers.The outcomes, the trends, the challenge. *J Am Dent Assoc.* Vol. 132(Suppl.):7S

Singhi AD, Califano J & Westra WH (2011). High-risk human papillomavirus in nasopharyngeal carcinoma. *Head Neck*

Sisk EA, Soltys SG, Zhu S, Fisher SG, Carey TE & Bradford CR (2002). Human papillomavirus and p53 mutational status as prognostic factors in head and neck carcinoma. *Head Neck,* Vol. 24, No. 9, pp. 841–9

Smith EM, Ritchie JM, Summersgill KF, Hoffman HT, Wang DH, Haugen TH, et al. (2004), Human papillomavirus in oral exfoliated cells and risk of head and neck cancer,. *J Natl Cancer Ins.* Vol. 96, pp. 449–55

Smith EM, Ritchie JM, Summersgill KF, Klussmann JP, Lee JH, Wang D et al. (2004). Age, sexual behavior and human papillomavirus infection in oral cavity and oropharyngeal cancers. *Int J Cancer,* Vol. 108, pp. 766-772

Snijders PJ, Scholes AG, Hart CA, et al. (1996). Prevalence of mucosotropic human papillomaviruses in squamous-cell carcinoma of the head and neck. *Int J Cancer,* Vol. 66, pp. 464–469

Snijders PJ, Steenbergen RD, Meijer CJ, Walboomers JM. (1997). Role of human papillomaviruses in cancer of the respiratory and upper digestive tract. *Clin Dermatol.,* Vol. 15, pp. 415–425

Strome SE, Savva A, Brissett AE, Gostout BS, Lewis J, Clayton AC, et al. (2002). Squamous cell carcinoma of the tonsils: a molecular analysis of HPV associations. *Clin Cancer Res,* Vol. 8, No. 4, pp. 1093–100

Sugiyama M, Bhawal U K, Kawamura M, Ishioka Y, Shigeishi H, Higashikawa K. et al. (2007). Human papillomavirus-16 in oral squamous cell carcinoma: Clinical correlates and 5-year survival British Journal of Oral and Maxillofacial Surgery, Vol. 45, pp. 116–122

Sugiyama M, Bhawal UK, Dohmen T, Ono S, Miyauchi M, Ishikawa T. (2003). Detection of human papillomavirus-16 and HPV-18 DNA in normal, dysplastic, and malignant oral epithelium. *Oral Surg Oral Med Oral Pathol Oral Radiol Endod.* Vol. 95, pp. 594–600

Syrjanen K, Syrjanen S, Lamberg M, Pyrhonen S & Nuutinen J (1983). Morphological and immunohistochemical evidence suggesting human papillomavirus (HPV) involvement in oral squamous cell carcinogenesis. *Int J Oral Surg,* Vol. 12, pp. 418-424

Syrjänen K & Syrjänen S. (2000). Papillomavirus infections in human disease, pp. 1-615, Wiley, New York

Syrjänen S (2004). HPV infections and tonsillar carcinoma. *J Clin Pathol,* Vol. 57, pp. 449-455

Syrjänen S (2005). Human papillomavirus (HPV) in head and neck cancer. *J Clin Virol. [Review],* Vol. 32, No. , pp. S59-66

St Guily JL, Clavel C, Okais C, Pretet JL, Beby-Defaux A, Agius G et al. (2011). Human papillomavirus genotype distribution in tonsil cancers. *Head Neck Oncol,* Vol. 3, pp. 6

St Guily JL, Borget I, Vainchtock A, Remy V & Takizawa C (2010). Head and neck cancers in France: an analysis of the hospital medical information system (PMSI) database. *Head Neck Oncol,* Vol. 2, pp. 22

Tang X, Jia L, Ouyang J, Takagi M. (2003). Comparative study of HPV prevalence in Japanese and north-east Chinese oral carcinoma. *J Oral Pathol Med.* Vol. 2, pp. 393–398

Torrente MC, Rodrigo JP, Haigentz M, Jr., Dikkers FG, Rinaldo A, Takes RP et al. (2011). Human papillomavirus infections in laryngeal cancer. *Head Neck,* Vol. 33, pp. 581-586

Tsai TC, Chen SL (2003). The biochemical and biological functions of human papillomavirus type 16 E5 protein. Arch Virol. Vol. 148, pp.1445–153

Tyan YS, Liu ST, Ong WR, Chen ML, Shu CH & Chang YS (1993). Detection of Epstein-Barr virus and human papillomavirus in head and neck tumors. *J Clin Microbiol,* Vol. 31, pp. 53-56 van Monsjou HS, Balm AJ, van den Brekel MM & Wreesmann VB (2010). Oropharyngeal squamous cell carcinoma: a unique disease on the rise? *Oral Oncol,* Vol. 46, pp. 780-785

Venuti A, Badaracco G, Rizzo C, Mafera B, Rahimi S & Vigili M (2004). Presence of HPV in head and neck tumours: high prevalence in tonsillar localization. *J Exp Clin Cancer Res,* Vol. 23, pp. 561-566

Vidal L & Gillison ML (2008). Human papillomavirus in HNSCC: recognition of a distinct disease type. *Hematol Oncol Clin North Am. [Review],* Vol. 22, No. 6, pp. 1125-42

Watts DH, Koutsky LA, Holmes KK, Goldman D, Kuypers J, Kiviat NB et al. (1998). Low risk of perinatal transmission of human papillomavirus: results from a prospective cohort study. *Am J Obstet Gynecol,* Vol. 178, pp. 365-73

Wiest T, Schwarz E, Enders C, Flechtenmacher C, Bosch FX (2002). Involvement of intact HPV16 E6/E7 gene expression in head and neck cancers with unaltered p53 status and perturbed pRb cell cycle control. *Oncogene,* Vol. 21, pp.1510-1517

Yang SW, Lee YS, Chen TA, Wu CJ & Tsai CN (2009). Human papillomavirus in oral leukoplakia is no prognostic indicator of malignant transformation. *Cancer Epidemiol,* Vol. 33, pp. 118-122

10

Implications of Human Papillomavirus Infections in the Biology of Head and Neck Cancers

Descamps Géraldine[1], Duray Anaëlle[1], Delvenne Philippe[2] and Saussez Sven[1]
[1]*Laboratory of Anatomy, Faculty of Medicine and Pharmacy, University of Mons*
[2]*Department of Pathology, CHU Sart-Tilman, University of Liège*
Belgium

1. Introduction

1.1 Epidemiology

Head and neck squamous cell carcinomas (HNSCCs) remain a significant cause of morbidity worldwide, with as many as 466831 and 168368 cases diagnosed in 2008 among men and women, respectively (Globocan, 2008; Grandis et al., 2004; Shah et al., 2003). HNSCCs constitute a collection of diseases that, despite their shared location and histology, can become different types of tumors that differ in pathogenesis, biology, sub-location and treatment and that can affect quality of life, including survival (Grandis et al., 2004; Shah et al., 2003). HNSCC patients in the early clinical stages (stages I and II) have similar survival rates, with a five-year survival between 70 and 90%, independent of the sub-location (Forastiere & Trotti, 1999). In contrast, HNSCC patients in the advanced clinical stages (stages III and IV) display completely different survival rates depending on the histological type of the tumor and its sub-location (Denis et al., 2004; Forastiere & Trotti, 1999). In 2008, Globocan data indicated that HNSCCs constituted the sixth and eighth most frequent cancer among men and women, respectively. Their frequency has varied over the last 20 years, with an increasing prevalence in women, which is highest in Europe, and a decreasing prevalence in men, which is highest in the USA. A comparison of global statistics with official data from Belgium reveals a strikingly increased incidence of HNSCCs in both sexes, with important regional differences. Indeed, Belgium has a higher incidence of HNSCC associated with smoking and alcohol consumption compared with other countries. In 2005, HNSCCs were the fourth most common cancer in men after prostate, lung and colorectal cancers and the eighth most common cancer in women after breast, colorectal, uterine, lung, melanoma, ovarian cancers and non-Hodgkin's lymphoma (Filleul et al., 2011). We can also observe inter-regional heterogeneity; in fact, the incidence is higher in men in Wallonia than in the Brussels region where the incidence of HNSCC in women rose. Finally, when we compare Belgian and French data, these cancers seem more frequent in French men than in

Belgian men, but there is an opposite trend among women, in which carcinomas of the larynx are more frequent in Belgium than in France.

1.2 Treatments of HNSCCs

The treatment of HNSCC patients in advanced disease stages combines surgery, radiation oncology, medical oncology, medical imaging and clinical pathology (Denis et al., 2004; Forastiere & Trotti, 1999; Grandis et al., 2004; Shah et al., 2003). This type of collaborative medical approach was initiated as early as 1970 when Fletcher and Evers reported the first convincing evidence showing the benefits of combining radiotherapy with surgery (Adelstein et al., 2003). In this context, cisplatin was investigated for the treatment of HNSCC in the early 1970s, and, from the late 1970s to the early 1990s, promising results were obtained with the use of various combinations of postoperative chemotherapy with radiotherapy in randomized (Al-Sarraf et al., 1998) and non-randomized studies (Jeremic et al., 2000). In the early 2000s, the Radiation Therapy Oncology Group (Denis et al., 2004) and the European Organization for Research and Treatment of Cancer (EORTC) (Cooper et al., 2004) conducted two randomized studies to test the relative efficacy of concurrent postoperative cisplatin administration and radiotherapy in the treatment of HNSCC. These two studies demonstrated that local control of the disease was significantly higher in the combined therapy group than in the group that received radiotherapy alone. Unfortunately, these combined treatments were frequently associated with adverse side effects. Although significant progress has been observed after combined treatments, a number of statements concerning HNSCCs currently remain valid: (i) almost two-thirds of HNSCC patients have advanced forms (stages III and IV) of the disease at diagnosis, (ii) 50% of HNSCC patients die within the two years following the initial diagnosis, and (iii) every year, 5% of the patients develop additional primary tumors. Therefore, novel approaches seem to be required to provide head and neck oncologists with a more effective armamentarium against this challenging disease (Bernier et al., 2004; Lang et al., 2004).

1.3 Risk factors for the development of HNSCC

Tobacco use and alcohol consumption are now well-established risk factors for the development of HNSCC; however, a proportion of HNSCC patients (15-20%) develop tumors even in the absence of exposure to these agents (Gillison et al., 2000) Moreover, Sturgis and Cinciripini reported that the overall incidence of HNSCC has declined in the United States over the past 20 years, which has been attributed to a decrease in smoking. Nevertheless, the study also demonstrated an increase in the frequency of tongue and pharyngeal cancers (Sturgis & Cinciripini, 2007). These findings suggest the importance of other risk factors, such as human papillomavirus (HPV), in the development of oropharyngeal and oral carcinomas.

2. HNSCC and HPV: incidence, biological pathways and impact on prognosis

Currently, persistent high-risk HPV (hr HPV) infection is widely accepted as the major cause of uterine cervical carcinoma with HPV 16 and 18 being the two most implicated types. These oncogenic papillomaviruses have also been related to others lesions, such as vulvar, vaginal, penile, anal and more recently, head and neck squamous cell carcinomas

(Chung & Gillison, 2009). Since 1983 when Syrjänen published the first study analyzing HPV infection in HNSCCs, the etiological role of HPV has become increasingly accepted. Indeed, although tobacco and alcohol exposure are established risk factors for HNSCCs, HPV infection may act synergistically with these carcinogenic agents. Presently, more than 120 human papillomaviruses have been identified by complete DNA sequence analysis. They are classified by family, genus, species and types according to several criteria. More precisely, types are determined on the basis of sequence homology to the gene encoding the L1 protein, which is the most conserved gene in the HPV genome (Aubin et al., 2007; de Villiers et al., 2004; de Villiers & Gunst, 2009). The genotypes are also more commonly used to refer the different types. However, in clinical practice, distinctions between HPV types include the type of epithelium infected (cutaneous *vs.* mucosal HPV) and the ability to effect cellular transformation. The capacity to transform epithelial cells is divided into high risk and low risk HPV: a benign proliferation is associated with the low-risk (lr) HPV type, and malignancy is associated with the high-risk (hr) HPV type (Nebesio et al., 2001; Syrjänen et al., 2011).

The human papillomavirus belongs to the highly diverse *Papillomaviridae* family. The HPV virion has a diameter of 55 nm and consists of circular double-stranded DNA containing approximately 8000 base pairs (bp). The HPV genome is encapsulated in a proteic capsid of 72 capsomers. Notably, the lack of envelope makes this virus resistant to environmental conditions, infectious for years and resistant to many therapeutics agents. The HPV genome consists of three major regions. The non-coding long control region (LCR) of 1000 bp contains the p97 promoter controlling E6 and E7 transcription, transcriptional regulatory elements and the binding sites for the E2 and E1 gene products (Neufcoeur et al., 2009; Ragin et al., 2007). The 3000bp region encodes two structural capsid proteins, namely, the late proteins L1 and L2. The icosahedral capsid can be constituted of L1 proteins alone or together with L2. The L1 capsid is comprised of 360 L1 molecules assembled as 72 pentameric capsomers, and the L1-L2 capsid contains 12 additional L2 molecules (Ishii et al., 2005). The six early proteins are encoded by a 4000bp region: two of the early proteins, E1 and E2, are regulatory proteins that modulate the replication and transcription of viral DNA and the expression of the other early genes; the early protein E4 acts in association with keratin filaments in host epithelial cells; the remaining three early proteins, E5, E6, and E7, are oncogenes involved in cellular transformation and maintenance of the malignant phenotype (Chung & Gillison, 2009; Doorbar & Myers, 1996).

2.1 Life cycle of the human papillomaviruses and molecular mechanisms of head and neck HPV carcinogenesis

The HPV life cycle is particularly complex. HPV infection requires abrasion in the stratified epithelium, providing access to the basal layer. Attachment of the virus to the host cell may be achieved through cell surface receptors or glycosaminoglycans, such as heparin sulfate. After this attachment, virions can be internalized via clathrin-dependent endocytosis and, after uncoating, the viral DNA is transported into the nucleus by the cytoskeleton. During this early infection, the virus maintains its genome as a nuclear episome at a low copy number (10-200 copies per cell) in the basal cell of the epithelium. This slight proliferation is limited in the basal cell layers, due to the expression of E1 and E2 proteins, which maintain the viral DNA as an episome (Chung & Gillison, 2009; Doorbar, 2005; Monsonégo, 2007). E1 is an ATP-dependent helicase initiating the viral replication in cooperation with E2 (Hughes & Romanos, 1993).

Moreover, E2 can act as a transcriptional repressor of E6 and E7 expression by binding to the non-coding region LCR, and it has a crucial role in the segregation of the viral genome during cell division (Psyrri & Dimaio, 2008; You et al., 2004). This initial infection is followed by a proliferative phase corresponding to an increased number of viral episomes. Indeed, normal epithelial cells differentiate from the basement membrane toward the apical surface. During this proliferative phase, the HPV genome may remain episomal or become integrated into the host genome. Next, the HPV DNA replicates to a high copy number and is encapsidated to produce virions only in terminally differentiated epithelial cells. Integration of the HPV genome into the host chromosome is thought to be a late event and to occur at random with a predilection for fragile chromosomal sites. This integration also leads to the loss of the E1 and E2 genomic sequences, releasing the HPV oncogenes from repression (Ragin et al., 2007). Overexpression of both E6 and E7 stimulate cell cycle progression with S-phase entry, leading to proliferation of squamous epithelial cells of the upper aerodigestive tract. These two oncogenes alter key tumor suppressor pathways. The third oncogene, E5, exerts its carcinogenic effects only during the early stages of infection because its gene sequence is deleted when HPV integrates the host genome (zur Hausen & de Villiers, 1994). However, this protein stimulates cell growth through binding to the epidermal growth factor receptor (EGFR), initiating cascades leading to upregulation of proto-oncogenes. The association of E7 with the retinoblastoma protein (pRb) is now well characterized. The pRb protein is a negative regulator of the cell cycle that prevents S-phase entry under normal conditions by associating with the E2F transcription factor. The association between pRb and E2F is broken upon HPV infection: E7 binds to pRb, leading to its degradation and the subsequent release of E2F, which stimulates cell proliferation. Note that the inactivation of pRb results in a reciprocal overexpression of the p16 protein, which is an inhibitor of cyclin-dependent kinases. Indeed, the Rb gene also regulates p16 by a negative feedback mechanism; consequently, the inactivation of pRb leads to p16 upregulation. The expression of this protein is elsewhere considered as a surrogate marker for HPV infection in both cervical and head and neck cancer (Klozar et al., 2010; Li et al., 1994). The E6 protein of hr HPVs binds simultaneously to a cellular ubiquitin ligase, known as the E6-associated protein (E6-AP), and to the tumor suppressor protein p53, resulting in its ubiquitination and subsequent proteolytic degradation. Normally, p53 regulates growth arrest and apoptosis after DNA damage and, depending on the damage incurred; p53 induces a prolonged cell cycle arrest or triggers apoptosis. Moreover, HPV infected cells avoid this process of cell death by E6-mediated inactivation of p53. This oncogene interferes with other pro-apoptotic proteins of both extrinsic and intrinsic apoptotic pathways, such as Bak, FADD and pro-caspase 8 (Garnett et al., 2006; Narisawa-saito & Kiyono, 2007; Thomas & Bank, 1999). Thus, these two oncoproteins are essential factors for HPV-induced cellular immortalization, transformation and carcinogenesis. Finally, expression of the late proteins L1 and L2 occurs in the upper layer, as cells differentiate and allow the encapsidation of the genome and the production of new infectious virions, which are released into the extracellular environment to re-initiate infection.

2.2 Epidemiology and incidence of HPV infection in head and neck region

In recent years, the relation between the presence of HPV DNA and the development of head and neck tumors from different anatomical sites was analyzed. Differences in prevalence were found from one site to another. For example, the meta-analysis directed by Kreimer considered more than 5000 tumors from 60 studies conducted on five continents; the authors showed that oropharyngeal tumors had the highest HPV prevalence (35.6%). Oral and laryngeal (including hypopharyngeal) carcinomas were infected in 23.5% and 24% of cases, respectively (Kreimer et al., 2005). Note that HPV16 accounted for 86.7% of all HPV-positive oropharyngeal tumors, compared with 68.2% in oral and 69.2% in laryngeal squamous cell carcinomas. Recently, Laco and colleagues also demonstrated this higher proportion in their study: 24 oral SCCs and 22 oropharyngeal SCCs (OPSCCs) were analyzed for HPV presence using the polymerase chain reaction (PCR). The results indicated that 82% of OPSCCs were HPV-positive, compared with 13% of OSCCs (Laco et al., 2011). The biological explanation for this higher HPV prevalence in tumors arising in oropharynx is becoming clearer. Both the tonsils and the base of tongue are lymphoid tissues that produce cytokines, which may affect HPV transcription and promote cell transformation (Klussmann et al., 2001). Furthermore, the tonsil epithelium presents morphological similarities to those of genital epithelia, such as deep invaginations of the tonsil surface that may facilitate viral particle retention. These invaginations, also called crypts, are flanked by stratified squamous epithelium, which facilitate viral access to basal cells. Additionally, both genital and tonsillar epithelia derive from the same endodermal embryonic layer (Ernoux et al., 2009).

As previously mentioned, reported rates of HPV positivity in HNSCCs vary widely. This inconsistency will be discussed with respect to anatomical site in a later chapter. However, this widespread variability must be interpreted with caution, but may be partially explained notably by differences in methodology of HPV detection. Indeed, according to several studies, multiple HPV detection methods are used, such as the polymerase chain reaction (PCR), *in situ* hybridization (ISH) and Southern hybridization. Among these techniques, numerous studies agree that PCR is the most sensitive. In fact, a review of the literature by Miller and White showed that HPV was identified with a higher frequency by using PCR (37.1%) than by using moderate- or low-sensitivity assays, such as Southern hybridization (27.2%) or ISH and immunohistochemistry (25.2%) (Miller & White, 1996). However, despite an increase in the use of PCR to detect HPV, variability in prevalence still exists and may be attributed to differences in the sensitivity of the PCR primer sets. Different consensus primer sets are used to detect and amplify HPV DNA, but the two most frequently used are the GP5+/GP6+ and the MY09/11 primers. Moreover, it seems that GP5+/GP6+ primers are more sensitive than MY09/11 for HPV detection in oral samples. Remmerbarch also recommends the PCR approach with nested GP5+/GP6+ primers (Remmerbach et al., 2004). Other explanations for the varying rates of prevalence could be the sample sources and collection methods (scalpel biopsy, swabs, brushings, and mouthwash). The geographical locations of the studies may also contribute to variations in HPV prevalence. Indeed, HPV prevalence in OSCCs is similar in Europe (16%) and North America (16.1%) but significantly greater in Asia (33%). For OPSCCs, the prevalence is significantly higher in North America (47%) compared with Europe (28.2%) (Kreimer et al., 2005). Finally, patient profiles, such as smokers *vs.* non-smokers and/or drinkers *vs.* non-drinkers, could also contribute to some variations. It turns out that the literature presents conflicting accounts of the association between smoking and/or drinking and HPV in the development of HNSCCs. Indeed, we can distinguish three distinct categories: studies showing that HPV is clearly associated with an increased risk of HNSCC in non-smokers, studies finding no difference in HPV-related carcinoma between smokers and non-smokers and studies providing evidence of an additive or synergistic effect between smoking and HPV-related HNSCC (Sinha et al., 2011). Fouret observed a higher prevalence of HPV in non-smokers, while an additive interaction was observed by Smith. HPV-positive smokers presented a greater risk of HNSCC compared with HPV-negative smokers or HPV-positive non-smokers (Fouret et al., 1997; Smith et al., 2004a). On the other hand, Paz found no statistical association between tumor HPV status and tobacco use (Paz et al., 1997). Biologically, smoking and alcohol can cause cellular and structural modifications in oral epithelia, which potentially increase the permeability to viral infection. These environmental agents are also known to suppress mediators of immune functions, facilitating HPV infection persistence (Pannone et al., 2011; Ragin et al., 2007; Sinha et al., 2011).

2.3 Prognosis of HPV positive head and neck squamous cell carcinoma

The significance of hr HPV infection and its impact on patient prognosis remains an important matter of debate, although a majority of studies have now confirmed an improved survival of HPV-positive patients compared with HPV-negative patients (Fakhry et al., 2008; Lindel et al., 2001; Lindquist et al., 2007). However, this strong positive prognostic factor is often confirmed in tonsillar and oropharyngeal carcinomas. Notably, the majority of studies that demonstrated increased survival were reporting on patients with oropharyngeal and/or tonsillar tumors (Ang et al., 2010; Lindel et al., 2001; Sedaghat et al., 2009). The meta-analysis by Ragin et al. examining the relationship between HPV and overall survival did not show any survival differences between HPV-positive and HPV-negative patients with cancer in non-oropharyngeal sites (Ragin et al., 2007). The same observation was made by Gillison et al., suggesting that these tumors may have an etiology distinct from that of tumors in non-oropharyngeal sites (Gillison et al., 2000). In fact, this subset of oropharyngeal HPV-positive cancers possesses distinct clinical features and outcomes, and it is particularly common in individuals who lack the traditional risk factors of tobacco and alcohol abuse. While it is unclear whether tobacco is a risk factor for HPV-induced oropharyngeal tumors, it seems that smoking has a negative impact on the survival of patients with HPV-positive tumors (Hafkamp et al., 2008). Nevertheless, there are reports in the literature on the prognostic significance of HPV infection describing a reduced influence on prognosis and other reports demonstrating no influence on prognosis. Indeed, two Swedish studies demonstrated that oral HPV infection was associated with a dramatically increased risk of OSCC development (Hansson et al., 2005; Rosenquist et al., 2007). Additionally, in 1994, Clayman et al. also showed that HPV detection significantly correlated with decreased survival (Clayman et al., 1994). On the other hand, other studies have failed to demonstrate an association between HPV positivity and prognosis (Duray et al., 2011a; Ernoux et al., 2011; Koskinen et al., 2003; Morshed et al., 2010). From a biological point of view, it is difficult to explain why patients with HPV infections have a worse survival than HPV-negative patients. One possible explanation is that HPV infected cells in locations with inflammatory activity may be stimulated to divide, facilitating tumor development (Dahlgren et al., 2004). Another hypothesis is that immunosuppression may favor HPV infection (Duray et al, 2010). In 2004, Kreimer reported that tonsillar HPV infection was strongly associated with HIV co-infection and immunosuppression (Kreimer et al., 2004). Recently, herpes simplex virus-2 (HSV2) infection was demonstrated to increase the risk of HPV infection (Moscicki et al., 2001). Furthermore, a study performed by Tung et al. reported the presence of HPV-16 or -18 and Epstein-Barr virus (EBV) in 80% of nasopharyngeal carcinoma samples (Tung et al., 1999). These co-infections might play an important role in the initiation of neoplastic transformation in human oral epithelial cells. HPV infections have also been implicated in several tumor cell immune escape mechanisms, such as the absence of an inflammatory response against tumor cells, the production of regulatory cytokines and the downregulation of Toll-like receptor 9 (Lepique et al., 2009).

3. HPV related head and neck carcinomas *versus* HPV non-related head and neck carcinomas: two different tumor entities

Head and neck tumors are now defined as two separate clinical entities: HPV-positive tumors and HPV-negative tumors. The tumors differ both clinically and molecularly. HPV-positive tumors present distinct histopathological features, including notably non-keratinizing basal cells and a prominent "koilocytic" morphology. These features were also associated with a basaloid morphology that is a morphologic variant of HNSCC (Williams et al., 1996). These HPV-positive tumors are also known to occur in a younger age group, to originate more frequently in the oropharynx (especially in the palatine tonsils and at the base of tongue), to be poorly differentiated because patients present with later-stage disease and to have a lower T-stage than HPV-negative tumors (Marur & Forastière, 2008). Another particularity concerns the overall survival, which seems to be better for HPV-infected patients. Indeed, the majority of studies agree with that of Gillison and colleagues, who found that the risk of dying from disease was reduced in patients with HPV-positive HNSCC (Gillison et al., 2000). HPV-positive and HPV-negative tumors also exhibit differences in tumor biology with HPV-positive tumors having fewer p53 mutations and displaying reduced association with tobacco and alcohol consumption. In fact, approximately one-third of the tumors harbor p53 mutations, but a marked difference in p53 mutation frequency is generally found when comparing HPV-positive and HPV-negative oropharyngeal tumors. Thus, this inverse association between p53 mutations and HPV detection in the oropharynx further suggests that HPV-positive and HPV-negative HNSCCs should be considered to be two distinct cancers with two parallel pathways: one driven by environmental agents (tobacco and alcohol) and another driven by infectious agents (high-risk HPVs). However, these two pathologic agents may interact and act synergistically to lead to the development of HNSCCs. All these observations frequently focus on the oropharynx, strengthening the etiologic role of HPV in oropharyngeal carcinomas. Nevertheless, the implication of HPV in non-oropharyngeal tumors is less firmly established (Gillison et al., 2000). Indeed, among HNSCC biopsies, the real HPV prevalence remains uncertain, due to the varying incidence rates reported in different studies.

4. Incidence of HPV in the general population and modalities of transmission

HPV infection of the oral cavity has not been studied extensively. In fact, the majority of studies on the oral and oropharyngeal cavities considered patients with benign or malignant lesions and did not include healthy patients. However, to establish the etiology and pathogenesis of HPV-associated lesions, it is important to investigate the prevalence of HPV in normal tissues. An overview of the literature describing HPV detection in normal head and neck mucosa in children and adults is shown in Table 1.

4.1 Incidence of HPV in normal oral mucosa

The prevalence of HPV DNA in normal oral mucosa ranges from 0% to 56.7% in healthy adults (Table 1). To date, several studies have also evaluated the presence of HPV infection in the healthy oral cavity of children. In fact, it is important to know the prevalence of HPV infections in childhood because HPV infection early in life could represent a risk factor for the development of head and neck cancer later in life. A prevalence of HPV infection in the oral cavities of children aged 0.3-11.6 years ranging from 0% to 47% has been reported (Syrjänen, 2010). The highest HPV prevalence rates by age group are detected before 1 year of age; the second peak occurs in adolescents aged 13-20 years (Smith et al., 2004b, 2007, 2010; Summersgill et al., 2001). According to the age studied, there are variations in the prevalence rate. In nasopharyngeal aspirates collected immediately after birth, the detection rate of HPV varies from 1.5% to 37% (Cason et al., 1995; Castellsague et al., 2009; Mazzatenta et al., 1996; Puranen et al., 1996, 1997; Rintala et al., 2005a, 2005b; Rombaldi et al., 2008; Sedlacek et al., 1989; Tenti et al., 1997, 1999; Watts et al., 1998). At the age of 1-4 days, Smith et al. in two studies found a low HPV incidence (from 0.9% to 1%) in the buccal swabs of neonates, whereas other studies showed a higher prevalence varying from 40% to 56% (Cason et al., 1995; Kaye et al., 1994; Pakarian et al., 1994; Tseng et al., 1998; Smith et al., 1995, 2004b). Similarly, the detection rate of HPV in infants between 6 weeks and 6 months after delivery varied between 0% and 62% (Cason et al., 2005; Fredericks et al., 1993; Kaye et al., 1994; Pakarian et al., 1994; Watts et al., 1998) and among 3-year-old children varied between 10% and 40% (Kojima et al., 2003; Puranen et al., 1996, 1997; Szydlowski et al., 2004). Mant et al. studied the acquisition and the clearance of HPV in the buccal mucosa of 4- to 9-year-old children and showed that, during a 30-month follow-up, 63% of 19 initially HPV-negative children acquired new HPV16 infection, while 40% of 22 initially HPV-positive children cleared the virus (Mant et al., 2003). In contrast, the Finnish Family HPV study found lower rates, which may be due to the fact that the children were younger and the detection method less sensitive. In fact, they found that, during the three-year follow-up, 42% of the children acquired incident infection, while 11% cleared their infection and 10% had persistent oral HPV infection (Rintala et al., 2005a, 2005b).

4.2 Incidence of HPV in normal tonsil

Regarding the literature, only a few studies have assessed the presence of HPV DNA in normal tonsillar tissues, with HPV detection rates varying from 0% to 24.4% in children/adolescents and 0% to 100% in adults (Table 1). In order to understand the epidemiology of HPV in the healthy population, we detected HPV in the palatine tonsils of children and adults who underwent tonsillectomy (recurrent tonsillitis, n=64) or sleep surgery (apnea: n=9; snoring: n=7). Among our series of 80 disease-free tonsils, 12.5% (10 cases) tested positive for hr HPV types [HPV16 (8 cases), HPV18 (1 case) and HPV31 (1 case)], 15% (12 cases) were positive for lr HPV types and 72.5% (58 cases) were negative. Among the hr HPV-positive tonsils, five were from children/adolescents and five were from adults (Duray et al., 2011b). By the end of 2002, Syrjänen compiled several studies from the United States, Japan, and Western Europe. In total, he determined an 8.5% (17 of 200) HPV positivity rate, either type 16 (12 cases) or type 6/11 (5 cases) (Syrjänen, 2004). A Greek study determined the presence of HPV DNA in children. They found 9 of 106 tonsils to be HPV-positive, with six cases having HPV-16, two cases having HPV-11 and one case having an untyped HPV (Mammas et al., 2006). Another study reported HPV-16 infection in 13 of 206 tonsils (6.3%) with 11 cases from children or young adults aged less than 25 years (Chen et al., 2005). These findings differed from those of several other studies in which low prevalence or no prevalence of oncogenic and non-oncogenic HPV was identified in the specimens studied (Brandsma & Abramson, 1989; Ernster et al., 2009; Klingenberg et al., 2010; Klussmann et al., 2001; Niedobitek et al., 1990; Ribeiro et al., 2006; Sisk et al., 2006; Snijders et al., 1992). In these anatomical sites, HPV-6 and -11 and HPV-16 and -18 were the most common types of lr and hr HPV, respectively (Table 1). According to the literature, prevalence rates of oral HPV in normal individuals vary substantially. It is believed that this great variation in HPV prevalence rates found in head and neck studies may be due to several factors, including the anatomical site, ethnic and geographical differences, the size of the cohorts, the sample collection methods (i.e., biopsy, lavages, scrapes), the materials used for testing (i.e., formalin-fixed biopsies, frozen or fresh biopsies, exfoliated fresh cells), and, probably most importantly, the HPV detection methods used (PCR, in situ hybridization, Southern blot hybridization). For example, using PCR and DNA hybridization techniques, the results showed a prevalence ranging from 0% to 81% (Castro et al., 2009; Ribeiro et al., 2006) in oral mucosa swabs of adults, whereas in biopsies, the rate was less variable with detection of HPV in 0% to 55% (Table 1). The disadvantages of oral rinsing and cytological scraping or brushing are that they collect superficial epithelial cells and that no additional tests were performed for validation (Klingenberg et al., 2010). Moreover, no viruses from latent infections in the basal or suprabasal layer cells are removed (Esquenazi et al., 2010).

4.3 Modalities of transmission of HPV

4.3.1 Sexual mode of transmission

It is now well established that, in the case of cervical cancer, HPV infection is a sexually transmitted disease, but little is known about transmission of oral HPV infection in the general population. In the literature, the majority of the studies evaluated the prevalence of HPV and the risk of sexual transmission in HNSCCs, but few studies tried to determine the frequency and the modalities of sexual and nonsexual HPV transmission in other groups, such as normal children and adult. In fact, Gillison and colleagues conducted a case-control study that compared 100 patients with oropharyngeal SCCs and 200 control patients, and they demonstrated that oral HPV infection was strongly associated with oropharyngeal carcinoma among patients who did not have the classical risk factors of tobacco and alcohol use. Moreover, these authors also demonstrated that a high lifetime number of oral sex or vaginal sex partners, engagement in casual sex, an early age at first intercourse, and the infrequent use of condoms were all associated with HPV-16-positive oropharyngeal cancer. These findings suggest that oral HPV infection is sexually acquired and is involved in the carcinogenesis of oropharyngeal cancer (D'Souza et al., 2007). More recently, they explored whether these sexual behaviors were associated with oral HPV infection in two distinct populations (a control patient population and a population of college-aged men). The first population (control group), which was enrolled in two case-control studies nested within a prospective cohort with HNSCC, consisted of patients at the Johns Hopkins outpatient otolaryngology clinic who were ≥ 18 years of age and had no history of cancer. The second population (college-aged men population) included male students who were > 17 years (women were excluded because some might have received the HPV quadrivalent vaccine). Oral HPV infection was detected in 4.8% of 332 control patients and in 2.9% of 210 college-aged men. Among the control group, the odds of developing oral HPV infection were significantly greater with increases in the lifetime number of oral or vaginal sex partners, whereas among the college-aged men, the odds of developing oral HPV infection were significantly greater with increases in the lifetime number of oral sex or open-mouth kissing partners, but not with increases in the lifetime number of vaginal sex partners. They concluded that oral HPV infection is sexually acquired and is transmitted by behaviors such as oral sex and open-mouth kissing (D'Souza et al., 2009). However, Smith et al. examined the prevalence of HPV in a large series of pregnant women to evaluate the concordance between infection of the cervix and the oral cavity. The lack of concordance in HPV types in either of the mucosal sites in pregnant women, between detection in the cervix and oral contact, and between females and males, suggests that the transmission of infection by auto-inoculation or by oral-genital sex between partners is low, suggesting that a number of issues remain unclear about the mechanisms of HPV transmission (Smith et al., 2004c). Another study also showed that despite a high frequency of oral-penile contact among young adults, the detection of oral HPV was rare, and no association between oral-penile contact and oral HPV infection was found (Winer et al. 2003).

4.3.2 Nonsexual mode of transmission

In children, the modalities of HPV transmission are difficult to explain. Gutman and colleagues described anogenital HPV disease in children after abusive sexual contact (Gutman et al., 1993). However, the high incidence of HPV infection observed in healthy children indicates that the transmission need not be sexual. To explain these pediatric HPV infections, several nonsexual modes of transmission can be proposed, including vertical transmission, horizontal transmission and autoinoculation. It can be due to a vertical transmission, which is divided into three subtypes depending on the assumed time of HPV transmission: (1) peri-conceptual transmission (time around fertilization) occurs theoretically via the infected oocyte or spermatozoon. Several studies showed the presence of HPV DNA in 8 to 64% of semen samples from asymptomatic men and also in seminal plasma and spermatozoa (Syrjänen, 2010). (2) Prenatal transmission (during pregnancy) has been proposed by studies reporting HPV DNA in amniotic fluid, placenta and cord blood samples. In placental samples, the rate of HPV DNA detection varied from 0% to 42.5% (Syrjänen, 2010). Rombaldi et al. observed an HPV infection in 23.3% of the cases studied and transplacental transmission in 12.2%. A significant correlation was also observed between placental HPV and the immunosupressive status of the mother (Rombaldi et al., 2008). Furthermore, Sarkola and colleagues found that HPV DNA was three times more prevalent among women who had smoked compared with never-smokers (Sarkola et al., 2008a). In amniotic fluid and cord blood, the prevalence of HPV varied from 15% to 65% and 0% to 13.5%, respectively. (3) Perinatal transmission occurs during birth and immediately thereafter. HPV transmission may be the result of close contacts between the fetus and infected cervical and vaginal cells of the mother during delivery. Using DNA sequencing, several authors have shown that the mother is the source of infection with evidence of virus transcription in some children (Cason et al., 1995; Kaye et al., 1996). Vertical transmission was considered when the maternal HPV type matches the HPV type isolated from the newborn/child. In 1989, Sedlacek et al. were the first to demonstrate HPV DNA in the nasopharyngeal secretions of infants delivered vaginally by mothers with genital HPV infection (Sedlacek et al., 1989). Since then, several authors evaluated the rate at which HPV is transmitted from mother to newborn/child, but this rate is extremely variable among studies. Medeiros and colleagues proposed the first systematic review on vertical HPV transmission, which included 2111 pregnant women and their 2113 newborns. They showed that pooled mother-to-child HPV transmission was 6.5% and was higher after vaginal delivery than after cesarean section. The authors also showed that the combined relative risk of mother-to-child HPV transmission was 7.3 (Medeiros et al., 2005). Rombaldi et al. determined the rate of maternal HPV transmission using PCR and nested multiple PCR on maternal cervical swabs and neonatal nasopharyngeal specimens. They reported that the perinatal transmission of HPV DNA occurred in 24.5% of the cases studied (Rombaldi et al., 2009). Other studies also suggest that vertical transmission is common, occurring in 40% to 80% of cases (Puranen et al., 1996; Rintala et al., 2005b; Tseng et al., 1998). These high rates of vertical HPV transmission were not confirmed by several studies, which found that the risk of vertical transmission to the oral or genital mucosa of newborns was rare (1-5%) (Smith et al., 1995, 2004b, 2010; Syrjänen & Puranen, 2000 Tenti et al., 1999; Watts et al., 1998). In two previous studies by Smith et al., only one mother/newborn pair was concordant for an HPV type, and among 203 infants, two had detectable HPV in oral or genital swabs (Smith et al., 1995, 2004b). Studies on persistent HPV infection showed that the concordance between mother/newborn infections was maintained between 37% to 83% at six weeks to six months after birth (Cason et al., 1995; Fredericks et al., 1993; Kaye et al., 1996), whereas Rintala et al. found that the prevalence declined to 10% in infants at 24 months of follow-up. This prospective cohort study assessed the dynamics of HPV transmission between parents and infants. They showed that the most common HPV profile was hr HPV in all family members, followed by HPV-positive mother-infant pairs, whereas HPV-positive father-infant pairs were less frequent. No such independent risk could be attributed to subclinical HPV infection in the father, but oral and genital HPV in the mother affected the risk of infant HPV (Rintala et al., 2005b). Thus, our results support the possibility of vertical transmission during pregnancy or perinatal transmission at the time of delivery. In other studies, the non-concordance of type-specific HPV between mother and newborn or the presence of oral HPV DNA in young children who were born to HPV-negative mothers suggest the existence of other transmission routes, such as the horizontal transmission of HPV. In these cases, HPV infection can be transmitted by milk during breastfeeding, by siblings via kissing, and by householders and friends via digital contacts (Syrjänen, 2010). There is one recent article showing the presence of HPV in 4% of 223 breast milk samples 3 days postpartum, regardless of the mother's oral or cervical HPV status (Sarkola et al., 2008b). Transmission via infected surfaces or other fomites, such as clothes, toys or eating utensils, is also possible. Autoinoculation can occur by scratching from one site of the body to another or by bathing (Myhre et al., 2003; Syrjänen & Puranen, 2000). HPV is known to multiply locally at the site of entry on the skin or mucous membranes; by deduction (logically) there is no viremia and no blood spread, but one study showed the presence of HPV in peripheral blood mononuclear cells (PBMCs) from HIV-infected pediatric patients and from healthy blood donors (Bodaghi et al., 2005).

Reference (year) (country)	Age range	Collected material (type of lesion)	Collection method	Technique(s)	Sample size	HPV positivity n (%)	Frequency LR (%) (type LR*)	Frequency HR (%) (type HR*)	Undetermined Type
Ernster et al. (2009) (USA)	Adults (≥21 years)	Tonsils (chronic tonsillitis, obstructive adenotonsillar hypertrophy, obstructive sleep apnea)	Tonsillectomy	PCR (type-specific HPV-16, -18)	226	0 (0%)	0 (0%)	0 (0%)	/
Mammas et al. (2006) (Greece)	Children (age ranged from 2 to 14 years)	Tonsils and adenoids (tonsillar and/or adenoid hyperplasia)	Tonsillectomy	PCR (GP5+/GP6+), HPV typing	106	9 (8.5%)	2/9 (22.2%) (**11**)	6/9 (66.7%) (**16**, 18, 33)	1/9 (11.1%)
Sisk et al. (2006) (USA)	Children (age range from 3 to 12 years)	Tonsils (hypertrophy or chronic tonsillitis)	Tonsillectomy	PCR (MY09/11), HPV typing	50	1 (2%)	1/50 (2%) (11)	0 (0%) (n.a.)	/
Chen et al. (2005) (Finland)	Young adults/adults (age ranged from 17 to 72 years) and children (age ranged from 1.5 to 16 years)	Tonsils (tonsillitis or tonsillar hypertrophy)	Tonsillectomy	PCR (MY09/11 and GP5+/GP6+)	206	13 (6.3%) (6 cases<17 years, 7 cases≥17 years)	n.a.	13/13 (100%) (**16**)	/
	Young adults/adults (age ranged from 18 to 74 years) and children (age ranged from 2 to 15 years)	Tonsillar exfoliated cells	Scrapes	PCR (MY09/11 and GP5+/GP6+)	174	1 (0.6%) (46 years)	n.a.	1/1 (100%) (**58**)	/
Strome et al. (2002) (USA)	Children (±5years)	Tonsils (tonsillar hyperplasia)	Biopsy	SB	48	3 (6.25%)	n.a.	3/3 (100%) (**16**)	/
Fukushima et al. (1994) (Japan)	Adults and children (age ranged from 1 to 82 years)	Tonsils (chronic tonsillitis)	Biopsy	PCR	38	5 (13.2%) (4, 19, 22, 24 and 41 years)	n.a.	5/5 (100%) (**16**, 18)	/
Smith et al. (1993) (USA)	n.a.	Tonsils (normal posterior tonsillar pilar)	Biopsy	PCR, SB	3	1 (33.3%)	1/1 (100%) (6, 11)	0 (0%)	/

Reference (year) (country)	Age range	Collected material (type of lesion)	Collection method	Technique(s)	Sample size	HPV positivity n (%)	Frequency LR (%) (type LR*)	Frequency HR (%) (type HR*)	Undetermined Type
Watanabe et al. (1993) (Japan)	Adults and children (age ranged from 4 to 46 years)	Tonsils (chronic tonsillitis)	Biopsy	PCR, SB	28	4 (14.3%)	n.a.	4/4 (100%) (**16**, 18)	/
Ribeiro et al. (2006) (Brazil)	Children (age ranged from 2 to 13 years)	Tonsils	Tonsillectomy	PCR (MY09/11)	100	0 (0%)	0 (0%)	0 (0%)	/
Tominaga et al. (1996) (Japan)	Adult (21 years)	Tonsillar condyloma acuminatum	Tonsillectomy	PCR	1	1 (100%)	1/1 (100%) (6/11)	0 (0%)	/
		Normal tonsillar mucosa	Tonsillectomy	PCR	3	3 (100%)	3/3 (100%) (6/11)	0 (0%)	/
Klussmann et al. (2001) (Germany)	Adults (age ranged from 20 to 65 years)	Tonsils (chronic tonsillitis)	Tonsillectomy	PCR	14	0 (0%)	0 (0%)	0 (0%)	/
Snijders et al. (1992) (Amsterdam)	n.a.	Tonsils (tonsillitis)	Biopsy	PCR	7	0 (0%)	0 (0%)	0 (0%)	/
Niedobitek et al. (1990) (The Netherlands)	Adults (age ranged from 47 to 80 years)	Tonsils (chronic inflammator disease)	Tonsillectomy	ISH	30	0 (0%)	0 (0%)	0 (0%)	/
Brandsma and Abramson (1989) (USA)	Adults (>35 years)	Tonsils (tonsillitis)	Tonsillectomy	SB	20	0 (0%)	0 (0%)	0 (0%)	/
Klingenberg et al. (2010) (Germany)	Adults and children (age ranged from 12 to 70 years)	Tonsils (chronic tonsillitis or snoring problems)	Biopsy	PCR	195	2 (1%)	0 (0%)	2/2 (100%) (**16/18**)	/
Kim et al. (2007) (Korea)	n.a.	Tonsils (chronic follicular tonsillitis)	Tonsillectomy	Real-time PCR	69	8 (11.6%)	n.a. (6, 11, 84)	3/8 (37.5%) (**16**, 58)	/

Reference (year) (country)	**Age range**	**Collected material (type of lesion)**	**Collection method**	**Technique(s)**	**Sample size**	**HPV positivity n (%)**	**Frequency LR (%) (type LR*)**	**Frequency HR (%) (type HR*)**	**Undetermined Type**
Duray et al. (2011) (Belgium)	Adults (age ranged from 18 to 57 years) and children/adolescents (age ranged from 1 to 17 years)	Tonsils (recurrent tonsillitis or apnea)	Tonsillectomy	PCR (GP5+/GP6+), real-time quantitative PCR	80	22 (27.5%) (11/35 adults, 11/45 children/adolescents)	12/22 (54.5%) (n.a.)	10/22 (45.5%) (**16**, 18, 31)	/
Giraldo et al. (2005) (Brazil)	Adults (women mean age 27.7±6.5 years)	Oral mucosa	Scrapes	PCR (MY09/11)	140	29 (20.7%)	n.a.	n.a.	/
Terai et al. (1999) (Japan)	Adults (age ranged from 22 to 48 years)	Oral mucosa	Scrapes	PCR, RFLP	30	17 (56.7%)	n.a.	n.a.	
Castro et al. (2009) (Brazil)	Women (age ranged from 14 to 51 years)	Oral mucosa	Scrapes	PCR (MY09/11)	30	0 (0%)	0 (0%)	0 (0%)	/
van Doornum et al. (1992) (The Netherlands)†	Adults	Buccal mucosa	Scrapes	PCR	176	0 (0%)	0 (0%)	0 (0%)	/
Badaracco et al. (1998) (Italy)†	Adults (women age ranged from 21 to 48 years)	Oral mucosa	Scrapes	PCR	29	11 (37.9%)	n.a.	n.a.	/
Cañadas et al. (2004) (Spain)	Women (sex workers)	Oral mucosa	Scrapes	PCR	188	15 (7.9%)	6/15 (40%) (**6**, 11)	4/15 (26.7%) (**16**, 18, 31, 33, 39)	5/15 (33.3%)
Rice et al. (2000) (United Kingdom)	Children (age ranged from 3 to 11 years)	Oral mucosa	Scrapes	PCR (MY09/11), HPV-16 nested PCR	267	157 (58.8%)	0 (0%)	157/157 (100%) (**16**)	/

Reference (year) (country)	Age range	Collected material (type of lesion)	Collection method	Technique(s)	Sample size	HPV positivity n (%)	Frequency LR (%) (type LR*)	Frequency HR (%) (type HR*)	Undetermined Type
Llamas-Martínez et al. (2008) (Spain)	Adults (mean age 42.8±16.7 years)	Oral mucosa	n.a.	PCR	30	7 (23.3%)	7/7 (100%) (**6**, 11)	0 (0%)	/
Saini et al. (2010) (Malaysia)	Adults (age ranged from 30 to 60 years & above) and children (age ranged from 1 to 18 years)	Oral mucosa	Scrapes	HC2 HR-HPV detection system	116 (70 women and 46 children)	5 (4.3%) (4 women, 5.7% ; 1 children, 2.2%)	0 (0%)	5/5 (100%) (n.a.)	/
Kellokoski et al. (1992a) (Finland)†	Adults	Oral mucosa	Scrapes	Dot blot hybridization	309	12 (3.8%)	n.a. (2, **6**, 7, **11**, 13)	n.a. (**16**)	/
Kellokoski et al. (1992b) (Finland)†	Adults	Oral mucosa	Biopsy	Southern blot hybridization, PCR	212 and 78	33 (15.6%) and 18 (23.1%)	n.a. (6, 11)	n.a. (16, 18)	/
Koch et al. (1997) (Danmark)	Children (age ranged from 0 to 17 years)	Oral mucosa	Scrapes	PCR	392	1 (0.25%)	0 (0%)	0 (0%)	1/1 (100%)
Esquenazi et al. (2010) (Brazil)	Adults (age ranged from 20 to 31 years)	Oral mucosa	Scrapes	PCR (GP5+/GP6+, MY09/11)	100	0 (0%)	0 (0%)	0 (0%)	/
Maitland et al. (1987) (United Kingdom)	Adults	Buccal mucosa	Biopsy	Hybridization	12	5 (41.6%)	0 (0%)	5/5 (100%) (**16**)	/
Scully et al. (1987) (United Kingdom)†	Adults	Oral mucosa	Biopsy	Hybridization	12	4 (41%)	n.a.	n.a.	/

Reference (year) (country)	Age range	Collected material (type of lesion)	Collection method	Technique(s)	Sample size	HPV positivity n (%)	Frequency LR (%) (type LR*)	Frequency HR (%) (type HR*)	Undetermined Type
Jenison et al. (1990) (Seattle)†	Adults and children	Oral mucosa	Scrapes	PCR	35 adults and 21 children	14 (40%) (adults), 9 (43%) (children)	6/14 (43%), 5/9 (55.5%) (**6**)	8/14 (57%), 4/9 (45.5%) (**16**)	/
Yeudall & Campo (1991) (United Kingdom)	Adults	Oral mucosa	Biopsy	PCR	25	2 (8%)	0/2 (0%)	2/2 (100%) (16, **18**)	/
Jalal et al. (1992) (England)†	Adults	Oral mucosa	Scrapes	PCR	48	25 (52%)	0 (0%)	25/25 (100%) (**16**)	/
Cruz et al. (1996) (The Netherlands)†	Adults	Normal gingiva	Biopsy	PCR	12	0 (0%)	0 (0%)	0 (0%)	/
Schwartz et al. (1998) (USA)	Adults (age ranged from 18 to 65 years)	Oral mucosa	Scrapes	PCR (MY09/11) and sequencing	435	40 (9.2%)	19/40 (47.5%) (**6**, **11**)	18/40 (45%) (**16**, **18**, **31/33/35**)	3/40 (7.5)
Smith et al. (1998) (USA)	Adults	Oral mucosa	Lavage	PCR	205	10 (4.8%)	n.a.	n.a.	
Hansson et al. (2005) (Sweden)	Adults (age ranged from 33 to 89 years)	Oral cavity	Mouthwash	PCR (MY09/11 and GP5+/6+) and DNA sequencing	320	14 (4.4%)	12/14 (85.7%) (**13**, 32, 54, 55, 62, 87, 10, 25, 75, **76**, RTRX9)	2/14 (14.3%) (**16**, 18, 33, 45, 58, 59, **67**, 68, 70)	/
Sugiyama et al. (2003) (Japan)†	Adults	Oral mucosa	Biopsy	PCR	44	16 (36.4%)	0 (0%)	16/16 (100%) (**16**)	/
Kansky et al. (2003) (Slovenia)†	Adults	Oral mucosa	Biopsy	PCR	61	4 (6.6%)	1/4 (25%) (11)	3/4 (75%) (16, 31, 68)	/

Reference (year) (country)	Age range	Collected material (type of lesion)	Collection method	Technique(s)	Sample size	HPV positivity n (%)	Frequency LR (%) (type LR*)	Frequency HR (%) (type HR*)	Undetermined Type
Zhang et al. (2004) (China)†	Adults	Oral mucosa	Biopsy	PCR	40	22 (55%)	0 (0%)	22/22 (100%) (**16/18**)	/
Smith et al. (2007) (USA)	Children/adolescents (age ranged from 2 weeks to 20 years)	Oral cavity/oropharynx	Scrapes	PCR, dot blot hybridization	1235	23 (1.9%)	13/23 (56.5%) (n.a.)	10/23 (43.5%) (n.a.)	/
Summersgill et al. (2001) (USA)	Children (≤ 20 years)	Oral mucosa	Scrapes (for younger children) or lavage	PCR (MY09/11), dot blot hybridization, sequencing	268	16 (6%) (11<7years and 5 between 13 and 20 years)	3/16 (18.75%) (**6**)	9/16 (56.25%) (**16**)	4/16 (25%)
Kurose et al. (2004) (Japan)	Adults and children (age ranged from 0 to ≥ 60 years)	Oral mucosa	Scrapes	PCR (MY09/11) and sequencing	662	4 (0.6%) (24, 48, 71 and 76 years)	2/4 (50%) (12, 71)	2/4 (50%) (16, 53)	/
Giovannelli et al. (2002) (Italy)	Adults (age ranged from 20 to 76 years)	Oral mucosa	Scrapes	PCR (MY09/11 and GP5+/6+) and sequencing	90	5 (5.5%)	0 (0%)	5/5 (100%) (16, **18**, 31, 33)	/
Cortezzi et al. (2004) (Brazil)	Adults (age ranged from 20 to 90 years)	Oral mucosa	Scrapes	PCR (GP5+/6+)	142	15 (10.6%)	1/15 (6.7%) (6/11)	14/15 (93.3%) (**16**, 51/45)	/
do Sacramento et al. (2005) (Brazil)	Adolescents/adults (age ranged from 16 to 52 years)	Oropharynx (tonsils, soft palate, base of the tongue, back wall of the pharynx)	Scrapes	PCR (MY09/11), dot blot hybrodization	50	7 (14%)	2/7 (28.6%) (61)	5/7 (71.4%) (16, 18, 52)	/
Sedlacek et al. (1989) (USA)†	Neonates	Oral pharyngeal cavity	Aspirates	Southern blot hybridization	45	15 (33.3%)	n.a.	n.a.	/
Puranen et al. (1996) (Finland)†	Children (age ranged from 0.3 to 11.6 years)	Oral cavity	Scrapes	PCR (MY09/11)	98	31 (31.6%)	n.a.	n.a.	/

Reference (year) (country)	**Age range**	**Collected material (type of lesion)**	**Collection method**	**Technique(s)**	**Sample size**	**HPV positivity n (%)**	**Frequency LR (%) (type LR*)**	**Frequency HR (%) (type HR*)**	**Undetermined Type**
Smith et al. (2010) (USA)	Newborns	Oral cavity	Scrapes	PCR (MY09/11), DNA hybridization, HPV typing	333	3 (0.9%)	1/3 (33.3%) (61)	2/3 (66.7%) (16, 51)	/
Kojima et al. (2003) (Japan)	Children (age ranged from 3 to 5 years)	Oral mucosa	Scrapes	PCR (consensus PCR L1C1/L1C2 and HPV-1003/1004), DNA sequencing	77	37 (48.1%)	40/52** (77%) (**1**, **2-6**, 8, 10, 11, 13, 20-24, 32, 34, 36-38, 42, 48, 50, 57, 60, 72, 75, **76**, 77, 80)	12/52** (23%) (**16**, 18, 31, 33, 52, 58, 59, 73)	

LR, low risk HPV type; HR, high risk HPV type; n.a., data not available; PCR, polymerase chain reaction; SB, Southern blotting.
Scrapes, term used for scrapes, brushes, swabs and smears.
*Column shows analyzed HPV-types mentioned in study (HPV type in bold represents most frequently found virus DNA).
**Data relate to # samples instead of subjects.
† Only abstract on free access

Table 1. Frequencies of HPV types present in normal head and neck mucosa (oral cavity and tonsils) of children and adults

5. Characteristics of infected benign and malignant head and neck lesions and prevalence site by site in head and neck region

5.1 The recurrent respiratory papillomatosis (RRP)

As briefly described previously, HNSCCs are characterized by varying rates of incidence and mortality around the world, such as higher rates in Southeast Asia and Eastern Europe (Kreimer et al., 2005). At present, it is known for certain that HPVs are the etiological agent of many benign and malignant tumors arising from epidermal tissues. Nearly thirty years ago, Gissmann and colleagues were the first team to detect DNA sequences from HPV types 6 and 11 in laryngeal papillomas (Gissmann et al., 1983). Laryngeal papillomatosis, also known as recurrent respiratory papillomatosis (RRP), is characterized by the recurrent growth of exophytic, wart-like lesions called papillomas, along the epithelium of the upper respiratory tract, such as the vocal cords, the arytenoids, the subglottis, the trachea and most commonly, the larynx (Lacey et al., 2006; Mammas et al., 2009). Although the RRPs are benign, their recurrent nature and location in the airways require frequent surgical removal and can cause significant morbidity and occasional mortality secondary to airway obstruction. Smoking and low-risk or high-risk HPV infections have also been proposed to be cofactors in the conversion of laryngeal papillomas into carcinomas (Doyle et al., 1994). These lesions were first described in the late 1800s by Sir Morrell Mackenzie, who recognized papillomas as distinct lesions of the laryngo-pharynx in children. RRPs are mostly caused by the low-risk HPV types 6 and 11, with a more aggressive disease course for the latter type. The disease is also categorized into juvenile onset (JORRP) and adult onset (AORRP) forms based on age at diagnosis. JORRP can be observed immediately during the postnatal period, but it is most commonly diagnosed between two and four years. In AORRP, the peak incidence ranges from 20 to 40 years of age, with dysphonia and hoarseness, and respiratory obstruction being the most common presenting symptoms in children and adults, respectively (Larson & Derkay, 2010). In cases of JORRP, lesions are suspected to originate from a perinatal infection of mothers with condylomatous lesions, which are an overwhelming risk factor. Thus, the virus is generally transmitted during gestation or during birth when the baby passes through the infected birth canal. In a Danish study, Silverberg and colleagues demonstrated that maternal condyloma during pregnancy increased the risk of JORRP in the child more than 200-fold (Silverberg et al., 2003). Moreover, 54% of childhood RRP patients were born to mothers with a history of vulvar condylomata at the time of delivery (Hallden & Majmudar, 1986). Among AORRP patients, the transmission mechanisms clearly vary. The infection probably results from sexual or non-sexual contact with an infected lesion. This evidence has been suggested by a case control study that showed AORRP patients were more likely to have more sexual partners and to have oral sex than controls (Kashima et al., 1992). Additionally, HPV is also able to form latent infections in healthy mucosa, suggesting that AORRP could be due to a reactivation of a latent HPV infection acquired during birth (Goon et al., 2007; Larson and Derkay, 2010). Thus, the relationship between HPV and laryngeal papillomatosis is well established. Indeed, it has been shown that 95% of solitary laryngeal papillomas in adults were positive for HPV (Lindeberg & Johansen, 1990). Moreover, Dickens et al. reported evidence that 59% of laryngeal papillomas showed the presence of the four most common subtypes, including the two low-risk dominant types 6 and 11 (Dickens et al., 1991). In general, the prevalence of RRP was estimated at between four to seven cases per million person-years, and the incidence is about 2 per 100,000 in adults and 4 per 100,000 in children

(Goon et al., 2007). A report in the United States estimated the number of new cases of childhood onset RRP was 1500 to 2500 each year (Derkay, 1995).

5.2 Implication of HPV in other benign lesions of the upper aerodigestive area

As in RRP, HPV is also involved in the development of different benign lesions occurring in the oral cavity, the pharynx, the larynx and the nasopharynx. Numerous studies have been conducted on benign tumors arising in the head and neck to evaluate the possible role of HPV in head and neck neoplasms. However, its implication in carcinogenesis is still controversial because of the different frequencies detected. Kashima et al. examined the diagnostic and prognostic relevance of HPV in 26 squamous papillomas and 29 inverted papillomas. They examined the presence of four HPV types using the PCR amplification technique. The proportion of tissue samples showing HPV infection was 15% and 24% for squamous papillomas and inverted papillomas, respectively, with HPV types 6 and 11 being the only two types detected in these lesions (Kashima et al., 1992). Four years later, HPV was detected with a prevalence of 81.8% in 22 cases of laryngeal squamous papillomas (LP) and 42.5% in 40 cases of nasal inverted papillomas (NIP). HPV types 6 and 11 were again implicated, with a slight bias for HPV 6 in LP and HPV 11 in NIP, suggesting that HPV may play a role in the development of both lesions, and that these viral types may exhibit relative differences in their tissue specificity (Shen et al., 1996). On the other hand, Hoffmann and colleagues had investigated whether HPV was implicated in sinunasal polyposis and found a positive signal in only 1 of the 39 investigated cases (2.6%) (Hoffmann et al., 2000). In oral and oropharyngeal areas, squamous cell papillomas are also benign tumors that occur mainly between 30 and 50 years of age but still represent about 8% of oral tumors in children (Castro & Filho, 2006). Many types of tumors can develop in the oropharynx and oral cavity, such as condiloma acuminata, the common wart and focal epithelial hyperplasia (FEH). Condiloma acuminata (CA) is often considered a sexually transmitted disease, but the trend is to consider that it may also be acquired by auto-inoculation or by maternal transmission (Castro & Filho, 2006; Syrjänen, 2003). HPV was detected in CA with a positivity rate varying between 75% to 85% for the two most frequent lr HPVs, HPV 6 and 11 (Chang et al., 1991; Syrjänen, 2003). Common warts, one of the most common skin lesions, are frequently located on the lips, hard palate, gums and tongue dorsum. HPV detection rates in oral warts have been shown to vary between 43% and 100% (Padayachee, 1994; Praetorius, 1997; Zeuss et al., 1991). Although the near 100% positivity of HPV 6 and 11 is well established for the majority of benign tumors, it has been shown that HPV 2 and HPV 57 were more prevalent in common oral warts (Padayachee, 1994). Finally, oral focal epithelial hyperplasia (FEH), also known as Heck's disease and characterized by multiple nodular elevations, is a third benign oral lesion that may be located in the oral mucosa, lower lips and tongue. Like for oral warts, HPV 6 and 11 are not the major types found in FEH. Indeed, HPV 13 and 32 have been identified in 75% to 100% of the cases (Praetorius, 1997). These two types were considered specific to focal epithelial hyperplasia, while HPV 32 was also found in other oral lesions (de Villiers, 1989). In 2002, Schwenger and colleagues showed that 100% of FEH cases tested were positive for HPV 13 and/or 32 (Schwenger et al., 2002). Moreover, in a recent Brazilian study, of sixteen benign tumors found among 86 examined oral lesions, 100% were positive for HPV (Lira et al., 2009). To confirm the great prevalence of HPV in benign laryngeal lesions, Arndt et al. assessed the presence of HPV genomes 6, 11, 16, 18, 31, 33 and 35 in 17 juvenile laryngeal papillomas (JLP), 27 adult laryngeal papillomas (ALP), 15 oral papillomas (OP) and 11 laryngeal leukoplakias (LL). The results showed 100% positivity for HPV 6 and 11 in JLP and ALP, 87% in OP and 63% in LL, whereas hr HPV 16, 18 and 33 were found in 22% of ALP, 20% of OP and 36% of LL, suggesting that the role of HPV in malignant transformation is less clear than in benign tumors (Arndt et al., 1997). In 2005, a combination of PCR and nested PCR was applied to improve the detection level of infected samples. Among 27 biopsies from different head and neck regions, such as the larynx, nasal cavities and sinuses, pharynx and oral cavity, 16 showed a positive result in either PCR or nested PCR or both, suggesting that this PCR system is a reliable tool for the detection of HPV DNA in benign lesions of the upper aerodigestive tract (Fisher et al., 2005). Conversely, in a retrospective study, 36 head and neck papillomata were tested for HPV 6, 11, 16 and 18 using PCR, and the results were not consistent with a role for HPV infection in the etiology of head and neck papillomata in adult patients. In fact, only 20% of benign tumors were positive for an HPV type (Campos-Bañales et al., 1995). Finally, in 2011, we assessed the presence of HPV DNA in a series of 39 laryngeal benign lesions (LBLs) from 20 cases of vocal nodules, 13 cases of chronic laryngitis and 6 cases of papillomas. The analysis was performed by PCR using the GP5+/GP6+ primers that amplify a conserved sequence located within the L1 region of the HPV genome. Next, all DNA extracts were tested for the presence of 18 different HPV genotypes using TaqMan-based real-time quantitative PCR. Four out of 39 specimens had insufficient tissue quantities for DNA extraction after pathological evaluation and were, therefore, excluded from further analyses. Note that PCR was also performed using β-globin primers to demonstrate the presence of amplifiable DNA in the tissue extracts. All 35 LBLs gave positive signals for β-globin. Among these 35 cases, we identified 27 lesions (77%) that were positive for HPV 16. In the hr HPV-negative subgroup (n=8), two specimens tested positive for HPV using the GP5+/GP6+ consensus primers and were considered infected with lr HPV types (Fig. 1). Only six benign lesions were negative in both GP5+/GP6+ and type-specific HPV PCR analyses (17%). Among the 27 hr HPV-positive lesions, 12 were both positive for GP5+/GP6+ and type-specific HPV (hr HPV+ group), whereas 15 were negative for GP5+/GP6+ and positive for type-specific HPV, which corresponds to the integrated HPV-positive group (int. hr HPV+) (Fig. 1) (Duray et al., 2011a).

This discrepancy observed in varying rates of incidence is mainly attributed to a variation in the sensitivity of the methods employed and in the epidemiological factors related to the group of patients examined. Indeed, the different methods have been classified in three categories according to the detection threshold of viral DNA copy number in the cell: techniques having a low sensitivity, such as immunohistochemistry and in situ hybridization; techniques with moderate sensitivity, such as Southern blot, dot blot and reverse dot blot hybridizations; and techniques displaying high sensitivity, such as the polymerase chain reaction, which can detect the virus in less than one copy per cell (Castro & Filho, 2005). Nevertheless, each method is limited by its sensitivity, its specificity, its practice and its cost, among other limiting factors. In conclusion, it is important to assess the efficacy of the different HPV detection techniques in order to establish HPV etiology in oral lesions.

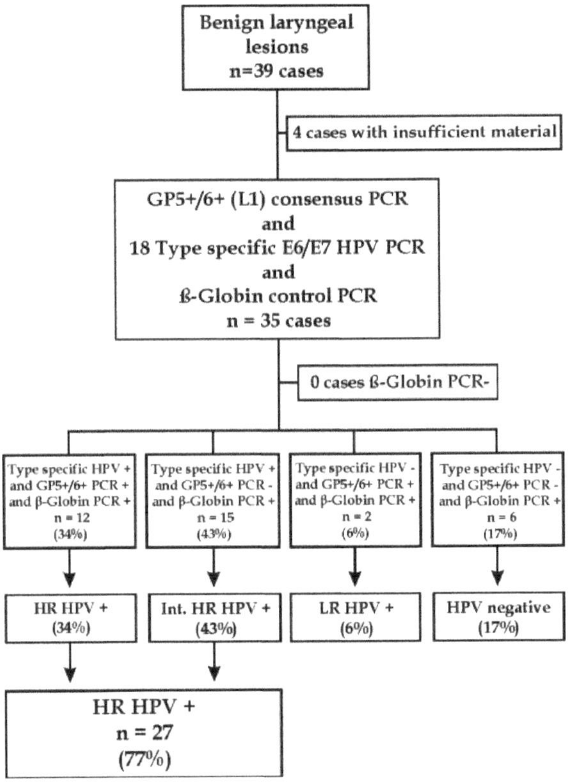

Fig. 1. HPV PCR results from 39 OSCC cases. Four samples could not be analyzed due to insufficient material, and β-globin could be amplified in all samples. Therefore, 35 cases in total were analyzed by type-specific real-time PCR and GP5+/GP6+ consensus PCR. Among these patients, 77% tested positive for infection with one or several types of hr HPV, 6% tested positive for lr HPV and 17% were HPV-negative.

5.3 Implication of HPV in malignant tumors of the upper aerodisgestive area

5.3.1 Incidence in hypopharyngeal tumors

HNSCC represents the sixth most common malignancy with an annual incidence of more than 600,000 cases worldwide and is responsible for approximately 350,000 deaths each year (Parkin et al., 2005). These cancers mainly comprise the hypopharyngeal, laryngeal, oropharyngeal and oral cancers. Depending on the anatomical location of the primary tumor, HNSCCs show an HPV prevalence of between 20% and 30% for hypo-, laryngeal and oral carcinomas and up to over 50% for tonsillar squamous cell carcinomas, especially Waldeyer's tonsillar ring (Deng et al., 2011). Furthermore, there is a persistent controversy on the role of HPV infection in HNSCC progression and on the influence of these infections on the final clinical outcome. Hypopharyngeal carcinoma is one of the less documented head and neck cancers in the literature. Indeed, few studies are exclusively devoted to hypopharyngeal cancers. Thus, the few cases available arise from certain studies that sometimes include hypopharyngeal cases in their cohort. Based on the literature, we observed a prevalence ranging from 0% to 82% (Ernoux et al., 2011; Hafkamp et al., 2003; Ringström et al., 2002). In fact, some authors failed to show prevalence higher than 10% (Gillison et al., 2000; Hafkamp et al., 2003; Ribeiro et al., 2011; Ringström et al., 2002; Stremlau et al., 1987), whereas others found prevalence greater than 50% (Arndt et al., 1992; Ernoux et al., 2011; Kleist et al., 2000; Koskinen et al., 2003; Tyan et al., 1993). Recently, we examined the presence of HPV DNA in a series of 75 patients with stage IV hypopharyngeal SCC (Ernoux et al., 2011). The same methods used previously to detect the virus in our paraffin-embedded samples (PCR using GP5+/GP6+ primers and subsequent TaqMan-based real-time quantitative PCR targeting type-specific sequences of 18 HPV types) were employed in the study. Of the 75 specimens, 8 had insufficient tissue for DNA extraction or quantitative PCR and were, therefore, excluded from further analysis (Fig. 2). Of the remaining 67 cases, another 6 from which were β-globin PCR-negative were also excluded from further analysis. Ultimately, 61 β-globin PCR-positive specimens were typed by quantitative real-time PCR using primers for 18 different HPV types (Fig. 2).

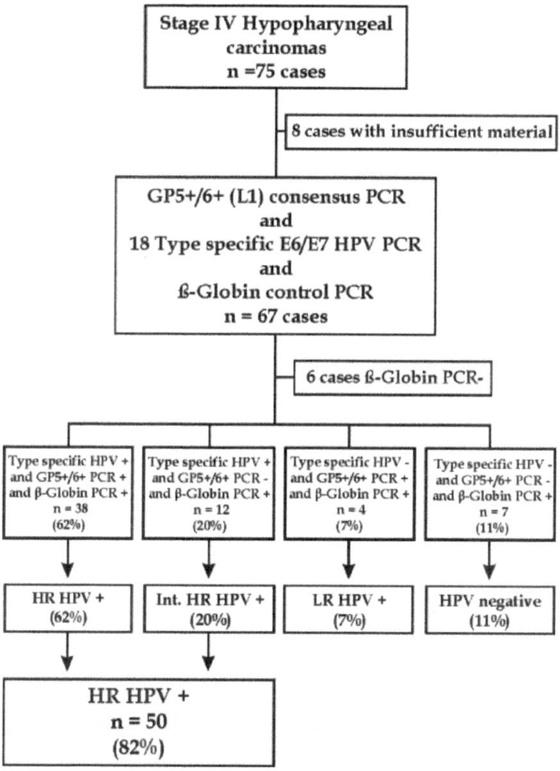

Fig. 2. HPV PCR results from 75 OSCC cases. Eight samples could not be analyzed due to insufficient material, and β-globin could not be amplified in six additional samples. Therefore, 61 cases in total were analyzed by type-specific real-time PCR and GP5+/GP6+ consensus PCR. Among these patients, 82% tested positive for infection with one or several types of hr HPV, 7% tested positive for lr HPV and 11% were HPV-negative.

From this homogeneous group of 61 HSCC tumor specimens, we identified 50 samples (82%) that tested positive for the following hr HPV types: HPV 16 (37 cases), 18 (4 cases), 33 (11 cases), 39 (1 case), 51 (5 cases), 53 (1 case), 58 (2 cases), 59 (1 case) and 66 (4 cases), four (7%) were positive for lr HPV types and seven (11%) were negative. Twelve samples were infected with multiple types of hr HPV. Among the 50 hr HPV-positive tumors, 38 were both GP5+/GP6+ positive and type-specific HPV-positive (hr HPV+ group). However, 12 tumors were GP5+/GP6+ negative and type-specific HPV-positive, corresponding to an integrated HPV+ group (int. hr HPV+) (Fig. 2).

This disagreement over HPV prevalence may be explained by the sensitivity of the methods used and the number of cases enrolled. Indeed, the use of different detection methods and HPV-specific probes, as well as varying numbers of tissue samples from different locations, has caused confusion over the frequency of HPV-positive lesions. Despite using the most sensitive method (PCR), we still observed a large variation in HPV detection rates, which can be explained by the relationship between results and sample sizes. In fact, the Kleist et al. study observed an 80% positivity among 5 samples, while Ribeiro et al. only detected HPV in 3.8% of cases among 78 tumors (Kleist et al., 2000; Ribeiro et al., 2011).

Concerning prognosis, statistical analysis did not reveal a significant correlation between hr HPV positivity and the proportion of disease-free patients. However, 32% (16/50 cases) of patients with hr HPV-positive tumors experienced relapse, compared with 8% of patients with HPV or lr HPV-positive tumors. The five-year disease-free survival was 88% in HPV negative and lr HPV-positive tumors *versus* 58% in hr HPV-positive tumors (Fig. 3).

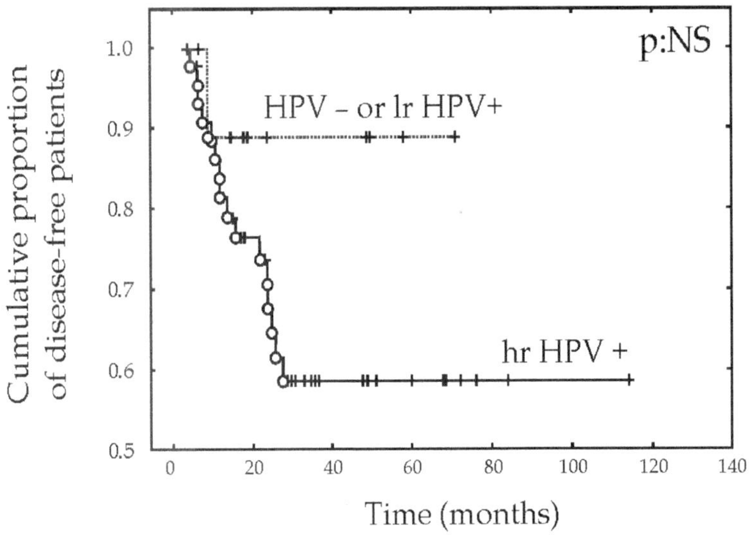

Fig. 3. Disease-free survival curves for high-risk HPV+ (hr HPV+) *versus* HPV negative and low-risk HPV+ (lr HPV+) patients. The *p*-value is not significant (NS)

As mentioned above, few publications have focused on HPV positivity in hypopharyngeal cancers. Evidently, our results are in accordance with a previous study by Morgan et al, who described for the first time that 75% of the 16 pharyngolaryngeal carcinomas in their series were HPV-positive (Morgan et al., 1991). Another study found a lower HPV positivity rate (46%) in tumors from 78 previously untreated patients with laryngeal and hypopharyngeal carcinomas (Clayman et al., 1994). The authors concluded that HPV-positive tumors represented a biologically distinct subset of tumors that had a worse prognosis than HPV negative tumors (Clayman et al., 1994). In contrast to our results, Paz et al. did not identify any HPV-positive tumors in a small series of seven hypopharyngeal carcinoma patients (Paz et al., 1997). Indeed, conclusions are difficult to draw, given the lack of interest in the prognostic outcomes of these cancers, but it would seem that HPV-associated hypopharyngeal carcinomas are characterized by a poorer prognosis, or a tendency towards having a poorer prognosis, than HPV-negative hypopharyngeal carcinomas (Clayman et al., 1994; Ernoux et al., 2011). Thus, HPV infection may be closely associated with the development of some hypopharyngeal carcinomas.

5.3.2 Incidence in laryngeal tumors

Laryngeal squamous cell carcinoma (LSCC) is the most frequent malignant tumor in the upper aerodigestive tract and is found predominantly in males. Although the relationship of HPV with SCC in the larynx is not well established, oncogenic HPVs have been proposed to be potential pathogenic factors. Studies focusing on HPV infections in LSCCs have reported wide variations in infection frequency that range from 0% to 85% (Almadori et al., 1996; Boscolo-Rizzo et al., 2009; Gallo et al., 2009; García-Milián et al., 1998; Koskinen et al., 2007; Lindeberg & Krogdahl, 1999; Rees et al., 2004). The prevalence varied widely with individual investigations. More than ten years ago, Brandwein et al. and Lie et al. reported that only 8% of LSCCs in the USA and Norway contained HPV DNA (Brandwein et al., 1993; Lie et al., 1996). Other authors also showed prevalence lower than 10%. In 1999, Lindeberg and Krogdahl demonstrated HPV infection in only one of 30 laryngeal carcinomas (Lindeberg & Krogdahl, 1999). More recently, in a cohort of 69 LSCC patients, 3 (4.4%) had HPV-positive samples, whereas other investigators did not find any HPV-positive samples among 68 LSCCs (Gallo et al., 2009; Koskinen et al., 2007). These findings support the view that the role of HPV in LSCC is less important in the larynx and also suggest the existence of other factors that play a more important role than viral infection in the carcinogenesis of these lesions. However, when we examine the few studies considering more than 80 patients with PCR-based analytical techniques, we observe higher percentages than previously demonstrated. Reports that include small sample sizes are subject to a potential selection bias. Indeed, the prevalence detected by Morshed et al. rose to 35.5%, but they did not find any significantly improved overall or disease-specific survival compared to patients with HPV-negative tumors (Morshed et al., 2008). In the same manner, high-risk HPV was found in 41 out of 110 LSCCs (37.3%) in a Brazilian study (de Oliveira et al., 2006). Larger samples being better, Syrjänen analyzed 116 LSCCs using *in situ* hybridization to demonstrate the presence of HPV DNA from types 6, 11, 16 and 30 in paraffin-embedded biopsies. A total of 15 of 116 (12.9%) tumors were shown to contain HPV DNA of at least one type (Syrjänen et al., 1987). This low prevalence can be explained by the use of a technique with lower sensitivity than PCR, which has the greatest sensitivity. Additionally, our study focused on HPV detection in a sample of 67 laryngeal SCCs revealed a 75% prevalence of high-risk HPV, as shown in Figure 4 (Duray et al., 2011a). To prevent false positives, precautions were taken to prevent tissue contamination. Our results may be explained by the fact that we used a sensitive (10-100 copies per PCR reaction) and type-specific real-time quantitative PCR analysis with a short amplification product (60-80 bp) that is more sensitive to the presence of degraded DNA, which is typically found in paraffin-embedded specimens.

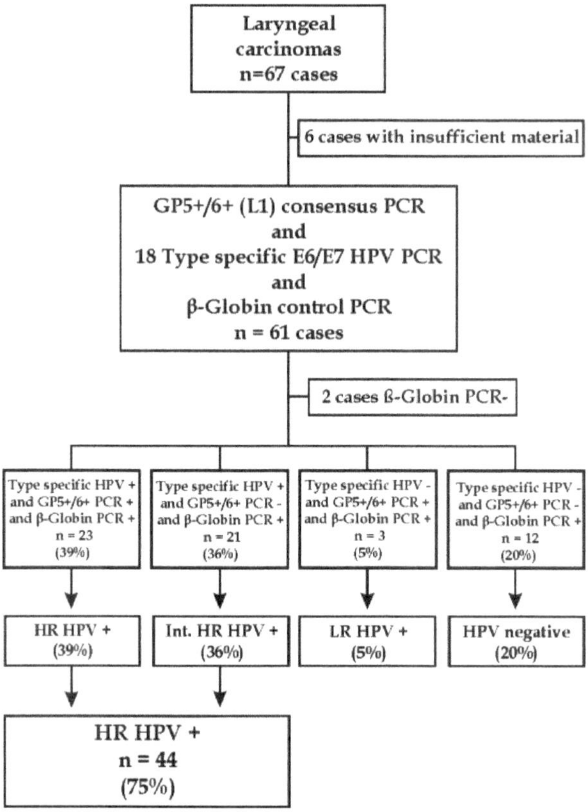

Fig. 4. HPV PCR results from 67 LSCC cases. Six samples could not be analyzed due to insufficient material, and β-globin could not be amplified in two additional samples. Therefore, 59 cases in total were analyzed by type-specific real-time PCR and GP5+/GP6+ consensus PCR. Among these patients, 75% tested positive for infection with one or several types of hr HPV, 5% tested positive for lr HPV and 20% were HPV-negative.

In this study, we also considered the prognostic value of the presence of hr HPV DNA in laryngeal carcinomas. We observed that positive hr HPV status did not correlate with the proportion of disease-free patients (Fig. 5). The five-year disease-free survival was 87% in HPV-negative or lr HPV-positive early-stage tumors *versus* 76% in hr HPV-positive early-stage tumors (Fig. 5A). The five-year disease-free survival was 60% in HPV-negative or lr HPV-positive late-stage tumors versus 58% in hr HPV-positive high-stage tumors (Fig. 5B). After grouping the early and late stages, the five-year disease-free survival was 77% in HPV-negative or lr HPV-positive laryngeal tumors versus 67% in hr HPV-positive laryngeal tumors (Fig. 5C). Similarly, Boscolo-Rizzo et al. found no significant differences in overall survival and disease-free survival between patients with HPV-positive tumors and patients with HPV-negative tumors (Boscolo-Rizzo et al., 2008). Although there is strong support in the literature for the association between HPV-positive tumors and better prognosis, especially in oropharyngeal carcinomas, other studies did not find an improved prognosis for HPV-associated tumors (Clayman et al., 1994; Dahlstrand et al., 2008; Ernoux et al., 2011).

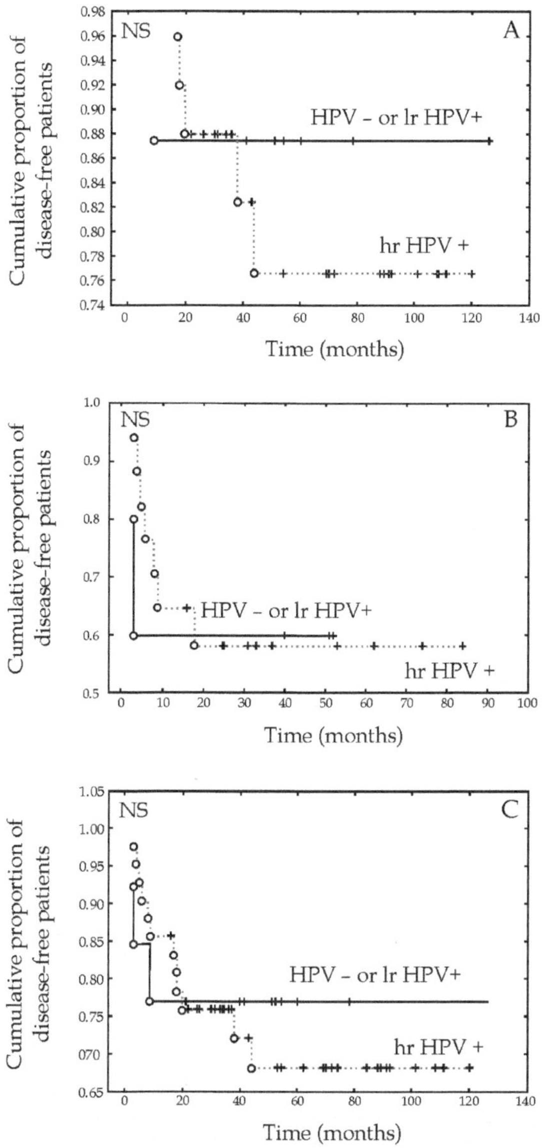

Fig. 5. Disease-free survival curves for high-risk HPV+ (hr HPV+) versus HPV- and low-risk HPV+ (lr HPV+) patients with low- (A) and high-stage (B) laryngeal carcinoma. (C) Disease-free survival curves for all stages together. The *p*-values were not significant (NS).

Although preliminary results may suggest biological oncogenic activity, the role of HPV infection in LSCCs has not been clearly established. Thus, in view of conflicting results, reports of the frequency of HPV infection in laryngeal carcinomas should be interpreted with caution, and despite low prevalence, there is no doubt that HPV is present in a subset of laryngeal carcinomas. Thus, we should not exclude the possibility of a causal relationship between HPV and some laryngeal tumors. Prospective studies with large numbers of patients and controls are required to confirm this hypothesis.

5.3.3 Incidence in oral tumors

Questions remain as to whether HPV is causally associated with cancer development at other sites in the upper aerodigestive tract. Its role continues to be a topic of debate, as a link with HNSCC was suggested more than 20 years ago (Syrjänen et al., 1983). Based on light microscopy examination, they observed koilocytosis, which is the presence of cytopathic HPV-induced alterations, in 35% of oral squamous cell carcinoma (OSCC) biopsies that were identical to those found in precancerous lesions and in uterine cervical carcinoma. Several meta-analyses have been dedicated to the relationship between HPV and OSCC (Kreimer et al., 2005; Miller & Johnstone, 2001; Syrjänen et al., 2011; Termine et al., 2008). The prevalence reported by these studies is quite different (23.5%, 33.7%, 38.1%, and 46.5%). This variability could be explained by different manner: Termine et al. included studies examining more than 40 specimens, and they calculated their prevalence exclusively on the basis of paraffin embedded (PE) specimens. On the other hand, Miller and Johnstone, similar to Kreimer et al., did not report HPV prevalence in PE and fresh frozen (FF) specimens separately. Miller and Johnstone were the first to publish a meta-analysis on HPV prevalence in normal and cancerous oral lesions. Pooled data from non-controlled studies published between 1982 and 1997 showed that HPV was 4.7 times more likely to be present in oral carcinomas when compared with normal mucosa (Miller & Johnstone, 2001). More recently, the interesting systematic review by Syrjänen et al. observed a pooled HPV detection rate of 33.7% in the OSCC group compared with 12% in the control group. The authors concluded that HPV infection significantly increases the risk for OSCC. It is important to note that the association of HPV with OSCC was significant only when HPV was detected in biopsy samples and that this significant association was completely lost when only exfoliated cells were used to analyze HPV in both cases and controls. Herrero et al. also showed that HPV DNA in exfoliated cells was not associated with HPV DNA detection in OSCC samples (Herrero et al., 2003). Thus, to obtain the most accurate results for the relationship between HPV and OSCC, future studies should only select biopsied tissues for HPV testing. In addition to the previously mentioned reviews, studies examining HPV infection in OSCC reported a wide range of detection rates from 0 to 61% (Herrero et al., 2003; Koskinen et al., 2003; Mishra et al., 2006; Ribeiro et al., 2011; Smith et al., 2004a). Varying sampling techniques together with widely divergent PCR methods across the studies explain most of this variability. Other criteria have also been considered: i) the specificity and size of PCR primers (e.g., GP5+/GP6+, MY09/11,...), ii) the geographical demographics, iii) the number of enrolled cases and iv) the prevalence of smoking and alcohol consumption in the studied population. A similar prevalence was detected by Zhao et al, who found 40.4% positivity (21 of 52 samples) with HPV 16 accounting for 63.5% and HPV 18 for 30.8%. Moreover, HPV had an independent prognostic effect on the overall survival of OSCC after adjusting for other factors, such as histological grade, TNM stage and tobacco use. Another characteristic was the significant correlation with improved survival in OSCC patients (Zhao et al., 2009). In 2001, Schwartz et al. also demonstrated that HPV16 presence was independently related to a favorable prognosis in a population of 254 OSCC patients (Schwartz et al., 2001). Gillison's well-controlled study found that oral cancers containing oncogenic HPV types had 74% less risk of disease-specific mortality (Gillison et al., 2000). On the other hand, many studies have also demonstrated that the prevalence of high-risk HPV types was low in OSCCs. Indeed, recently, only 2% of the PE tissues analyzed tested positive in Lopes study (Lopes et al., 2011). Almost the same observation was made by several studies using qPCR techniques (Boy et al., 2006; Ha et al., 2002; Koskinen et al., 2003). Furthermore, a meta-analysis suggested that the association between HPV and cancer was strongest for the tonsils, intermediate for the oropharynx and weakest for the mouth and larynx (Hobbs et al., 2006). In contrast, a Hungarian study demonstrated that 31 of 65 (48%) oral cancer cases had evidence of HPV using qPCR methods, reflecting the impact of geographical variation (Szarka et al., 2009). In fact, geographical origin is a well-known variability factor regarding HPV prevalence, with Asia having the highest worldwide frequency and Africa having the lowest (Termine et al., 2008). A hypothesis was suggested that OSCC HPV prevalence could be biased and overestimated because of a non-precise assignment of the anatomical site resulting in a "contamination" of the OSCC cohort with oropharyngeal cancers (Lopes et al., 2011). Once again, the detection methods remain the argument of choice to compare the different results obtained. In fact, two teams recently proposed two methods for HPV detection: *in situ* PCR and *in situ* PCR ISH. These methods combine the sensitivity of solution PCR with the subcellular localization provided by traditional ISH (Koyama et al., 2007; Uobe et al., 2001). Nevertheless, there are currently insufficient data in the literature to support the adequacy of these techniques. Finally, in our study, the prevalence of HPV infection reached 70%, with 44% being hr HPV-positive and 26% being lr HPV-positive (Fig. 6) (Duray & Descamps et al., in revision). The high incidence of HPV in our samples may also be explained by the fact that a very sensitive PCR (GP5+/GP6+ primers: 10–100 copies per reaction) was combined with a type-specific real-time quantitative PCR analysis and a short amplification product (60–80 bp). To a similar end, Termine et al. demonstrated that PCR-based studies resulted in higher prevalence rates compared with studies using *in situ* hybridization (Termine et al., 2008). Our results confirmed this finding because almost 65% of HPV+ specimens where also positive using ISH, whereas the ISH/PCR correspondence was excellent for the negative specimens.

Moreover, high-risk HPV positivity was associated with shorter disease-free survival in our cohort of 147 OSCC patients. The five-year disease-free survival was 76% for patients with HPV-negative tumors versus 40% for patients with HPV-positive tumors (p=0.007) (Fig. 7A). Furthermore, the five-year disease-free survival was 48% for patients with lr HPV-positive tumors versus 37% for patients with hr HPV-positive tumors (p=0.015) (Fig. 7B). These data suggest that HPV infection was significantly associated with a worse prognosis. Moreover, Cox multivariate analyses combining the HPV status with clinical variables (TNM staging and node status) demonstrated that only HPV status had an independent impact on patient prognosis (p=0.01; hazard ratio=2.81). An analysis of viral loads in infected patients did not show any statistically significant relationship between TNM staging and risk of recurrence.

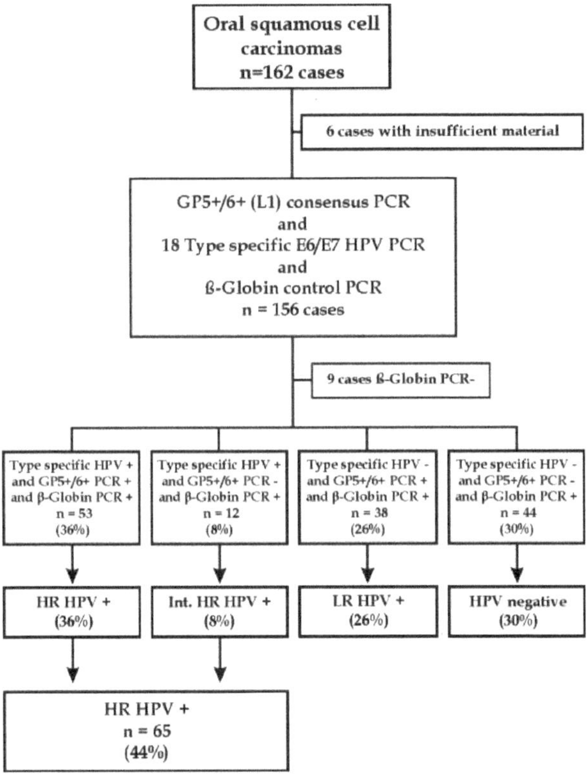

Fig. 6. HPV PCR results from 162 OSCC cases. Six samples could not be analyzed due to insufficient material, and β-globin could not be amplified in nine additional samples. Therefore, 147 cases in total were analyzed by type-specific real-time PCR and GP5+/GP6+ consensus PCR. Among these patients, 44% tested positive for infection with one or several types of hr HPV, 26% tested positive for lr HPV and 30% were HPV-negative.

Although a majority of studies demonstrated an improved outcome for OSCC patients, the meta-analysis by Ragin and Taioli examining the relationship between HPV and overall survival did not show any survival differences between HPV-positive and HPV-negative patients with cancers at non-oropharyngeal sites (Ragin & Taioli, 2007). The same observation was made by Gillison et al., suggesting that these tumors may have an etiology distinct from that of tumors at non-oropharyngeal sites (Gillison et al., 2008). The poor prognosis reported in the hr HPV-positive population in this study has been demonstrated in other studies. Indeed, two Swedish studies demonstrated that oral HPV infection was associated with a dramatically increased risk of developing OSCC (Hansson et al., 2005; Rosenquist et al., 2007). Additionally, in 1994, Clayman et al. also showed that HPV detection was significantly correlated with decreased survival (Clayman et al., 1994). Other studies have failed to demonstrate an association between HPV positivity and prognosis (Ernoux et al., 2011; Morshed, 2010). We hypothesize that immunosuppression may favor HPV infection (Duray et al., 2010). In 2004, Kreimer reported that tonsillar HPV infection was strongly associated with HIV co-infection and immunosuppression (Kreimer et al.,

2004). Recently, herpes simplex virus-2 (HSV2) infection was demonstrated to increase the risk of HPV infection (Moscicki et al., 2001). Furthermore, a study performed by Tung et al. reported the presence of HPV 16 or 18 and Epstein Barr virus (EBV) in 80% of nasopharyngeal carcinoma samples (Tung et al., 1999). These co-infections may play an important role in the initiation of neoplastic transformation in human oral epithelial cells. In conclusion, the effect of HPV on oral cancer remains contentious. Thus, to formally confirm the role of HPV as an etiological agent in OSCC, sample processing and PCR analysis protocols should be standardized to allow a more precise comparison of the results. Furthermore, future studies should report separately the type-specific prevalence rates. This information would be very useful in order to evaluate the long-term effects of the recent HPV vaccines.

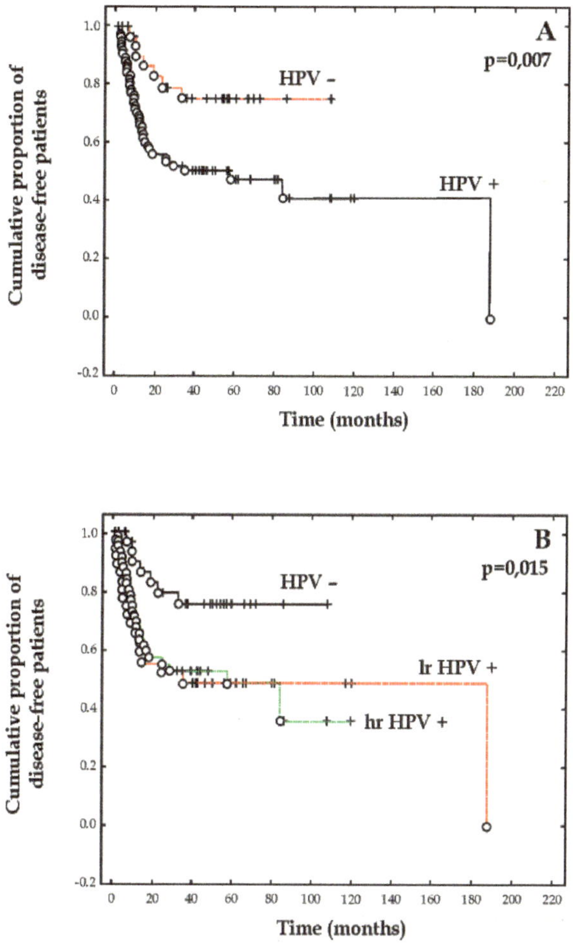

Fig. 7. The HPV+ subgroup (and specifically the hr HPV + subgroup) is associated with a worse prognosis ($p = 0.007$ and $p = 0.015$). Standard survival time analyses were performed using Kaplan-Meier curves, the Gehan-Wilcoxon text and the Log-rank test.

5.3.4 Incidence in oropharyngeal tumors

During the past several years, an increased incidence of oropharyngeal squamous cell carcinoma (OSCC), the head and neck cancer in which HPV is commonly found, was observed. In 2007, Sturgis and Cinciripini proposed a possible emerging epidemic of HPV-associated cancers (Sturgis & Cinciripini, 2007). Indeed, accumulating molecular and epidemiological data now show that hr HPV types are responsible for a subset of OSCCs (D'Souza et al., 2007; Lindquist et al., 2007). Therefore, the International Agency for Research on Cancer (IARC) recognized HPV as a risk factor for oropharyngeal cancer. In the United States, the prevalence of HPV in OSCC has evolved over the last 30 years. Based on data from Colorado, the percentage rose from 33% during the 1980s to 70% in the 1990s and 82% during 2000 to 2004 (Ernster et al., 2007). During the 2000s, different prevalence rates were reported, ranging from 63% to 92% among oropharynx, tongue and tonsil cases (Brown et al., 2011). Tonsillar cancer is the most common oropharyngeal cancer, followed by cancer of the base of the tongue, and these two cancers accounts for 90% of all OSCCs (Dahlstrand & Dalianis, 2005). In Stockholm, as in the USA, HPV prevalence among tonsil cases increased over the years from 23% in 1970 up to 83% in 2003 to 2007 (Nasman et al., 2009). In contrast, in Beijing, the prevalence of tonsillar cancers is particularly low, with rates of 0.1% in men and 0.0 in women. Interestingly, in places with a marked Western influence, such as Hong-Kong and Taiwan, rates of tonsillar cancer were 6 to 12 times higher than in Beijing (Marklund & Hammarstedt, 2011). Large variations in incidence rates are also observed. In Europe, the highest rates were seen in France, particularly in Somme region, where the rates were as high as 6.4% for men (Parkin et al., 2002). Similar to HNSCC, the prognosis for OSCC is generally low in the more advanced stages with an overall five-year survival rate of approximately 25% (Licitra et al., 2002). Nevertheless, in HPV infected OSCC, a major feature noted in almost all studies is that HPV is a favorable prognostic factor for clinical outcome independently of tumor stage, age, gender and grade of differentiation. In fact, patients with HPV DNA-positive tumors appear to have a significant prognostic advantage compared with patients having HPV-negative tumors (Ang et al., 2010). However, previous studies have suggested that the presence of HPV DNA in tumor tissue was not a sufficient factor to indicate an involvement of the viral genes in tonsillar carcinomas. Good indicators reflecting an active involvement of HPV are the levels of viral E6-E7 mRNA (Cuschieri et al., 2008). Thus, E6 and E7 expression are regularly assessed with success, suggesting an active involvement of HPV in the etiology of tumors (Lindquist et al., 2007). Recently, an interesting study provided strong evidence that HPV status was an independent prognostic factor for overall survival among patients with OSCC, which may confirm that HPV-positive and HPV-negative OSCC constitute two distinct clinical entities with different causes, risk factor profiles and survival outcomes. To validate this hypothesis, future clinical trials should be designed specifically for patients with HPV-positive or HPV-negative OSCC (Ang et al., 2010). Concerning this improved survival, Lindquist et al. observed a difference between HPV patients who smoked and did not smoke. In fact, patients with HPV-positive tonsillar cancer who had never smoked had a better prognosis than those who were smokers, which is in accordance with the studies of Ang and Rotnaglova (Ang et al., 2010; Lindquist et al., 2007; Rotnaglova et al., 2010). These observations may be explained by an immune response induced by HPV but abrogated by smoking. A different option, also suggested by Ang et al, is that smoking and HPV are associated with different categories of tumors and that smoking induces additional genetic alterations in these tumors (Ramqvist & Dalianis, 2010, Ang et al., 2010). Some investigators have suggested that the better clinical outcome can be attributed either to higher radiosensitivity of HPV-positive tumors or to active antiviral cellular immune responses in infected patients (Dahlstrand & Dalianis, 2005). Treatment of patients with advanced disease often includes both oncological and surgical treatment, as both carry acute side effects, such as difficulties in swallowing or talking, dry mouth and jawbone necrosis. Oncological treatment has fortunately evolved towards the development of altered fractionation radiotherapy, integration of chemotherapy with radiotherapy and the introduction of targeted biological therapy. The combined modality treatment and the intensified fractionation have improved the outcome for head and neck cancer patients in general (Bourhis et al., 2006; Pignon et al., 2009). As a result of this intensified therapy, patients have substantial chronic side effects. It is therefore important to differentiate patients who do and do not need intensified treatment to increase patient survival times and quality of life. The improved response to oncological treatment for OSCC HPV-positive patients may also be explained by the presence of an intact p53-mediated apoptotic response in HPV-positive tumors and by immunological factors related to HPV infection (Spanos et al., 2009). In conclusion, HPV-positive OSCC is recognized as a distinct subset of head and neck squamous cell carcinomas having a favorable outcome. Patients with HPV-positive tonsillar carcinomas may also benefit from a less aggressive treatment, but this conclusion will need to be validated by further studies in order not to compromise existing, excellent treatment outcomes in patients with HPV-dependent tumors.

6. Impact of HPV on the immune system of head and neck cancers

6.1 The escape of HPV in the immune system

The contradiction between the studies examining the correlation between HPV infection and prognosis may result from differences in immune status among HNSCC patients. In fact, a persistent HPV infection that can lead to the development of cancer requires immune tolerance. Therefore, HPV has developed several mechanisms to avoid detection by the host immune defense system. In the case of infection by a virus, it is important to distinguish between the mechanisms used by tumor cells to evade immune attack and those used by HPV. The infectious cycle of HPV is itself an immune evasion mechanism because viral gene expression and viral protein synthesis are confined to keratinocytes, which are programmed to die; thus, HPV replication does not cause cell death and does not present a danger signal to the immune system (Stanley, 2006, 2009). Without cell lysis, there is little or no release of the proinflammatory cytokines important for the activation and migration of dendritic cells (Stanley, 2006, 2009). Even if there is no cell death, keratinocytes should be activated to induce type I interferon responses, which have anti-viral, anti-proliferative, anti-angiogenic and immune-stimulatory properties. Several data suggest that E6 and E7 oncogenes have evolved mechanisms to interact with components of the interferon pathway and to downregulate the effects of type I IFN (Stanley, 2009). For instance, the virus maintains a low level of viremia, there is no blood-borne phase and only minimal amounts of replicating virus are exposed to the immune system. As a result of these facts, the virus is practically invisible to the host (Kanodia et al., 2007; Stanley, 2009). HPV is able to dysregulate the antigen processing machinery (APM) by downregulating peptide-MHC complexes, which are essential for recognition of infected cells by T cells. In particular, the E7 oncoprotein of HPV-16 and -18 repress the promoter for MHC class I heavy chain expression, and HPV-18 E7 is also able to repress the promoter that regulates expression of TAP1 (transporter associated with antigen protein 1) and LMP2 genes (Georgopoulos et al., 2000). HPV-16 E5 induces alkalinization of the Golgi complex, leading to disruption of trafficking, including transport of the MHC class I complex (Ashrafi et al., 2005). In HPV-positive benign laryngeal lesions, there is a decrease of MHC class I and TAP-1 expression, and the low expression of TAP-1 was associated with rapid recurrence of the disease (Bonagura et al., 1994; Vambutas et al., 2000). Another way in which HPV may suppress immune responses is via the modulation of chemokine (suppression of MCP-1 expression, downregulation of IL-8 expression) and pro-inflammatory cytokine (downregulation of IL-18 expression) expression and via skewing the cytokine profile in favor of a Th2 response (IL-4, -5, -6, -10, -13) instead of a Th1 cytokine expression (IL-2, IFN-γ) (Kanodia et al., 2007). Moreover, the E6 and E7 oncoproteins downregulate toll-like receptor 9 (TLR9), which induces proinflammatory genes essential for induction of immune responses (Hasan et al., 2007). The failure of the immune system to recognize HPV may also be explained by the fact that HPV16 E7 protein has widespread similarity to several human proteins, such as xeroderma pigmentosum group G complementing protein (XPGC) and the retinoblastoma binding protein 1 (RBP-1); thus, the immune system does not recognize them as foreign molecules but as self molecules (O'Donovan et al., 1993; Scherly et al., 1993).

6.2 Defects in the immune system of HNSCC patients

Patients suffering from head and neck cancers exhibit deficits in the humoral and cellular immune systems, which have been shown to be correlated with a worse prognosis. The strategies employed by head and neck cancers to escape the immune system are varied: they can directly inhibit the immune response by producing soluble mediators or they can target the APM via downregulation of HLA class I and/or other components of the APM (Duray et al., 2010). In the first steps of carcinogenesis, there is an increase of Langerhans cells, whereas in invasive carcinomas, a decrease was observed (Fig.8). The accumulation of macrophages in the peritumoral area seems to play a protumoral role by secreting VEGF and stimulating angiogenesis (Duray et al., 2010) (Fig.8). Antitumor responses of HNSCC patients are compromised in the presence of functional defects or apoptosis of T-cells, both circulating and tumor-infiltrating. Functional assays with tumor-infiltrating lymphocytes TILs isolated from the tumor bed have identified a number of defects, such as (i) absent or low expression of the CD3 zeta chain (CD3ζ), which is the key signaling molecule in the T-cell receptor pathway (Whiteside, 2005), (ii) decreased proliferation in response to mitogens or IL-2 (Whiteside, 2005), (iii) the inability to kill tumor cell targets (Hathaway et al., 2005; Hoffmann et al., 2004), (iv) an imbalance in the cytokine profile, with a striking absence of IL-2 and/or IFN-γ production (Reichert et al., 1998a), and (v) evidence of pronounced apoptotic features in a considerable proportion of TILs (Whiteside, 2005; Young et al., 1996). Several studies demonstrated the involvement of the Fas/FasL signaling pathway, the mitochondrial pathway, TRAIL, and TNF-α in the apoptosis of T cells in HNSCC patients (Duray et al., 2010). Furthermore, changes in the expression of the ζ chain of TILs are biologically significant because the absence or low expression of this chain in TILs in patients with stage III or IV HNSCC predicts a poor survival compared with patients expressing a normal ζ chain (Reichert et al., 1998b; Whiteside, 1999). Another study showed that patients with more aggressive tumors or with a recurrence within the preceding two years expressed the lowest levels of the ζ chain (Kuss et al., 1999). Various studies showed an increased abundance of T regulatory cells Tregs in TILs and peripheral blood, and their immunosuppressive action could be another mechanism employed by the tumor cells to escape antitumor immunity. Lau et al. demonstrated an increase of Tregs in patients with nasopharyngeal carcinoma, and their suppression of the proliferation of CD4-positive/CD25-negative T cells could explain the decreased antitumor immunity of T cells (Lau et al., 2007) (Fig.8).

6.3 Effects of HPV on the immune system of patients with benign or malignant lesions of the upper aerodisgestive area

Considering the high HPV prevalence in the population, it remains unclear why a very small fraction of HPV-exposed individuals develop RRP. To better understand this result, Bonagura and colleagues studied the differences between RRP patients infected with HPV-6 or -11 and healthy individuals who were also infected with HPV but never developed RRP. They provided evidence that there are several immune alterations in patients with RRP, such as (i) an adaptative immune response induces a Th2-like/T-regulatory phenotype. In fact, patients with RRP displayed elevated levels of Th2-like chemokines (CCL17, CCL18, CCL22) and cytokines (IL-4, IL-10), whereas levels of TH1-like chemokines (CCL19, CCL21) and cytokines (IL-12, IL-18, IFN-γ) were downregulated. In papillomas, there is an enrichment of Tregs, which suppress Th1-like responses to HPV. (ii) Interestingly, the expression of IL-4 by CD4-positive T cells was increased in papillomas, whereas the expression of IFN-γ was reduced. An expression of IL-10 by CD4-positive T cells was also observed in the blood (PBMCs) of patients with RRP. These findings suggest that CD4-positive T cells express TH2-like cytokines and reduce Th1-like T-cell function. (iii) A decrease of CD4-positive and CD8-positive T cell Vβ repertoires. Moreover, they showed that HPV-11 E6 can suppress T-cell alloreactivity and that natural killer cells are dysfunctional in RRP. Furthermore, they also proposed an inhibitory cycle of immunocytes that support the development of RRP. In response to HPV proteins, memory Th2-like T cells express IL-4 and IL-10, and T-regulatory cells express IL-10 and TGF-β, inducing resting macrophages to become alternatively activated macrophages. These macrophages express TH2-like chemokines (CCL17, CCL18) and cytokine (IL-10) that induce naïve CD4-positive T cells to become Tregs and memory TH2-like T cells. Together, these cells form a cycle of inhibitory immunocytes that block the function of the effector helper type I CD4-positive T-cells (TH1-like). As a result, HPV infection is not cleared, and papillomas will recur (Bonagura et al., 2010). A correlation between the severity of laryngeal papillomas and an increase of CD83-positive dendritic cells exists, and this enhancement may be due to an impaired migration of matured DC (Kovalenko et al., 2009). These observations suggest that patients with RRP have a perturbation in their cellular immune response (or have a defect in their cellular immunity) and are, therefore, unable to eliminate their disease with an effective HPV-specific T-cell response. This immune imbalance may influence the development and severity of respiratory papillomatosis (Bonagura et al., 1999).

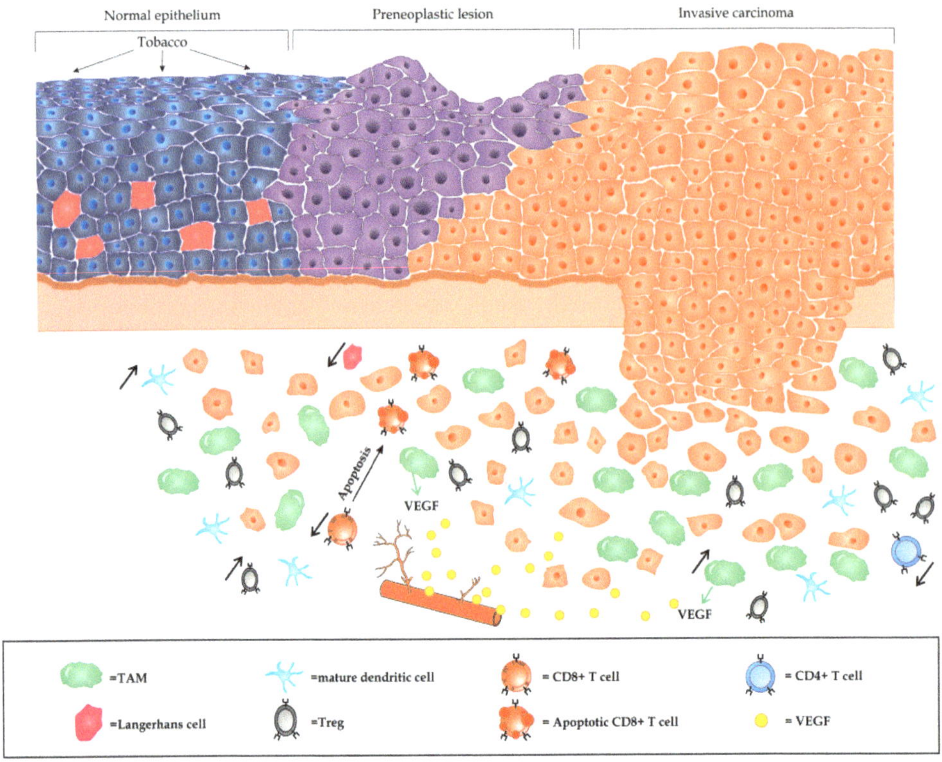

Fig. 8. Description of immunosuppressive mechanisms during the head and neck tumor progression: in the normal epithelia of the upper aerodigestive tracts, LCs are present in the suprabasal layers. When mucosae of these areas are exposed to tobacco, the number of LCs increases whereas these cells decrease in invasive carcinomas. The mature DCs are prominent in the peritumoral area and correlated positively with the expression of VEGF. DCs are also more abundant in patients with metastasis. A higher level of TAM is observed in HNSCCs and these cells constitute a source of VEGF which play a crucial role in angiogenesis. HNSCCs can induce the apoptosis of CD8+ T cells using the mitochondrial and/or Fas/FasL pathways. Tregs can induce apoptosis of CD8+ T cells and inhibition of the proliferation of CD4+ T cells.

There are few data on the interaction between the host immune system and HPV infection in HNSCCs, meaning that the role of innate and adaptative immunity in the development and progression of HPV-positive HNSCCs is largely unknown. As mentioned previously, in several studies, HPV positive HNSCC cancer was associated with a favorable outcome. From these results, some authors supported the hypothesis that the immune response may play a positive role in HPV-positive HNSCC prognosis, but in those cases, an intact immune system is necessary. An increased frequency of T cells specific for peptides derived from the oncogenic HPV E7 protein was observed in HNSCC patients positive for HPV16 compared with HNSCC patients negative for HPV or with healthy volunteers (Albers et al., 2005; Hoffmann et al., 2006). Therefore, antiviral immunity exists against E7 oncogenic protein, but these T cells are unable to eliminate the tumor (Hoffmann et al., 2006), perhaps due to immune escape of tumor cells from cytotoxic T cells (CTL) recognition (Albers et al., 2005). In fact, using immunohistochemistry, a reduced expression of APM components and HLA class I antigens was observed in HPV16-positive HNSCCs compared with adjacent normal squamous epithelium, which is consistent with the suggestion of a phenomenon of immune escape during viral carcinogenesis (Albers et al., 2005). Thus, further studies are necessary to explain this type of tumor resistance. Williams et al. investigated whether HPV-specific immune mechanisms can result in tumor clearance. For that, they generated HPV-positive and HPV-negative tonsil cell lines by transducing primary mouse tonsil epithelial cells, which are able to form squamous cell cancers in mice. When they examined immune-competent and immune-incompetent mice with or without HPV, they observed a difference in growth and survival patterns. In fact, in the immune-competent mouse group, about one-third of the HPV-positive mice cleared their tumors, compared with none of the HPV-negative mice. Moreover, by comparing the survival of the mice that did not clear their tumors, they observed that mice injected with HPV-positive cells had a significantly better survival than mice injected with HPV-negative cells. In the mouse group lacking B- and T-cell immunity, there was no difference in the tumor growth pattern or survival between the HPV-positive and HPV-negative groups. Therefore, the difference in growth between HPV-positive and HPV-negative mice is immune mediated. The data indicated that CD4-positive and CD8-positive T cells were required to mount this immune response. They also showed that the immune clearance capacity could be transferred from a cleared mouse into an immunodeficient mouse. In fact, the splenocytes from cleared mice and HPV-positive tumor cells were injected into an immunodeficient mouse, and they observed that all treated mice developed and cleared tumors (Williams et al., 2009). In another animal model of HPV-associated cancer, the authors tried to better understand why HPV-positive cancer may represent an advantage in survival, as has been shown in several studies, and they compared how these cancers responded to therapies usually used for the treatment of HNSCC with responses of HPV-negative tumors. Thus, they looked at the effect of radiation and cisplatin co-therapy on HPV-positive and HPV-negative cancer cells *in vivo* and in immunocompetent and immunodeficient mouse models. *In vitro*, HPV-positive cells were more resistant to radiation and cisplatin therapy compared with HPV-negative cells, whereas *in vivo*, HPV-positive tumors were more sensitive to radiotherapy compared with HPV-negative tumors. Furthermore, cisplatin was able to clear HPV-positive tumors, but not HPV- tumors, in mice. In immunodeficient mice, neither radiation nor cisplatin was able to cure their tumors. They also showed that, after an adoptive transfer of wild-type immune cells into immunodeficient mice, the clearance of HPV-positive tumors was restored upon cisplatin therapy. These findings suggested that an intact immune system was essential for tumor clearance with radiation and cisplatin therapy. Moreover, the findings indicate that survival does not seem to be due to increased epithelial sensitivity to these therapies and that radiation and cisplatin induce an immune response to this antigenic cancer (Spanos et al., 2009). More recently, Wansom and collaborators tried to understand better the clinical importance of adaptive immunity in patients with HPV16-positive oropharyngeal cancer and to examine whether it affects patient outcome. They showed that the percentage of CD8 cells was significantly higher and the CD4:CD8 ratio was significantly lower in HPV16-positive oropharyngeal patients. In comparing smokers and nonsmokers, the percentage of

CD8 cells was similar in the two groups, suggesting that the difference in CD8 levels was associated with HPV status and not with tobacco consumption. This elevated percentage of CD8 cells was associated with a response to induction chemotherapy and complete tumor response after chemoradiotherapy. These results (high percentage of CD8 cells and low CD4:CD8 ratio) were also associated with an improved overall survival. The mechanism by which there is an increase of T cells in the peripheral blood of HPV-positive patients has not been elucidated. One hypothesis suggested by the authors is that HPV-16-positive tumors have increased antigenicity through the E7 antigen, causing enhanced stimulation of the immune system, which more readily identifies tumor cells as foreign. This hypothesis is supported by a study led by Smith et al., in which the intralymphatic immunization of mice bearing E7-expressing tumors with E7 peptide resulted in a considerable expansion of E7-specific CD8 cells, which are effective in suppressing disease progression (Smith et al., 2009). In another animal model, the DNA vaccine with HSP70 fused to HPV-16 E7 has been demonstrated to dramatically increase the frequency of E7-specific CD8-positive T cells and to enhance the antitumor effects against E7-expressing tumor cells (Chen et al., 2000). All of these data support the idea that the clearance of HPV-positive tumor cells is antigen-dependent. Thus, the authors concluded that circulating CD8 cell levels may be a prognostic factor, and improved adaptive immunity may play a favorable role in the prognosis of patients with HPV16-positive tumors (Wansom et al., 2010).

7. Acknowledgement

Students supported by a grant from the FNRS (Bourse Télévie)

GD and AD contributed equally.

8. References

Adelstein, DJ., Li, Y., Adams, GL., Wagner, H Jr., Kish, JA., Ensley, JF., Schuller, DE. & Forastiere, AA. (2003). An intergroup phase III comparison of standard radiation therapy and two schedules of concurrent chemoradiotherapy in patients with unresectable squamous cell head and neck cancer. *Journal of Clinical Oncology,* Vol.21, No.1, (January 2003), pp. 92-98

Albers, A., Abe, K., Hunt, J., Wang, J., Lopez-Albaitero, A., Schaefer, C., Gooding, W., Whiteside, TL., Ferrone, S., DeLeo, A. & Ferris, RL. (2005). Antitumor activity of human papillomavirus type 16 E7-specific T cells against virally infected squamous cell carcinoma of the head and neck. *Cancer Research,* Vol.65, No.23, (December 2005), pp. 11146-11155

Almadori, G., Cadon,i G., Cattani, P., Posteraro, P., Scarano, E., Ottaviani, F., Paludetti, G. & Maurizi, M. (1996). Detection of human papillomavirus DNA in laryngeal squamous cell carcinoma by polymerase chain reaction. *European Journal of Cancer,* Vol.32A, No.5, (May, 1996), pp. 783-788

Al-Sarraf, M., LeBlanc, M., Giri, PG., Fu, KK., Cooper, J., Vuong, T., Forastiere, AA., Adams, G., Sakr, WA., Schuller, DE. & Ensley, JF. (1998). Chemoradiotherapy versus radiotherapy in patients with advanced nasopharyngeal cancer: phase III randomized Intergroup study 0099. *Journal of Clinical Oncology,* Vol.16, No.4, (April 1998), pp. 1310-1317

Ang, KK., Harris J., Wheeler, R., Weber, R., Rosenthal, DI., Nguyen-Tân, PF., Westra, WH., Chung, CH., Jordan, RC., Lu, C., Kim, H., Axelrod, R., Silverman, CC., Redmond, KP. & Gillison, ML. (2010). Human papillomavirus and survival of patients with oropharyngeal cancer. *The New England Journal of Medicine,* Vol.363, No.1, (July 2010), pp. 24-35

Arndt, O., Zeise, K., Bauer, I. & Brock, J. (1992). Type 6/11 and 16/18 squamous epithelial cancers of the upper respiratory tract and digestive system. An in situ hybridization study. *Laryngo-Rhino-Otologie,* Vol.71, No.10, (October 1992), pp. 500-504

Arndt, O., Johannes, A., Zeise, K. & Brock, J. (1997). High-risk HPV types in oral and laryngeal papilloma and leukoplakia. *Laryngo-Rhino-Otologie,* Vol.76, No.3, (March 1997), pp. 142-149

Ashrafi, GH., Haghshenas, MR., Marchetti, B., O'Brien, PM. & Campo, MS. (2005). E5 protein of human papillomavirus type 16 selectively downregulates surface HLA class I. *International Journal of Cancer,* Vol.113, No.2, (January 2005), pp. 276-283

Aubin, F., Pretet, JL., Mougin, C. & Riethmuller, D. (2007). Human papillomavirus infection. *Annales de Dermatologie et de Vénéréologie,* Vol.134, No.1, (January 2007), pp. 94-99

Badaracco, G., Venuti, A., Di Lonardo, A., Scambia, G., Mozzetti, S., Benedetti Panici, P., Mancuso, S. & Marcante, ML. (1998). Concurrent HPV infection in oral and genital mucosa. *Journal of Oral Pathology & Medicine,* Vol.27, No.3, (March 1998), pp. 130-134

Bernier, J., Domenge, C., Ozsahin, M., Matuszewska, K., Lefèbvre, JL., Greiner, RH., Giralt, J., Maingon, P., Rolland, F., Bolla, M., Cognetti, F., Bourhis, J., Kirkpatrick, A. & van Glabbeke, M. (2004). Postoperative irradiation with or without concomitant chemotherapy for locally advanced head and neck cancer. *The New England Journal of Medicine,* Vol.350, No.19, (May 2004), pp. 1945-1952

Bodaghi, S., Wood, LV., Roby, G., Ryder, C., Steinberg, SM. & Zheng, ZM. (2005). Could human papillomaviruses be spread through blood? *Journal of Clinical Microbiology,* Vol.43, No.11, (November 2005), pp. 5428-5434

Bonagura, VR., Siegal, FP., Abramson, AL., Santiago-Schwarz, F., O'Reilly, ME., Shah, K., Drake, D. & Steinberg, BM. (1994). Enriched HLA-DQ3 phenotype and decreased class I major histocompatibility complex antigen expression in recurrent respiratory papillomatosis. *Clinical and Diagnostic Laboratory Immunology,* Vol.1, No.3, (May 1994), pp. 357-360

Bonagura, VR., Hatam, L., DeVoti, J., Zeng, F. & Steinberg, BM. (1999). Recurrent respiratory papillomatosis :altered $CD8^+$ T-cell subsets and T_H1/T_H2 cytokine imbalance. *Clinical Immunology,* Vol.93, No.3, (December 1999), pp. 302-311

Bonagura, VR., Hatam, LJ., Rosenthal, DW., DeVoti, JA., Lam, F., Steinberg, BM. & Abramson, AL. (2010). Recurrent respiratory papillomatosis : a complex defect in immune responsiveness to human papillomavirus-6 and -11. *Acta Pathologica, Microbiologica et Immunologica Scandinavica,* Vol.118, No.6-7, (June 2010), pp. 455-470

Boscolo-Rizzo, P., Da Mosto, MC., Fuson, R., Frayle-Salamanca, H., Trevisan, R. & Del Mistro, A. (2008). HPV-16 E6 L83V variant in squamous cell carcinomas of the upper aerodigestive tract. *Journal of Cancer Research and Clinical Oncology,* Vol.135, No.4, (April 2009), pp. 559-566

Bourhis, J., Overgaard, J., Audry, H., Ang, KK., Saunders, M., Bernier, J., Horiot, JC., Le Maître, A., Pajak, TF., Poulsen, MG., O'Sullivan, B., Dobrowsky, W., Hliniak, A.,

Skladowski, K., Hay, JH., Pinto, LH., Fallai, C., Fu, KK., Sylvester, R. & Pignon, JP. (2006). Hyperfractionated or accelerated radiotherapy in head and neck cancer: a meta-analysis. *The Lancet*, Vol.368, No.9538, (September 2006), pp. 843-854

Boy, S., Van Rensburg, EJ., Engelbrecht, S., Dreyer, L., van Heerden, M. & van Heerden, W. (2006). HPV detection in primary intra-oral squamous cell carcinomas--commensal, aetiological agent or contamination? *Journal of Oral Pathology & Medicine*, Vol.35, No.2, (February 2006), pp. 86-90

Brandsma, JL. & Abramson, AL. (1989). Association of papillomavirus with cancers of the head and neck. *Archives of Otolaryngology-Head & Neck Surgery*, Vol.115, No.5, (May 1989), pp. 621-625

Brandwein, MS., Nuovo, GJ. & Biller, H. (1993). Analysis of prevalence of human papillomavirus in laryngeal carcinomas. Study of 40 cases using polymerase chain reaction and consensus primers. *Annals of Otology, Rhinology and Laryngology*, Vol.102, No.4 Pt 1, (April 1993), pp. 309-313

Brown, LM., Check, DP. & Devesa, SS. (2011). Oropharyngeal cancer incidence trends: diminishing racial disparities. *Cancer Causes & Control*, Vol.22, No.5, (May 2011), pp. 753-763

Campos-Bañales, ME., Pérez-Piñero, B., Barrios del Pino, Y., Salido Ruiz, E., Rivero Suárez, J., Ruiz Casals, E. & López Aguado, D. (1995). DNA papillomavirus detection in head and neck benign proliferative lesions. *Anales otorrinolaringológicos ibero-americanos*, Vol.22, No.5, (1995), 487-494

Cañadas, MP., Bosch, FX., Junquera, ML., Ejarque, M., Font, R., Ordoñez, E. & De Sanjosé, S. (2004). Concordance of prevalence of human papillomavirus DNA in anogenital and oral infections in a high-risk population. *Journal of Clinical Microbiology*, Vol.42, No.3, (March 2004), pp. 1330-1332

Cason, J., Kaye, JN., Jewers, RJ., Kambo, PK., Bible, JM., Kell, B., Shergill, B., Pakarian, F., Raju, KS. & Best, JM. (1995). Perinatal infection and persistence of human papillomavirus types 16 and 18 in infants. *Journal of Medical Virology*, Vol.47, No.3, (November 1995), pp. 209-218

Cason, J. & Mant, CA. (2005). High-risk mucosal human papillomavirus infections during infancy & chilhood. *Journal of Clinical Virology*, Vol.32, Suppl.1, (March 2005), pp. S52-S58

Castellsagué, X., Drudis, T., Cañadas, MP., Goncé, A., Ros, R., Pérez, JM., Quintana, MJ., Muñoz, J., Albero, G., de Sanjosé, S. & Bosch, FX. (2009). Human papillomavirus (HPV) infection in pregnant women and mother-to-child transmission of genital HPV genotypes : a prospective study in Spain. *BMC Infectious Diseases*, Vol.9, No.74, (May 2009), pp. 1-12

Castro, TP. & Bussoloti, Filho I. (2005). Prevalence of human papillomavirus (HPV) in oral cavity and oropharynx. *Brazilian Journal of Otorhinolaryngology*, Vol.72, No.2, (March-April 2006), pp. 272-282

Castro, TM., Bussoloti Filho, I., Nascimento, VX. & Xavier, SD. (2009). HPV detection in the oral and genital mucosa of women with positive histopathological exam for genital HPV, by means of the PCR. *Brazilian Journal of Otorhinolaryngology*, Vol.75, No.2, (March-April 2009), pp. 167-171

Chang, F., Syrjänen, S., Kellokoski, J. & Syrjänen, K. (1991). Human papillomavirus (HPV) infections and their associations with oral disease. *Journal of Oral Pathology & Medicine*, Vol.20, No.7, (August 1991), pp. 305-317

Chen, CH., Wang, TL., Hung, CF., Yang, Y., Young, RA., Pardoll, DM. & Wu, TC. (2000). Enhancement of DNA vaccine potency by linkage of antigen gene to an HSP70 gene. *Cancer Research*, Vol.60, No.4, (February 2000), pp. 1035-1042

Chen, R., Sehr, P., Waterboer, T., Leivo, I., Pawlita, M., Vaheri, A. & Aaltonen, LM. (2005). Presence of DNA of Human papillomavirus 16 but no other types in tumor-free tonsillar tissue. *Journal of Clinical Microbiology*, Vol.43, No.3, (March 2005), pp. 1408-1410

Chung, CH. & Gillison, ML. (2009). Human papillomavirus in head and neck cancer: its role in pathogenesis and clinical implications. *Clinical Cancer Research,* Vol.15, No.2, (November 2009), pp. 6758-6762

Clayman, GL., Stewart, MG., Weber, RS., el-Naggar, AK. & Grimm, EA. (1994). Human papillomavirus in laryngeal and hypopharyngeal carcinomas. Relationship to survival. *Archives of Otolaryngology Head & Neck Surgery,* Vol.120, No.7, (July 1994), pp. 743-748

Cooper, JS., Pajak, TF., Forastiere, AA., Jacobs, J., Campbell, BH., Saxman, SB., Kish, JA., Kim, HE., Cmelak, AJ., Rotman, M., Machtay, M., Ensley, JF., Chao, KS., Schultz, CJ., Lee, N. & Fu, KK. (2004). Postoperative concurrent radiotherapy and chemotherapy for high-risk squamous-cell carcinoma of the head and neck. *The New England Journal of Medicine,* Vol.350, No.19, (May 2004), pp. 1937-1944

Cortezzi, SS., Provazzi, PJ., Sobrinho, JS., Mann-Prado, JC., Reis, PM., de Freitas, SE., Filho, JF., Fukuyama, EE., Cordeiro, JA., Cury, PM., Maniglia, JV., Villa, LL., Tajara, EH. & Rahal, P. (2004). Analysis of human papillomavirus prevalence and TP53 polymorphism in head and neck squamous carcinomas. *Cancer Genetics and Cytogenetics,* Vol.150, No.1, (April 2004), pp. 44-49

Cruz, IB., Snijders, PJ., Steenbergen, RD., Meijer, CJ., Snow, GB., Walboomers, JM. & van der Waal, I. (1996). Age-dependence of human papillomavirus DNA presence in oral squamous cell carcinomas. *European Journal of Cancer Part B : Oral Oncology,* Vol.32B, No.1, (January 1996), pp. 55-62

Cuschieri, K. & Wentzensen, N. (2008). Human papillomavirus mRNA and p16 detection as biomarkers for the improved diagnosis of cervical neoplasia. *Cancer Epidemiology,* Biomarkers & Prevention, Vol.17, No.10, (October 2008), pp. 2536-2545

Dahlgren, L., Dahlstrand, HM., Lindquist, D., Högmo, A., Björnestål, L., Lindholm, J., Lundberg, B., Dalianis, T. & Munck-Wikland, E. (2004). Human papillomavirus is more common in base of tongue than in mobile tongue cancer and is a favorable prognostic factor in base of tongue cancer patients. *International Journal of Cancer,* Vol.112, Vol.6, (December 2004), pp. 1015-1019

Dahlstrand, HM. & Dalianis, T. (2005). Presence and influence of human papillomaviruses (HPV) in Tonsillar cancer. *Advances in Cancer Research,* Vol.93, (2005), pp. 59-89

Dahlstrand, H., Näsman, A., Romanitan, M., Lindquist, D., Ramqvist, T. & Dalianis, T. (2008). Human papillomavirus accounts both for increased incidence and better prognosis in tonsillar cancer. *Anticancer Research,* Vol.28, No.2B, (March-April 2008), pp. 1133-1138

Deng, Z., Hasegawa, M., Matayoshi, S., Kiyuna, A., Yamashita, Y., Maeda, H. & Suzuki, M. (2011). Prevalence and clinical features of human papillomavirus in head and neck squamous cell carcinoma in Okinawa, southern Japan. *European Archives of Oto-Rhino-Laryngology,* ahead of print, (February 2011)

Denis, F., Garaud, P., Bardet, E., Alfonsi, M., Sire, C., Germain, T., Bergerot, P., Rhein, B., Tortochaux, J. & Calais, G. (2003). Final results of the 94-01 French Head and Neck Oncology and Radiotherapy Group randomized trial comparing radiotherapy alone with concomitant radiochemotherapy in advanced-stage oropharynx carcinoma. *Journal of Clinical Oncology,* Vol.22, No.1, (January 2004), pp. 69-76

de Oliveira, DE., Bacchi, MM., Macarenco, RS., Tagliarini, JV., Cordeiro, RC. & Bacchi, CE. (2006). Human papillomavirus and Epstein-Barr virus infection, p53 expression, and cellular proliferation in laryngeal carcinoma. *American Journal of Clinical Pathology,* Vol.126, No.2, (August 2006), pp. 284-293

Derkay, CS. (1995). Task force on recurrent respiratory papillomas. A preliminary report. *Archives of Otolaryngology Head & Neck Surgery,* Vol.121, No.12, (December 1995), pp. 1386-1391

de Villiers, EM. (1989). Heterogeneity of the human papillomavirus group. *The Journal of Virology,* Vol.63, No.11, (November 1989), pp. 4898-4903

de Villiers, EM., Fauquet, C., Broker, TR., Bernard, HU. & zur Hausen H. (2004). Classification of papillomaviruses. *Virology,* Vol.324, No.1, (June 2004), pp. 17-27

de Villiers, EM. & Gunst, K. (2009). Characterization of seven novel human papillomavirus types isolated from cutaneous tissue, but also present in mucosal lesions. *Journal of General Virology,* Vol.90, Pt8, (August 2009), pp. 1999-2004

Dickens, P., Srivastava, G., Loke, SL. & Larkin, S. (1991). Human papillomavirus 6, 11, and 16 in laryngeal papillomas. *The Journal of Pathology,* Vol.165, No.3, (November 1991), pp. 243-246

Doorbar, J. & Myers, G. (1996). The E4 protein, In: *Human papillomaviruses: a compilation and analysis of nucleic acid and amino acid sequences,* Myers, G., Delius, H., Icenogel, J., Bernard, H-U., Baker, C., Halpern, A., Wheeler, C., (Ed), pp. 58-80, Los Alamos National Laboratory, New Mexico

Doorbar, J. (2005). The papillomavirus life cycle. *Journal of Clinical Virology,* Vol.32, Suppl 1, (March 2005), pp. S7-15

do Sacramento, PR., Babeto, E., Colombo, J., Cabral Ruback, MJ., Bonilha, JL., Fernandes, AM., Pereira Sobrinho, JS., de Souza, FP., Villa, LL. & Rahal, P. (2006). The prevalence of human papillomavirus in the oropharynx in healthy individuals in a brazilian population. *Journal of Medical Virology,* Vol.78, No.5, (May 2006), pp. 614-618

Doyle, DJ., Henderson, LA., Lejeune, FE Jr. & Miller, RH. (1994). Changes in human papillomavirus typing of recurrent respiratory papillomatosis progressing to malignant neoplasm. *Archives of Otolaryngology Head & Neck Surgery,* Vol.120, No.11, (November 1994), pp. 1273-1276

D'Souza, G., Kreimer, AR., Viscidi, R., Pawlita, M., Fakhry, C., Koch, WM., Westra, WH. & Gillison ML. (2007). Case-control study of human papillomavirus and oropharyngeal cancer. *The New England Journal of Medicine,* Vol.356, No.19, (May 2007), pp. 1944-1956

D'Souza, G., Agrawal, Y., Halpern, J., Bodison, S. & Gillison, ML. (2009). Oral sexual behaviors associated with prevalent oral human papillomavirus infection. *The Journal of Infectious Diseases,* Vol.199, No.9, (May 2009), pp. 1263-1269

Duray, A., Demoulin, S., Hubert, P., Delvenne, P. & Saussez, S. (2010). Immune suppression in head and neck cancers: a review. *Clinical and Developmental Immunology,* (2010), pp. 1-15

Duray, A., Descamps, G., Arafa, M., Decaestecker, C., Remmelink, M., Sirtaine, N., Ernoux-Neufcoeur, P., Mutijima, E., Somja, J., Depuydt, CE., Delvenne, P. & Saussez, S. (2011a). High incidence of high-risk HPV in benign and malignant lesions of the larynx. *International Journal of Oncology*, Vol.39, No.1, (July 2011), pp. 51-59

Duray, A., Descamps, G., Bettonville, M., Sirtaine, N., Ernoux-Neufcoeur, P., Guenin, S., Mouallif, M., Depuydt, E., Delvenne, P. & Saussez, S. (2011b). High prevalence of high-risk human papillomavirus in palatine tonsils from healthy children and adults. *Otolaryngology-Head and Neck Surgery*, add Vol.145, No.2, (August 2011), pp. 230-235

Duray, A., Descamps, G., Decaestecker, C., Remmelink, M., Sirtaine, N., Lechien, J., Ernoux-Neufcoeur, P., Bletard, N., Somja, J., Depuydt, C., Delvenne, P. & Saussez, S. (2011). HPV DNA strongly correlates with a poorer prognosis in oral cavity carcinoma. *The Laryngoscope*, in revision

Ernoux-Neufcoeur, P., Arafa, M., Decaestecker, C., Duray, A., Remmelink, M., Leroy, X., Herfs, M., Somja, J., Depuydt, CE., Delvenne, P. & Saussez, S. (2010). Combined analysis of HPV DNA, p16, p21 and p53 to predict prognosis in patients with stage IV hypopharyngeal carcinoma. *Journal of Cancer Research & Clinical Oncology*, Vol.137, No.1, (January 2011), pp. 173-181

Ernster, JA., Sciotto, CG., O'Brien, MM., Finch, JL., Robinson, LJ., Willson, T. & Mathews, M. (2007). Rising incidence of oropharyngeal cancer and the role of oncogenic human papilloma virus. *The Laryngoscope*, Vol.117, No.12, (December 2007), pp. 2115-2128

Ernster, JA., Sciotto, CG., O'Brien, MM., Robinson, LJ. & Willson, T. (2009). Prevalence of oncogenic human papillomavirus 16 and 18 in the palatine tonsils of the general adult population. *Archives of Otolaryngology-Head & Neck Surgery*, Vol.135, No.6, (June 2009), pp. 554-557

Esquenazi, D., Bussoloti Filho, I., Carvalho Mda, G. & de Barros, FS. (2010). The frequency of human papillomavirus findings in normal oral mucosa of healthy people by PCR. *Brazilian Journal of Otorhinolaryngology*, Vol.76, No.1, (February 2010), pp. 78-84

Fakhry, C., Westra, WH., Li, S., Cmelak, A., Ridge, JA., Pinto, H., Forastiere, A. & Gillison, ML. (2008). Improved survival of patients with human papillomavirus-positive head and neck squamous cell carcinoma in a prospective clinical trial. *The Journal of the National Cancer Institute*, Vol.100, No.4, (February 2008), pp. 261-269

Filleul, O., Preillon, J., Crompot, E., Lechien, J. & Saussez, S. (2011). Incidence of head and neck cancers in Belgium : comparison with worldwide and french data. *Bulletin du Cancer*, Vol.98, No.10, (October 2011), pp. 1173-1183

Fischer, M. (2005). Investigation of a broad-spectrum PCR assay for human papillomaviruses in screening benign lesions of the upper aerodigestive tract. ORL: *Journal for Oto-Rhino-Laryngology and Its Related Specialties*, Vol.67, No.4, (November 2005), pp. 237-241

Forastiere, AA. & Trotti, A. (1999). Radiotherapy and concurrent chemotherapy : a strategy that improves locoregional control and survival in oropharyngeal cancer. *Journal of the National Cancer Institute*, Vol.91, No.24, (December 1999), pp. 2065-2066

Fouret, P., Monceaux, G., Temam, S., Lacourreye, L. & St Guily, JL. (1997). Human papillomavirus in head and neck squamous cell carcinomas in nonsmokers. *Archives of Otolaryngology Head and Neck Surgery*, Vol.123, No.5, (May 1997), pp. 513-516

Fredericks, BD., Balkin, A., Daniel, HW., Schonrock, J., Ward, B. & Frazer, IH. (1993). Transmission of human papillomaviruses from mother to child. *Australian and New Zealand Journal of Obstetrics and Gynaecology*, Vol.33, No.1, (February 1993), pp. 30-32

Fukushima, K., Ogura, H., Watanabe, S., Yabe, Y. & Masuda, Y. (1994). Human papillomavirus type 16 DNA detected by the polymerase chain reaction in non-cancer tissues of the head and neck. *European Archives of Oto-Rhino-Laryngology*, Vol.251, No.2, (1994), pp. 109-112

Gallo, A., Degener, AM., Pagliuca, G., Pierangeli, A., Bizzoni, F., Greco, A. & de Vincentiis, M. (2009). Detection of human papillomavirus and adenovirus in benign and malignant lesions of the larynx. *Otolaryngology Head and Neck Surgery*, Vol.141, No.2, (August 2009), pp. 276-281

García-Milián, R., Hernández, H., Panadé, L., Rodríguez, C., González, N., Valenzuela, C., Araña, MD. & Perea, SE. (1998). Detection and typing of human papillomavirus DNA in benign and malignant tumours of laryngeal epithelium. *Acta oto-laryngologica*, Vol.118, No.5, (September 1998), pp. 754-758

Garnett, TO., Filippova, M. & Duerksen-Hughes, PJ. (2006). Accelerated degradation of FADD and procaspase 8 in cells expressing human papilloma virus 16 E6 impairs TRAIL-mediated apoptosis. *Cell Death and Differentiation*, Vol.13, No.11, (November 2006), pp. 1915-1926

Georgopoulos, NT., Proffitt, JL. & Blair, GE. (2000). Transcriptional regulation of the major histocompatibility complex (MHC) class I heavy chain, TAP1 and LMP2 genes by the human papillomavirus (HPV) type 6b, 16 and 18 E7 oncoproteins. *Oncogene*, Vol.19, No.42, (October 2000), pp. 4930-4935

Gillison, ML., Koch, WM., Capone, RB., Spafford, M., Westra, WH., Wu, L., Zahurak, ML., Daniel, RW., Viglione, M., Symer, DE., Shah, KV. & Sidransky, D. (2000). Evidence for a causal association between human papillomavirus and a subset of head and neck cancers. *Journal of the National Cancer Institute*, Vol.92, No.9, (May 2000), pp. 709-720

Gillison, ML., D'Souza, G., Westra, W., Sugar, E., Xiao, W., Begum, S. & Viscidi, R. (2008). Distinct risk factor profiles for human papillomavirus type 16-positive and human papillomavirus type 16-negative head and neck cancers. *Journal of the National Cancer Institute*, Vol.100, No.6, (March 2008), pp. 407-420

Giovannelli, L., Campisi, G., Lama, A., Giambalvo, O., Osborn, J., Margiotta, V. & Ammatuna, P. (2002). Human papillomavirus DNA in oral mucosal lesions. *The Journal of Infectious Diseases*, Vol.185, No.6, (March 2002), pp. 833-836

Giraldo, P., Gonçalves, AKS., Pereira, SAS., Barros-Mazon, S., Gondo, ML. & Witkin, SS. (2006). Human papillomavirus in the oral mucosa of women with genital human papillomavirus lesions. *European Journal of Obstetrics & Gynecology and Reproductive Biology*, Vol. 126, No.1, (May 2006), pp. 104-106

Gissmann, L., Wolnik, L., Ikenberg, H., Koldovsky, U., Schnürch, HG. & zur Hausen, H. (1983). Human papillomavirus types 6 and 11 DNA sequences in genital and laryngeal papillomas and in some cervical cancers. *Proceedings of the National Academy of Sciences of the United States of America*, Vol.80, No.2, (January 1983), pp. 560-563

Globocan 2008, In: *International Agency for Research on Cancer*, 16th May 2011, Available from: http://globocan.iarc.fr/.

Goon, P., Sonnex, C., Jani, P., Stanley, M. & Sudhoff, H. (2007). Recurrent respiratory papillomatosis: an overview of current thinking and treatment. *European Archives of Oto-Rhino-Laryngology,* Vol.265, No.2, (February 2008), pp.147-151

Grandis, JR., Pietenpol, JA., Greenberger, JS., Pelroy, RA. & Mohla, S. (2004). Head and neck cancer : meeting summary and research opportunities. *Cancer Research,* Vol.64, No.21, (November 2004), pp. 8126-8129

Gutman, LT., Herman-Giddens, ME. & Phelps, WC. (1993). Transmission of human genital papillomavirus disease : comparison of data from adults and children. *Pediatrics,* Vol.91, No.1, (January 1993), pp. 31-38

Ha, PK., Pai, SI., Westra, WH., Gillison, ML., Tong, BC., Sidransky, D. & Califano, JA. (2002). Real-time quantitative PCR demonstrates low prevalence of human papillomavirus type 16 in premalignant and malignant lesions of the oral cavity. *Clinical Cancer Research,* Vol.8, No.5, (May 2002), pp. 1203-1209

Hafkamp, HC., Speel, EJ., Haesevoets, A., Bot, FJ., Dinjens, WN., Ramaekers, FC., Hopman, AH. & Manni, JJ. (2003). A subset of head and neck squamous cell carcinomas exhibits integration of HPV 16/18 DNA and overexpression of p16INK4A and p53 in the absence of mutations in p53 exons 5-8. *International Journal of Cancer,* Vol.107, No.3, (November 2003), pp. 394-400

Hafkamp, HC., Manni, JJ., Haesevoets, A., Voogd, AC., Schepers, M., Bot, FJ., Hopman, AH., Ramaekers, FC. & Speel, EJ. (2008). Marked differences in survival rate between smokers and nonsmokers with HPV 16-associated tonsillar carcinomas. *International Journal of Cancer,* Vol.122, No.12, (June 2008), pp. 2656-2664

Hallden, C. & Majmudar, B. (1986). The relationship between juvenile laryngeal papillomatosis and maternal condylomata acuminata. *The Journal of Reproductive Medicine,* Vol.31, No.9, (September 1986), pp. 804-807

Hansson, BG., Rosenquist, K., Antonsson, A., Wennerberg, J., Schildt, EB., Bladström, A. & Andersson, G. (2005). Strong association between infection with human papillomavirus and oral and oropharyngeal squamous cell carcinoma: a population-based case-control study in southern Sweden. *Acta Oto-Laryngologica,* Vol.125, No.12, (September 2005), pp. 1337-1344

Hasan, UA., Bates, E., Takeshita, F., Biliato, A., Accardi, R., Bouvard, V., Mansour, M., Vincent, I., Gissmann, L., Iftner, T., Sideri, M., Stubenrauch, F. & Tommasino, M. (2007). TLR9 expression and function is abolished by the cervical cancer-associated human papillomavirus type 16. *Journal of Immunology,* Vol.178, No.5, (March 2007) pp. 3186-3197

Hathaway, B., Landsittel, DP., Gooding, W., Whiteside, TL., Grandis, JR., Siegfried, JM., Bigbee, WL. & Ferris, RL. (2005). Multiplexed analysis of serum cytokines as biomarkers in squamous cell carcinoma of the head and neck patients. *The Laryngoscope,* Vol.115, No.3, (March 2005) pp. 522-527

Herrero, R., Castellsagué, X., Pawlita, M., Lissowska, J., Kee, F., Balaram, P., Rajkumar, T., Sridhar, H., Rose, B., Pintos, J., Fernández, L., Idris, A., Sánchez, MJ., Nieto, A., Talamini, R., Tavani, A., Bosch, FX., Reidel, U., Snijders, PJ., Meijer, CJ., Viscidi, R., Muñoz, N., Franceschi, S. & IARC Multicenter Oral Cancer Study Group. (2003). Human papillomavirus and oral cancer: the International Agency for Research on Cancer multicenter study. *Journal of the National Cancer Institute,* Vol.95, No.23, (December 2003), pp. 1772-1783

Hobbs, CG., Sterne, JA., Bailey, M., Heyderman, RS., Birchall, MA. & Thomas, SJ. (2006). Human papillomavirus and head and neck cancer: a systematic review and meta-analysis. *Clinical Otolaryngology*, Vol.31, No.4, (August, 2006), pp. 259-266

Hoffmann, M., Kahn, T., Goeroegh, T., Lohrey, C., Gottschlich, S., Meyer, J., Rudert, H. & Maune, S. (2000). Tracing human papillomavirus DNA in nasal polyps by polymerase chain reaction. *Acta oto-laryngologica*, Vol. 120, No.7, (October 2000), pp. 872-875

Hoffmann, TK., Bier, H. & Whiteside, TL. (2004). Targeting the immune system : novel therapeutic approaches in squamous cell carcinoma of the head and neck. *Cancer Immunology*, Vol.53, No.12, (December 2004), pp. 1055-1067

Hoffmann, TK., Arsov, C., Schirlau, K., Bas, M., Friebe-Hoffmann, U., Klussmann, JP., Scheckenbach, K., Balz, V., Bier, H. & Whiteside, T.L. (2006). T cells specific for HPV16 E7 epitopes in patients with squamous cell carcinoma of the oropharynx. *International Journal of Cancer*, Vol.118, No.8, (April 2006), pp. 1984-1991

Hughes, FJ. & Romanos, MA. (1993). E1 protein of human papillomavirus is a DNA helicase/ATPase. *Nucleic Acids Research*, Vol.21, No.25, (December 1993), pp. 5817-5823

Ishii, Y., Ozaki, S., Tanaka, K. & Kanda, T. (2005). Human papillomavirus 16 minor capsid protein L2 helps capsomeres assemble independently of intercapsomeric disulfide bonding. *Virus Genes*, Vol.31, No.3, (December 2005), pp. 321-328

Jalal, H., Sanders, CM., Prime, SS., Scully, C. & Maitland, NJ. (1992). Detection of human papillomavirus type 16 DNA in oral squames from normal young adults. *Journal of Oral Pathology & Medicine*, Vol.21, No.10, (November 1992), pp. 465-470

Jenison, SA., Yu, XP., Valentine, JM., Koutsky, LA., Christiansen, AE., Beckmann, AM. & Galloway, DA. (1990). Evidence of prevalent genital-typa human papillomavirus infections in adults and children. *The Journal of Infectious Diseases*, Vol.162, No.1, (July 1990), pp. 60-69

Jeremic, B., Shibamoto, Y., Milicic, B., Nikolic, N., Dagovic, A., Aleksandrovic, J., Vaskovic, Z. & Tadic, L. (2000). Hyperfractionated radiation therapy with or without concurrent low-dose daily cisplatin in locally advanced squamous cell carcinoma of the head and neck: a prospective randomized trial. *Journal of Clinical Oncology*, Vol.18, No.7, (April 2000), pp. 1458-1464

Kanodia, S., Fahey, LM. & Kast, WM. (2007). Mechanisms used by human papillomaviruses to escape the host immune response. *Current Cancer Drug Targets*, Vol.7, No.1, (February 2007), pp. 79-89

Kansky, AA., Poljak, M., Seme, K., Kocjan, BJ., Gale, N., Luzar, B. & Golouh, R. (2003). Human papillomavirus DNA in oral squamous cell carcinomas and normal oral mucosa. *Acta Virologica*, Vol.47, No.1, (2003), pp. 11-16

Kashima, HK., Shah, F., Lyles, A., Glackin, R., Muhammad, N., Turner, L., Van Zandt, S., Whitt, S. & Shah, K. (1992). A comparison of risk factors in juvenile-onset and adult-onset recurrent respiratory papillomatosis. *The Laryngoscope*, Vol.102, No.1, (January 1992), pp. 9-13

Kashima, HK., Kessis, T., Hruban, RH., Wu, TC., Zinreich, SJ. & Shah, KV. (1992). Human papillomavirus in sinonasal papillomas and squamous cell carcinoma. *The Laryngoscope*, Vol.102, No.9, (September 1992), pp. 973-976

Kaye, JN., Cason, J., Pakarian, FB., Jewers, RJ., Kell, B., Bible, J., Raju, KS. & Best, JM. (1994). Viral load as a determinant for transmission of human papillomavirus type 16 from mother to child. *Journal of Medical Virology*, Vol.44, No.4, (December 1994), pp. 415-421

Kaye, JN., Starkey, WG., Kell, B., Biswas, C., Shanti Raju, K., Best, JM. & Cason, J. (1996). Human papillomavirus type 16 in infants : use of DNA sequence analyses to determine the source of infection. *Journal of General Virology*, Vol.77, No.6, (June 1996), pp. 1139-1143

Kellokoski, J., Syrjänen, S., Yliskoski, M. & Syrjänen, K. (1992a). Dot blot hybridization in detection of human papillomavirus (HPV) infections in the oral cavity of women with genital HPV infections. *Oral Microbiology and Immunology*, Vol.7, No.1, (February 1992), pp. 19-23

Kellokoski, JK., Syrjänen, SM., Chang, F., Yliskoski, M. & Syrjänen, KJ. (1992b). Southern blot hybridization and PCR in detection of oral human papillomavirus (HPV) infections in women with genital HPV infections. *Journal of Oral Pathology & Medicine*, Vol.21, No.10, (November 1992), pp. 459-464

Kim, SH., Koo, BS., Kang, S., Park, K., Kim, H., Lee, KR., Lee, MJ., Kim, JM., Choi, EC. & Cho, NH. (2007). HPV integration begins in the tonsillar crypt and leads to the alteration of p16, EGFR and c-myc during tumor formation. *International Journal of Cancer*, Vol.120, No.7, (April 2007), pp. 1418-1425

Kleist, B., Poetsch, M., Bankau, A., Werner, E., Herrmann, FH. & Lorenz, G. (2000). First hints for a correlation between amplification of the Int-2 gene and infection with human papillomavirus in head and neck squamous cell carcinomas. *Journal of Oral Pathology & Medicine*, Vol.29, No.9, (October 2000), pp. 432-437

Klingenberg, B., Hafkamp, HC., Haesevoets, A., Manni, JJ., Slootweg, PJ., Weissenborn, SJ., Klussmann, JP. & Speel, EJ. (2010). p16 INK4A overexpression is frequently detected in tumour-free tonsil tissue without association with HPV. *Histopathology*, Vol.56, No.7, (June 2010), pp. 957-967

Klozar, J., Tachezy, R., Rotnáglová, E., Koslabová, E., Saláková, M. & Hamsíková, E. (2010). Human papillomavirus in head and neck tumors: epidemiological, molecular and clinical aspects. *Wiener Medizinische Wochenschrift*, Vol.160, No.11-12, (June 2010), pp. 305-309

Klussmann, JP., Weissenborn, SJ., Wieland, U., Dries, V., Kolligs, J., Jungehuelsing, M., Eckel, HE., Dienes, HP., Pfister, HJ. & Fuchs, PG. (2001). Prevalence, distribution, and viral load of human papillomavirus 16 DNA in tonsillar carcinomas. *Cancer*, Vol.92, No.11, (December 2001), pp. 2875-2884

Koch, A., Hansen, SV., Nielsen, NM., Palefsky, J. & Melbye, M. (1997). HPV detection in children prior to sexual debut. *International Journal of Cancer*, Vol.73, No.5, (November 1997), pp. 621-624

Kojima, A., Maeda, H., Kurahashi, N., Sakagami, G., Kubo, K., Yoshimoto, H. & Kameyama, Y. (2003). Human papillomaviruses in the normal oral cavity of children in Japan. *Oral Oncology*, Vol.39, No.8, (December 2003), pp. 821-828

Koskinen, WJ., Chen, RW., Leivo, I., Mäkitie, A., Bäck, L., Kontio, R., Suuronen, R., Lindqvist, C., Auvinen, E., Molijn, A., Quint, WG., Vaheri, A. & Aaltonen, LM. (2003). Prevalence and physical status of human papillomavirus in squamous cell carcinomas of the head and neck. *International Journal of Cancer*, Vol.107, No.3, (November 2003), pp. 401-406

Koskinen, WJ., Brøndbo, K., Mellin Dahlstrand, H., Luostarinen, T., Hakulinen, T., Leivo, I., Molijn, A., Quint, WG., Røysland, T., Munck-Wikland, E., Mäkitie, AA., Pyykkö, I.,

Dillner, J., Vaheri, A. & Aaltonen, LM. (2007). Alcohol, smoking and human papillomavirus in laryngeal carcinoma: a Nordic prospective multicenter study. *Journal of Cancer Research and Clinical Oncology,* Vol.133, No.9, (September 2007), pp. 673-678

Kovalenko, S., Lukashenko, P., Romanovskaya, A., Soldatski, IL., Bakanov, SI., Pfister, H. & Gerein, V. (2008). Distribution and density of CD1a+ and CD83+ dendritic cells in HPV-associated laryngeal papillomas. *International Journal of Pediatric Otorhinolaryngology,* Vol.73, No.2, (February 2009), pp. 249-256

Koyama, K., Uobe, K. & Tanaka, A. (2007). Highly sensitive detection of HPV-DNA in paraffin sections of human oral carcinomas. *Journal of Oral Pathology & Medicine,* Vol.36, No.1, (January 2007), pp. 18-24

Kreimer, AR., Alberg, AJ., Daniel, R., Gravitt, PE., Viscidi, R., Garrett, ES., Shah, KV. & Gillison, ML. (2004). Oral human papillomavirus infection in adults is associated with sexual behavior and HIV serostatus. *American Journal of Infectious Diseases,* Vol.189, No.4, (February 2004), pp. 686-698

Kreimer, AR., Clifford, GM., Boyle, P. & Franceschi, S. (2005). Human papillomavirus types in head and neck squamous cell carcinomas worldwide: a systematic review. *Cancer Epidemiology, Biomarkers & Prevention,* Vol.14, No.2, (February 2005), pp. 467-475

Kurose, K., Terai, M., Soedarsono, N., Rabello, D., Nakajima, Y., Burk, RD. & Takagi, M. (2004). Low prevalence of HPV infection and its natural history in normal oral mucosa among volunteers on Miyako Island, Japan. *Oral Surgery, Oral Medicine, Oral Pathology, Oral Radiology & Endodontics,* Vol.98, No.1, (July 2004), pp. 91-96

Kuss, I., Saito, T., Johnson, JT. & Whiteside TL. (1999). Clinical significance of decreased ζ chain expression in peripheral blood lymphocytes of patients with head and neck cancer. *Clinical Cancer Research,* Vol.5, No.2, (February 1999), pp. 329-334

Lacey, CJ., Lowndes, CM. & Shah, KV. (2006). Chapter 4: Burden and management of non-cancerous HPV-related conditions: HPV-6/11 disease. *Vaccine,* Vol.24, No.3, (August 2006), pp. 35-41

Laco, J., Vosmikova, H., Novakova, V., Celakovsky, P., Dolezalova, H., Tucek, L., Nekvindova, J., Vosmik, M., Cermakova, E., Ryska, A. (2011). The role of high-risk human papillomavirus infection in oral and oropharyngeal squamous cell carcinoma in non-smoking and non-drinking patients: a clinicopathological and molecular study of 46 cases. *Virchows Archiv,* Vol.458, No.2, (February 2011), pp. 179-187

Lang, K., Menzin, J., Earle, CC., Jacobson, J. & Hsu, MA. (2004). The economic cost of squamous cell cancer of the head and neck: findings from linked SEER-Medicare data. *Archives of Otolaryngology Head & Neck Surgery,* Vol.130, No.11, (November 2004), pp. 1269-1275

Larson, DA., & Derkay, CS. (2010). Epidemiology of recurrent respiratory papillomatosis. *Acta Pathologica, Microbiologica and Immunologica Scandinavica,* Vol.118, No.6-7, (June 2010), pp. 450-454

Lau, KM., Cheng, SH., Lo, KW., Lee, SA., Woo, JK., van Hasselt, CA., Lee, SP., Rickinson, AB. & Ng, MH. (2007). Increase in circulating Foxp3+ CD4+ CD25high regulatory T cells in nasopharyngeal carcinoma patients. *British Journal of Cancer,* Vol.96, No.4, (February 2007), pp. 617-622

Lepique, AP., Daghastanli, KR., Cuccovia, IM. & Villa, LL. (2009). HPV16 tumor associated macrophages suppress antitumor T cell responses. *Clinical Cancer Research,* Vol.15, No.13, (July 2009), pp. 4391-4400

Li, Y., Nichols, MA., Shay, JW. & Xiong, Y. (1994). Transcriptional repression of the D-type cyclin-dependent kinase inhibitor p16 by the retinoblastoma susceptibility gene product pRb. *Cancer Research,* Vol.54, No.23, (December 1994), pp. 6078-6082

Licitra, L., Bernier, J., Grandi, C., Merlano, M., Bruzzi, P. & Lefebvre, JL. (2002). Cancer of the oropharynx. *Critical Reviews in Oncology/Hematology,* Vol.41, No.1, (January 2002), pp. 107-122

Lie, ES., Karlsen, F. & Holm, R. (1996). Presence of human papillomavirus in squamous cell laryngeal carcinomas. A study of thirty-nine cases using polymerase chain reaction and in situ hybridization. *Acta oto-laryngologica,* Vol.116, No.6, (November 1996), pp. 900-905

Lindeberg, H. & Johansen, L. (1990). The presence of human papillomavirus (HPV) in solitary adult laryngeal papillomas demonstrated by in-situ DNA hybridization with sulphonated probes. *Clinical Otolaryngology and Allied Sciences,* Vol.15, No.4, (August 1990), pp. 367-371

Lindeberg, H. & Krogdahl, A. (1999). Laryngeal cancer and human papillomavirus: HPV is absent in the majority of laryngeal carcinomas. *Cancer Letters,* Vol.146, No.1, (September 1999), pp. 9-13

Lindel, K., Beer, KT., Laissue, J., Greiner, RH. & Aebersold, DM. (2001). Human papillomavirus positive squamous cell carcinoma of the oropharynx: a radiosensitive subgroup of head and neck carcinoma. *Cancer,* Vol.92, No.4, (August 2001), pp. 805-813

Lindquist, D., Romanitan, M., Hammarstedt, L., Näsman, A., Dahlstrand, H., Lindholm, J., Onelöv, L., Ramqvist, T., Ye, W., Munck-Wikland, E. & Dalianis, T. (2007). Human papillomavirus is a favourable prognostic factor in tonsillar cancer and its oncogenic role is supported by the expression of E6 and E7. *Molecular Oncology,* Vol.1, No.3, (December 2007), pp. 350-355

Lira, RC., Miranda, FA., Guimarães, MC., Simões, RT., Donadi, EA., Soares, CP. & Soares, EG. (2009). BUBR1 expression in benign oral lesions and squamous cell carcinomas: correlation with human papillomavirus. *Oncology Reports,* Vol.23, No.4 (April 2010), pp. 1027-1036

Llamas-Martínez, S., Esparza-Gómez, G., Campo-Trapero, J., Cancela-Rodríguez, P., Bascones-Martínez, A., Moreno-López, LA., García-Núñez, JA. & Cerero-Lapiedra, R. (2008). Genotypic determination by PCR-RFLP of human papillomavirus in normal oral mucosa, oral leukoplakia and oral squamous cell carcinoma samples in Madrid (Spain). *Anticancer Research,*Vol.28, No.6A, (November-December 2008), pp. 3733-3742

Lopes, V., Murray, P., Williams, H., Woodman, C., Watkinson, J. & Robinson, M. (2011). Squamous cell carcinoma of the oral cavity rarely harbours oncogenic human papillomavirus. *Oral Oncology,* ahead of print, (June 2011)

Maitland, NJ., Cox, MF., Lynas, C., Prime, SS., Meanwell, CA. & Scully, C. (1987). Detection of human papillomavirus DNA in biopsies of human oral tissue. *British Journal of Cancer,* Vol.56, No.3, (September 1987), pp. 245-250

Mammas, IN., Sourvinos, G., Michael, C. & Spandidos, DA. (2006). Human papilloma virus in hyperplastic tonsillar and adenoid tissues in children. *The Pediatric Infectious Disease* Journal, Vol.25, No.12, (December 2006), pp. 1158-1162

Mammas, IN., Sourvinos, G. & Spandidos, DA. (2009). Human papilloma virus (HPV) infection in children and adolescents. *European Journal of Pediatrics,* Vol.168, No.3, (March 2009), pp. 267-273

Mant, C., Kell, B., Rice, P., Best, JM., Bible, JM. & Cason, J. (2003). Buccal exposure to human papillomavirus type 16 is a common yet transitory event of childhood. *Journal of Medical Virology,* Vol. 71, No.4, (December 2003), pp. 593-598

Marklund, L. & Hammarstedt, L. (2010). Impact of HPV in Oropharyngeal Cancer. *Journal of Oncology,* (2011)

Marur, S. & Forastiere, AA. (2008). Head and neck cancer: changing epidemiology, diagnosis, and treatment. *Mayo Clinic Proceedings,* Vol.83, No.4, (April 2008), pp. 489-501

Mazzatenta, C., Fimiani, M., Rubegni, P., Andreassi, L., Buffi, P. & Messina, C. (1996). Vertical transmission of human papillomavirus in cytologically normal women. *Genitourin Medicine,* Vol.72, No.6, (December 1996), pp. 445-452

Medeiros, LR., de Moraes Ethur, A.B., Hilgert, JB., Zanini, RR., Berwanger, O., Bozzetti, MC. & Mylius, LC. (2005). Vertical transmission of the human papillomavirus : a systematic quantitative review. *Cadernos Saude Publica,* Vol.21, No.4, (July-Augustus 2005), pp. 1006-1015

Miller, CS. & White, DK. (1996). Human papillomavirus expression in oral mucosa, premalignant conditions, and squamous cell carcinoma: a retrospective review of the literature. *Oral Surgery, Oral Medicine, Oral Pathology, Oral Radiology & Endodontics,* Vol.82, No.1, (July 1996), pp. 57-68

Miller, CS. & Johnstone, BM. (2001). Human papillomavirus as a risk factor for oral squamous cell carcinoma: a meta-analysis, 1982-1997. *Oral Surgery, Oral Medicine, Oral Pathology, Oral Radiology & Endodontics,* Vol.91, No.6, (June 2001), pp. 622-635

Mishra, A., Bharti, AC., Varghese, P., Saluja, D. & Das, BC. (2006). Differential expression and activation of NF-kappaB family proteins during oral carcinogenesis: Role of high risk human papillomavirus infection. *International Journal of Cancer,* Vol.119, No.12, (December 2006), pp. 2840-2850

Monsonégo, J. (2007). *Traité des infections et pathologies génitales à papillomavirus,* Springer, 9782287720642, Paris

Morgan, DW., Abdullah, V., Quiney, R. & Myint, S. (1991). Human papilloma virus and carcinoma of the laryngopharynx. *The Journal of Laryngology and Otology,* Vol.105, No.4, (April 1991), pp. 288-290

Morshed, K., Polz-Dacewicz, M., Szymański, M. & Polz, D. (2008). Short-fragment PCR assay for highly sensitive broad-spectrum detection of human papillomaviruses in laryngeal squamous cell carcinoma and normal mucosa: clinico-pathological evaluation. *European Archives of Oto-Rhino-Laryngology,* Vol.265, No.Suppl 1, (July 2008), pp. 89-96

Morshed, K. (2010). Association between human papillomavirus infection and laryngeal squamous cell carcinoma. *Journal of Medical Virology,* Vol.82, No.6, (May 2010), pp. 1017-1023

Moscicki, AB., Hills, N., Shiboski, S., Powell, K., Jay, N., Hanson, E., Miller, S., Clayton, L., Farhat, S., Broering, J., Darragh, T. & Palefsky, J. (2001). Risks for incident human papillomavirus infection and low-grade squamous intraepithelial lesion development in young females. *The Journal of the American Medical Association,* Vol.285, No.23, (June 2001), pp. 2995-3002

Myhre, AK., Dalen, A., Berntzen, K. & Bratlid, D. (2003). Anogenital human papillomavirus in non-abused preschool children. *Acta Paediatrica,* Vol.92, No.12, (December 2003), pp. 1445-1452

Narisawa-Saito, M. & Kiyono, T. (2007). Basic mechanisms of high-risk human papillomavirus-induced carcinogenesis: roles of E6 and E7 proteins. *Cancer Science,* Vol.98, No.10, (October 2007), pp. 1505-1511

Näsman, A., Attner, P., Hammarstedt, L., Du, J., Eriksson, M., Giraud, G., Ahrlund-Richter, S., Marklund, L., Romanitan, M., Lindquist, D., Ramqvist, T., Lindholm, J., Sparén, P., Ye, W., Dahlstrand, H., Munck-Wikland, E. & Dalianis, T. (2009). Incidence of human papillomavirus (HPV) positive tonsillar carcinoma in Stockholm, Sweden: an epidemic of viral-induced carcinoma? *International Journal of Cancer,* Vol.125, No.2, (July 2009), pp. 362-366

Nebesio, CL., Mirowski, GW. & Chuang, TY. (2001). Human papillomavirus: clinical significance and malignant potential. *International Journal of Dermatology,* Vol.40, No.6, (June 2001), pp. 373-379

Neufcoeur, PE., Arafa, M., Delvenne, P. & Saussez, S. (2009). Involvement of human papillomavirus in upper aero-digestive tracts cancers. *Bulletin du Cancer,* Vol.96, No.10, (October 2009), pp. 941-950

Niedobitek, G., Pitteroff, S., Herbst, H., Shepherd, P., Finn, T., Anagnostopoulos, I. & Stein, H. (1990). Detection of human papillomavirus type 16 DNA in carcinomas of the palatine tonsil. *Journal of Clinical Pathology,* Vol.43, No.11, (November 1990), pp. 918-921

O'Donovan, A. & Wood, RD. (1993). Identical defects in DNA repair in xeroderma pigmentosum group G and rodent ERCC group 5. *Nature,* Vol.363, No.6425, (May 1993), pp. 185-188

Padayachee, A. (1994). Human papillomavirus (HPV) types 2 and 57 in oral verrucae demonstrated by in situ hybridization. *Journal of Oral Pathology & Medicine,* Vol.23, No.9, (October 1994), pp. 413-417

Pakarian, F., Kaye, J., Cason, J., Kell, B., Jewers, R., Derias, NW., Raju, KS. & Best, JM. (1994). Cancer associated human papillomaviruses: perinatal transmission and persistence. *British Journal of Obstetrics and Gynaecology,* Vol.101, No.6, (June 1994), pp. 514-517

Pannone, G., Santoro, A., Papagerakis, S., Lo Muzio, L., De Rosa, G. & Bufo, P. (2011). The role of human papillomavirus in the pathogenesis of head & neck squamous cell carcinoma: an overview. *Infectious Agents and Cancer,* Vol.6, No.4, (March 2011)

Parkin, DM., Whelan, SL., Ferlay, J., Teppo, L., Thomas, D. & Thomas, DM. (2002). *Cancer Incidence in Five Continents* (vol.8), IARC, 9283224272, Lyon

Parkin, DM., Bray, F., Ferlay, J. & Pisani, P. (2005). Global cancer statistics, 2002. CA: *A Cancer Journal for Clinicians,* Vol.55, No.2, (March-April 2005), pp. 74-108

Paz, IB., Cook, N., Odom-Maryon, T., Xie, Y. & Wilczynski, SP. (1997). Human papillomavirus (HPV) in head and neck cancer. An association of HPV 16 with squamous cell carcinoma of Waldeyer's tonsillar ring. *Cancer,* Vol.79, No.3, (February 1997), pp. 595-604

Pignon, JP., le Maître, A., Maillard, E. & Bourhis, J. (2009). Meta-analysis of chemotherapy in head and neck cancer (MACH-NC): an update on 93 randomised trials and 17,346 patients. *Radiotherapy & Oncology,* Vol.92, No.1, (July 2009), pp. 4-14

Praetorius, F. (1997). HPV-associated diseases of oral mucosa. *Clinics in Dermatology,* Vol.15, No.3, (May 1997), pp. 399-413

Psyrri, A. & DiMaio, D. (2008). Human papillomavirus in cervical and head-and-neck cancer. *Nature Clinical Practice Oncology,* Vol.5, No.1, (January 2008), pp. 24-31

Puranen, M., Yliskoski, M., Saarikoski, S., Syrjänen, K. & Syrjänen, S. (1996). Vertical transmission of human papillomavirus from infected mothers to their newborn babies and persistence of the virus in childhood. *American Journal of Obstetrics & Gynecology,* Vol.174, No2, (February 1996), pp. 694-699

Puranen, MH., Yliskoski, MH., Saarikoski, SV., Syrjänen, KJ. & Syrjänen, SM. (1997). Exposure of an infant to cervical human papillomavirus infection of the mother is common. *American Journal of Obstetrics & Gynecology,* Vol.176, No.5, (May 1997), pp. 1039-1045

Ragin, CC., Modugno, F. & Gollin, SM. (2007). The epidemiology and risk factors of head and neck cancer: a focus on human papillomavirus. *Journal of Dental Research,* Vol.86, No.2, (February 2007), pp. 104-114

Ragin, CC. & Taioli, E. (2007). Survival of squamous cell carcinoma of the head and neck in relation to human papillomavirus infection: review and meta-analysis. *International Journal of Cancer,* Vol.121, No.8, (October 2007), pp. 1813-1820

Ramqvist, T. & Dalianis, T. (2010). Oropharyngeal cancer epidemic and human papillomavirus. *Emerging Infectious Diseases Journal,* Vol.16, No.11, (November 2010), pp. 1671-1677

Rees, L., Birchall, M., Bailey, M. & Thomas, S. (2004). A systematic review of case-control studies of human papillomavirus infection in laryngeal squamous cell carcinoma. *Clinical Otolaryngology and Allied Sciences,* Vol.29, No.4, (August 2004), pp. 301-306

Reichert, TE., Rabinowich, H., Johnson, JT. & Whiteside, TL. (1998a). Mechanisms responsible for signaling and functional defects. *Journal of Immunotherapy,* Vol.21, No.4, (July 1998), pp. 295-306

Reichert, TE., Day, R., Wagner, EM. & Whiteside, TL. (1998b). Absent or low expression of the ζ chain in T cells at the tumor site correlates with poor survival in patients with oral carcinoma. *Cancer Research,* Vol.58, No.23, (December 1998), pp. 5344-5347

Remmerbach, TW., Brinckmann, UG., Hemprich, A., Chekol, M., Kühndel, K. & Liebert, UG. (2004). PCR detection of human papillomavirus of the mucosa: comparison between MY09/11 and GP5+/6+ primer sets. *Journal of Clinical Virology,* Vol.30, No.4, (August 2004), pp. 302-308

Ribeiro, KMX., Alvez, JM., Pignatari, SSN. & Weckx, LLM. (2006). Detection of human papilloma virus in the tonsils of children undergoing tonsillectomy. *The Brazilian Journal of Infectious Diseases,* Vol.10, No.3, (June 2006), pp. 165-168

Ribeiro, KB., Levi, JE., Pawlita, M., Koifman, S., Matos, E., Eluf-Neto, J., Wunsch-Filho, V., Curado, MP., Shangina, O., Zaridze, D., Szeszenia-Dabrowska, N., Lissowska, J., Daudt, A., Menezes, A., Bencko, V., Mates, D., Fernandez, L., Fabianova, E., Gheit, T., Tommasino, M., Boffetta P., Brennan, P. & Waterboer, T. (2011). Low human papillomavirus prevalence in head and neck cancer: results from two large case-control studies in high-incidence regions. *International Journal of Epidemiology,* Vol.40, No.2, (April 2011), pp. 489-502

Rice, PS., Mant, C., Cason, J., Bible, JM., Muir, P., Kell, B. & Best, JM. (2000). High prevalence of human papillomavirus type 16 infection among children. *Journal of Medical Virology*, Vol.61, No.1, (May 2000), pp. 70-75

Ringström, E., Peters, E., Hasegawa, M., Posner, M., Liu, M. & Kelsey, KT. (2002). Human papillomavirus type 16 and squamous cell carcinoma of the head and neck. *Clinical Cancer Research*, Vol.8, No.10, (October 2002), pp. 3187-3192

Rintala, MA., Grénman, SE., Järvenkylä, ME., Syrjänen, KJ. & Syrjänen, SM. (2005a). High-risk types of human papillomavirus (HPV) DNA in oral and genital mucosa of infants during their first 3 years of life : experience from the finnish HPV family study. *Clinical Infectious Diseases*, Vol.41, No.12, (December 2005), pp. 1728-1733

Rintala, MA., Grénman, SE., Puranen, MH., Isolauri, E., Ekblad, U., Kero, PO. & Syrjänen. (2005b). Transmission of high-risk human papillomavirus (HPV) between parents and infant : a prospective study of HPV in families in Finland. *Journal of Clinical Microbiology*, Vol.43, No.1, (January 2005), pp. 376-381

Rombaldi, RL., Serafini, EP., Mandelli, J., Zimmermann, E. & Losquiavo, KP. (2008). Transplacental transmission of human papillomavirus. *Virology Journal*, Vol.5, No.106, (September 2008), pp. 1-14

Rombaldi, RL., Serafini, EP., Mandelli, J., Zimmermann, E. & Losquiavo, KP. (2009). Perinatal transmission of human papillomavirus DNA. *Virology Journal*, Vol.6, No.83, (June 2009), pp. 1-12

Rosenquist, K., Wennerberg, J., Annertz, K., Schildt, EB., Hansson, BG., Bladström, A. & Andersson, G. (2007). Recurrence in patients with oral and oropharyngeal squamous cell carcinoma: human papillomavirus and other risk factors. *Acta Oto-Laryngologica*, Vol.127, No.9, (September 2007), pp. 980-987

Rotnáglová, E., Tachezy, R., Saláková, M., Procházka, B., Košl'abová, E., Veselá, E., Ludvíková, V., Hamšíková, E. & Klozar J. (2011). HPV involvement in tonsillar cancer: prognostic significance and clinically relevant markers. *International Journal of Cancer*, Vol.129, No.1, (July 2011), pp. 101-110

Saini, R., Khim, TP., Rahman, SA., Ismail, M. & Tang, TH. (2010). High-risk human papillomavirus in the oral cavity of women with cervical cancer, and their children. *Virology Journal*, Vol.16, No.7, (June 2010), pp. 1-7

Sarkola, ME., Grénman, SE., Rintala, MA., Syrjänen, KJ. & Syrjänen, SM. (2008a). Human papillomavirus in the placenta and umbilical cord blood. *Acta Obstetricia et Gynecologica Scandinavica*, Vol.87, No.11, (2008), pp. 1181-1188

Sarkola, M., Rintala, M., Grénman, S. & Syrjänen, S. (2008b). Human papillomavirus DNA detected in breast milk. *Pediatric Infectious Disease Journal*, Vol.27, No.6, (June 2008), pp. 557-558

Scherly, D., Nouspikel, T., Corlet, J., Ucla, C., Bairoch, A. & Clarkson, SG. (1993). Complementation of the DNA repair defect in xeroderma pigmentosum group G cells by a human cDNA related to yeast RAD2. *Nature*, Vol.363, No.6425, (May 1993), pp. 182-185

Schwartz, SM., Daling, JR., Doody, DR., Wipf, GC., Carter, JJ., Madeleine, MM., Mao, EJ., Fitzgibbons, ED., Huang, S., Beckmann, AM., McDougall, JK. & Galloway, DA. (1998). Oral cancer risk in relation to sexual history and evidence of human papillomavirus infection. *Journal of the National Cancer Institute*, Vol.90, No.21, (November 1998), pp. 1626-1636

Schwartz, SR., Yueh, B., McDougall, JK., Daling, JR. & Schwartz, SM. (2001). Human papillomavirus infection and survival in oral squamous cell cancer: a population-based study. *Otolaryngology Head and Neck Surgery,* Vol.125, No.1, (July 2001), pp. 1-9

Schwenger, JU., von Buchwald, C. & Lindeberg, H. (2002). Oral focal epithelial hyperplasia. Any risk of confusion with oral condylomas? *Ugeskrift for Laeger,* Vol.164, No.37, (September 2002), pp. 4287-4290

Scully, C., Maitland, NJ., Cox, MF. & Prime, SS. (1987). Human papillomavirus DNA and oral mucosa. *Lancet*, Vol.7, No.1(8528), (February 1987), pp. 336

Sedaghat, AR., Zhang, Z., Begum, S., Palermo, R., Best, S., Ulmer, KM., Levine, M., Zinreich, E., Messing, BP., Gold, D., Wu, AA., Niparko, KJ., Kowalski, J., Hirata, RM., Saunders, JR., Westra, WH. & Pai, SI. (2009). Prognostic significance of human papillomavirus in oropharyngeal squamous cell carcinomas. *The Laryngoscope,* Vol.119, No.8, (August 2009), pp. 1542-1549

Sedlacek, TV., Lindheim, S., Eder, C., Hasty, L., Woodland, M., Ludomirsky, A. & Rando, RK. (1989). Mechanism for human papillomavirus transmission at birth. *American Journal of Obstetrics & Gynecology*, Vol.161, No.1, (July 1989), pp. 55-59

Shah, JP. & Patel, SG. (2003). *Head and neck surgery and oncology*. New York : Mosby, pp. 232-236, 352

Shen, J., Tate, JE., Crum, CP. & Goodman, ML. (1996). Prevalence of human papillomaviruses (HPV) in benign and malignant tumors of the upper respiratory tract. *Modern Pathology,* Vol.9, No.1, (January 1996), pp. 15-20

Silverberg, MJ., Thorsen, P., Lindeberg, H., Grant, LA. & Shah, KV. (2003). Condyloma in pregnancy is strongly predictive of juvenile-onset recurrent respiratory papillomatosis. *Obstetrics & Gynecology,* Vol.101, No.4, (April 2003), pp. 645-652

Sinha, P., Logan, HL. & Mendenhall, WM. (2011). Human papillomavirus, smoking, and head and neck cancer. *American Journal of Otolaryngology,* ahead of print, (May 2011)

Sisk, J., Schweinfurth, JM., Wang, XT. & Chong, K. (2006). Presence of human papillomavirus DNA in tonsillectomy specimens. *The Laryngoscope,* Vol.116, No.8, (August 2006), pp. 1372-1374

Smith, EM., Pignatari, SS., Gray, SD., Haugen, TH. & Turek, LP. (1993). Human papillomavirus infection in papillomas and nondiseased respiratory sites of patients with recurrent respiratory papilomatosis using the polymerase chain reaction. *Archives of Otolaryngology-Head & Neck Surgery*, Vol.119, No.5, (May 1993), pp. 554-557

Smith, EM., Johnson, SR., Cripe, T., Perlman, S., McGuinness, G., Jiang, D., Cripe, L. & Turek, LP. (1995). Perinatal transmission and maternal risks of human papillomavirus infection. *Cancer Detection and Prevention,* Vol.19, No.2, (1995), pp. 196-205

Smith, EM., Hoffman, HT., Summersgill, KS., Kirchner, HL., Turek, LP. & Haugen, TH. (1998). Human papillomavirus and risk of oral cancer. *Laryngoscope*, Vol.108, No.7, (July 1998), pp. 1098-1013

Smith, EM., Ritchie JM., Summersgill KF., Klussmann JP., Lee JH., Wang D., Haugen TH. & Turek LP. (2004a). Age, sexual behavior and human papillomavirus infection in oral cavity and oropharyngeal cancers. *International Journal of Cancer,* Vol.108, No.5, (February 2004), pp. 766-772

Smith, EM., Ritchie, JM., Yankowitz, J., Swarnavel, S., Wang, D., Haugen, TH. & Turek, LP. (2004b). Human papillomavirus prevalence and types in newborns and parents : concordance and modes of transmission. *Sexually Transmitted Diseases*, Vol.31, No.1, (January 2004), pp. 57-62

Smith, EM., Ritchie, JM., Yankowitz, J., Wang, D., Turek, LP. & Haugen, TH. (2004c). HPV prevalence and concordance in the cervix and oral cavity of pregnant women. *Infectious Diseases in Obstetrics and Gynecology*, Vol.12, No.2, (June 2004), pp. 45-56

Smith, EM., Swarnavel, S., Ritchie, JM., Wang, D., Haugen, TH. & Turek, LP. (2007). Prevalence of human papillomavirus in the oral cavity/oropharynx in a large population of children and adolescents. *The Pediatric Infectious Disease Journal*, Vol.26, No.9, (September 2007), pp. 836-840

Smith, KA., Meisenburg, BL., Tam, VL., Pagarigan, RR., Wong, R., Joea, DK., Lantzy, L., Carillo, MA., Gross, TM., Malyankar, UM., Chiang, CS., Da Silva,DM., Kündig, TM., Kast, WM., Qiu, Z. & Bot, A. (2009). Lymph node-targeted immunotherapy mediates potent immunity resulting in regression of isolated or metastatic human papillomavirus-transformed tumors. *Clinical Cancer Research*, Vol.15, No.19, (October 2009), pp. 6167-6176

Smith, EM., Parker, MA., Rubenstein, LM., Haugen, TH., Hamsikova, E. & Turek, LP. (2010). Evidence for vertical transmission of HPV from mothers to infants. *Infectious Diseases in Obstetrics and Gynecology*, (2010), pp. 1-7

Snijders, PJ., Cromme, FV., van den Brule, AJ., Schrijnemakers, HF., Snow, GB., Meijer, CJ. & Walboomers, JM. (1992). Prevalence and expression of human papillomavirus in tonsillar carcinomas, indicating a possible viral etiology. *International Journal of Cancer*, Vol.51, No.6, (July 1992), pp. 845-850

Spanos, WC., Nowicki P., Lee, DW., Hoover, A., Hostager, B., Gupta, A., Anderson, ME. & Lee, JH. (2009). Immune response during therapy with cisplatin or radiation for human papillomavirus-related head and neck cancer. *Archives of Otolaryngology Head & Neck Surgery*, Vol.135, No.11, (November 2009), pp. 1137-1146

Stanley, MA. (2006). Immune responses to human papillomavirus. *Vaccine*, Vol.24, Suppl1, (March 2006), pp. S1/16-S1/22

Stanley, MA. (2009). Immune responses to human papilloma viruses. *Indian Journal of Medical Research*, Vol.130, No.3, (September 2009), pp. 266-276

Stremlau, A., Zenner, HP., Gissmann, L. & zur Hausen, H. (1987). Demonstration and organizational structure of the DNA of human papillomaviruses in laryngeal and hypopharyngeal carcinomas. *Laryngologie, Rhinologie, Otologie*, Vol.66, No.6, (June 1987), pp. 311-315

Strome, SE., Savva, A., Brissett, AE., Gostout, BS., Lewis, J., Clayton, AC., McGovern, R., Weaver, AL., Persing, D. & Kasperbauer, JL. (2002). Squamous cell carcinoma of the tonsils : a molecular analysis of HPV associations. *Clinical Cancer Research*, Vol.8, No.4, (April 2002), pp. 1093-1100

Sturgis, EM. & Cinciripini, PM. (2007). Trends in head and neck cancer incidence in relation to smoking prevalence: an emerging epidemic of human papillomavirus-associated cancers? *Cancer*, Vol.110, No.7, (October 2007), pp. 1429-1435

Sugiyama, M., Bhawal, UK., Dohmen, T., Ono, S., Miyauchi, M. & Ishikawa, T. (2003). Detection of human papillomavirus-16 and HPV-18 DNA in normal, dysplastic, and malignant oral epithelium. *Oral Surgery, Oral Medicine, Oral Pathology, Oral Radiology & Endodontics*, Vol.95, No.5, (May 2003), pp. 594-600

Summersgill, KF., Smith, EM., Levy, BT., Allen, JM., Haugen, TH. & Turek, LP. (2001). Human papillomavirus in the oral cavities of children and adolescents. *Oral and Maxillofacial Pathology*, Vol.91, No.1, (January 2001), pp. 62-69

Syrjänen, K., Syrjänen, S., Lamberg, M., Pyrhönen, S. & Nuutinen, J. (1983). Morphological and immunohistochemical evidence suggesting human papillomavirus (HPV) involvement in oral squamous cell carcinogenesis. *International Journal of Oral & Maxillofacial Surgery*, Vol.12, No.6, (December 1983), pp. 418-424

Syrjänen, S., Syrjänen, K., Mäntyjärvi, R., Collan, Y. & Kärjä, J. (1987). Human papillomavirus DNA in squamous cell carcinomas of the larynx demonstrated by in situ DNA hybridization. *ORL: Journal for Oto-Rhino-Laryngology and Its Related Specialties*, Vol.49, No.4, (1987), pp. 175-186

Syrjänen, S. & Puranen, M. (2000). Human papillomavirus infections in children : the potential role of maternal transmission. *Critical Reviews in Oral Biology & Medicine*, Vol.11, No.2, (2000), pp. 259-274

Syrjänen, S. (2003). Human papillomavirus infections and oral tumors. *Medical Microbiology and Immunology*, Vol.192, No.3, (August 2003), pp. 123-128

Syrjänen, S. (2004). HPV infections and tonsillar carcinoma. *Journal of Clinical Pathology*, Vol.57, No.5, (May 2004), pp. 449-455

Syrjänen, S. (2010). Current concepts on human papillomavirus infections in children. *Acta Pathologica, Microbiologica et Immunologica Scandinavica*, Vol.118, No.6-7, (June 2010), pp. 494-509

Syrjänen, S., Lodi, G., von Bültzingslöwen, I., Aliko, A., Arduino, P., Campisi, G., Challacombe, S., Ficarra, G., Flaitz, C., Zhou, HM., Maeda, H., Miller, C. & Jontell, M. (2011). Human papillomaviruses in oral carcinoma and oral potentially malignant disorders: a systematic review. *Oral Diseases*, Vol.17, Suppl.1, (April 2011), pp. 58-72

Szarka, K., Tar, I., Fehér, E., Gáll, T., Kis, A., Tóth, ED., Boda, R., Márton, I. & Gergely, L. (2009). Progressive increase of human papillomavirus carriage rates in potentially malignant and malignant oral disorders with increasing malignant potential. *Oral Microbiology and Immunology*, Vol.24, No.4, (August 2009), pp. 314-318

Szydlowski, J., Durzynski, L., Myga, M., Grzegorowski, M. & Gozdzicka-Józefiak, A. (2004). Human papillomavirus DNA presence of the upper respiratory tract mucosa of healthy children. *Otolaryngologia Polska*, Vol.58, No.1, (2004), pp. 211-215

Tenti, P., Zappatore, R., Migliora, P., Spinello, A., Maccarini, U., De Benedittis, M., Vesentini, N., Marchitelli, G., Silini, E. & Carnevali, L. (1997). Latent human papillomavirus infection in pregnant women at term : a case-control study. *Journal of Infectious Diseases*, Vol.176, No.1, (July 1997), pp. 277-280

Tenti, P., Zappatore, R., Migliora, P., Spinillo, A., Belloni, C. & Carnevali, L. (1999). Perinatal transmission of human papillomavirus from gravidas with latent infections. *Obstetrics & Gynecology*, Vol.93, No.4, (April 1999), pp. 475-479

Terai, M., Hashimoto, K., Yoda, K. & Sata, T. (1999). High prevalence of human papillomaviruses in the normal oral cavity of adults. *Oral Microbiology and Immunology*, Vol.14, No.4, (August 1999), pp. 201-205

Termine, N., Panzarella, V., Falaschini, S., Russo, A., Matranga, D., Lo Muzio, L. & Campisi, G. (2008). HPV in oral squamous cell carcinoma vs head and neck squamous cell carcinoma biopsies: a meta-analysis (1988-2007). *Annals of Oncology*, Vol.19, No.10, (October, 2008), pp. 1681-1690

Thomas, M. & Banks, L. (1999). Human papillomavirus (HPV) E6 interactions with Bak are conserved amongst E6 proteins from high and low risk HPV types. *Journal of General Virology*, Vol.80, Pt 6, (June 1999), pp. 1513-1517

Tominaga, S., Fukushima, K., Nishizaki, K., Watanebe, S., Masuda, Y. & Ogura H. (1996). Presence of human papillomavirus type 6f in tonsillar condyloma acuminatum and clinically normal tonsillar mucosa. *Japanese Journal of Clinical Oncology*, Vol.26, No.6, (December 1996), pp. 393-397

Tseng, CJ., Liang, CC., Soong, YK. & Pao, CC. (1998). Perinatal transmission of human papillomavirus in infants : relationship between infection rate and mode of delivery. *Obstetrics & Gynecology*, Vol.91, No.1, (January 1998), pp. 92-96

Tung, YC., Lin, KH., Chu, PY., Hsu, CC. & Kuo, WR. (1999). Detection of human papilloma virus and Epstein-Barr virus DNA in nasopharyngeal carcinoma by polymerase chain reaction. *The Kaohsiung Journal of Medical Sciences*, Vol.15, No.5, (May 1999), pp. 256-262

Tyan, YS., Liu, ST., Ong, WR., Chen, ML., Shu, CH. & Chang, YS. (1993). Detection of Epstein-Barr virus and human papillomavirus in head and neck tumors. *Journal of Clinical Microbiology*, Vol.31, No.1, (January 1993), pp. 53-56

Uobe, K., Masuno, K., Fang, YR., Li, LJ., Wen, YM., Ueda, Y. & Tanaka, A. (2001). Detection of HPV in Japanese and Chinese oral carcinomas by in situ PCR. *Oral Oncology*, Vol.37, No.2, (February 2001), pp. 146-152

Vambutas, A., Bonagura, VR. & Steinberg, BM. (2000). Altered expression of TAP-1 and major histocompatibility complex class I in laryngeal papillomatosis: correlation of TAP-1 with disease. *Clinical and Diagnostic Laboratory Immunology*, Vol.7, No.1, (January 2000), pp. 79-85

Van Doornum, GJ., Hooykaas, C., Juffermans, LH., van der Lans, SM., van der Linden, MM., Coutinho, RA. & Quint, WG. (1992). Prevalence of human papillomavirus infections among heterosexual men and women with multiple sexual partners. *Journal of Medical Virology*, Vol.37, No.1, (May 1992) pp. 13-21

Wansom, D., Light, E., Worden, F., Prince, M., Urba, S., Chepeha, DB., Cordell, K., Eisbruch, A., Taylor, J., D'Silva, N., Moyer, J., Bradford, CR., Kurnit, D., Kumar, B., Carey, TE. & Wolf, GT. (2010). Correlation of cellular immunity with human papillomavirus 16 status and outcome in patients with advanced oropharyngeal cancer. *Archives of Otolaryngology-Head & Neck Surgery*, Vol.136, No.12, (December 2010), pp. 1267-1273

Watanabe, S., Ogura, H., Fukushima, K. & Yabe, Y. (1993). Comparison of virapap filter hybridization with polymerase chain reaction and southern blot hybridization methods for detection of human papillomavirus in tonsillar and pharyngeal cancers. *European Archives of Oto-Rhino-Laryngology*, Vol.250, No.2, (1993), pp. 115-119

Watts, DH., Koutsky, LA., Holmes, KK., Goldman, D., Kuypers, J., Kiviat, NB. & Galloway, DA. (1998). Low risk of perinatal transmission of human papillomavirus : results from a prospective cohort study. *American Journal of Obstetrics and Gynecology*, Vol.178, No.2, (February 1998), pp. 365-373

Whiteside, TL. (1999). Signaling defects in T lymphocytes of patients with malignancy. *Cancer Immunology Immunotherapy*, Vol.48, No.7, (October 1999), pp. 346-352

Whiteside, TL. (2005). Immunobiology of head and neck. *Cancer and Metastasis Reviews*, Vol.24, No.1, (January 2005), pp. 95-105

Williams, GR., Lu, QL., Love, SB., Talbot IC. & Northover, JM. (1996). Properties of HPV-positive and HPV-negative anal carcinomas. *The Journal of Pathology,* Vol.180, No.4, (December 1996), pp. 378-382

Williams, R., Lee, DW., Elzey, BD., Anderson, ME., Hostager, BS. & Lee, JH. (2009). Preclinical models of HPV+ and HPV- HNSCC in mice : an immune clearance of HPV+ HNSCC. *Head and Neck,* Vol.31, No.7, (July 2009), pp. 911-918

Winer, RL., Lee, S-K., Hughes, JP., Adam, DE., Kiviat, NB. & Koutsky, LA. (2003). Genital human papillomavirus infection : incidence and risk factors in a cohort of female university students. *American Journal of Epidemiology,* Vol.157, No.3, (February 2003), pp. 218-226

Yeudall, WA. & Campo, MS. (1991). Human papillomavirus DNA in biopsies of oral tissues. *Journal of General Virology,* Vol.72, No.1, (January 1991), pp. 173-176

You, J., Croyle, JL., Nishimura, A., Ozato, K. & Howley, PM. (2004). Interaction of the bovine papillomavirus E2 protein with Brd4 tethers the viral DNA to host mitotic chromosomes. *Cell,* Vol.117, No.3, (April 2004), pp. 349-360

Young, MRI., Wright, MA., Lozano, Y., Matthews, JP., Benefield, J. & Prechel, MM. (1996). Mechanisms of immune suppression in patients with head and neck cancer: influence on the immune infiltrate of the cancer. *International Journal of Cancer,* Vol.67, No.3, (July 1996), pp. 333-338

Zeuss, MS., Miller CS. & White DK. (1991). In situ hybridization analysis of human papillomavirus DNA in oral mucosal lesions. *Oral Surgery, Oral Medicine, Oral Pathology, Oral Radiology and Endodontology,* Vol.71, No.6, (June 1991), pp. 714-720

Zhang, ZY, Sdek, P., Cao, J. & Chen, WT. (2004). Human papillomavirus type 16 and 18 DNA in oral squamous cell carcinoma and normal mucosa. *International Journal of Oral and Maxillofacial Surgery,* Vol.33, No.1, (January 2004), pp. 71-74

Zhao, D., Xu QG., Chen XM. & Fan, MW. (2009). Human papillomavirus as an independent predictor in oral squamous cell cancer. *International Journal of Oral Science,* Vol.1, No.3, (September 2009), pp. 119-125

zur Hausen, H. & de Villiers, EM. (1994). Human papillomaviruses. *Annual Review of Microbiology,* Vol.48, (1994), pp. 427-447

11

The Role of Human Papillomavirus in Head and Neck Cancers

Lucinei Roberto Oliveira[1], Andrielle Castilho-Fernandes[2], Alícia Greyce Turatti Pessolato[2], Régia Caroline Peixoto Lira[2], João Paulo Oliveira-Costa[2], Luciana Souza Chavasco[1], Fabiana Alves Miranda[2], Ivan de Oliveira Pereira[1], Edson Garcia Soares[2] and Alfredo Ribeiro-Silva[2]

1. Introduction

Tobacco and alcohol are well-established risk factors for head and neck squamous cell carcinomas (HNSCC), but it can also develop in individuals not exposed to them. However, only a small proportion of tobacco exposed individuals have developed HNSCC, and there is an emerging tumoral population who lack exposure to these mentioned risk factors, suggesting that others factors can play a role in head and neck carcinogenesis. Over the past two decades, the role of high-risk human papilloma virus (HPV) has been studied through several studies worldwide, and data supporting its role as a causative agent in the development and progression of a subset of HNSCC has been controversial, with considerable variability in frequency depending on the population studied, tumor localization, quality of samples and technical resources utilized for HPV detection. As is the case in cervical and anogenital carcinomas, the most frequently detected high-risk HPVs in HNSCC are the 16 and 18 genotypes. The tonsils and oropharynx are the specific sites associated with higher risk of HPV oncogenic transformation, and investigations suggest that HPV infection in these anatomic sites is an independent risk factor for carcinogenesis. The establishment and maintenance of HPV genomes in the squamous epithelium and HPV-related HNSCC cancer is believed to be originated by oncogenic potential of HPV integration into host DNA genome and their ability to manipulate cell cycle regulators, resulting in deregulated expression of oncoproteins such as E6, which promotes degradation of the tumor suppressor protein p53, allowing cells to evade cell cycle checkpoints, and also E7, which binds to retinoblastoma protein (pRb) and could promote the entrance in S1 phase of cell cycle, leading to disruption of normal cell cycle controls. Following cell division, infected cells leave the basal layer, migrate towards the suprabasal regions and begin to differentiate. Increased understanding of cervical pathogenesis has led to confirmation of HPV as an etiological agent for cancers and consequently to the development of preventive vaccines targeting HPV antigens for the control of cervical cancer. The HPV vaccine was developed as a result of the achievement of core technologies able to produce virus-like

[1] *Vale do Rio Verde University, Brazil*
[2] *Ribeirao Preto Medical School, University of Sao Paulo, Brazil*

particles (VLPs). The recombinant DNA was used to generate VLPs able to mimicking the natural virus and eliciting high-titers of virus neutralizing antibodies. With the progress through advanced stages of clinical trials and further exploration of combinatorial strategies, there is a great promise for significant advances also in the field of therapeutic HPV vaccine development. We recently conducted a study with the purpose of investigate the presence of HPV in a Brazilian population sample of HNSCC patients. In cases with positive specimens, the analysis was extended to clinicopathological profile characterization and to the correlation between patient survival and HPV DNA presence in primary HNSCC tumors as well as in their corresponding matched samples of recurrences, lymph nodal metastasis and necropsies. This research was conducted on the medical files of patients with head and neck tumors, the histopathological diagnosis of HNSCC was confirmed and paraffin-embedded specimens were selected for investigation. Moreover, in this chapter we discuss the current status of HPV vaccines as well as the main associated factors that interfere on establishment of strategies that better could act to control the infections and development of malignant neoplasias.

2. Historical aspects

One of the earliest manifestations of HPV infection was observed during an autopsy performed in 1974 on the embalmed body of an ancient Egyptian worker from 12th century BC who had a wart on the sole of his foot (Onon, 2010, as cited in McCaffery, 1974). The Ancient Greeks and Romans had already recognized that genital warts could be sexually transmitted (Onon, 2010, as cited in Claude Moore Health Sciences Library, 2011); however, the viral origin of warts was only confirmed in the 19th century (Onon, 2010, as cited in Ciuffo, 1907). By the early 1970s, the herpes simplex virus type 2 was thought to be the sexually transmitted etiologic factor that was responsible for cervical cancer (Onon, 2010, as cited in Klein, 1973). However, Harald Zur Hausen, a young German professor of virology, was not convinced of this hypothesis, and in 1976, he postulated that papilloma viruses play a role in cancer of the cervix. Papilloma viruses have now been well established as the cause of almost 100% of cervical carcinomas (Kumaraswamy & Vidhya, 2011).

The link between HPV and HNSCC was first studied by Syrjänen et al. (1983) in a light microcopy examination of 40 biopsy specimens from oral squamous cell carcinomas (OSCC), when the authors observed changes that are characteristic of HPV infection in 16 of the lesions. Recently, several studies have addressed the presence and prevalence of HPV in these types of tumors (Kumaraswamy & Vidhya, 2011). However, although the discovery of HPV has suggested that the virus may be a possible etiologic factor of oral pre-cancer and cancer, this association has not been as consistent as in cervical cancers.

3. Head and neck cancer

Head and neck malignancies compose a heterogeneous group and are believed to originate from sequential mutations that can occur as a consequence of progressive genetic instability and/or environmental factors, such as tobacco and alcohol consumption. These pathologies include a number of different types of cancer that arise from a variety of sites in the upper aerodigestive tract. Analysis of these tumors has revealed a heterogeneous neoplastic process that involves numerous sites with unique sets of epidemiologic, histopathologic, and treatment considerations. Approximately 40% of head and neck cancers occur in the oral cavity, 15% occur in the pharynx, 25% occur in the larynx and the remaining tumors occur in other sites (Dobrossy, 2005). The most frequent histological type is the squamous cell carcinoma, which occurs in over 95% of cases. Squamous cell carcinomas originate from the epithelial surface of the oral cavity, oropharynx, hypopharynx, and larynx and affect approximately 500.000 patients worldwide each year (Popović et al., 2010). Low survival rates have been presented across several studies worldwide and reflect the need for more careful attention to HNSCCs. Because the mortality rates have essentially remained unchanged over the last several decades, considerable interest lies in discovering prognostic markers to guide therapeutic planning.

4. HPV

Papillomaviruses are a family of pathogens that infect exclusively the epithelial tissues of amphibians, reptiles, birds and mammals (Franceschi, 2007). The viruses are grouped according to the anatomic site of infection and their preference for either cutaneous or mucosal squamous epithelium. The cutaneous types, or beta papillomaviruses, are usually found in the general population and cause common warts. In contrast, the alpha, or mucosotropic, papillomaviruses have been implicated in mucosal infections (Snow & Laudadio, 2010; Vidal & Gillison, 2008). The mucosotropic group of human papillomavirus comprises 15 species and infects the anogenital tract, upper aerodigestive tract and other head and neck mucosa. Because they are sexually transmitted and play important roles in diseases, these viruses have received much attention and research and clinical investment (Chow et al., 2010).

The HPV genome is a small (55 nm), double-stranded DNA molecule of approximately 8.000 base pairs, and it contains three identified regions: a late region (L) containing two genes, L1 and L2, which encode the viral capsid proteins; an early region (E) encoding proteins involved in viral DNA replication and the control of viral transcription, such as E1 and E2, and the main transforming genes E6, E7 and E5; and a long control region (LCR), found between the L and E regions, which contains several binding sites for nuclear and viral transcriptional factors, promoter sequences and an open reading frame (ORF) region (Fernandes et al., 2009). The early and late gene regions are both protein-encoding, but the LCR is non-encoding. The LCR possesses numerous binding sites for many repressors and activators of transcription, suggesting that this region may play a role in determining the range of hosts for specific HPV types (Tanzi et al., 2009).

Traditionally, the papillomaviruses have been classified by type and by the ORF L1 region because this region is greatly conserved along the viral genome and has been used to detect new types of papillomavirus for more than 15 years. However, other genomic regions can also be used (i.e., E6 and E7). Each genotype is characterized as being more than 10% different from all other genotypes in their specific regions of DNA sequences. Differences of 2% to 10% define a subtype and less than 2% define a viral variant. Closely related types (approximately 80-90% identical) are classified as members of the same species, and they tend to share important biological properties, such as tissue tropism, disease manifestation, and pathogenicity (Chow et al., 2010; De Villiers et al., 2004). Currently, well over 120 different genotypes of HPVs have been isolated, sequenced and phylogenetically characterized. Thirty-three percent of these 120 genotypes are known to infect the human genital tract (De Villiers et al., 2004; Hennessey et al., 2009, as cited in Longworth & Laimins, 2004; Martinez et al., 2007). Mucosotropic HPVs can be further classified into non-oncogenic, or low-risk, types or as potentially oncogenic, or high-risk, types. Mucosal and genital HPVs can be divided into low-risk (HPVs 6, 11, 40, 42, 43, 44, 54, 61, 70, 72, 81) and high-risk (HPVs 16, 18, 31, 33, 35, 51, 52) types according to their presence in malignant lesions (Bosch et al., 2002; Muñoz et al., 2003). HPVs 31, 33, 35, 51 and 52 are sometimes regarded as "intermediate risk" viruses because they are more common in mild or severe dysplastic lesions than in carcinomas (Fernandes et al., 2009).

The late region units L1 and L2 encode for viral capsid proteins during the late stages of virion assembly (Park et al., 1995). The protein encoded by L1 is highly conserved among different papilloma virus species; accordingly, antibodies against the bovine papilloma virus have been used to identify HPV capsid proteins in human tissues. The minor capsid protein encoded by L2 has more sequence variations than that of the L1 protein; hence, the L2 protein has been a source of antigen for specific types of HPV antibodies. The E1 and E2 region units encode proteins that are vital for extrachromosomal DNA replication and completion of the viral life cycle. The E2 protein is modular and contains an N-terminal activation domain that is important for viral transcription and replication and for interaction with host chromosomes during mitosis. The E2 region also encodes two proteins, one of which inhibits transcription of the early region, while the other increases the transcription of the early region (Ward et al., 1989). The HPV E5 proteins are small, extremely hydrophobic, and located mainly at the endosomal membranes, Golgi apparatus and, to a lesser extent, the plasma membranes. Moreover, E5 proteins are traditionally known to interact with the transmembrane domain of the EGF receptor and to modulate its concentration and phosphorylation (Villa et al., 2002). When present, E5 interacts with various transmembrane proteins, such as the EGF receptors, platelet-derived growth factor β, and colony stimulating factor-1 (Talbert-Slagle & DiMaio, 2009).

The multiplicity of functions of the three small papillomavirus oncoproteins, E5, E6 and E7, continues to be amazing. Specifically, more than a dozen protein-protein interactions between E6 and cellular proteins have been published (Villa et al., 2002). In the protein-encoding regions, the E6 and E7 ORF are considered to play the most important roles. These units encode for oncoproteins that allow viral replication and the immortalization and transformation of the cell that host the HPV DNA (Doorbar et al., 1991).

Mucosal high-risk E6 proteins are best known for their ability to associate with the cellular tumor suppressor p53. The association of E6 with p53 leads to degradation of p53 via recruitment of an ubiquitin ligase, E6-AP, and results in the inhibition of the transcriptional regulatory activities of the p53 protein in tissue culture cells (Gonzalez et al., 2001; Jones & Münger, 1997). Similarly, the high-risk HPV E7 proteins are best known for their ability to associate with the cellular tumor suppressor pRb, and this association can promote pRb degradation (Jones & Münger, 1997) through a proteasome-mediated pathway that disrupts the capacity of pRb to bind and inactivate functionally cellular E2F transcription factors (Gonzalez et al., 2001). In addition to binding pRb, high-risk E7 proteins can bind to other pocket proteins (p107 and p130) that are related to pRb and interact with different members of the E2F family of transcription factors (Dyson et al., 1992). The inactivation of pocket proteins by E7 is necessary but not sufficient to elicit the transforming potential of E7 (Phelps et al., 1992). High-risk E7 is also purported to complex with cyclins (Dyson et al.,

1992) and to inactivate the cyclin associated kinase inhibitors p21 and p27 (Jones & Münger, 1997). Thus, E7 can associate with and/or alter the activities of multiple cellular factors that normally contribute to the regulation of the cell cycle. The oncogenic properties of E6 and E7 and their effects on p53 and pRb have provided the general basis for further investigations of the role of HPV in carcinogenesis. The research examining the actions of these two oncoproteins has shown how they can subvert key cell cycle and regulatory processes, such as cyclins, cyclin-dependent kinases (CDKs) and cyclin-dependent kinase inhibitors (CDIs), to transform and immortalize the host cells (Southern & Herrington, 2000).

Proving the importance of p53 and pRb in cell cycle progression, the repression of HPV 16 E6 and E7 expression by dual shRNA transfection has been shown to be capable of restoring the p53 and pRb tumor suppressor pathways and activating apoptosis (Psyrri et al., 2009, Rampias et al., 2009). Thus, the demonstration of this tumor suppressor inactivation by the E6 and E7 HPV oncoproteins has provided a basic explanation for how the high-risk HPV types exert their oncogenic effects on cervical cells.

5. The route of cellular conquest by HPV

Unlike other viruses, HPV does not infect or replicate in antigen-presenting cells of the epithelium nor induce cell lysis, so there is no chance for antigen-presenting cells to present antigens derived from the virion to the immune system. Despite the observation that more than 50% of infections present seroconversion in the patients, the production of antibodies usually occurs only months after the initial infection (Vidal & Gillison, 2008, as cited in Tindle, 2002). The life cycle of papillomaviruses is closely tied to the epithelial differentiation process. Infection occurs exclusively in squamous epithelial cells (keratinocytes) with preference for the keratinocyte stem cell as the initial target of HPV infection (Vidal & Gillison, 2008). The route of entry for HPV infection is microtraumas or small wounds in the skin or mucosal surface. These breaks in the epithelial surface allow the virus to access and persist in the nuclei of infected basal layer cells of the epithelium. Until now, no single receptor has been definitively identified and established as being responsible for HPV entry. Some reports have suggested that a6 integrin may be a candidate receptor because it is expressed primarily during wound healing. The glycosaminoglycan heparin, a polysaccharide expressed on the cell surface, may also play a role in the attachment necessary for the initiation of HPV infection (Vidal & Gillison, 2008).

HPV uses the host cell DNA machinery to maintain the production of viral progeny. This mechanism of viral-induced cell growth is very well known and is analogous to other viruses that disrupt the control of cell growth (Hebner & Laimins, 2006). Following cell division, as the basal cells divide into squamous epithelial cells, HPV establishes its DNA genome in the host cell nuclei, replicates and reaches a high copy number. Infected cells then leave the basal layer, migrate toward the suprabasal regions and begin to differentiate. In the basal layer phase, the HPV genome is maintained at a low copy number, providing a type of stock of viral DNA for further use in cell divisions. At the same time, 'early' viral genes (E5, E6 and E7) are expressed, resulting in enhanced proliferation of the infected cells and their lateral expansion. While the basal cells and viral DNA divide, some daughter cells may be maintained in the basal layers, whereas other daughter cells move toward the upper layers of the epithelium and begin to differentiate. During the process in which the infected cells enter into the suprabasal layers, the viral genome replicates to a higher copy number;

'late' viral gene (L1 and L2) expression is initiated; and structural proteins, as such capsid proteins, are formed. Subsequently, virions are assembled and released as the upper layer of epithelium is shed, as shown in Figure 1 (Fehrmann & Laimins, 2003; Scheurer et al., 2005; Vidal & Gillison, 2008).

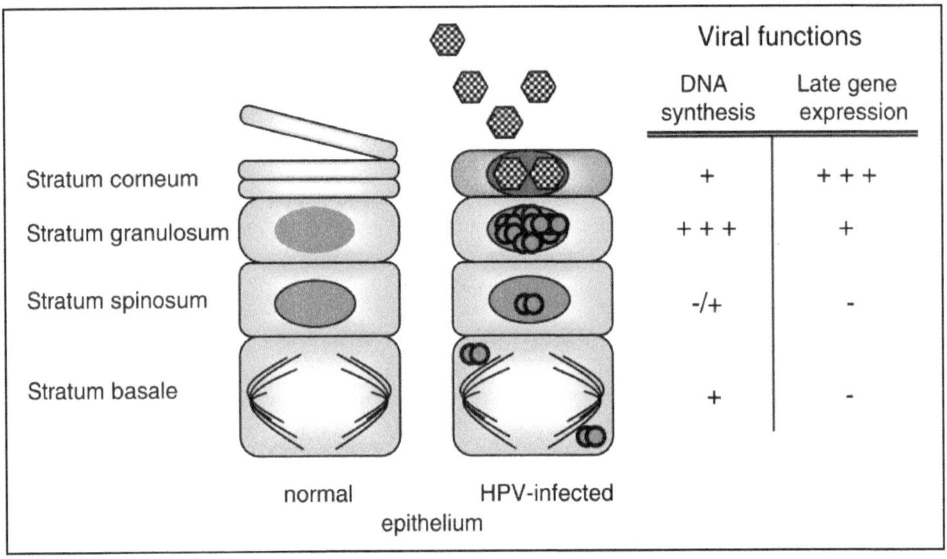

Fig. 1. Representation of normal and HPV-infected epithelium according to the cellular differentiation and the differentiation-dependent viral functions (Adapted from Fehrmann & Laimins, 2003).

HPV replication occurs through two mechanisms. The first mechanism occurs in the basal layer cells where the viral genome is distributed to daughter cells. In this mechanism, viral genome integration ensures a persistent infection in the proliferative cells from the basal layer and is associated with a higher risk of malignant cellular transformation. In the second mechanism, which is known as episomal or vegetative, HPV replication occurs in the more differentiated layers of the epithelium and the integration of viral DNA into the host cell genome is not necessary. Despite the fact that the replication processes and gene expression are controlled by the cell differentiation process, much about this mechanism is still unknown, and cervical cancer serves as a model for understanding HPV pathogenesis in other sites, such as in head and neck cancers (Zur Hausen, 2002). During cervical infection, the viral genome frequently integrates into the host cell genome. This integration occurs preferentially at fragile sites. The integration of viral DNA most likely disrupts the E2 coding region, causing the loss of the role of E2 in transcriptional control; therefore, the expression of the E6 and E7 oncoproteins becomes deregulated (Vidal & Gillison, 2008).

In tonsillar carcinomas, the absence of integrated HPV DNA does not suppress the expression of viral oncogenes, indicating that viral DNA integration is not an essential step for carcinogenesis and that the virus continues to be present in an episomal form (Hebner & Laimins, 2006; Vidal & Gillison, 2008). The mechanism used by HPV to remain in cancer tissue as an episomal form and produce high copy numbers is still unclear. However, some observations have shown that the oncoprotein E2 may serve as an 'anchor' that links episomal HPV to the cellular mitotic spindles (Psyrri et al., 2009).

6. How does HPV reach the head and neck sites?

Generational changes have occurred in sexual practices around the world, where the young people are having their first sexual experience at an earlier age, with greater numbers of sexual partners and with a higher probability of engaging in oral sex compared to individuals from earlier decades (Heck et al., 2010). These differences in sexual behavior can also be seen between patients with HPV-positive HNSCCs, especially among those with the high-risk type HPV-16 (Gillison et al., 2008).

In oropharyngeal cancers (OPCs) that are positive for HPV, a frequent association with sexual behavior has been found (D'Souza et al., 2007). An investigation of more than 5000 cases of head and neck cancer and more than 6000 control cases from 12 different countries has indicated that a history of six or more lifetime sexual partners and four or more oral sex partners increases the odds of developing OPC. In cancer at the base of tongue, this association was found among individuals who have two sexual partners compared to those with only one, while little evidence has indicated any association between sexual practice and cancers of the oral cavity or of the larynx. Additionally, an increased risk of tonsillar cancer is associated with a history of four or more oral sex partners (3-fold increased risk), age at sexual debut < 18 years among men (2-fold increased risk) and in husbands of women who presented cervical dysplasia or cancer (Lajer & Von Buchwald, 2010). In addition to oral sexual activity, open-mouthed kissing has been found to be associated with oral HPV infections. Because this practice is common among young people in many countries, it may contribute to HPV circulation and increase the risk of HPV infection among individuals who might not otherwise be exposed. The prevalence of HPV in control patients from the studies of oral cancer varies from 5% to 9%; however, the same sexual behaviors associated with HNSCC can increase the odds of HPV infection in this population. Interestingly, in patients with HNSCCs, heavier smoking and alcohol use is associated with risky sexual behaviors, but this association is not observed in control individuals without cancer (D'Souza et al., 2009).

No difference was noticed between men and women according the outcomes of oral sex or number of oral sex partners and lifetime sexual partners, and the prevalence of oral HPV was found to be similar between heterosexual and bisexual women. In contrast, the presence of oral HPV infection is unlikely in virgins and women who have sex with women, which suggests that oral HPV is more likely to be associated with sexual exposure to male partners than to female partners (Ragin et al., 2011).

7. HPV and oral lesions

In the oral cavity, 24 types of HPV (1, 2, 3, 4, 6, 7, 10, 11, 13, 16, 18, 30, 31, 32, 33, 35, 45, 52, 55, 57, 59, 69, 72 and 73) have been associated with benign lesions and 12 types (2, 3, 6, 11, 13, 16, 18, 31, 33, 35, 52 and 57) with malignant lesions (Bouda et al., 2000; Kojima et al., 2002). The low-risk HPV types cause benign oral hyperplasias that are usually painless and non-ulcerated (Cleveland, 2011). Verruca vulgaris (caused by HPV 2, HPV 4 and other HPV types) usually occurs on the lips, hard palate and gingiva. Condyloma acuminata or genital warts (caused by HPV 6 and HPV 11) may also affect the oral mucosa and are found more commonly on keratinized mucosa (Cleveland et al., 2011; D'Souza et al., 2007; Dayyani et al., 2010). Notwithstanding, since the first report of the presence of HPV DNA in head and neck cancer, 65 high-risk types have been consistently detected at different sites; however, these types are specifically found in transcriptionally active tumor cells (Vidal & Gillison, 2008). According to data from a review, 99% of HPV infections in head and neck cancers are by high-risk types 16, 18, 31 and 33 (Kreimer et al., 2005). Additionally, several others HPV types (6, 11, 35, 45, 51, 52, 56, 58, 59 and 68) have rarely been detected in head and neck cancer. Infection with HPV 33 accounts for up to 10% of positive head and neck cancers; however, the HPV 16 type is by far the most common type detected in head and neck cancer (Fakhry et al., 2008; Kreimer et al., 2005; Snow & Laudadio, 2010), and oropharyngeal tumors are more likely to have HPV 16 than other types at head and neck sites. The genotype 16 accounts for 78% to 100% of positive oropharyngeal cases, while HPV-18 accounts for only 1% of cases (Kreimer et al., 2005). Seropositivity for HPV 16 has a greater association with an increased risk of OPC (OR = 14.4) than with the development of oral cavity cancer (OR = 3.6). This association is particularly strong in individuals without a history of smoking or drinking (OR = 33.6) (Hennessey et al., 2009). An interesting prevalence profile of the HPV types has been observed in some investigations in the countryside of Sao Paulo state in Brazil, where a higher prevalence of HPV 18 than HPV 16 was found in oral and cervical carcinomas. Furthermore, the presence of HPV 18 was found to be associated with metastasis to the lymph nodes and shorter patient survival (Guimarães et al., 2010; Lira et al., 2010; Mazon et al., 2011).

The results from recent studies have suggested that some of these cancers, primarily those that originate in the oropharynx (and, more specifically, at the base of the tongue and the tonsils), are associated with high-risk HPV infection (Lopes et al., 2011). This association is strengthened by the fact that the same oncogenic HPV types detected in cervical carcinomas have been identified in head and neck cancers. In recent oral cancer guidelines published by the American Dental Association (ADA), HPV was recognized as a risk factor for OPCs, but whether HPV is also responsible for some oral cavity cancers was questioned (Rethman, 2010).

Several head and neck tumors have been analyzed for the presence of HPV, and HPV DNA has been found in different proportions of tumors from different head and neck sites (Kreimer et al., 2005; Syrjanen, 2005). Some evidence has indicated that some subtypes of HPV are linked to head and neck cancer, especially those arising from some oropharyngeal subsites (e.g., tonsil and the base of the tongue) (Gillespie et al., 2009). The overall HPV prevalence in HNSCC ranges from 3% to 40% and could vary more according to the specific site. HPV has been found in 4-80% of oral cancers, 15-85% of tonsillar cancers, approximately 24% of non-tumor site-specific HNSCC and 14-57% of OPCs (IARC, 2007; Kreimer et al., 2005; Machado et al., 2010; Syrjanen, 2005; Termine et al., 2008). Brazilian observations in the countryside of Sao Paulo state have found a low prevalence of HPV in tumors of the larynx (Miranda et al., 2009) and an increase in the presence of HPV DNA in oral cavity cancers during the past two decades (Lira et al., 2010; Mazon et al., 2011; Oliveira et al., 2008). The wide variation in HPV prevalence can be attributed to different detection techniques, small sample numbers, differences in the lesions and sampling techniques and epidemiological characteristics of the populations studied (Feller et al., 2010). Among the many methods to detect HPV infections, both polymerase chain reaction (PCR) and in situ hybridization assays have been well validated.

Because of the high sensitivity of the PCR assay, it may detect not only oncogenic infections but also productive infections, virions or laboratory artifacts, which are common problems in HPV screening for cervical cancer (Leemans et al., 2011). The following additional techniques can also provide data regarding the presence of HPV: light and electron microscopy, ELISA, gene expression by DNA microarray, Dot blot, Southern blot, hybrid capture and ligase chain reaction for probe amplification. Despite the existence of innumerable options for HPV detection in HNSCC, a standardization of procedures for routine application has yet to be developed (Feller et al., 2010; Kumaraswamy & Vidhya, 2011; Snow & Laudadio, 2010).

A global consensus exists regarding the increasing risk of OPCs with HPV, mainly in the tonsils and at the base of the tongue (Attner et al., 2010; Heck et al., 2010). A survey of the Surveillance, Epidemiology and End Results (SEER) database revealed that the incidence rates for HPV at the base of the tongue and in the tonsils increased by 2% and 4%, respectively, between 1973 and 2001 in younger US populations (ages 20-44 years). At the same time, the incidence in all other oral and pharyngeal sites remained constant or decreased (Gillespie et al., 2009). Other countries, such as Sweden, have seen a similar increase in the incidence of tonsil cancer from 1997-2002; HPV could be isolated in 23% of specimens in the 1970s, 28% in the 1980s, 57% in the 1990s and 68% in specimens since 2000 (Hammarstedt et al., 2006). A review of 60 studies of HPV prevalence, which was published in 2005, observed an overall prevalence of 26% of HPV in HNSCCs, with a greater percent at the oropharynx (36%) (Kreimer et al., 2005). Similar numbers were obtained from the results of a recent meta-analysis that included more than 5000 patients. Among all HNSCCs, 22% of cases presented HPV infection, and the subgroup of OPCs presented a prevalence of 41% (Dayyani et al., 2010). In the USA, approximately 40-80% of OPC cases are associated with HPV, whereas in Europe, the proportion ranges from 90% in Sweden to 20% in populations that contain a great number of heavy smokers (Marur et al., 2010).

Confirming the importance of HPV infection in HNSCC, the 2007 International Agency for Research on Cancer (IARC) monograph on HPV found sufficient evidence for HPV carcinogenicity in the oral cavity and oropharynx and limited evidence for HPV carcinogenicity in the larynx (IARC, 2007). Currently, the identification of distinct epidemiological profiles in HPV-positive and HPV-negative HNSCCs is possible. Although studies have shown no concordance regarding some of these epidemiological aspects, we may have to look at HPV-positive and HPV-negative HNSCCs in a separate manner in the future, including scientific, diagnostic, epidemiological and clinical aspects and the management of treatment. The main factors studied are heavy or no tobacco/marijuana exposure, heavy or mild alcohol consumption, poor or intact dentition, low or high oral sex exposure, age > 50 years or < 45 years, lower or higher socioeconomic status and deceasing or increasing incidence (Gillespie et al., 2009). The epidemiological trend suggests that HPV-positive HNSCC occurs more often in younger patients (age < 50 years), which differs from the typical characteristics of head and neck cancer (which is more frequent in men above 40 years old). The tumors associated with the presence of HPV usually appear strawberry-like and exophytic on gross inspection and occur more frequently in the tonsil and the base of tongue with a basaloid aspect, poor differentiation and cystic changes within metastatic lymph nodes

(Gillespie et al., 2009). In addition, gene expression profiles are known to be different in HPV-positive OPCs compared with HPV-negative cases (Lajer & Von Buchwald, 2010).

8. HPV in oropharyngeal cancer

The OPCs comprises tumors arising in posterior regions of oral cavity, and its incidence has been increasing, especially between individuals aged 40 to 55 years. It is accepted that a great part of OPCs, especially in lingual and palatine tonsils, are originated by HPV infection. Compared to non-contaminated individuals, the relative risk is 15- to 200- fold in HPV infected patients, and may not show a history of known risk factors for OPC, such tobacco and alcohol consumption, highlighting a different pattern for non-HPV-related OPC (Marur et al., 2008). Moreover, the presence of HPV is also associated to positive cervical lymph nodes of patients in different sites of HNSCCs, but mainly in oropharynx (Goldenberg et al., 2008; Lira et al., 2010; Machado et al., 2010).

Although oral and oropharyngeal HPV infections are primarily sexually acquired, other methods of contamination such as mouth to mouth contact between partners and between family members, besides autoinoculation, are also potential routes where HPV infection of oropharyngeal sites can be established. As oral and oropharyngeal subclinical HPV infection is not uncommon, it is possible that the epithelium may serve as a reservoir of virus (Feller et al., 2010).

The most common morphological presentation of HPV-related OPC is different of non-HPV tumors. The HPV OPCs usually are not associated with dysplasia of surface epithelium, show lobular growth, are usually infiltrated by lymphocytes and have prominent basaloid morphology. Two microscopic features of HPV-related OPCs are likely to cause diagnostic ambiguity. First, HPV-related HNSCC is customarily misperceived as a poorly differentiated carcinoma based on the immature appearance of the tumor cells. In point of fact, the appearance of the tumor cells closely emulates the appearance of the reticulated epithelium—the specialized epithelium lining the tonsillar crypts from which HPV-related cancers arise. Thus, HPV-related OPCs are in fact highly differentiated. Clinically, HPV-related tumors present mostly at an early T stage, but show an advanced nodal stage, generally presenting as stage III or IV tumors, although HPV-related OPCs usually have a better prognosis when compared to non-HPV tumors. Despite the HPV-associated OPC patients have a relatively better disease-free survival rate, some individuals develop recurrence of their cancers after treatment and dies from recurrent disease. Based in this condition, screening tests could be beneficial for the detection of disease persistence or of early disease, using unique markers associated with HPV infection (Feller et al., 2010).

9. HPV in laryngeal cancer

The relative frequency of HPV genotypes in carcinoma of the larynx is still unknown; several studies have demonstrated variable frequencies ranging from 8 to 58.8% (Hobbs et al., 2006; Psyrri et al., 2008). The larynx forms of contamination and transmission of the virus are sometimes speculative. Infections of the larynx, pharynx and esophagus can occur, especially at birth when the newborn passes through the birth canal and comes in contact with the fluid-contaminated site. Together with oral-genital transmission, puerperal infection is one explanation for the presence of HPV in the oral cavity, larynx and esophagus (Zur Hausen, 1996).

The potential oncogenic importance of low-risk types of HPV in the development of laryngeal papillomas is well established, and the predominant types are HPV 6 and 11 (Herrero et al. 2003; Madkan et al., 2007), which are pathogens of laryngeal papillomatosis. According to the clinical characteristics and natural history of disease, four different forms of laryngeal papillomas exist, namely isolated juvenile papillomatosis, juvenile multiple, adult and adult isolated multiple (Madkan et al. 2007; Torrente & Ojeda, 2007). More recently, this nomenclature has been replaced by recurrent respiratory papillomatosis (RRP), which more accurately describes the extent of the disease and its tendency to recur (Muenscher et al., 2008). Juvenile-onset laryngeal papillomas are associated with HPV transmitted by vertical transmission from a mother with active or latent anogenital infection. More than 30% of mothers with genital warts gave birth to children who developed juvenile-onset laryngeal papillomatosis. This disease occurs most commonly in first-born children and those who were delivered vaginally to young mothers with genital warts. Cases of children with laryngeal papillomatosis who were born by cesarean section are rare. The progression of papillomas is slow, causing the progressive symptoms of shortness of breath, persistent cough and dysphonia. Juvenile laryngeal papillomatosis affects both sexes equally. The most worrisome aspect of the disease is the spread of the virus thorough the tracheobronchial tree, progressing to pulmonary papillomatosis and often resulting in an uncontrollable and fatal infection. Another important event is the malignant transformation of laryngeal papillomas, which despite being a rare event, occurs in approximately 3-7% of cases.

The laryngeal papillomas of adult onset generally affect individuals with a higher number of sexual partners and greater frequency of orogenital contacts. The oral-genital transmission hypothesis is based on the fact that laryngeal papillomatosis and genital warts have the same associated HPV infections (HPV 6 and 11). The area of transition from cuboidal and cylindrical epithelium in the larynx and uterine cervix may favor the occurrence of HPV in this location (Torrente & Ojeda, 2007).

The premalignant lesions of the larynx are defined as morphologically altered tissue in which the occurrence of cancer is more likely than in apparently normal tissues. The detection of HPV DNA in premalignant lesions shows that HPV infection can be involved in the development of some lesions. Premalignant oral lesions usually develop as a result of several factors, such as tobacco and alcohol, and the synergistic interaction of HPV infection with these factors may play a role in the progression to cancer (Torrente & Ojeda, 2007). However, although HPV has been found in a large proportion of laryngeal cancers, more epidemiological and experimental studies are needed to clarify the role of HPV in laryngeal carcinomas.

10. Interaction between traditional risk factors and HPV infection in HNSCCs

Smoking and alcohol consumption are characteristics of patients with oral, oropharyngeal, hypopharyngeal, and laryngeal cancer. However, in the last 30 years, the presence of HPV associated with the increase in the incidence of HNSCCs at specific sites has suggested that the HPV infection can be a potential risk factor, independent of tobacco abuse and ethanol consumption (Blomberg et al., 2011; Chaturvedi et al., 2008; D'Souza et al., 2007; Hammarstedt et al., 2006; Klozar et al., 2010).

Several clarifying findings have recently been made in the scene of HPV in the head and neck. The traditional prototype of an OSCC patient used to be an older man who had smoked and consumed alcohol for many years. However, this profile no longer represents patients who are now diagnosed with oral cancer. The patients now are usually younger (< 60 years) Caucasians with no history of smoking or alcohol drinking (D'Souza et al., 2007; Gillison et al., 2008). The main risk factors, tobacco and alcohol, have been supplanted by other risk factors associated with HPV and sexual behavior, which include the number of sexual partners, a history of oral-genital and oral-anal sex. As a biomarker, the detection of HPV infection is emerging as a powerful method for identifying oral cancer. The presence and progress of the disease affects the selection of patients for specific treatments and tumor surveillance (Westra, 2009, as cited in Begum et al., 2003).

Whether the use of tobacco or alcohol and HPV are synergistic in the etiopathogenesis of oral and oropharyngeal cancers is not yet clear (Feller et al., 2010). Notably, many studies of HPV infection and exposure to tobacco have concluded that patients with tumors containing HPV DNA are characterized by moderate or no consumption of tobacco and alcohol, unlike individuals in the typical head and neck cancer patient population (D'Souza et al., 2007; Hafkamp et al., 2008; Klussmann et al., 2003). In research performed by Koch et al. (1999) a 2-fold higher rate of HPV-associated tumors was observed in noncurrent smokers compared to current smokers, although the group classified as noncurrent smokers included both never and former smokers (Sinha et al., 2011). However, small sized groups, weak statistical evidence, and inconsistent definitions of smoking status could limit some of these studies. No consensus exists regarding the definition of current, never or former smokers or the criteria of light vs. heavy smoking (Sinha et al., 2011).

In contrast, most of the studies that have noted a positive association between tobacco and HPV infection have had large sample sizes and adequate controls, which support consistent conclusions. A study that evaluated 201 cases of HNSCC using an ELISA assay to assess anti-HPV virus-like particles observed no interaction with alcohol in the oral cavity or oropharynx cancer, but a significant interaction between HPV and tobacco among oropharyngeal cases was obtained (Herrero et al., 2003; Smith et al., 2010). Other information provided by these studies is the influence of smoking intensity on disease survival. Heavy smoking of more than 20 pack-years has been associated with an increased hazard ratio of death (hazard ratio, 1.79) in patients with HPV-positive OPC compared to patients who smoke less than 20 pack-years (Gillison et al., 2009).

Although much of our understanding of HPV in HNSCCs is based on the model of cervical cancer, the degree of interaction between smoking and HPV in this type of cancer is still not well known. Biologically, smoking can suppress the mediators of immune function, facilitating the persistence of HPV infection and the development of cancer (Sinha et al., 2011). The DNA damage caused by smoking may impede the cell's ability to recuperate from mutagenic insults; together with an increase in p53 mutations, this impairment can produce fragile sites or "hot spots" of DNA breakage, which facilitates the integration of the virus into the host DNA (Sinha et al., 2011). Thus, genetic or epigenetic alterations caused by tobacco have also been postulated to accelerate disease progression in HPV-infected individuals (Maxwell et al., 2010; Sinha et al., 2011).

11. What can HPV tell us about prognosis and treatment?

Due to locoregional recurrences, distant metastases and second primary tumors, no substantial improvement in survival has been observed in patients with HNSCCs in recent decades (Leemans et al., 2011). Because multivariate analyses have pointed to HPV status as significant prognostic information in addition to the traditional established factors, the data suggest that HPV is the most important independent prognostic factor in HNSCC (Hannisdal et al., 2010; Lajer & Von Buchwald, 2010). HPV-infected HNSCCs have favorable prognoses upon treatment compared with HPV-negative tumors at a similar clinical stage (Leemans et al., 2011). Most investigations that have evaluated HPV infection and survival agree that HPV-positive patients have a significantly better survival (5-year survival of approximately 70%) than HPV-negative patients (5-year survival of approximately 35%) (Fakhry et al., 2008; Klozar et al., 2008; Vidal & Gillison, 2008). A prospective multicentric study has shown that individuals presenting HPV-positive OPCs had better response rates to chemotherapy than individuals with no HPV infection (Fakhry et al., 2008). Numerically, in the same study, the overall 2-year survival rate for those presenting HPV-positive tumors was 95% (95% CI = 87%-100%), compared with a 2-year survival rate of 62% (95% CI = 49%-74%) for those without HPV infection (Henessey et al., 2009). In other multicenter prospective trials evaluating treatment responses in oropharyngeal or laryngeal carcinomas, the HPV-positive OPCs were found to have higher response rates to chemotherapy (82% versus 55%) than HPV-negative cases (Fakhry et al., 2008). Other similar findings have been obtained in treatment response to radiotherapy associated with the presence and titer of the high-risk HPV 16 (Dayyani et al., 2010; Vidal & Gillison, 2008). This improved survival is more pronounced in OPCs (Dayyani et al., 2010; Hannisdal et al., 2010), and even in investigations with no significant associations, there is a tendency toward HPV positivity in patients with longer survival.

Although the improved prognosis conferred by HPV seems to be independent of the treatment strategy, the mechanism responsible for this survival difference is still unclear. Several hypotheses have been proposed, which include the fact that patients presenting HPV-related HNSCCs are usually non-smokers and non-drinkers and do not show comorbid disorders. Moreover, despite the lack of conclusion regarding the correlation of HPV positivity in some HNSCC sites with p53 status, an enhanced radiosensitivity of HPV-positive tumors due to an improved apoptotic response secondary to the absence of mutations in TP53 of HPV-positive tumors has been proposed, as has immune surveillance to viral-specific tumor antigens (Vidal & Gillison, 2008) and lack of field cancerization characteristics of individuals with tobacco- and alcohol-related HNSCCs (Hennessey et al., 2009).

12. Our results regarding HPV infection in Brazilian oral squamous cell carcinoma patients

The true prevalence of HPV DNA in OSCC and its role as a possible oncogenic agent are still controversial. We performed a study that aimed to investigate the HPV frequency in Brazilian patients with OSCC in order to establish a clinicopathological profile and its possible influence on prognosis (Oliveira et al., 2008). We examined the correlation between patient survival and HPV expression in primary tumors (PTs), and their matched samples (MSs) of recidives, lymph nodal metastasis (LNM) or necropsies. Eighty-seven PTs and their corresponding 87 MSs were tested for HPV infection through PCR using general and type-specific HPV primers. For HPV DNA detection, we utilized the GP5+/GP6+ (Bioneer Inc.) consensus general primer pair to amplify a 150-bp fragment from the L1 gene of general HPV types (GP5+, 5'-TTTGTTACTGTGGTAGATACTAC-3'; GP6+, 5'-GAAAAATAAACTGTAAATCATATTC-3'). After, PCR was then performed on the HPV-positive DNA samples to determine if they contained genotypes 16 and 18, using specific primers targeting ~100 bp in the E7 ORF: HPV-16E7.667 (5'-GATGAAATAGATGGTCCAGC-3'), HPV-16E7.774 (5'-GCTTTGTACGCACAACCGAAGC-3'), HPV-18E7.696 (5'-AAGAAAACGATGAAATAGATGGA-3') and HPV-18E7.799 (5'-GGCTTCACACTTACAACACA-3') (Bioneer Inc.). Of the 87 patients investigated, 17 (19.5%) were found to have HPV DNA in their tumors. An investigation of all the paraffin-embedded specimens revealed the presence of HPV DNA in 18 of the 174 samples (10.4%), 10 (11.5%) from PTs and 8 (9.2%) from MSs. Notwithstanding, no virus infection was detected in the corresponding PT of 7 (8.1%) MSs, and only a patient demonstrated HPV DNA positivity in both samples. The HPV genotypes 16 and 18 were detected in 4 (22.2%) and 3 (16.7%) of the positive samples, respectively. Infection with both genotypes was found in 6 (33.3%) investigated samples, and the HPV genotype was unidentified in 5 (27.8%) samples. The tongue was the most prevalent infected anatomical site. Our main result was a significant number of positive HPV samples among non-smoking patients, and albeit a possible influence of HPV on tumoral induction cannot be ruled out, the low frequency of HPV positive OSCC cases found in our investigation does not suggest that this virus has the same etiological influence on patients as tobacco consumption does, and although we cannot rule out a possible transient role for HPV in the induction of OSCC, we think that the occasional detection of HPV in OSCC resulting from the incidental colonization of tumoral lesions might reflect the true involvement of HPV in most investigations.

13. HPV vaccine

In many countries, vaccines against some HPV types are administered to girls and young women with the goal of protecting them against HPV-induced cervical cancer (Villa et al., 2005; Muñoz et al., 2010). The introduction of HPV vaccines has also drawn more attention to the fact that HPV is associated not only with cervical cancer and genital warts but also with other tumors, such as head and neck and anogenital cancers (Zur Hausen, 2006).

Although the majority of HPV vaccine research has focused on cervical cancer, some vaccine developers have targeted other diseases related to different strains of HPV, including two types of HPV (6 and 11) that can cause genital warts and recurrent respiratory papillomatosis in the larynx. Vaccines against these other strains have attracted the interest of vaccine developers because these vaccines may qualify for orphan drug status and fast-track licensing in the United States (Nventa Biopharmaceuticals Corporation, 2005; Path, 2006).

Emerging results from vaccine trials have suggested that some cross-protection is possible. Vaccines against cervical cancer also have the potential to prevent other cancers that are caused by the same types of HPV, including a subset of head and neck cancers (notably the OPC) (Herrero et al., 2003, Kreimer et al., 2005), and half or more of anogenital cancers outside the cervix, including cancer of the vulva, vagina, penis, and anus (Daling et al., 2005, Gross & Pfister 2004). Theoretically, these vaccines should also work against the same viruses at other anatomical sites. If proven to do so, this approach would represent a major conceptual breakthrough, not only in prevention of these diseases, but equally importantly, by providing the 'missing link' in the chain of evidence for the final proof of HPV etiology of these tumors (Syrjänen, 2010).

13.1 Types of HPV vaccines

The development of prophylactic and therapeutic vaccines targeting HPV antigens for the control of tumors caused by HPV is increasing worldwide. These upcoming vaccines are part of a new generation of vaccines that employ genetic engineering, using the ability to manipulate and transfer genes from one organism to another (Path, 2006).

Prophylactic vaccines work primarily by stimulating humoral immunity and inactivating HPV before the virus infects the host cells (Zinkernagel, 2003). This strategy requires high levels of antibodies at mucosal surfaces over long periods of time (Path, 2006). Maintaining these high levels is difficult, so it is recommended that prophylactic vaccines should also stimulate a cellular immune response that is capable of eliminating early stages of infection in host cells (Duggan-Keen et al., 1998; Galloway, 1998).

In contrast, therapeutic vaccines aim to generate cell-mediated immune responses using killer T cells that actively destroy HPV-infected cells and may exert immediate effects on lowering HPV-related disease incidence. To be effective, therapeutic HPV vaccines must prompt cell-mediated immunity because antibodies cannot reach and eliminate the virus once it has been incorporated into host cells (Ling et al., 2000; Chu, 2003; Maclean et al., 2005). This type of vaccine could help people who are already infected with HPV. Used alone or in combination with standard therapies, a therapeutic vaccine could help prevent the progression of low-grade disease and cause existing lesions to regress, avoiding the recurrence of cancer lesions after treatment (Chu, 2003; Stanley, 2003).

In a broad revision, Path (2001) described the existence of five types of HPV vaccines: recombinant live vector vaccines; protein and peptide vaccines; virus-like particles (VLPs); "naked" DNA vaccines; and edible vaccines (in which plants are genetically engineered to express HPV antigens in fruits and vegetables, leading to immunization through ingestion of the modified foods).

The following three categories of HPV proteins represent potential targets for vaccines, each of which is expressed during different stages of infection and disease:

1. The capsid proteins L1 and L2 compose the outside coat of HPV particles. These proteins interact with the surface molecules of epithelial cells during early stages of infection to gain entry for the viral DNA. Because L1 and L2 are present during the initial infection, they are ideal targets for a prophylactic vaccine (Lowy & Schiller, 1998). However, once HPV has integrated into the tumor cells, the capsid proteins are not always present and they are not reliable targets for a therapeutic vaccine.
2. The oncoproteins E6 and E7 continue to be expressed during later stages of disease and are the primary targets of therapeutic vaccines. These proteins bind the human tumor suppressor genes p53 and pRB (Duggan-Keen et al., 1998) and are involved in the malignant transformation of HPV-infected cells (Van Driel et al., 1999).
3. The proteins E1 and E2 are necessary for HPV replication within cells before the virus integrates into the host DNA (Duggan-Keen et al., 1998; Van Driel et al., 1999). Because E1 and E2 are expressed at higher levels than E6 and E7 at the early stages of HPV infection,

they may represent the best targets for a therapeutic vaccine designed to treat the early stages of disease, such as low-grade dysplasias (Tindle, 1996; Lowy & Schiller, 1998).

13.2 The HPV prophylactic vaccines

The current HPV prophylactic vaccines are based on VLPs (Van Monsjou et al., 2010). At present, two prophylactic HPV vaccines are commercially available: the bivalent (HPV 16/18) vaccine Cervarix® (GlaxoSmithKline, Middlesex, UK) and the quadrivalent (HPV 6/11/16/18) Gardasil® (Merck, NJ, USA). Licensed globally, these two vaccines have produced great expectations that they will prevent infections and tumors induced by different HPV types (Syrjänen, 2010).

The US Food and Drug Administration (FDA) approved Gardasil for females ages 9-26 in 2006. In October 2009, the FDA approved Cervarix for use in females ages 10-25 and approved Gardasil for use in males ages 9-26 to prevent genital warts and to prevent the spread of cervical cancer. Moreover, the FDA (2010 and 2010a) has proclaimed that the dosing and administration schedule should be 0.5 mL administered intramuscularly (preferably in a deltoid muscle) on a 3-dose schedule. The second dose should be administered 1 to 2 months later, and the third dose should be administered 6 months after the first dose.

These vaccines target the HPV major capsid protein L1 and can assemble to form VLP morphologically resembling native virions to generate robust antibody responses and prevent HPV infection. However, Gardasil and Cervarix differ in their adjuvants, which are substances added to a vaccine to enhance its impact by stimulating immune responses. In Gardasil, each type of VLP is purified and adsorbed on an aluminum-containing adjuvant (amorphous aluminum hydroxyphosphate sulfate), which is widely used. In contrast, Cervarix is formulated with a novel adjuvant, AS04, developed by the Corixa Corporation to strengthen and prolong the immune response to vaccines. Like aluminum hydroxide, AS04 includes MPL® (3-deacylated monophosphoryl lipid A), which is a derivative of the lipid A molecule found in gram-negative bacteria and a potent immune system stimulant because it primes innate immunity and may stimulate adaptive immunity and enhance antibody titers (Ma; Roden; Wu, 2010).

Although clinical trials of Gardasil and Cervarix have been extremely promising, these first generation VLP vaccines may not be the ideal vaccine candidates, especially in low-resource settings. Researchers are now actively working to develop other prophylactic HPV vaccines that may be effective against a broader range of HPV types and have a longer shelf life.

13.3 The HPV therapeutic vaccines and its perspectives

Immunotherapy offers an attractive alternative treatment strategy because it can address both the underlying HPV infection and the visible lesions. Moreover, immunotherapy can target all HPV-associated lesions, regardless of location, and induce long-lasting immunity, thus preventing recurrence (Chu, 2003; Stanley, 2003).

A judgment of whether therapeutic HPV vaccine candidates have a real effect on disease has been difficult because most trials have not been placebo-controlled. The vaccines have also shown, at best, limited efficacy in eradicating established tumors, although the fact that they have mostly been tested in advanced stage cancer patients with compromised immune systems may have limited their impact (Brinkman et al., 2005).

Perhaps the most effective HPV vaccine strategy calls for a vaccine that possesses both prophylactic and therapeutic properties. A chimeric vaccine of this type could both prevent new HPV infections and clear existing infections. Moreover, such a vaccine would benefit and could be administered to both sexually inexperienced young individuals and older individuals who already harbor HPV (Franceschi, 2005). Opportunities for primary and secondary prevention should be assessed, including the use of HPV vaccines to prevent infection and therapeutic vaccines in the adjuvant setting for locoregional recurrence and distant disease (Marur et al. 2010). Combined with the fact that no therapeutic vaccines currently exist for other diseases, this goal makes therapeutic HPV vaccine development a challenging task.

The eventual routine of HPV prophylactic vaccination will most likely have an impact not only on the incidence of cervical and anogenital cancers in women and men but also on the incidence of some groups of head and neck tumors, as in OPC. The increasing proportion of HPV-positive head and neck cancers underlines the increasing importance of routine prophylactic vaccination against HPV, and together with tobacco and alcohol control, this vaccination could have a decisive position in the prevention of head and neck cancer (Klozar et al., 2010). Vaccines directed against HPV 16, which accounts for 80-90% of all HPV-positive HNSCC, currently exist in Europe and USA (Dahlstrand & Dalianis, 2005; Sturgis & Cinciripini, 2007; Hammarstedt et al., 2006; Lindquist et al., 2007; Mellin et al., 2002; Gillison et al., 2008; Ang et al., 2010; Marur et al., 2010; Näsman et al., 2009; Attner et al., 2010).

14. Final considerations

Several aspects still remain to be discovered in the field of head and neck cancers and HPV infection, but the epidemiological analysis of the last decade demonstrates a rapid increase in the incidence of HPV-associated HNSCCs, and sufficient evidence now exists for a causal role of HPV in HNSCC. The genomic detection of HPV DNA, primarily in OPCs, provides stronger support for a viral etiology in HNSCC. Although some synergies between HPV oncogenes and other carcinogens have been hypothesized, non-smoking and non-drinking patients and those who sexually debut at a younger age have an increased risk of HPV-positive HNSCCs but show a favorable prognosis. Specifically in oral mucosa, some authors have suggested that the occasional finding of HPV DNA in OSCC specimens might not result from viral infection but rather from an incidental HPV colonization. However, a relative HPV contribution to oral carcinogenesis may occur in a subgroup of patients, mainly in areas where tobacco use is less common.

Targeted therapy for HNSCCs now demands more predictive biomarkers, such as the HPV infection status and mutation status of crucial genes, which could contribute to personalized treatment for individual patients and decrease the inherent morbidities. However, for a better understanding of whether the HPV status of tumors has real therapeutic implications in affecting the clinical outcome, upcoming clinical trials should be significantly standardized in their design and performed on HNSCCs that have been adequately selected and classified with respect to the different head and neck anatomical sites. Moreover, we suggest that other methodologies should be utilized to improve HPV detection and that additional population studies should be performed to confirm these findings.

We believe that the increasing proportion of HPV-positive HNSCCs highlights the importance of vaccination against HPV. Although detection of the true effects of HPV vaccination on cancer incidence will probably continue for several decades, monitoring the current effects of HPV vaccination is crucial, not only in cervical cancer, but also in head and neck cancer.

15. References

Ang, K.K.; Harris, J.; Wheeler, R.; Weber, R.; Rosenthal, D.I.; Nguyen-Tân, P.F. et al. (2010). Human Papillomavirus and Survival of Patients with Oropharyngeal Cancer. The New England Journal of Medicine, 363, 1, pp. 24-35, DOI: 10.1056/NEJMoa0912217.

Attner, P.; Du, J.; Näsman, A.; Hammarstedt, L.; Ramqvist, T.; Lindholm, J. et al. (2010). The role of human papillomavirus in the increased incidence of base of tongue cancer. International Journal of Cancer, 126, 12, pp. 2879-2884, DOI: 10.1002/ijc.24994.

Blomberg, M.; Nielsen, A.; Munk, C. & Kjaer, S.K. (2011). Trends in head and neck cancer incidence in Denmark, 1978–2007: Focus on human papillomavirus associated sites. International Journal of Cancer, 129, 6, pp. 733-741, DOI: 10.1002/ijc.25699.

Bosch, F.X.; Lörincz, A.; Muñoz, N.; Meijer, C.J. & Shah, K.V. (2002). The causal relation between human papillomavirus and cervical cancer. J Clin Pathol, 55, pp. 244-265.

Bouda, M.; Gorgoulis, V.G.; Kastrinakis, N.G.; Giannoudis, A.; Tsoli, E.; Danassi-Afentaki, D. et al. (2000). "High risk" HPV types are frequently detected in potentially malignant and malignant oral lesions, but not in normal oral mucosa. Modern Pathology, 13, 6, pp. 644-653.

Brinkman, J.A.; Caffrey, A.S.; Muderspach, L.I.; Roman, L.D. & Kast, W.M. (2005). The impact of anti-HPV vaccination on cervical cancer incidence and HPV-induced cervical lesions: consequences for clinical management. European Journal of Gynaecological Oncology, 26, 2, pp.129–142.

Chaturvedi, A.K.; Engels, E.A.; Anderson, W.F. & Gillison, M.L. (2008). Incidence trends for human papillomavirus-related and -unrelated oral squamous cell carcinomas in the United States. Journal of Clinical Oncology, 26, 4, pp. 612-619, DOI: 10.1200/JCO.2007.14.1713

Chow, L.T.; Broker, T.R. & Steinberg, B.M. (2010). The natural history of human papillomavirus infections of the mucosal epithelia. APMIS, 118, 6-7, pp. 422–449, DOI: 10.1111/j.1600-0463.2010.02625.x

Chu, R.N. (2003). Therapeutic vaccination for the treatment of mucosotropic human papillomavirus-associated disease. Expert Opinion on Biological Therapy, 3, 3, pp. 477–486.

Cleveland, J.L.; Junger, M.L.; Saraiya, M.; Markowitz, L.E.; Dunne, E.F. & Epstein, J.B. (2011). Implications for dentistry cell carcinomas in the United States: papillomavirus and oropharyngeal squamous. J Am Dent Assoc, 142, pp. 915-924.

D'Souza, G.; Agrawal, Y.; Halpern, J.; Bodison, S. & Gillison, M.L. (2009). Oral sexual behaviors associated with prevalent oral human papillomavirus infection. Journal of Infectious Diseases, 199, 9, pp. 1263-1269, DOI: 10.1086/597755.

D'Souza, G.; Kreimer, A.; Viscidi, R.; Pawlita, M.; Fakhry, C.; Koch, W.M. et al. (2007). Case-control study of human papillomavirus and oropharyngeal cancer. N Engl J Med, 356, pp. 944-1956.

Dahlstrand, H.M. & Dalianis, T. (2005). Presence and influence of human papillomaviruses (HPV) in tonsillar cancer. Adv Cancer Res, 93, pp. 59–89. DOI: 10.1016/S0065-230X(05)93002-9.

Daling, J.R.; Madeleine, M.M.; Johnson, L.G.; Schwartz, S.M.; Shera, K.A.; Wurscher, M.A. et al. (2005). Penile cancer: importance of circumcision, human papillomavirus and smoking in situ and invasive disease. International Journal of Cancer, 116, 4, pp. 606-616.

Dayyani, F.; Etzel, C.J.; Liu, M.; Ho, C.H.; Lippman, S.M. & Tsao, A.S. (2010). Meta-analysis of the impact of human papillomavirus (HPV) on cancer risk and overall survival in head and neck squamous cell carcinomas (HNSCC). Head & Neck Oncology, 2 , pp. 15, DOI: 10.1186/1758-3284-2-15.

Dayyani, F.; Etzel, C.J.; Liu, M.; Ho, C.H.; Lippman, S.M. & Tsao, A.S. (2010). Meta-analysis of the impact of human papillomavirus (HPV) on cancer risk and overall survival in head and neck squamous cell carcinomas (HNSCC). Head & Neck Oncology., 2, 7, pp 2-15.

De Villiers, E.M.; Fauquet, C.; Broker, T.R.; Bernard, H.U. & Zur Hausen, H. (2004). Classification of papillomaviruses. Virology, 324, 1, pp. 17-27, DOI: 10.1016/j.virol.2004.03.033.

Dobrossy L. (2005). Epidemiology of head and neck cancer: magnitude of the problem. Cancer and Metastasis Rev, 24, 1, pp. 9-17.

Doorbar, J.; Ely, S.; Sterling, J.; McLean, C. & Crawford L. (1991). Specific interaction between HPV 16 E1-E4 and cytokeratins results in collapse of the epithelial cell intermediate filament network. Nature, 352, pp. 824-827.

D'Souza, G.; Kreimer, A.R.; Viscidi, R.; Pawlita, M.; Fakhry, C.; Koch, W.M. et al. (2007). Case-control study of human papillomavirus and oropharyngeal cancer. The New England journal of medicine, 356, 19, pp. 1944-1956.

Duggan-Keen, M.F.; Brown, M.D.; Stacey, S.N. & Stern, P.L. (1998). Papillomavirus vaccines. Frontiers in Bioscience, 3, pp. 1192-1208.

Dyson, N.; Guida, P.; McCall, C. & Harlow, E. (1992). Adenovirus E1A makes two distinct contacts with the retinoblastoma protein. J Virol., 66, 7, pp. 4606-4611.

Fakhry, C.; Westra, W.H.; Li, S.; Cmelak, A.; Ridge, J.A.; Pinto, H. et al. (2008). Improved survival of patients with human papillomavirus-positive head and neck squamous cell carcinoma in a prospective clinical trial. Journal of the National Cancer Institute, 100, 4, pp. 261-269, DOI: 10.1093/jnci/djn011.

Fehrmann, F. & Laimins, L.A. (2003). Human papillomaviruses: targeting differentiating epithelial cells for malignant transformation. Oncogene, 22, 33, pp. 5201-5207, DOI: 10.1038/sj.onc.1206554.

Feller, L.; Wood, N.H.; Khammissa, R.A. & Lemmer, J. (2010). Human papillomavirus-mediated carcinogenesis and HPV-associated oral and oropharyngeal squamous cell carcinoma. Part 2: Human papillomavirus associated oral andoropharyngeal squamous cell carcinoma. Head & Face Medicine, pp. 6-15, DOI: 10.1186/1746-160X-6-15.

Fernandes, J.V.; Meissner, R.V.; Carvalho, M.G.F.; Fernandes, T.A.A.M.; Azevedo, P.R.M. & Villa, L.L. (2009). Prevalence of HPV infection by cervical cytologic status in Brazil. International Journal of Gynecology & Obstetrics, 105, 1, pp. 21-24.

Food and Drug Administration (FDA) (2010). Licensure of Bivalent Human Papillomavirus Vaccine (HPV2, Cervarix) for Use in Females and Updated HPV Vaccination Recommendations from the Advisory Committee on Immunization Practices (ACIP). MMWR Morbidity and Mortality Weekly Report., 59, 20, pp. 626-629.

Food and Drug Administration (FDA) (2010). Licensure of Quadrivalent Human Papillomavirus Vaccine (HPV4, Gardasil) for Use in Males and Guidance from the Advisory Committee on Immunization Practices (ACIP). MMWR Morbidity and Mortality Weekly Report. , 59, 20, pp. 630-632.

Franceschi, S. (2005). The International Agency for Research on Cancer (IARC) commitment to cancer prevention: the example of papillomavirus and cervical cancer. Recent Results in Cancer Research. 166, pp. 277–297.

Galloway, DA. (1998). Is vaccination against human papillomavirus a possibility? Lancet, 351(suppl III), pp. 22-24.

Gillespie, M.B.; Rubinchik, S.; Hoel, B. & Sutkowski, N. (2009). Human Papillomavirus and Oropharyngeal Cancer: What You Need to Know in 2009. Current Treatment Options in Oncology, 10, 5-6, pp. 296-307, DOI: 10.1007/s11864-009-0113-5.

Gillison, M.L. (2008). Human papillomavirus-related diseases: oropharynx cancers and potential implications for adolescent HPV vaccination. J Adolesc Health. 43(4 suppl), pp. S52-S60.

Gillison, M.L.; D'Souza, G.; Westra, W.; Sugar, E.; Xiao, W.; Begum, S. & Viscidi, R. (2008). Distinct risk factor profiles for human papillomavirus type 16-positive and human papillomavirus type 16-negative head and neck cancers. Journal of the National Cancer Institute, 100, 6, pp. 407–420, DOI: 10.1093/jnci/djn025.

Gillison, M.L.; Harris, J.; Westra, W.; Chung, C.; Jordan, R.; Rosenthal, D. et al. (2009). Survival outcomes by tumor human papillomavirus (HPV) status in stage III-IV oropharyngeal cancer (OPC) in RTOG 0129. Journal of Clinical Oncology, Vol. 27, No. 15s (Jun 2009), suppl. Abstr 6003.

Gillison, M.L.; Koch, W.M.; Capone, R.B.; Spafford, M.; Westra, W.H.; Wu, L. et al. (2000). Evidence for a causal association between human papillomavirus and a subset of head and neck cancers. J Natl Cancer Inst. 92, pp. 709–20. DOI: 10.1093/jnci/92.9.709.

Goldenberg, D.; Begum, S.; Westra, W.H.; Khan, Z.; Sciubba, J.; Pai, S.I. et al. (2008). Cystic lymph node metastasis in patients with head and neck cancer: an HPV-associated phenomenon. Head & Neck, 30, 7, pp. 898–903, DOI: 10.1002/hed.20796.

Gonzalez, S.L.; Stremlau, M.; He, X.; Basile, J.R. & Münger, K. (2001). Degradation of the retinoblastoma tumor suppressor by the human papillomavirus type 16 E7 oncoprotein is important for functional inactivation and is separable from proteasomal degradation of E7. Virology, 75, 16, pp. 7583-7591.

Gross, G. & Pfister, H. (2004). Role of human papillomavirus in penile cancer, penile intraepithelial squamous cell neoplasias and in genital warts. Medical Microbiology and Immunology (Berlin), 193, 1, pp. 35–44.

Guimarães, M.C.; Soares, C.P.; Donadi, E.A.; Derchain, S.F.; Andrade, L.A.; Silva, T.G. et al. (2010). Low Expression of Human Histocompatibility Soluble Leukocyte Antigen-G

(HLA-G5) in Invasive Cervical Cancer With and Without Metastasis, Associated With Papilloma Virus (HPV). Journal of Histochemistry & Cytochemistry, 58, 5, pp. 405–411, DOI: 10.1369/jhc.2009.954131.

Hafkamp, H.C.; Manni, J.J.; Haesevoets, A.; Voogd, A.C.; Schepers, M.; Bot, F.J. et al. (2008). Marked differences in survival rate between smokers and nonsmokers with HPV 16-associated tonsillar carcinomas. International Journal of Cancer, 122, 12, pp. 2656–2664, DOI: 10.1002/ijc.23458.

Hammarstedt, L.; Lindquist, D.; Dahlstrand, H.; Romanitan, M.; Dahlgren, L.O.; Joneberg, J. et al. (2006). Human papillomavirus as a risk factor for the increase in incidence of tonsillar cancer. International Journal of Cancer, 119, 11, pp. 2620-2623, DOI: 10.1002/ijc.22177.

Hannisdal, K.; Schjølberg, A.; De Angelis, P.M.; Boysen, M. & Clausen, O.P. (2010). Human papillomavirus (HPV)-positive tonsillar carcinomas are frequent and have a favourable prognosis in males in Norway. Acta Oto-laryngologica, 130, 2, pp. 293-299.

Hebner, C.M. & Laimins, L.A. (2006). Human papillomaviruses: basic mechanisms of pathogenesis and oncogenicity. Reviews in Medical Virology, 16, 2, pp. 83–97, DOI: 10.1002/rmv.488.

Heck, J.E.; Berthiller, J.; Vaccarella, S.; Winn, D.M.; Smith, E.M.; Shan'gina, O.; Schwartz, S.M. et al. (2010). Sexual behaviours and the risk of head and neck cancers: a pooled analysis in the International Head and Neck Cancer Epidemiology (INHANCE) consortium. International Journal of Epidemiology, 39, 1, pp. 166–181, DOI:10.1093/ije/dyp350.

Hennessey, P.T.; Westra, W.H. & Califano, J.A. (2009). Human papillomavirus and head and neck squamous cell carcinoma: recent evidence and clinical implications. Journal of Dental Research, 88, 4, pp. 300-306, DOI: 10.1177/0022034509333371.

Hennessey, P.T.; Westra, W.H. & Califano, J.A. (2009). Human papillomavirus and head and neck squamous cell carcinoma: recent evidence and clinical implications. J Dent Res., 88, 4, pp. 300-306.

Herrero, R. (2003). Human papillomavirus and cancer of the upper aerodigestive tract. J. Natl. Cancer Inst. Monographs, 31, pp. 47-51.

Herrero, R.; Castellsagué, X.; Pawlita, M.; Lissowska, J.; Kee, F.; Balaram, P.; Rajkumar, T. et al. (2003). Human papillomavirus and oral cancer: the international agency for research on cancer multicenter study. Journal of the National Cancer Institute, 95, 23, pp. 1772-1783, DOI: 10.1093/jnci/djg107.

Hobbs, C.G.; Sterne, J.A.; Bailey, M.; Heyderman, R.S.; Birchall, M.A. & Thomas, S.J. (2006). Human papillomavirus and head and neck cancer: a systematic review and meta-analysis. Clin. Otolaryngol., 31, 4, pp. 259-266.

International Agency for Research on Cancer (IARC). (2007). Human papillomaviruses, in: IARC monographs on the evaluation of carcinogenic risks to humans, 90, Lyon: IARC, 2007. Accessed June, 2011. Available from: <http://monographs.iarc.fr>.

Jones, D.L. & Münger, K. (1997). Analysis of the p53-mediated G1 growth arrest pathway in cells expressing the human papillomavirus type 16 E7 oncoprotein. J Virol, 71, 4, pp. 2905-2912.

Jones, S.R.; Myers, E.N. & Barnes, L. (1984). Benign neoplasm of the larynx. Otolaryngol. Clin. North Am., 17, pp. 151–178.

Klozar, J.; Kratochvil, V.; Salakova, M.; Smahelova, J.; Vesela, E.; Hamsikova, E. et al. (2008). HPV status and regional metastasis in the prognosis of oral and oropharyngeal cancer. European Archives of Oto-Rhino-Laryngology, 265, Suppl 1, pp. 75-82, DOI: 10.1007/s00405-007-0557-9.

Klozar, J.; Tachezy, R.; Rotnáglová, E.; Koslabová, E.; Saláková, M. & Hamsíková, E. (2010). Human papillomavirus in head and neck tumors: epidemiological, molecular and clinical aspects. Wiener Medizinische Wochenschrift, 160, 11-12, pp. 305-309, DOI: 10.1007/s10354-010-0782-5.

Klussmann, J.P.; Weissenborn, S.J.; Wieland, U.; Dries, V.; Eckel, H.E.; Pfister, H.J. & Fuchs, P.G. (2003). Human papillomavirus-positive tonsillar carcinomas: a different tumor entity? Medical Microbiology and Immunology (Berl), 192, 3, pp. 129-132, DOI: 10.1007/s00430-002-0126-1.

Koch, W.M.; Lango, M.; Sewell, D.; Zahurak, M. & Sidransky, D. (1999). Head and neck cancer in nonsmokers: a distinct clinical and molecular entity. Laryngoscope, 109, 10, pp. 1544-1551.

Kojima, A.; Maeda, H.; Sugita, Y.; Tanaka, S. & Kameyama, Y. (2002). Human papillomavirus type 38 infection in oral squamous cell carcinomas. Oral Oncology, 38, 6, pp. 591-596, DOI: 10.1016/S1368-8375(01)00112-9.

Kreimer, A.R.; Clifford, G.M.; Boyle, P. & Franceschi, S. (2005). Human papillomavirus types in head and neck squamous cell carcinomas worldwide: a systematic review. Cancer Epidemiology Biomarkers & Prevention, 14, 2, pp. 467-475, DOI: 10.1158/1055-9965.

Kumaraswamy, K. L. & Vidhya, M. (2011). Human papilloma virus and oral infections: An update. Journal of Cancer Research and Therapeutics, 7, 2, pp. 120-127, DOI: 10.4103/0973-1482.82915.

Lajer, C.B. & Von Buchwald, C. (2010). The role of human papillomavirus in head and neck cancer. APMIS, 118, 6-7, pp. 510-519, DOI: 10.1111/j.1600-0463.2010.02624.x.

Leemans, C.R.; Braakhuis, B.J. & Brakenhoff, R.H. (2011). The molecular biology of head and neck cancer. Nature Reviews Cancer, 11, 1, pp. 9-22, DOI: 10.1038/nrc2982.

Lindquist, D.; Romanitan, M.; Hammarstedt, L.; Nasman, A.; Dahlstrand, H.; Lindholm, J. et al. (2007). Human papillomavirus is a favourable prognostic factor in tonsillar cancer and its oncogenic role is supported by the expression of E6 and E7. Mol Oncol. 1, pp. 350-355. DOI: 10.1016/j.molonc.2007.08.005

Ling, M.; Kanayama, M.; Roden, R. & Wu, T.C. (2000). Preventive and therapeutic vaccines for human papillomavirus-associated cervical cancers. Journal of Biomedical Science. 7, pp. 341-356.

Lira, R.C.; Miranda, F.A.; Guimarães, M.C.; Simões, R.T.; Donadi, E.A.; Soares, C.P. & Soares, E.G. (2010). BUBR1 expression in benign oral lesions and squamous cell carcinomas: Correlation with human papillomavirus. Oncology Reports, 23, 4, pp. 1027-1036, DOI: 10.3892/or_00000729.

Lopes, V.; Murray, P.; Williams, H.; Woodman, C.; Watkinson, J. & Robinson M. (2011). Squamous cell carcinoma of the oral cavity rarely harbours oncogenic human papillomavirus. Oral Oncology, 47, 8, pp. 698-701.

Lowy, D.R. & Schiller, J.T. (1998). Papillomaviruses and cervical cancer: pathogenesis and vaccine development. Journal of the National Cancer Institute Monographs, 23, pp. 27-30.

Lowy, D.R. & Schiller, J.T. (1998). Papillomaviruses: prophylactic vaccine prospects. Biochimica et Biophysica Acta, 1423, pp. M1-M8.

Machado, J.; Reis, P.P.; Zhang, T.; Simpson, C.; Xu, W.; Perez-Ordonez, B. et al. (2010). Low prevalence of Human Papillomavirus in oral cavity carcinomas. Head & Neck Oncology, 2, pp. 6, DOI: 10.1186/1758-3284-2-6.

Maclean, J.; Rybicki, E.P. & Williamson, A. (2005). Vaccination strategies for the prevention of cervical cancer. Expert Review of Anticancer Therapy, 5, 1, pp. 97–107.

Madkan, V.K.; Cook-Norris, R.H.; Steadman, M.C.; Arora, A.; Mendoza, N. & Tyring, S.K. (2007). The oncogenic potential of human papillomaviruses: a review on the role of host genetics an environmental cofactors. Brit. J. Dermatol., 157, pp. 228–241.

Martinez, I.; Wang, J.; Hobson, K.F.; Ferris, R.L. & Khan, S.A. (2007). Identification of differentially expressed genes in HPV-positive and HPV-negative oropharyngeal squamous cell carcinomas. European Journal of Cancer, 43, 2, pp. 415-432, DOI: 10.1016/j.ejca.2006.09.001.

Marur, S. & Forastiere, A.A. (2008). Head and neck cancer: changing epidemiology, diagnosis, and treatment. Mayo Clin Proc., 83, 4, pp. 489-501.

Marur, S., D'Souza, G., Westra, W.H. & Forastiere, A.A. (2010). HPV-associated head and neck cancer: a virus-related cancer epidemic. The Lancet Oncology, 11, 8, pp. 781 - 789, DOI: 10.1016/S1470-2045(10)70017-6.

Maxwell, J.H.; Kumar, B.; Feng, F.Y.; McHugh, J.B.; Cordell, K.G.; Eisbruch, A. et al. (2010). HPV-positive/p16-positive/EBV-negative nasopharyngeal carcinoma in white North Americans. Head & Neck, 32, 5, pp. 562–567, DOI: 10.1002/hed.21216.

Mazon, R.C.; Gerbelli, T.R.; Neto, C.B.; de Oliveira, M.R.B.; Donadi, E.A.; Goncalves, M.A.G. et al. (2011). Abnormal cell-cycle expression of the proteins p27, mdm2 and cathepsin B in oral squamous-cell carcinoma infected with human papillomavirus. Acta histochemica, 113, 2, pp. 109–116, DOI: 10.1016/j.acthis.2009.08.008.

Mellin, H.; Dahlgren, L.; Munck-Wikland, E.; Lindholm, J.; Rabbani, H.; Kalantari, M. et al. (2002). Human papillomavirus type 16 is episomal and a high viral load may be correlated to better prognosis in tonsillar cancer. Int J Cancer., 102, pp. 152–8. DOI: 10.1002/ijc.10669.

Miranda, F.A.; Hassumi, M.K.; Guimarães, M.C.; Simões, R.T.; Silva, T.G.; Lira, R.C. et al. (2009). Galectin-3 Overexpression in Invasive Laryngeal Carcinoma, Assessed by Computer-assisted Analysis. Journal of Histochemistry & Cytochemistry, 57, 7, pp. 665-673, DOI: 10.1369/jhc.2009.952960.

Muenscher, A.; Feucht, H.H.; Kutta, H.; Tesche, S. & Wenzel, S. (2008). Integration of human papilloma virus type 26 in laryngeal cancer of a child. Auris Nasus Larynx., doi:10.1016/j.anl.2008.05.011.

Muñoz, N.; Bosch, F.X.; De Sanjosé, S.; Herrero, R.; Castellsague, X.; Shah, K.V. et al. (2003). Epidemiologic classification of human papillomavirus types associated with cervical cancer. N Engl J Med, 348, pp. 518-527.

Muñoz, N.; Kjaer, S.K.; Sigurdsson, K.; Iversen, O.E.; Hernandez-Avila, M.; Wheeler, C.M. et al. (2010). Impact of human papillomavirus (HPV)-6/11/16/18 vaccine on all HPV-associated genital diseases in young women. J Natl Cancer Inst. 102:325–39. DOI: 10.1093/jnci/djp534.

Näsman, A.; Attner, P.; Hammarstedt, L.; Du, J.; Eriksson, M.; Giraud, G. et al. (2009). Incidence of human papillomavirus (HPV) positive tonsillar carcinoma in

Stockholm, Sweden: an epidemic of viral-induced carcinoma? International Journal of Cancer, 125, 2, pp. 362-366, DOI: 10.1002/ijc.24339.

NCI. Vaccine Therapy With or Without Imiquimod in Treating Patients With Grade 3 Cervical Intraepithelial Neoplasia. [cited; Available from: http://clinicaltrials.gov/ ct2/show/NCT00788164

Nventa Pharmaceuticals Corporation website (formerly Stressgen Biotechnologies). (2005). Heat shock proteins and the immune system. San Diego, Calif. Available at: http://www.nventacorp.com/pdf/CoValFusionsHspE7-20060718.pdf. Accessed July 24, 2011.

Oliveira, L.R.; Silva, A.R.; Ramalho, L.N.Z.; Simões, A.L. & Zucoloto, S. (2008). HPV infection in Brazilian oral squamous cell carcinoma patients and its correlation with clinicopathological outcomes. Molecular Medicine Reports, 1, 1, pp. 123-129.

Onon, T.S. (2010). History of human papillomavirus, warts and cancer: What do we know today? Best Practice & Research Clinical Obstetrics and Gynaecology, [epub ahead of print], DOI: 10.1016/j.bpobgyn.2011.05.001.

Park, T-W.; Fujiwara, H. & Wright, T.C. (1995). Molecular biology of cervical cancer and its precursors. Cancer, 76, pp. 1902-1913.

Phelps, W.C.; Münger, K.; Yee, C.L.; Barnes, J.A. & Howley, P.M. (1992). Structure-function analysis of the human papillomavirus type 16 E7 oncoprotein. J Virol, 66, 4, pp. 2418-2427.

Popović, B.; Jekić, B.; Novaković, I.; Luković, L.; Konstantinović, V.; Babić, M. & Milašin, J. (2010). Cancer genes alterations and HPV infection in oral squamous cell carcinoma. International Journal of Oral and Maxillofacial Surgery, 39, 9, pp. 909-915.

Program for Appropriate Technology in Health (PATH). (2001). Proceedings. Presented at: Meeting of the HPV Strategies for Developing Countries Expert Working Group, Bill & Melinda Gates Foundation, January 18-19, Seattle, Wash.

Program for Appropriate Technology in Health (PATH). (2006). Current and Future HPV Vaccines: Promise and Challenges.

Psyrri, A. & Dimaio, D. (2008). Human papillomavirus in cervical and head-and-neck cancer. Nat. Clin. Pract. Oncol., 5, 1, pp. 24-31.

Psyrri, A.; Gouveris, P. & Vermorken, J.B. (2009). Human papillomavirus-related head and neck tumors: clinical and research implication. Current Opinion in Oncology, 21, 3, pp. 201–205, DOI:10.1097/CCO.0b013e328329ab64.

Ragin, C.; Edwards, R.; Larkins-Pettigrew, M.; Taioli, E.; Eckstein, S.; Thurman, N.; Bloome, J. & Markovic, N. (2011). Oral HPV Infection and Sexuality: A Cross-Sectional Study in Women. International Journal of Molecular Science, 12, 6, pp. 3928-3940, DOI: 10.3390/ijms12063928.

Rampias, T.; Sasaki, C.; Weinberger, P. & Psyrri, A. (2009). E6 and e7 gene silencing and transformed phenotype of human papillomavirus 16-positive oropharyngeal cancer cells. J Natl Cancer Inst, 101, 6, pp. 412-23.

Rethman, M.P.; Carpenter, W.; Cohen, E.E., et al. (2010). American Dental Association Council on Scientific Affairs Expert Panel on Screening for Oral Squamous Cell Carcinomas. Evidence-based clinical recommendations regarding screening for oral squamous cell carcinomas. JADA, 141, 5, pp. 509-520.

Scheurer, M.E.; Tortolero-Luna, G. & Adler-Storthz, K. (2005). Human papillomavirus infection: biology, epidemiology, and prevention. International Journal of Gynecological Cancer, 15, 5, pp. 727-746.

Sinha, P.; Logan, H.L. & Mendenhall, W.M. (2011). Human papillomavirus, smoking, and head and neck cancer. American Journal of Otolaryngology-Head and Neck Medicine and Surgery, [epub ahead of print], DOI: 10.1016/j.amjoto.2011.02.001.

Smith, E.M.; Rubenstein, L.M.; Haugen, T.H.; Hamsikova, E. & Turek, L.P. (2010). Tobacco and alcohol use increases the risk of both HPV-associated and HPV-independent head and neck cancers. Cancer Causes Control, 21, 9, pp. 1369-1378, DOI: 10.1007/s10552-010-9564-z.

Snow, A.N. & Laudadio, J. (2010). Human Papillomavirus Detection in Head and Neck Squamous Cell Carcinomas. Advances in Anatomic Pathology, 17, 6, pp. 394-403, DOI: 10.1097/PAP.0b013e3181f895c1.

Southern, S.A. & Herrington, C.S. (2000). Disruption of cell cycle control by human papillomavirus with special reference to cervical carcinoma. Int J Gynecol Cancer, 10, pp. 263-274.

Stanley, M. (2003). Genital human papillomavirus infections—current and prospective therapies. Journal of the National Cancer Institute Monographs. 31, pp. 117124.

Sturgis, E.M. & Cinciripini, P.M. (2007). Trends in head and neck cancer incidence in relation to smoking prevalence: an emerging epidemic of human papillomavirus-associated cancers? Cancer, 110, pp. 1429-1435. DOI: 10.1002/cncr.22963.

Syrjänen, S. (2005). Human papillomavirus (HPV) in head and neck cancer. Journal of Clinical Virology, 32, Suppl 1, pp. S59-S66, DOI: 10.1016/j.jcv.2004.11.017.

Syrjänen, S. (2010). The role of human papillomavirus infection in head and neck cancers. Annals of Oncology 21 (Supplement 7), pp. 243-245.

Syrjänen, S.; Syrjänen, K.; Mantyjarvi, R.; Collan, Y. & Karja, J. (1987). Human papillomaviruse DNA in squamous cell carcinomas of the larynx demonstrated by in situ DNA hybridization. J. Otorhinolaryngol .Relat. Spec., 49, pp. 175-186.

Talbert-Slagle, K. & DiMaio, D. (2009). The bovine papillomavirus E5 protein and the PDGF β receptor: It takes two to tango. Virology, 384, 2, pp. 345-351.

Tanzi, E.; Amendola, A.; Bianchi, S.; Fasolo, M.M.; Beretta, R. et al. (2009). Human papillomavirus genotypes and phylogenetic analysis of HPV-16 variants in HIV-1 infected subjects in Italy. Vaccine, 27, 1, pp. 17-23.

Termine, N.; Panzarella, V.; Falaschini, S.; Russo, A.; Matranga, D.; Lo, M.L. & Campisi G. (2008). HPV in oral squamous cell carcinoma vs head and neck squamous cell carcinoma biopsies: a meta-analysis (1988-2007). Annals of Oncology, 19, 10, pp. 1681-1690, DOI: doi: 10.1093/annonc/mdn372.

Tindle, R. (1996). Human papillomavirus vaccines for cervical cancer. Current Opinion in Immunology, 8, 5, pp. 643-650. Available online at www.biomednet.com/library/fulltext/JIMM.im8502.

Torrente, M.C. & Ojeda, J.M. (2007). Exploring the relation between human papillomas virus and larynx cancer. Acta Otolaryngol., 127, 9, pp. 900-906.

Van Driel, W.J.; Kenter, G.G.; Fleuren, G.J.; Melief, C.J. & Trimbos, B.J. (1999). Immunotherapeutic strategies for cervical squamous carcinoma. Current Therapeutic Issues in Gynecologic Cancer, 13, 1, pp. 259-271.

Van Monsjou, H.S.; Balm, A.J.M.; Van den Brekel, M.M. & Wreesmann, V.B. (2010). Oropharyngeal squamous cell carcinoma: A unique disease on the rise? Oral Oncology, 46, pp. 780–785

Vidal, L. & Gillison, M.L. (2008). Human papillomavirus in HNSCC: recognition of a distinct disease type. Hematology / Oncology Clinics of North America, 22, 6, pp. 1125-1142, DOI: 10.1016/j.hoc.2008.08.006.

Villa, L.L.; Bernard, H.U.; Kast, M.; Hildesheim, A.; Amestoy, G. & Franco, E.L. (2002). Past, present, and future of HPV research: highlights from the 19th International Papillomavirus Conference-HPV2001. Virus Research, 89, pp. 163-173.

Villa, L.L.; Costa, R.L.; Petta, C.A.; Andrade, R.P.; Ault, K.A.; Giuliano, A.R. et al. (2005). Prophylactic quadrivalent human papillomavirus (types 6, 11, 16, and 18) L1 virus-like particle vaccine in young women: a randomized double-blind placebo-controlled multicentre phase II efficacy trial. Lancet Oncol., 6, pp. 271–278. DOI: 10.1016/S1470-2045 (05)70101-7.

Ward, P.; Coleman, D.V. & Malcolm, D.B. (1989). Regulatory mechanisms of the papillomaviruses. Trends Genet, 5, pp. 97-98.

Westra, W.H. (2009). The Changing Face of Head and Neck Cancer in the 21st Century: The Impact of HPV on the Epidemiology and Pathology of Oral Cancer. Head and Neck Pathology, 3, 1, pp. 78–81, DOI: 10.1007/s12105-009-0100-y.

Zinkernagel, R.M. (2003). On natural and artificial vaccinations. Annual Review of Immunology, 21, pp. 515–546.

Zur Hausen, H. (1996). Papillomavirus infections: a major cause of human cancers. Biochim Biophys Acta, 1288, 2, pp.55-78.

Zur Hausen, H. (2002). Papillomaviruses and cancer: from basic studies to clinical application. Nature Reviews Cancer, 2, 5, pp. 342-350, DOI: 10.1038/nrc798.

Zur Hausen, H. (2006). Infections causing human cancer. Weinheim (Germany): Wiley-VCH Verlag, pp. 145–243.

12

The Impact of Human Papillomavirus on Cancer Risk in Penile Cancer

Angela Adamski da Silva Reis and Aparecido Divino da Cruz
Federal University of Goiás/Biological Sciences Institute/
Department of Biochemistry and Molecular Biology
Pontifical Catholic University of Goiás - Department of Biology/
Núcleo de Pesquisas Replicon
Brazil

1. Introduction

Infection with human papillomavirus (HPV) is necessary for the development of the cervical cancer. Although, the relationship between HPV and cervical cancer is well documented and well established in the literature, the relationship between men and HPV-associated cancers is just emerging (Palefsky,2010).

The HPV has been shown to play a causative role in anal, head, neck, oral and penile carcinomas. The latter is a rare tumor accounting of a 1 per 100.000 incidence rate in Western countries, including Europe and North America, and representing less than 1% of all male cancers. On the contrary, the incidence in some emerging countries is much higher, reaching 18% to 20% of all male tumors (Salvioni et al., 2009). General socioeconomic factors and access to health-care systems might contribute to the discrepancies in this incidence.

The incidence rate increases with age, although the disease has also been reported in young men. Early diagnosis may be not only lifesaving but also essential to functionally and esthetically acceptable treatment. Many patients still seek medical attention at a late stage, when a conservative therapeutic approach is no longer feasible. Awareness of penile cancer and its prevention are at the heart of the recent controversies about circumcision and about the necessity to treat HPV infections (Micali et al., 2006).

There has been little progress in managing penile cancer during the past decade. The overall survival figures remain unchanged and its etiopathogenesis is still not fully understood (Chaturvedi, 2010; Dillner et al., 2000). Researchers have focused their investigation on a potential association between HPV infection and penile cancer development. However, this association is not absolute and other factors are implicated in the initiation and progression of the disease. The following chapter focuses on the natural history of penile cancer, addressing the probable mechanism by which HPV leads to malignant transformation of the penile epithelium, the relationship of genital HPV for risk penile cancer, and the preventive strategies to reduce HPV infection in men.

2. The role of human papillomavirus infection in etiology of penile cancer

Among men and women, cancers of the anogenital tract and their precursor lesions have been strongly linked to infection with sexually transmitted HPV (Wilkin & Chiasson, 2004). HPV causes virtually all cervical cancers and the virus is found in association with at least 90% of cervical carcinomas (de Sanjosé et al., 2007; Moscicki et al., 2006). The variability in HPV-attributable proportions for non cervical cancers arises partially from differences in HPV detection methods across studies as well as from true geographic differences in HPV distribution world-wide (Chaturvedi, 2010). Despite the reported variability, 90%-93% of anal cancers, 12%-63% of oropharyngeal cancers, 36%-46.9% of penile cancers, 40%-64% of vaginal cancers, and 40%-51% of vulvar cancers are potentially attributable to HPV infection (Caltellsagué et al., 2002; Chaturvedi 2010; Gillison, 2008; Giuliano et al., 2008; Giuliano et al., 2010; Miralles-Guri et al., 2009). See fig. 1 to identify average prevalence of HPV infection associated with anatomical cancer sites.

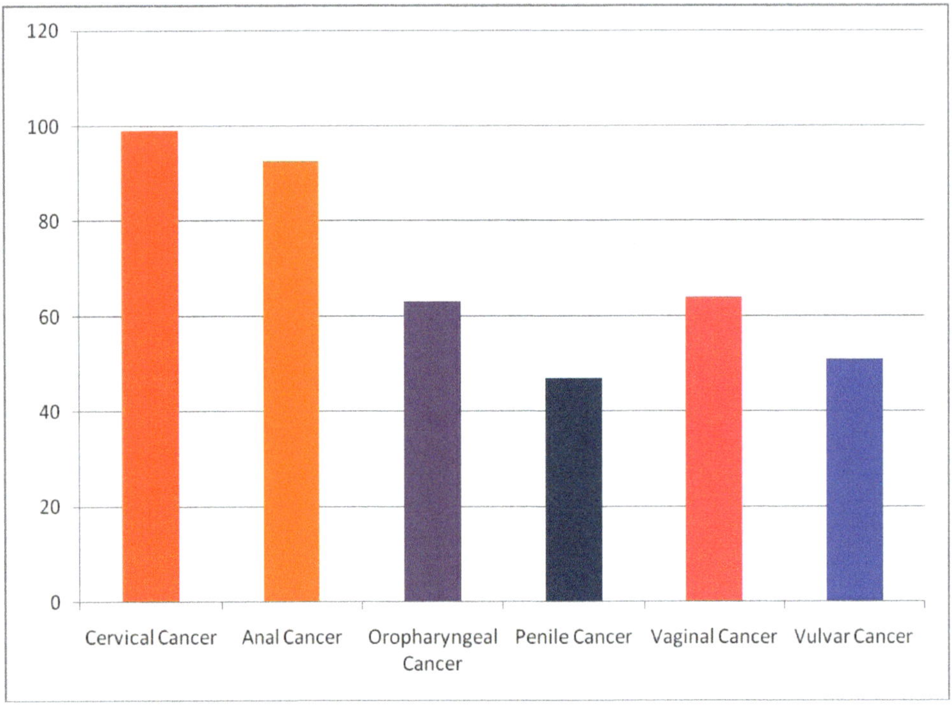

Fig. 1. HPV DNA prevalence among cases of cancer

Acquisition of HPV is very common, particularly among sexually active young adults, and incidence of infection with oncogenic HPV types appears to be higher than the incidence of infection with non-oncogenic types (Baseman & Koutskyl, 2005). Oncogenic HPV types 16 and 18 and history of other concurrent sexually transmitted diseases were found to be significantly associated with progression to cervical cancer (Cavalcanti et al., 2000). Carcinoma of the uterine cervix is the sixth most common cancer among women worldwide, with very high mortality rates in developing countries. It was observed more than 20 years ago that some types of HPV were more frequent in malignant than in benign lesions, and infection with high-risk types of HPV is now considered the major risk factor for the development of cancer of the uterine cervix (Villa, 2006).

The advent of screening to identify and treat cervical cancer precursor lesions and cervical intraepithelial neoplasia (CIN) has led to a substantial reduction in the incidence of cervical cancer in those countries where routine screening is in place. Conversely, most cervical cancer-related mortality occurs in countries where there is no routine cervical screening. On the other hand, it is clear that HPV infection in men is a serious clinical issue (Palefsky, 2010). The role of men in HPV infection of women was investigated in early epidemiological studies using questionnaires that addressed the sexual behavior of the husbands or sexual partners of women with and without cervical cancer. More recent studies had, in addition, been able to detect the presence of HPV DNA in exfoliated cells from the penile shaft, the coronal sulcus, and the distal urethra (Bosch et al., 2006). Squamous Cell Cancers (SCC) of the penis have a low association with HPV, whereas warty/basaloid cancers are strongly associated with HPV. Depending on the proportion of samples that are squamous vs warty/basaloid in any given report, the proportion of penile cancers associated with HPV varies considerably (Palefsky, 2010).

HPV positivity is higher in penile intraepithelial neoplasias (PIN1/2/3) and in the basaloid histological type, ranging from 75 to 80% and decreasing to a range between 30 to 60% in invasive SCC. Cancers of the penis are largely SCC (IARC 2007; Rubin et al., 2001). Provide that identification of HPV implies a casual role of the virus with the carcinogenic process, the attributable fraction of penile cancer related to HPV could estimated to be 40%-50% of penile cancer and molecular studies have confirmed the role of the HPV 16 and 18 (Miralles-Guri, 2009). On the other hand, the majority of studies included at least one case of cancer with HPV 6 or 11, which in several studies were more common than HPV 18 (Levi et al., 1998; Miralles-Guri et al., 2009; Rubin et al., 2001). HPV 31 and 33 were detected only rarely (IARC 2007).

The epidemiologic association of HPV with penile cancer fulfills the criteria for causality: strength and consistency of the association, with increased risk of these cancers among HPV-infected individuals; specificity of the association; temporality of the association, with HPV infection preceding the development of cancer by several years; biologic gradient of increasing risk with increasing exposure to HPV infection; coherence, plausibility, and experimental evidence of oncogenic potential of HPVs; analogy of the association of HPV with increased risk of penile cancer; and experimental evidence through the necessity for consistent expression of HPV oncogenes for maintenance of the malignant phenotype (Chatuverti, 2010).

2.1 Epidemiology and natural history of penile cancer

Penile cancer prevalence varies according to geographic region, socioeconomic status and ethnic origin. Penile squamous cell carcinoma (SCC) is a relatively rare disease and accounts for less than 0.5% of all cancers in men worldwide (Backes et al., 2009). In Europe and United States penile cancer incidence rates vary from 0.1 to 1.5 per 100,000 men (Backes et al., 2009; Bigot, 2011; Curado et al., 2007; Reis et al., 2010a). In 2010, there were about 1,250 new cases of penile cancer in the United States, resulting in 310 deaths, with an incidence rate of 0.3 to 1.8 per 100,000 men (Lawindy et al., 2011). The estimated lifetime direct medical cost for incident penile cancer was $ 4.4 million in 2003 and an estimated 240 associated deaths occurred in 2005 (Smith et al., 2010).

The wide variation of penile SCC prevalence is likely explained by the large variance in risk factors, in particular, the practice of neonatal circumcision (Minhas et al., 2010). The incidence is very low among Jewish populations that commonly practice neonatal circumcision (0.1 per 100,000) [Morris et al., 2011; Pow-Sang et al., 2010]. Typical SCC is the most frequent type of invasive penile cancer, representing about 95% of all cases (Hernandez et al., 2008; Pizzocaro et al., 2010). Penile cancer is much more common in African, Asian, and South American countries, constituting about 10% of the malignant diseases in those countries and thus posing a considerable public health concern (Lawindy et al., 2011). Penile SCC is a common male cancer with an incidence of 2–5 per 100,000 men, constituting up to 10–22% of all male cancers in some regions in Central and South America (Goiania, Brazil), Asia (Chiang Mai, Thailand) and Africa (Kyadondo, Uganda) than in other parts of the world (Parkin et al., 2003; Tornesello et al., 2008). Higher incidence rates are found in some countries such as Uganda (4.4/100,000) and Paraguay (4.2/100,00) [Lawindy et al., 2011; Pow-Sang & Astigueta, 2009].

Brazil has one of the highest rates of penile cancer in the world, 6-14 per 100,000 males per year, comprising 2-6% of all males malignancies with 7% of cases occurring in men aged under 35 y.o. and 39% in men older than 66 y.o. Among cases, 87% are uncircumcised. All tumors seen in men circumcised in childhood were of low grade, whereas 12% of those circumcised in adulthood had high-grade tumors (Favorito et al., 2008). At least in two Brazilian States (Maranhão and Pernambuco), penile cancer is reportedly the 2nd highest cause of carcinoma death in men, second only to lung cancer. At the main oncology hospital in Recife-Pernambuco, in the Northeast region of Brazil, on average one or two men each week need to undergo penile amputation due to cancer, with very poor prognosis (Morris et al.,2011).

Despite the large Brazilian migration from the Northeast to the Southeast, motived mainly by the population seeking for life opportunities in the most developed economic region in the country. Koifman (2011) reported that penile cancer was more prevalent in patients born in the state of Rio de Janeiro. According to the data from the Brazilian Ministry of Health, there is an estimated 850 partial or complete penile surgical procedures performed in the context of malignancy yearly within Brazil, with approximately 50% of these procedures being performed in the North and Northeast regions of the country (Favorito et al., 2008).

The presence of an intact foreskin has been identified as an important risk factor for developing penile cancer (Lawindy et al., 2011). Circumsicion protects against HPV infection, in a cohort study involving men in the USA, Mexico and Brazil, both low-risk and high-risk HPV types were less frequent in circumcised men (Giulliano et al., 2011). Male circumcision is the commonly performed surgical procedure in the world. The surgical technique is determined by social circumstances, together with the indication for the operation and the patient's age. There is no therapeutic male circumcision, which by definition does not treat an underlying pathological process. The motivations underling the procedure may be religious, cultural, social or prophylactic (Perera et al., 2010).

In most cases, the reason for circumcision is of religious or cultural origin. Both Jewish and Islamic laws promote male circumcision. Jewish male infants are circumcised on the eighth day, according to Biblical teaching, whereas among Muslims variations in the timing of circumcision do exist, with some communities delaying the procedure until the age of 10 years. Ritual circumcision is also performed in several African tribes as a ceremony of passage into adulthood (Micali et al., 2006).

Circumcision is the most common operation performed in males in the United States, where approximately 60% of male infants are routinely circumcised in the neonatal nursery, in most cases due to parental choice and nonreligious reasons. In Canada, approximately 48% of males are circumcised (Micali et al., 2006). In Australia the annual incidence of penile cancer was 0.8 per 100,000 men, which is similar to the US figure. As in the USA, over two-thirds of older men in Australia are circumcised. However, since the 1970s, Australia experienced a decline on the number of infant male circumcision. Thus, an increase on penile cancer has been expected in that population (Morris et al., 2011).

In most of Europe, in South and Central America, and in most Asian countries, including the People's Republic of China, Taiwan, Japan, and North Korea, male circumcision is uncommon. In a medical setting, postnatal circumcision is regarded as both a treatment for phimosis and a possible prophylactic measure for the prevention of penile cancer and other infectious or inflammatory conditions (Micali et al., 2006). In countries where circumcision is not practiced routinely, such as those in South America and parts of Africa, penile cancer can be ten times more common than in high-income countries, representing 10-22% of all male cancer (Morris et al., 2011).

The first suggestion linking circumcision and penile cancer was reported in 1932, when, among, 1.103 penile cancer cases in USA, none where Jewish despite 3% of the population being Jewish (Wolbarst, 1932). Circumcision as a measure to prevent penile cancer has been repeatedly related by different investigators. Maden et al. (1993) found that the risk of penile cancer was 3.2 times larger among men who had never been circumcised in comparison to men circumcised at birth and 3.0 times higher among men circumcised after the neonatal period. Schoen et al. (2000) reported that of 89 men with invasive penile cancer whose circumcision status was known, 2 (2.3%) had been circumcised as newborns and 87 had not been circumcised. The relative risk of invasive penile cancer for uncircumcised to circumcised men was 22:1. In a population-based case-control study in western Washington state carried by Daling et al. (2005), men who had not been circumcised in childhood had a 1.5 fold increased risk of developing penile cancer. Morris & Rose (2007) reported circumcision as a biomedical imperative for the 21st century, not only for the reduction of penile cancer, but also for a decrease in urinary tract infections, inflammatory dermatoses, and sexually transmitted diseases.

Studies have consistently reported neonatal or childhood circumcision to be associated with reduced risk of penile cancer, which geographically corresponds to reduced rates of penile SCC in populations that culturally practice neonatal circumcision (Maden et al., 1993; Micali et al., 2006; Morris et al., 2011; Perera et al., 2010; Tseng et al., 2001). The protective effect of childhood circumcision, but not of adulthood circumcision, seems to be attributable to the elimination of inflammatory conditions related to poor genital hygiene, such as phimosis and balanitis (Pizzacaro et al., 2009). On the other hand, the preventive effect of newborn circumcision on SCC development is still unclear. It occurs only if circumcision is performed at birth or early in life, whereas late or adult circumcision seems to be ineffective in risk reduction.

Beyond lack of circumcision there are others factors related with penile cancer such as phimosis. A history of phimosis also imposes a significant risk for the development of penile cancer, which is. Approximately 25% - 60% of patients with penile cancer have phimosis (Lawindy et al., 2011). Precancerous lesions are found in an additional 15% to 20% of patients with phimosis (Pow Sang et al., 2002). Thus, phimosis is considered one of the strongest risk factors for penile cancer. The relative risk of penile cancer among men with phimosis was 64.6. The frequency of phimosis in men with penile carcinoma is high, ranging from 44% to 85%. Phimosis leads invariably to retention of the normally desquamated epidermal cells and urinary products (smegma) resulting in conditions of chronic irritation with or without bacterial inflammation of the prepuce and the glans. However, there is no supporting evidence of the role of smegma as a carcinogen. Therefore, much debate still exist regarding this risk factor, as smegma is not yet believed to contribute to the development of penile cancer (Lawindy et al., 2011).

In a meta-analysis reported by Larke et al. (2011), four studies evaluated the association between phimosis and penile cancer (OR range 4.9-37.2). The effect of childhood/adolescent circumcision on invasive penile cancer may be largely mediated through elimination of phimosis, since there was no evidence of an association of circumcision with invasive disease when analyses were restricted to individuals with no history of phimosis. Morris et al., (2011) related that 45-85% of men with penile cancer have a history of phimosis and causes dysplastic (pre-cancerous) changes in the skin of the preputial sac. The authors demonstrated 52% of penile cancer with a long foreskin had phimosis. These findings have led to conclusion that circumcision in early childhood by elimination phimosis may help prevent penile cancer. Thus, the phimosis is a stronger risk factor for invasive disease compared to *in situ* cancer which further supports the argument that circumcision acts through prevention of phimosis and that some *in situ* cancers develop through a different pathway to invasive cancer (Daling et al., 2005; Larke et al., 2011).

Poor genital hygiene in uncircumcised men, even in the absence of phimosis, may also lead to the retention of microorganisms and secretions, including smegma. Whether good standards of genital personal hygiene in uncircumcised males may provide the same level of protection of circumcision against penile SCC has been questioned. Although a lower incidence of penile SCC, even among uncircumcised individuals, is noted in countries and communities with a high standard of genital hygiene and widespread diffusion of private bathing facilities (Micali et al., 2006).

Smith et al. (2010) reported that flat penile lesions are much more frequent in uncircumcised men and associated with higher prevalence of HPV and higher viral loads. The authors suggest that circumcision reduces the prevalence of HPV associated flat lesions and may ultimately reduce male to female HPV transmission. The increased risk of HPV infection among uncircumcised men observed and has important implications regarding HPV associated malignancies in men and their female partners. However, despite some favorable medical evidence, the promotion of circumcision as a mean of controlling HPV and other sexually transmitted infections remains controversial (Hernandez et al., 2008; Van Howe, 2007).

HPV infection alone is insufficient to cause epithelial malignancy in men. Unlike cervical cancer, evidences suggest that HPV infection is not a necessary cause of penile cancer with HPV prevalence ranging between 15 and 71% among penile cancer tissues (Rubin et al., 2001). Daling et al., (2005) measured the percentage of HPV DNA-positive tumors in their study and concluded that there was a consistent association between HPV infection and the development of most penile cancers.

The role of circumcision in penile cancer prevention is unclear: it could possibly be ascribed to a lower baseline risk of disease due to a decrease in the amount of susceptible tissue, prevention of potential cofactors with HPV (such as phimosis) from promoting disease or another mechanism.

However, male circumcision has been widely debated as a preventive measure for sexually transmitted infection human immunodeficiency virus/acquired immune deficiency syndrome (HIV/AIDS), urinary tract infection and penile cancer (Gray et al., 2010; Perera et al., 2010). Individuals with HIV/AIDS are at increased risk of HPV-associated cancers. This increased risk among persons with HIV or AIDS is consistent with a high incidence and persistence of HPV infections (Chaturvedi et al., 2009). On the other hand, circumcision can be considered an important cofactor in the natural history of HPV infection, since it may influence the risks of the acquisition and transmission of HPV as well as of cervical cancer. Castellsague et al., (2002) has provided epidemiologic evidence that male circumcision is associated with a reduced risk of genital HPV infection in men and with a reduced risk of cervical cancer in women with high-risk sexual partners. Thus, male circumcision may potentially reduce exposure of female partners to HPV infection.

Early age at first sexual intercourse, high lifetime number of female sexual partners, smoking, and lack of condom use are identified risk factors for penile SCC (Maden et al., 1993; Reis et al., 2010a). Some studies have also identified chronic smoking as an associated risk factor for the development of penile cancer (Pow-Sang et al., 2010). Tseng et al. (2001) found that the incidence of penile cancer among men who had ever smoked cigarettes was 2.4 times that of men who had never smoked. Harish & Ravi (1995) found a significant association between smoking or chewing tobacco and the development of penile carcinoma. In 503 men and age-matched controls, a multivariate analysis demonstrated a significant association and dose-dependent relationship. Maden et al. (1993) found that the risk of penile cancer among men who smoked at diagnosis was 2.8 times that of men who had never smoked, and lifetime smoking of >45 pack-years of cigarettes elevated the risk to 3.2 times that of men who had never smoked.

The efficacy of latex condoms for reducing risk of contracting sexually acquired HPV infection is not well established, although some degree of protection is likely provided. *In vitro* studies demonstrated the impermeability of latex condoms to HPV during conditions simulating sexual intercourse. Thus, condom use could be effective in reducing HPV-associated outcomes such as genital warts, cervical, anal and penile cancers (Shew & Fortenberry, 2005).

The incidence of penile cancer is lower compared to that of cervical cancer (Curado et al., 2007), likely due to the lower susceptibility of the penis to the malignant transformation virus-induced as compared to the cervix. Additionally, penile cancer, like cervical cancer, is caused by high-risk HPV, but penile cancer is 10 times less common than cervical cancer (Morris et al., 2007). In a large case series, HPV DNA was positive in invasive penile cancer in 40% to 50% of cases. Thus, many studies have shown a strong correlation of the presence of HPV types 16 and 18 with penile carcinoma (Daling et al., 2005; Gentile et al., 2006; Pascual et al., 2007; Senba et al., 2006; Tornesello et al., 2008; Villa & Lopes., 1986).

2.1.1 Human papillomavirus infection in men who have sex with men

HPV infection is considered to be a sexually transmitted disease, and the risk of HPV infection is increased by certain sexual behaviours (Sirera et al., 2006). HPV associated malignancies have been reported to occur in excess among patients with HIV or AIDS (Frisch et al.,2000). Co-infection with HIV and HPV has been investigated in studies due to the increased risks of warts and malignant neoplasias in the anal and genital tracts. Several studies conducted in men infected with HIV focus on the anal canal due to the high rates of HPV infection, anal intraepithelial neoplasia (AIN) and anal cancer. On the other hand, few studies have examined the penile region for HPV infections in men infected with HIV (Silva et al., 2011).

HPV infection is an independent risk factor for acquiring human immunodeficiency virus (HIV) infection and some forms of cancer. Men who have sex with men (MSM) may be difficult to identify in general practice because many of them do not self identify as homosexuals or bisexuals or are still having sex with women as they develop their sexual identity. The incidence of anal cancer among MSM is higher than cervical cancer rates among women. HPV has been definitively associated with more than 85% of all cancerous or precancerous anal lesions worldwide (Dietz & Nyberg, 2011).

The vast majority of HPV infections in immunocompetent individuals is transient, and the amount of persistent infections is rather low. This contrasts to immunosuppressed individuals, as patients with HIV infection exhibits high rates of persistent HPV infection. Consequently, these individuals have a high risk for HPV-associated malignant disease. Within the last decade, sufficient data were published to conclude that AIN and anal cancer continuously increase in HIV-positive MSM despite the use of highly active antiretroviral therapy. In contrast, only limited data are currently available on HPV-associated diseases at other anatomical sites of HIV-positive MSM, for example, oral cavity or penis (Kreuter &Wieland, 2009).

Giuliano et al. (2011) designed a cohort study to estimate the incidence and clearance of type-specific genital HPV in men and to assess associated factors. The incidence of a new genital HPV infection was 38.4 per 1000 person in 1159 men studied (95% CI 34.3–43.0). Oncogenic HPV infection was significantly associated with having a high number of lifetime female sexual partners (hazard ratio 2.40, 1.38–4.18, for at least 50 partners *vs* not more than one partner), and number of male partners who carried out anal intercourse (2.57, 1.46–4.49, for at least three male partners *vs* no recent partners). The median duration of HPV infection was 7.52 months (6.80-8.61) for any HPV and 12.19 months (7.16-18.17) for HPV 16. Clearance of oncogenic HPV infection decreased in men with a high number of lifetime female partners (0.49, 0.31–0.76, for at least 50 female partners *vs* not more than one partner), and in men in Brazil (0.71, 0.56–0.91) and Mexico (0.73, 0.57–0.94) compared with the USA.

Clearance of oncogenic HPV was more rapid with increasing age (1.02, 1.01–1.03). The results from that study provided much needed data about the incidence and clearance of HPV infection in men. These data are essential for the development of realistic cost-effectiveness models for male HPV vaccination internationally.

Current data on the spread of HPV infection to the different body parts implicated in sexual practices in both MSM and heterosexual men are limited. A cross-sectional study was carried out to evaluate the prevalence of HPV infection in the anus, mouth and penis in this specific population. The authors found the prevalence of penile HPV infection in HIV-positive men was 36% (95% CI, 26–48%), with a prevalence of 38% (95% CI, 25–53%) in MSM and 32% (95% CI, 14–55%) in heterosexual men, p= 0.43. (Sirera et al., 2006). The first study to address HPV DNA persistence and clearance in the genital area among men infected and non-infected with HIV. The authors observed that more men infected with HIV presented with multiple HPV types compared to the men seronegative to HIV. This finding may be attributed to the two groups' different immunodeficiency levels. Multiple infections with different types of HPV including high-risk HPVs are more frequent in men who are infected with HIV (Silva et al., 2011). However, there are few available studies on the persistence and elimination of HPV infection in men, such as HPV associated with penile carcinoma.

2.2 Mechanism of neoplastic transformation in cells

Papillomaviruses (PV) are small, non-enveloped, double-stranded DNA viruses that infect mucosal and cutaneous epithelia in a wide variety of higher vertebrates in a species-specific manner and induce cellular proliferation. PV isolates are traditionally described as "types". PV types have been detected in all carefully examined mammals and birds, with the possible exception of laboratory mice. In the only extensively studied host, humans, more than 100 human PV (HPV) types have been described based on the isolation of complete genomes, but independent studies indicate that many more exist, with a yet larger number presumed to exist based on the detection of subgenomic amplicons (Bernard et al., 2010, de Villiers et al., 2004). From the HPV types identified, approximately half of them infect the genital tract (Bosch et al., 2008). Many of these HPV types have been shown to be ubiquitous and globally distributed (de Villiers et al., 2004).

HPV are small DNA viruses that infect epithelial tissues. Whether cutaneous or mucosal, the more than 100 types of HPV described have in common a circular DNA genome of about 8.000 base pairs. A double-stranded circular DNA genome encodes approximately eight open-reading frames (ORFs). These small genomes are organized into an early, a late, and a long control region. The products of 3 genes from the early control region, genes *E6, E5* and *E7,* are essential in the HPV-induced processes of cellular transformation and immortalization (Moddy & Laimins, 2010), and 2 genes from the late control region, genes *L1* and *L2,* encode the viral capsid proteins (Villa, 2006). The figure 1 shows the general organization of the HPV genome (Ghittoni et al., 2010; Villa, 2006).

The process by which HPV facilitates tumor initiation and fosters tumor progression is an exceptional model to understand the development of many human cancers and also allows identification of additional signaling pathways targeted in malignant progression (Moddy & Laimins, 2010). An explanation for this is that the expression of viral genes *E6* and *E7* is increased in cells with integrated high risk HPV genome, and these genes products, the oncoproteins E6 and E7, respectively bind and inactivate cell tumor suppressor proteins p53 and pRb (Ghittoni et al., 2010).

The association between HPV and human cancer was first proposed more than three decades ago by Harald zur Hausen (2002). Subsequently, his group isolated several mucosal HPV types from cervical lesions, including the high-risk HPV16 (Bosch et al., 2008). Additionally, several studies have demonstrated the direct role of HPV infection in the development of several human cancers (Bosch et al., 2008; Caltellsagué et al., 2002; Gillison et al., 2008; Giuliano et al., 2008; Giuliano et al., 2010). HPV 16 and HPV 18 are the most frequently found HPV types in cervical cancers worldwide (Bosch et al., 2008; Munoz et al., 2003).

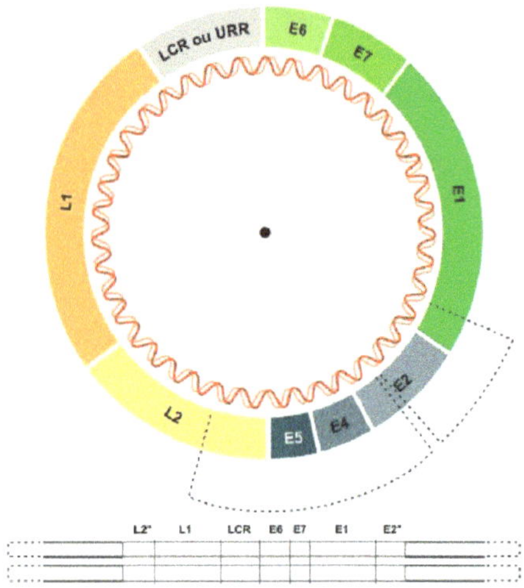

Function of viral proteins
E1: viral replication
E2: viral replication and transcription
E4: destabilization of cytokeratin network
E5: mediates mitogenic signal of growth factors
E6: major oncoprotein
E7: major oncoprotein
L1: major viral coat protein
L2: minor viral coat protein

Fig. 1. The genome of the HPV. The diagram indicates the ORFs of the early (E) and Late (L) genes, and the long control region (LCR). Functional of viral proteins.

For this reason, the majority of the biological studies were focused on these two HPV types (Moddy & Laimins, 2010; Villa, 2006). High-risk HPVs are also associated with many vulvar, anal, and penile carcinomas and contribute to oral cancer (Parkin & Bray, 2006). On the other hand, carcinomas from different anatomical sites, in contrast to cervical cancer, appear to be preferentially associated with HPV 16 (Chaturvedi, 2010; Gillison, 2008; Miralles-Guri et al., 2009). For instance, in the subset of penile cancer attributed to HPV infection, HPV 16 was found in 60,23% of cases (Miralles-Guri et al., 2009).

HPV-associated cancers are intimately linked to HPV persistence and the accumulation of chromosomal rearrangements in the infected tissue (Moody & Laimins, 2010). Studies suggest an association between HPV infection and penile cancer. The mechanism by which HPV leads to malignant transformation is likely mediated through two viral genes *E6* and *E7*, which are actively transcribed in HPV infected cells (Pow-Sang & Astigueta, 2009). The products of the early genes, *E6* and *E7*, of the high-risk HPV types play a key role in both events. Indeed, these proteins have developed a number of strategies to evade host immune surveillance allowing viral persistence, and to alter cell cycle and apoptosis control, facilitating the accumulation of DNA damage and mutations. Often, the oncoproteins target the same cellular pathways with different mechanisms, showing a strong synergism in promoting cellular transformation and neutralizing the immune response (Ghittoni et al., 2010).

In cervical carcinogenesis, recombination between HPV and chromossomal DNA is frequent and likely necessary for cancer progression. Moreover, DNA methylation, specifically on the *L1* gene, has been accepted as an important biomarker for cancerous progression in the cervix. The term DNA methylation refers to the transfer of a methyl group to cytosines that are part of CpG dinucleotides (meCpGs), which results in the binding of meCpG specific transcriptional repressors, for example MeCP2. In undifferentiated cervical cells, HPV-16 acquires a low and sporadically distributed CpG methylation, which disappears completely upon differentiation. During carcinogenesis, upon integration of HPV-16 and 18 into cellular DNA, the *L1* gene, and to a lower extent adjacent long control region (LCR) sequences, become hypermethylated, a fate of HPV DNA shared with most unrelated external DNA sequences that enter mammalian cells. The same mechanisms apparently occur during penile carcinogenesis, according with the study of Kalantari et al. (2008), which investigated the properties of HPV genomes in penile carcinomas from Brazilian patients. Their observations of frequent viral DNA methylation, chromosomal integration, and the prevalence of high-risk variants suggest that HPV dependent carcinogenesis of the penis and cervix follow similar etiological and epidemiological parameters.

A single nucleotide polymorphism (SNP) in codon 72 of *TP53* has attracted wide attention over the past decade. The most common polymorphism at codon 72 results in a non-conservative change of arginine to proline within a proline-rich region of p53, in a domain known to be important for growth suppression and apoptotic functions (Tornesello et al., 2008), may be involved in multiple steps of carcinogenesis and may also account for genetic differences in susceptibility to cancer (Reis et al., 2010b; Tornesello et al., 2008, Almeida et al., 2008). It has been demonstrated that the *TP53* polymorphism distribution varies according to ethnic and geographical backgrounds, like most human genetic polymorphisms (Reis et al., 2010b).

Storey et al. (1998) found that women who are homozygous for *TP53*Arg are seven times more susceptible to HPV-associated squamous carcinoma of the cervix than are heterozygous women. Since then, many groups have reported an effect of the *TP53* codon 72 polymorphism on cervical cancer and others carcinomas. A meta-analysis of several studies on *TP53* polymorphism at codon 72 confirmed that arginine homozygous genotype is associated with an increased risk of invasive cervical cancers, but not with squamous intraepithelial lesions, supporting the hypothesis that the polymorphism may have a main role in the progression of HPV-related cancers, rather than in the tumor initiation (Koushik et al., 2004). On the other hand, very few studies have been designed to investigate *TP53* polymorphisms in penile carcinomas.

In a case-control study, Tornesello et al. (2008) analyzed the polymorphism of the gene *TP53* at codon 72 and found the polymorphism associated with increased risk for 78 penile SCC biopsies (n = 17 from Uganda and n = 61 from Italy). Despite, significant differences in arginine and proline allele distribution were observed when the cases were stratified by

HPV status. Thus, no evidence of association between homozygosity for p53 arginine and HPV-related or HPV-unrelated penile SCC was observed among Ugandan or Italian populations. In another study, the *TP53* Arg/Arg genotype did not appear to represent a risk factor for the development of genital SCC in men, and no correlation was found between the *TP53* polymorphism at codon 72 and the presence of HPV DNA in the tumour tissue (Humbey et al., 2003).

The role of several tumour suppressor genes and cellular oncoproteins has been characterized by studying HPV E6 and E7 and or other related viral oncoproteins. The knowledge of HPV and cancer association obtained during the past three decades is extremely relevant. Worldwide, this knowledge has led to clinical and scientific achievements such as the generation, commercialization, and distribution of cervical cancer high-risk HPV vaccines. As a consequence of research studies on virus and cancer association, the Nobel Prize in Physiology or Medicine 2008 was awarded to Dr. Harald zur Hausen for his discovery of HPV causing cervical cancer (Ghittoni et al., 2010).

Certainly, the expression of viral oncoproteis is needed to induce and maintain the neoplastic phenotype of cervical cancer cells. The similarity of the tissues leads one to assume that a similar mechanism may play a role in the development of HPV-induced penile cancer (Kayes et al., 2007). Provided that identification of HPV implies a causal role of the virus with the carcinogenic process, the attributable fraction of penile cancer related to HPV has been estimated at 47%. The etiology of penile carcinomas is likely to be heterogeneous, co-existing both HPV related and HPV-independent pathways. Based on cervical cancer studies, penile cancer could also arise from initial HPV infection which persists over time, causing genetics alterations within the infected penile epithelium, leading to the cancer development. However, the molecular mechanisms underneath HPV-induced penile cancer remain to be completely understood (reviewed in Miralles-Guri et al., 2009).

2.3 High risk HPV-associated penile cancer

Molecular biology techniques with different sensitivity and specificity have facilitated the characterization of the entire HPV genome, where different functional regions are identified, as a profile of their gene expression. The techniques of Southern blotting and *in situ* hybridization have been used extensively in the past to identify viral sequences in tissues. Additionally, polymerase chain reaction (PCR) and its variants have been recognized as the most appropriate method to identify and type HPV genomes because of its higher sensitivity and specificity (Campisi et al., 2007).

The most studies in penile cancer use PCR consensus primers for HPV DNA detection, such GP5+/6 and My9/11. However, a small set of PCR studies included the SPF10 primers to identify HPV genomes. Almost all studies used previously stored formalin-fixed and paraffin-embedded samples (Table 1). However, sample preparation and fixation lead to DNA degradation, decreasing PCR efficiency and reducing the size of amplifiable DNA (Miralles-Guri et al., 2009).

When using PCR as a strategy to identify viral genome, false-negative results may occur due to variations of the primer binding sites on target DNA, which in turn would lead to lower amplification signals of some HPV genotypes. Because of this problem, the PCR method may not detect all HPV genotypes present in the sample. Recently, studies involving genotyping of HPV with genotype-specific oligonucleotides and DNA microarray analysis have been reported. A novel DNA biochip is described based on a plastic substrate, onto which small polymer droplets and single-stranded DNA are printed in the form of microarrays. After DNA isolation, PCR and biochip read-outs were compared, the chip allowed for genotyping of the most common virus strains, which, according to current prevalence studies, cover 85–95% of all infections. Following the biochip approach, as little as 10 virus copies can be detected within a short exposure time. Even using paraffin-embedded material and 104 copies per PCR are sufficient to allow rapid and reliable HPV genotyping (Brandstetter et al., 2010). The biochip technique has become more successful for early cervical and non-cervical cancer diagnosis and might become the methodology of choice for HPV detection in the near future.

As HPV E6 and E7 expression is necessary for the induction and the maintenance of the transformed phenotype, HPV-associated tumors are valuable tools to investigate important aspects of human carcinogenesis. Molecular evidence for a causal association includes the presence of HPV genomes in tumor cells, integration and specificity of HPV genomes, high HPV viral load in tumors, and elevated and constitutive expression of E6 and E7 oncogenes in tumor cells (Chaturvedi, 2010). Presence of HPV was found to be a risk factor for penile SCCs (Rubin et al., 2001; Gregoire et al., 1995). Several molecular techniques with different sensitivity and specificity have been used for HPV detection and genotyping among the different epidemiological studies. Considering that the incidence of penile and cervical cancers is high in the same geographical areas, it is reasonable to assume that both types of cancer share the same etiological factors. However, less than half of penile cancers are related to HPV infection (Gross & Pfister, 2004; Rubin et al., 2001) whereas the virus is found in almost all cervical SCCs (Chaux et al., 2010).

Additionally, studies have reported a heterogeneous prevalence of high risk HPV types, suggesting that only a subset of cases can be attributed to viral infection (See table 1). In the two recent studies of the HPV type distribution in penile carcinoma, a global HPV prevalence was found to be approximately 46.9% and 47,9%, (Backes et al., 2009; Miralles-Guri et al., 2009). About half of the penile tumors were associated with HPV 16 (64.07%) and 18 (9.70%) with little presence of other genotypes, 45 (1.45%), 33 (0.97%) and 31 (0.36%), respectively. As expected, the literature confirmed a higher prevalence of HPV 16 and 18 in penile tumors (73.78%). This finding was in agreement across of all 36 studies presented in table 1.

Virtually all of the studies in Table 1 used PCR to detect HPV DNA, a method slightly more sensitive than southern blotting and *in situ* hybridization. The higher the sensitivity of the method used, the more likely the prevalence of HPV is closer to the real prevalence associated with penile cancer. The relatively wide range of HPV prevalence in penile tumors in the published literature confirms that in addition to geographic differences. The greatest percentage of studies used PCR consensus primers for HPV DNA detection, such as GP5+/6+ and MY09/11.

In the study of Gregoire et al. (1995), HPV DNA was detected in 26 (22.2%) of 117 specimens. In 23 (88.5%) of the 26 HPV-positive specimens, only HPV type 16 was identified. HPV DNA was frequently associated with SCC in areas showing basaloid and/or warty changes virus DNA was more often associated with high-grade tumors (p=0.0278) exhibiting aggressive growth (p=0.0382) localized to the penile glans (p=0.0324). Stepwise logistic regression analysis revealed that only tumor histopathology was a significant predictor of an HPV association. Heidman et al. (2007) detecetd HPV DNA in 46 of 83 (55%) and HPV16 was the predominant type, appearing in 24 (52%) of 46 of penile SCCs. In a case control study in Denmark, of the 37 penile SCC patients whose tumor tissues were PCR-examined for the presence of HPV DNA, 24 (65%) were high-risk HPV positive, and 1 (3%) was positive to a low-risk HPV type (HPV 6) [Madsen et al., 2008].

Author	Year	Country	Sample	Method	Cases	HPV	HPV 16	HPV 18	HPV 31	HPV 33	HPV 45
Villa & Lopes	1986	Brazil	Frozen	Southern Blot (SB)	18	8	0	7	0	0	0
Kiyabu et al.	1989	USA	PE	PCR TS	5	2	2	0	0	0	0
Varma et al.	1991	USA	PE	PCR TS 6/11/16	30	23	15	0	0	0	0
Wiener et al.	1992	USA	FFPE	PCR TS 16/18 / SB	29	9	8	1	0	0	0
Sarkar et al.	1992	USA	FFPE	PCR TS 6/11/16/18	12	9	9	0	0	0	0
Iwasawa et al.	1993	Japan	FFPE	PCR TS 16/18	111	70	68	2	0	0	0
Suzuki et al.	1994	Japan	Fresh /PE	PCR TS	13	7	4	0	1	2	0
Chan et al.	1994	China	PWE	PCR TS 16/18	41	6	2	2	0	0	0
Cupp et al.	1995	USA	FFPE	PCR My9/11 TS 16/18	45	23	17	2	0	0	0
Gregoire et al.	1995	USA/ Paraguay	FFPE	PCR TS 6/11/16/18 SB	117	26	23	0	0	0	0
Cubilla et al.	1998	USA /Paraguay	FFPE	PCR TS	11	0	0	0	0	0	0
Nasca et al.	1999	Italy	FFPE	PCR TS	4	3	2	0	0	0	0
Poblet et al.	1999	Spain	FFPE	PCR TS	2	2	2	0	0	0	0
Levi et al.	1998	Brazil	Frozen	PCR My9/11 TS 16/18	50	28	16	3	0	0	0
Picconi et al.	2000	Argentina	FFPE	PCR GP5+/6+	38	27	6	8	0	0	0
Bezzera et al.	2001	Brazil	FFPE	PCR TS	82	25	13	4	0	0	1
Gil et al.	2001	Brazil	FFPE	My9/11 PCR TS	55	17	3	0	0	0	0
Rubin et al.	2001	USA/ Paraguay	FFPE	PCR SPF	142	60	36	2	0	0	4
Perceau et al.	2003	France	FFPE	PCR GP5+/6+ TS	17	6	3	0	0	0	0

Author	Year	Country	Sample	Method	Cases	HPV	HPV 16	HPV 18	HPV 31	HPV 33	HPV 45
Liegl et al.	2004	Austria	FFPE	PCR TS	5	5	5	0	0	0	0
Nascimento et al.	2004	Brazil	Fresh /PE	My9/11 PCR TS	16	10	1	0	0	1	0
Daling et al.	2005	USA	FFPE	My9/11	94	75	65	0	0	0	0
Salazar et al.	2005	Mexico	FFPE	PCR TS 16	46	28	28	0	0	0	0
Gentile et al.	2006	Italy	FFPE	PCR My9/11 GP5+/6+	11	8	5	2	0	0	0
Lont et al.	2006	Nerther-lands	FFPE	PCR GP5+/6+	171	50	38	3	0	2	3
Dorfman et al.	2006	Venezuela	FFPE	My9/11	5	5	0	0	0	0	0
Senba et al.	2006	Thailand	FFPE	PCR SPF	65	53	1	36	0	0	0
Protzel et al.	2007	Germany	FFPE	PCR TS 6/11/16/18	18	4	3	0	0	0	0
Pascual et al.	2007	Spain	FFPE	PCR My9/11 GP5+/6+	49	38	32	4	0	0	0
Heidman et al.	2007	Nerther-lands	FFPE	-	83	46	24	3	0	1	2
Guerrero et al.	2008	Spain	FFPE	PCR GP5+/6+	24	11	11	0	0	0	0
Yanagawa et al.	2008	Japan	FFPE	PCR - RFLP	25	3	3	0	0	0	0
Scheiner et al.	2008	Brazil	frozen	PCR My9/11	80	58	12	1	2	2	2
Madsen et al.	2008	Denmark	-	PCR GP5+/6+ TS	37	25	24	0	0	0	0
Prowse et al.	2008	UK	FFPE	PCR SPF	26	14	11	0	0	0	0
Tornesello et al.	2008	Uganda /Italy	FFPE	PCR My9/11 GP5+/6+	78	40	36	0	0	0	0
Total					1655	824	528	80	3	8	12

PE=paraffin-embedded
FFPE= formalin-fixed paraffin- embedded
PCR TS= polymerase chain reaction type specific
PCR-RFLP= polymerase chain reaction – restriction fragment length polymorphism

Table 1. Prevalence for HPV in 36 studies (n=1.644) Adapted from Backes et al., 2009; Miralles-Guri et al., 2009.

The objective of the Senba et al. (2006) study was to determine the relation between penile cancer and the prevalence of HPV genotypes in northern Thailand. Eighty-eight specimens of penile tissue (65 malignant, 1 pre-malignant, and 22 benign cases) were examined to determine the association of HPV infection. HPV DNA was detected in 81.5% of cases of penile cancer using PCR. The high-risk HPV16, most commonly associated with penile cancer in previous reports, was found in only one case in this study. The most prevalent genotype was the high-risk HPV-18, found in 55.4% of the cases (32.3% single and 23.1% multiple infection) followed by the low-risk HPV-6, found in 43.1% of the cases (24.6% single and 18.5% multiple infection). In this study, penile cancer was found to be highly correlated with HPV DNA.

Several studies have confirmed a predominance of penile cancer in the North and Northeast of Brazil which are regions with lower human development indexes (Favorito et al., 2008; Koifman et al., 2011; Reis et al., 2010a). Scheiner et al. (2008) in Rio de Janeiro, Brazil found that HPV infection may have contributed to malignant transformation in a large proportion of their penile cancer cases but only inguinal metastasis was a prognostic factor impacting survival of those patients. In another Brazilian study the patients having HPV type-16 in their tumors were submitted to major surgical procedures to remove the primary tumor (p=0.04). The relative risk of death for patients with HPV type-16 was 7.59 times greater than that for the virus negative group. Also, patients presenting HPV type 16 in the tumor presented a lower tendency for survival (without statistical significance). Coilocitosis was detected in 12 patients, presenting a significant correlation with the presence of HPV type-16 (p=0.026). The authors concluded the infection by HPV was strongly associated with penile epidermoid carcinoma (30.9%). The presence of HPV type-16 in the tumors was associated with increased tumor-related mortality. No HPV 18 was detected in their samples (Gil et al., 2001). The presence of genomic DNA of HPV 16 and 18 in penile cancers identified by Southern blotting (Villa & Lopes, 1986) and polymerase chain reaction (PCR) (Bezerra et al., 2001) assays also in Brazil.

In a case control study to analyze the genetic susceptibility involving *TP53* polymorphism, 78 penile SCC biopsies (n= 17 from Uganda, n= 61 from Italy) and blood samples from 150 healthy controls (n = 57 from Uganda, n = 93 from Italy) were collected. Among Uganda cases the heterozygous, proline homozygous and arginine homozygous genotype frequency was 41.2%, 52.9% and 5.9%, respectively, and among controls was 40.3%, 54.4%, and 5.3%, respectively (P = 0.9917). Conversely, among Italian cases genotype distribution was 42.6%, 4.9%, and 52.5%, and among controls was 34.4%, 7.5%, and 58.1%, respectively (p=0.5343). No significant differences in arginine and proline allele distribution were observed when the cases were stratified by HPV status. Therefore, no evidence of association between homozygosity for p53 arginine and HPV-related or HPV-unrelated penile squamous cell carcinoma was observed among Ugandan or among Italian populations (Tornesello et al., 2008).

Poblet et al. (1999) described two cases of penile SCC in HIV-positive patients with distinctive clinicopathologic characteristics. The tumors appeared in patients infected with HIV and were located in the glans of the penis. Histologically, the tumors were well-differentiated, infiltrating, penile SCC. The entire spectrum from benign condyloma to infiltrative SCC was present in the two patients. The reported cases suggest a synergic interaction of HPV and HIV in the carcinogenic process of some penile carcinoma. In fact, the immune system efficiency is a key to control HPV replication, which was evident in the increased incidence of lesions caused by HPV and recurrent infections in the group seropositive for HIV. However, the cellular and molecular mechanisms responsible for protection from and elimination of HPV infection are not fully established (Silva et al., 2011). Based on cervical cancer studies, penile cancer could also arise from an initial HPV infection which persists over time and causes genetic alterations, leading to an interference of the cell division cycle and apoptosis. The International Agency for Research on Cancer (IARC) has concluded that there is sufficient evidence to classify HPV infection as a Group I carcinogen for cancers of the cervix, anus, oropharynx, penis, vagina, and vulva (IARC, 2007). However, epidemiologic and molecular data in support of a causal association are currently sparse and do not extend beyond detection of HPV genomes in tumor cells in these cancers (Chaturvedi et al. 2010).

The most serious consequences of genital HPV infections in women are high-grade squamous intraepithelial lesions, which can progress to invasive cervical cancer (IARC, 2007). Numerous studies have investigated the potential risk factors for HPV among heterosexual men, men who have sex with men (MSM), and men with HIV/AIDS. Universal HPV risk factors described have included the number of lifetime sex partners, frequency of condom use, race/ethnicity, educational level, presence of a concomitant sexually transmitted infections (STIs) [especially HIV/AIDS infection], and a positive history of tobacco use.

High-risk male populations, most notably MSM and HIV/AIDS-infected males, as a community, characteristically have a lifestyle that may incorporate psychosocial, physical, and sexual practices that place them at greater risk for STIs such as HPV infections. This population falls increasingly vulnerable to HPV-associated cancers because of frequent high-risk behaviors, increased likelihood of concomitant infections, and a current lack of male cancer screening guidelines (Kreuter et al., 2009). However, studies have shown that uncircumcised men have an additional anatomical risk factor as there is a lower incidence of HPV infection and HPV-associated penile cancer in circumcised men, especially in those men who were circumcised at a younger age (Castellsague et al.,2002).

Studies have demonstrated that HPV infection in the penis is highly prevalent among heterosexual men who are seronegative for HIV, with rates ranging from 52% to 72% (Giuliano et al., 2008; Silva et al., 2011). In a recent longitudinal study to assess the persistence and clearance of HPV DNA from the penis of men infected and non-infected with HIV, the results demonstrated 66% of men without HIV infection presented with some type of HPV. The vast majority of such infections are transient, and virus elimination occurs rapidly in immunocompetent individuals (Silva et al., 2011)

The quadrivalent HPV vaccine was licensed in 2006 for use in women aged 9 to 26 to prevent infection with HPV serotypes (6, 11, 16 and 18) to prevent HPV related cervical cancer. The immunization protocol covers the most prevalent HPV serotypes (Garland et al., 2007). In 2009, the vaccine approval was extended to boys and men aged 9 to 26 based on prevention of infection with serotypes 6 and 11, and subsequent prevention of genital warts. In 2010, the vaccine received an additional indication for prevention of anal cancer in men and women. However, given multiple etiologies and the low incidence of penile cancer, vaccination also will likely provide marginal benefit on a population level. Nevertheless, the vaccine should decrease penile cancer caused by HPV 16 and 18, which are the most common subtypes associated with penile carcinomas. Vaccination is likely to have a more substantial benefit for benign HPV-related diseases of the penis, such as condyloma acuminata, which are far more common in any population (Barroso et al., 2011).

When considering the impact of a vaccine on cancer incidence, it is useful to consider the past experience with Hepatitis B virus (HBV) (Franceschi et al., 2002). Like HPV, HBV is the cause of cancer, specifically hepatocellular carcinoma - in chronically infected individuals. Unlike HPV, however, HBV is also associated with acute disease at the time of infection and substantial morbidity and mortality from causes other than cancer (Plummer & Franceschi, 2002). In the case of HPV vaccination, it is likely that secular trends in cervical cancer incidence or mortality will provide convincing evidence of its effectiveness. Thus, a decline in the incidence and in the mortality rates from cervical and non-cervical cancers is expected in many populations after the introduction of screening and immunization programs.

2.4 Prevention for penile cancer

Two HPV vaccines were developed, a quadrivalent vaccine that provides protection against HPV types 6, 11, 16, and 18 and a bivalent vaccine that protects against HPV types 16 and 18. The quadrivalent and bivalent vaccine were approved by the U.S. Food and Drug Administration (FDA) for the prevention of HPV associated cervical cancer, adenocarcinoma *in situ*, cervical intraepithelial neoplasia (CIN) grades 1-3, vulvar intraepithelial neoplasia, vaginal intraepithelial neoplasia grades 2/3, vaginal cancer, vulvar cancer, and genital warts in women aged 9-26 years (Chaturvadi et al., 2010). The quadrivalent Gardasil™ (Merck and Co. Inc - Whitehouse Station, NJ) vaccine is currently approved for sale in 85 countries. Cervarix®, the HPV vaccine produced by GlaxoSmith Kline, has been approved in the European Union, Australia, and Kenya, with applications pending elsewhere (Agosti and Goldie, 2007). According to the researchers, the vaccine was 89% effective in preventing infection with HPV types 16 and 18, and 100% effective in preventing the diseases associated with these types (Chaturvadi et al., 2010).

The L1 virus-like particles (VLP) for specific HPV types is a highly efficacious vaccine antigen in humans. Clinical trials of multivalent L1 VLP vaccines intended to be disseminated in public health programs have shown safety, immunogenicity, and high efficacy (Bosch & Harper, 2006). Studies have shown that serologic diagnosis of HPV infection using genetically engineered HPV capsids (VLPs) correlates well with HPV DNA presence in cervical smears. The L1 VLP vaccines are unlikely to be effective as a treatment of women currently positive for a persistent HPV infection of the same type. Because the vaccines are prophylactic and not therapeutic, vaccination is not effective in clearing either established infections or pre-existing disease. Although the duration of protection is as yet unknown, current data indicated that both vaccines are immunogenic and efficacious for up to 4 years after vaccination (Chaturvadi et al., 2010). The antibodies produced recognized type-specific conformational epitopes present on VLPs, particularly against the viral capsid protein L1 and the humoral response against HPV, i.e., the production of IgG, is stable over time (Chatuverti et al., 2010; Villa, 2006). Both the quadrivalent and the bivalent prophylactic vaccines have demonstrated high efficacy (90%-98%) against persistent HPV infection and vaccine type-related CIN 2 or above (Paavonen et al., 2007). Additionally, both vaccines are safe and immunogenic among adolescent males aged 10-18 years and 9-15 years, respectively. The quadrivalent vaccine has demonstrated high efficacy in preventing persistent HPV infection (85.6%), external genital lesions (90.4%), condyloma (89.4%), and PIN (100%) among adolescent boys and young men aged 16 to 26 years (Chaturvadi et al., 2010).

Some studies have demonstrated a strong association between lifetime number of sexual partners and genital HPV acquisition. The acquisition of new sexual partners continues throughout all age groups. In addition, studies have shown consistently that the risk of cervical cancer can be predicted as much by a woman's own sexual behaviour as by the sexual behaviour of her husband/partner. The presence of HPV DNA in the penis and urethra of her sexual partner(s) is directly related to her HPV carrier status and, therefore, her increased risk of developing cervical cancer (Castellsague et al., 2009).

Jasen & Shaw (2004) presented three major issues to be resolved in order to take full advantage of the promise of HPV vaccines. First, the global infrastructure must be reinforced to accommodate the logistics of delivery of a new vaccine to a, perhaps, non pediatric population. This is a rather tall order, and in practice, this may become a pediatric vaccine in developing countries even if the developed world makes a different choice. There are no adolescent vaccination programs in most parts of the world. The World Health Organization's Expanded Program for Immunization delivers the "basic six" vaccines (diphtheria, tetanus, pertussis, polio, measles and BCG) to a large fraction of the world's birth cohort. If effective immunity could be shown to last into adulthood, then pediatric administration may be the easier solution for developing countries. Second, the capacity for producing HPV vaccines on a global scale must be created. The "chicken-and-egg" aspect of this problem might not be as obvious to those outside the vaccine industry. In order to justify the capital and other ancillary investments necessary to create manufacturing capacity approximately ten times greater than one might normally contemplate, there must be some reasonable assurance of a market for the product. This is tightly linked to the third issue, funding. In most of the world, vaccines are paid for by governmental or international donor agencies. Until recently, the vaccines provided through such funding mechanisms have been "traditional" vaccines such as the "basic six" mentioned above.

To deliver an HPV vaccine for cervical cancer to the women in greatest need, many of whom live in the very poorest countries around the world, one can only hope that industry, governments, and donor organizations will make similar efforts and alliances to guarantee the proper deliver of the vaccines for those who truly need them. Clinical studies to date have focused on women because they suffer most from the pathology of HPV infection. Men, however, are considered important vectors in the chain of HPV infection and dissemination. With the notable exception of penile warts and some cases of penile and anal cancer, there is little obvious pathology associated with HPV in heterosexual males, making HPV very difficult to be detected in that population. This is partly because of the lack (until recently) of an acceptable method of sampling. MSM how practice anal intercourse are subjected to development of anal intraepithelial neoplasia. The anal epithelium has a transition zone similar to that of the cervix, and this is the most frequent site of HPV infection in this group. Since vaccines work best when given to large proportions of the population, vaccination trials to show some efficacy in men are also being considered (Jansen & Shaw, 2004).

As a consequence of the recent licensing of the quadrivalent and the bivalent HPV vaccines, important questions have emerged regarding investment policies for vaccination programs. The decision for an individual country, such as Brazil, over others developing countries, to introduce a new public health intervention must take into consideration multiple factors. These include the disease burden, effectiveness of the intervention, the financial costs required to initiate and sustain the program, the cost-effectiveness of the intervention, the programmatic capacity and infrastructure necessary to successfully deliver the intervention, and the likelihood of cultural acceptability, political will and public support (Goldie et al., 2007).

The quadrivalent vaccine also dominates the bivalent vaccine as it lacks cross-reactivity against non-16/18 oncogenic HPV types and it also reducces the incidence rates of on genital warts (Dee &Howel, 2010). In a recent study, Malasya (2011) reported for the cost-effectiveness analysis, the cost per life year saved vaccine compared to no vaccine, as $12,866 and $12,827 for the quadrivalent and the bivalent vaccines, respectively. Comparing the bivalent to the quadrivalent vaccine, the cost-effectiveness ratio (ICER) is $12,488, showing that the bivalent vaccine saves more lives per cost. However, the cost per Quality-Adjusted Life Years (QALY) saved for the quadrivalent vaccine compared to no vaccine was estimated as $9,071, while it was $10,392 for the bivalent vaccine, with the quadrivalent vaccine dominating the bivalent vaccine due to the additional QALY effect on the reduction of genital warts (Lee et al., 2011).

A study also investigated the cost-effectiveness of HPV vaccination in France, using a quadrivalent HPV vaccine. This study compared screening plus vaccination at age 14 years with screening alone. The ICER for the addition of vaccination to screening was €13,809/QALY when considering all direct healthcare costs. This is somewhat higher than the finding of €9,706/QALY for the bivalent vaccine,. Although it should be noted that no study undertook a direct head-to-head comparison of the two products and the results may therefore not be directly comparable (Bergeron et al., 2008).

For a country like Brazil, the clinical benefits of an HPV 16/18 vaccine is likely to be substantial. The most influential factor on cost-effectiveness is the vaccine cost. If the cost per vaccinated woman is less than I$ 25,00 implying a per dose cost of approximately I$ 5,00 vaccination is likely to be extremely cost-effective in Brazil. The most effective strategy, within a framework that would still be potentially cost-effective in Brazil, would be vaccination before age 12, followed by screening three times per lifetime between ages 35 and 45. Assuming a coverage rate of 70%, this strategy would be expected to prevent more than 100,000 cases of invasive cervical cancer over a 5-year period. Finally, vaccination strategies we have identified as cost-effective may be unaffordable in low and even middle income countries without international financial aid. The results from the studies carried out in North America and Europe can provide guidance to the global community by helping to identify health investments of highest priority and with the greatest promise and best effectiveness to the population at risk (Goldie et al., 2007).

After a vaccination campaign begun, the population will be a mixture of younger, vaccinated women and older unvaccinated women. The impact of vaccination is not seen in the population as a whole until the vaccinated group dominates in the high-risk age group (Bosch & Harper,2006). Thus, screening programs will be required to complement vaccine programs for many decades, providing the epidemiological means to understand the actual effect of the vaccination on the selected group. On the other hand, educational actions to prevent cervical and non cervical cancers, which are part of basic health actions, should be implemented as a professional commitment to the population's quality of life and a health care quality, emphasizing patients' autonomy in self-care.

Recently, a Brazilian study aimed to evaluate the applicability of an educational booklet that contained information for the general population about promotion and prevention of infections and neoplasic diseases caused by the HPV. The study was arranged in two phases. First, the booklet was given to 2000 volunteers who evaluated the applicability of the booklet without previous education or discussion about the subject. The educational material was published and 2000 copies were distributed during a health social event. In the event, the booklet raised the interest of the general public and gave the volunteers a chance to participate in a study that investigated the presence of the HPV as part of the genital microbiote. In a second phase, a detailed analysis of the data was made and the booklet revealed applicable. The authors concluded that managing and presenting the information beforehand is an important step to promote and improve preventive campaigns and strategies aimed to the population at large regarding HPV infection and its potential role on carcinogenesis (Reis et al., 2010c).

Education should not only be considered an extra activity, but an effective action to redirect health promotion practices as a whole. Reis et al. (2010c) suggested that preventive knowledge about the natural history of cervical and non cervical cancers and, including the feasibility of HPV vaccination programs for both sexes, will decrease the incidence of HPV associated cancers and has the potential to be of great significance to health management of high-risk female and male populations.

Proper condom use as a primary prevention measure for STI should remain a top priority for health official campaigns. The preventive strategies should keep on focusing primarily on the increase of STI. This knowledge is proven powerful to elicit individual awareness responsible for influencing individual risk perception amongst those sexually active. However, the campaigns must understand that modifying individual risk perception does not effectively translate into changes of preventive behaviors. To reach the public health goal of reducing STI prevalence, barriers to engaging in STI prevention need to be addressed, including education strategies.

3. Conclusion

Penile SCC is a severe and uncommon disease with devastating medical psychological consequences for the patients. The disease is mainly related to poor hygiene, sexual history, and smoking. Male circumcision has been used as a preventive measure for sexually transmitted infection with positive impact on the reduction of penile cancer incidence rates when neonatally performed. Penile cancer development is facilitated by phimosis. In general, penile SCC imposes an increase in the relative risk of invasive disease compared to an *in situ* cancer. The understanding of the natural history of penile cancer is fundamental to promote effective preventive strategies. Globalization and promiscuity are expected to be the major causes leading to the increase of penile SCC incidence. The oncoproteins of high risk HPV types target cellular pathways promoting cellular transformation and neutralizing the immune response. FDA recently approved and licensed the first vaccine for HPV-6, -11, -16, and -18 for early prevention in teenagers and young adults. Vaccination is likely to have a more substantial benefit for prevent cervical and non cervical cancers. Novel preventive strategies are important to complement the immunization programs that should always take educational strategy as an important step on primary prevention.

4. Acknowledgment

This chapter was written by two researchers of the HPV Study Group in Goiânia-GO, Brazil (A.A.S.R. and A.D.C.). The authors thank R. S. Santos, L.P. Barcelos and A.A.P. de Paula for their assistance in the preparation of the chapter and S. Quail for English support.

5. References

Agosti, J.M. & Goldie, S.J. (2007). Introducing HPV vaccine in developing countries-key challenges and issues. *The New England Journal of Medicine*, Vol. 356, No. 9, (May 2007), pp. 1908-1910, ISSN 0028-4793

Almeida, P.S.; Manoel, W.J.; Reis, AA.; Silva E.R. & Saddi,V.A. (2008). TP53 codon 72 polymorphism in adult soft tissue sarcomas. *Genetics and Molecular Research*, Vol. 7, No. 4, (May 2008), pp. 1344-1352, ISSN 1676-5680

Backes, D.M.; Kurman, R.J.; Pimenta, J.M. & Smith, J.S. (2009). Systematic review of human papillomavirus in invasive penile cancer. *Cancer Causes Control*, Vol. 20, No. 4, (April 2009), pp. 449-457, ISSN 0957-5243

Barroso, L.F. & Wilkin, T. (2011). Human Papillomavirus Vaccination in Males: The State of the Science. *Current Infectious Disease Reports*, Vol. 13, No. 1, (January 2011), pp.175–181, ISSN 1523-384

Baseman, J.G. & Koutskyl, L.A. (2005). The epidemiology of human papillomavirus infections. *Journal of Clinical Virology* , Vol. 32, No. 1001, (March 2005), pp. S16–S24, ISSN 1386-6532

Benard, V.B.; Johnson,C.J.; Thompson, T.D.; Roland,K.B.; Lai,S.M.; Cokkinides,V. Tangka, F.; Hawkins, N.A.; Lawson, H. & Weir, H.K. (2008). Examining the Association Between Socioeconomic Status and Potential Human Papillomavirus-associated Cancers. *Cancer*,Vol. 113, Supp. 10, (November 2008), pp. 2910–2918, ISSN 1097-0142

Bergeron, C.; Largeron, N.; McAllister, R.; Mathevet, P. & Remy, V. (2008). Cost-effectiveness analysis of the introduction of a quadrivalent human papillomavirus vaccine in France. *International Journal of Technology Assessment in Health Care*, Vol. 24, No. 1, (January 2011), pp. 10–19, ISSN 0266-4623

Bezzera, A.L.; Lopes, A. & Landman, G. (2001). Clinicopsthologic features and human papillomavirus DNA prevalence of wartyand squamous cell carcinoma of the penis. *The American Journal of Surgical Pathology*, Vol. 25, No. 5, (May 2001), pp. 673-678, ISSN 0147-5185

Bigot, P. (2011). Le point sur les lésions dermatologiques du pénis: comment repérer les lésions précancéreuses du pénis? *Progrès en Urologie*, Vol. 21, Supp. 2, (March 2011), pp.S50-S52, ISSN 1166-7087

Bosch, F.X. Quiao, YL. & Castellsagué, X. (2006). Chapter 2: The epidemiology of human papillomavirus infection and its association with cervical cancer. *Journal of Infection*, Vol. 94, Supp. 1, (January 2006), pp. S8–S21, ISSN 0020-7292

Bosch, F.X.; Burvhell, A.N.; Schiffman, M.; Giuliano, A.R.; de Sanjosé, S.; Bruni, L.; Tortolero-Luna, G.; Kjaer, S.K. & Muñoz, N. (2008). Epidemiology and Natural History of Human Papillomavirus Infections and Type-Specific Implications in Cervical Neoplasia. In: ICO Monograph Series on HPV and Cervical Cancer: General Overview, *Vaccine*, Vol. 26, Supp. 10, (August 2008), pp. K1–K16, ISSN 0264-410X

Bosch, X. & Harper, D. (2006). Prevention strategies of cervical cancer in the HPV vaccine era. *Gynecologic Oncology*, Vol. 103, No. 1, (August 2006), pp. 21–24, ISSN 0090-8258

Brandstetter, T.; Böhmer, S.; Prucker, O.; Bissé, E.; zur Hausen, A. Alt-Mörbe, J. & Rühe, J. (2010). A polymer-based DNA biochip platform for human papilloma virus genotyping. *Journal of Virological Methods*, Vol. 163, No. 1, (January 2010), pp. 40-48, ISSN 0166-0934

Campisi, G.; Panzarella, V.; Giuliani, M.; Lajolo, C.; Di Fede, O.; Falaschini, S.; Di Liberto, C.; Scully, C. & Lo Muzio, L. (2007). Human papillomavirus: Its identikit and controversial role in oral oncogenesis, premalignant and malignant lesions (Review). *International Journal Of Oncology*, Vol. 30, No. 4, (April 2007), pp. 813-823, ISSN 1019-6439

Castellsagué, X.; Bosxh, F.X. & Muñoz, N. (2002). Environmental co-factors in HPV carcinogenesis. *Virus Research*, Vol. 89, No. 2, (February2002), pp. 191-199, ISSN 0168-1702

Castellsagué, X.; Schneider,A.; Kaufmann, A.M. & Bosch, F.X. (2009). HPV vaccination against cervical cancer in women above 25 years of age: key considerations and current perspectives. *Gynecologic Oncology*, Vol. 115, No. 3, (March 2009), pp. S15–S23, ISSN 0090-8258

Cavalcanti, S.M.B.; Zardo, L.G.; Passos, M.R.L. & Oliveira, L.H.S. (2000). Epidemiological Aspects of Human Papillomavirus Infection and Cervical Cancer in Brazil. *Journal of Infection*, Vol. 40, No. 1, (January 2000), pp. 80–87, ISSN 0163-4453

Chan, K.W.; Lam, K.Y. ; Chan, A.C; Lau, P. & Srivastava, G. (1994). Prevalence of human papillomavirus types 16 and 18 in penile carcinoma: a study of 41 cases using PCR. *Journal of Clinical Pathology*, Vol. 47, No. 9, (February 1994) pp. 823-826, ISSN 0021-9746

Chaturvedi, A.K. (2010). Beyond Cervical Cancer: Burden of Other HPV-Related Cancers Among Men and Women. *Journal o f Adolescent Health*, Vol. 46, Supp. 4, (April 2010), pp. S20–S26, ISSN 1054-139X

Chaturvedi, A.K.; Madeleine, M.M.; Biggar, R.J. & Engels, E.A. (2009). Risk of Human Papillomavirus - Associated Cancers Among Persons With AIDS. *Journal of the National Cancer Institute*, Vol. 101,No. 16, (August 2009), pp. 1120 - 1130, ISSN 0027-8874

Chaux, A.; Lezcano, C.; Cubilla, A.L.;Tamboli, P.; Ro, J. & Ayala, A. (2010). Comparison of Subtypes of Penile Squamous Cell Carcinoma From High and Low Incidence Geographical Regions. *International Journal of Surgical Pathology*, Vol. 18, No. 4, (August, 2010), pp. 268–277, ISSN *1066-8969*

Cubilla, A.L.; Reuter, V.E. & Gregoire, L. (1998). Basaloid squamous cell carcinoma: a distinctive human papillomavirus-related penile neoplasm: a report of 20 cases. *American Journal of Surgical Pathology*, Vol. 22, No. 6, (June 1998), pp. 755-761, ISSN 0147-5185

Cupp, M.R.; Malek, R.S. & Goellner, J.R. (1995). The detection of human papillomavirus deoxyribonucleic acid in intraepithelial, in situ, verrucous and invasive carcinoma of the penis. *The Journal of Urology*, Vol.154, No. 5, (May 1995), pp. 1024-1029, ISSN 0022-5347

Curado, M.P.; Edwards, B.; Shin, H.R.; Storm, H.; Ferlay, J.; Heanue, M. & Boyle, P. (Ed(s).)(2007). *Cancer incidence in five continents* . IARC Scientific Publications, Vol. IX, No. 160, ISBN 978-92-832-2162-3, Lyon, France

Daling, J.R.; Madeleine, M.M.; Johnson, L.G.; Schwartz, S.M. Shera, K.A., Wurscher, M.A.; Carter, J.J.; PorterP.L.; Galloway, D.A.; McDougall, J.K. & Krieger, JN. (2005). Penile cancer: importance of circumcision, human papillomavirus and smoking in situ and invasive disease. *International Journal of Cancer,* Vol. 116,No. 4, (Aril 2005), pp. 606-616, ISSN 0020-7136

de Sanjosé, S. Diaz, M. Castellsagué, X. Clifford, G. Bruni, L. Muñoz, N. & Bosch F.X. (2007) Worldwide prevalence and genotype distribut ion of cervical human papillomavirus DNA in women with normal cytology: a meta-analysis. *The Lancet Infectious Disease,* Vol. 7, No. 7, (July 2007), pp. 453-459, ISSN 1473-3099

de Villiers, E-M.; Fauquet, C.; Broker, T.R.; Bernard, H-U. & zur Hausen, H. (2004). Classification of papillomavirus. *Virology,* Vol. 324, No. 1, (June 2004), pp. 17- 27, ISSN 0042-6822

Dee, A. & Howell, F.A. (2010). cost-utility analysis of adding a bivalent or quadrivalent HPV vaccine to the Irish cervical screening programme. *The European Journal of Public Health,* Vol. 20, No. 2, (October 2010), pp. 213–9, ISSN 1101-1262

Dietz, C.A. & Nyberg, C.R. (2011).Genital, oral, and anal human papillomavirus infection in men who have sex with men. *The Journal of the American Osteopathic Association,* Vol. 111, Supp. 2, (March 2011), pp. S19-25, ISSN 0098-6151

Dillner, J.; Krogh, V.; Horenblas, S. & Meijer, C.J. (2000). Etiology of squamous cell carcinoma of the penis. *Scandanavian Journal of Urology and Nephrology Supplement,* Vol. 205, (May 2000), pp. 189-193, ISSN 0300-8886

Dorfman, S.; Cavazza, M. & Cardoso, J. (2006). Penile cancer associated with so-called low-risk human papillomavirus. Report of fivecases from rural Venezuela. *Tropical Doctor,* Vol. 36, No. 4, (April 2006) pp. 232-233, ISSN 0049-4755

Favorito, L.A.; Nardi, A.C.; Ronalsa, M.; Zequi, S.C.; Sampaio, J.B. & Glina, S. (2008). Epidemiologic Study on Penile Cancer in Brazil. *International Brazilian Journal of Urology,* Vol. 34, No. 5, (September/October 2008), pp. 587-593, ISSN 1677-5538

Franceschi, S; Castellsague, S; Maso, L.D.; Smith, J.S.; Plummer, M.; Ngelangel, C.; Chichareon, S.; Eluf-Neto, J.; Shah, K.V.; Snijders, P.J.F.; Meijer, C.J.L.M.; Bosch, F.X. & Muñoz, N. (2002). Prevalence and determinants of human papillomavirus genital infection in men. *British Journal of Cancer,* Vol. 86, No. 3, (March 2002), pp. 705 - 711, ISSN 0007-0920

Frisch, M.; Biggar, R.J. & Goedert, J.J. (2000). Human Papillomavirus-Associated Cancers in Patients With Human Immunodeficiency Virus Infection and Acquired Immunodeficiency Syndrome. *Journal of the National Cancer Institute,* Vol. 92, No. 18, (September 2000), pp. 1500-1510, ISSN 0027-8874

Garland, S. M.; Cuzick, J.; Domingo, E.J.; Goldie, S.J., Kim, Y-T.; Konno, R.;Parkin, DM; Qiao, Y-L.; Sankaranarayanan, R.; Stern, P.L.; Tay, S.K. & Bosch, F.X. (2007). Recommendations for Cervical Cancer Prevention in Asia Pacific. *Vaccine,* Vol. 26S, No. 19, (May 2007), pp. M89–M98, ISSN 0264-410X

Gentile, V.; Vicini, P.; Giacomeli, L .; Cardillo, M.R.; Pierangeli, A. & Degener, A.M. (2006). Detection of human papillomavirus DNA, p53 and Ki67 expression in penile carcinomas. *International Journal of immunopathology Pharmacology,* Vol. 19, No. 1, (January/March 2006), pp. 209-215, ISSN 0394-6320

Ghittoni, R.; Accardi, R.; Hasan, U.; Gheit, T.; Sylla, B. & Tommasino, M. (2010). The biological properties of E6 and E7 oncoproteins from human papillomaviruses. *Virus Genes,* Vol. 40, No. 1, (February 2010), pp. 1–13, ISSN 0920-8569

Gil, A.O.; Pompeo, A.C.L.; Goldstein, P.J.; Saldanha, L.B.; esquita, J.L.B. & Arap, S. (2001). *Brazilian Journal of Urology,* Vol. 27, No. 5, (September 2001), pp. 461-468, ISSN 1677-5538

Gillison, M.L. (2008). Human Papillomavirus-Related Diseases: Oropharynx Cancers and Potential Implications for Adolescent HPV Vaccination. *Journal of Adolescent Health*, Vol. 43, No. 4, (April 2008), pp. S52-S60, ISSN 1054-139X

Giuliano, A.R.; Tortolero-Luna, G.; Ferrer, E.; Burchell, A.N.; de Sanjosé, S.; Kjaer, S.K.; Muñoz, N.; Schiffman, M. & Bosch, F.X. (2008). Epidemiology of Human Papillomavirus Infection in Men, Cancers other than Cervical and Benign Conditions. *Vaccine*, Vol. 26, Supp. 10, (August 2008), pp. K17–K28, ISSN 0264-410X

Giuliano, A.R. Anic, G. &Nyitray, A.G. (2010). Epidemiology and pathology of HPV disease in males. *Gynecologic Oncology*, Vol. 117, No. 2, (February 2010), Supp. 1, pp. S15-S19, ISSN 0090-8258

Giuliano, A.R.; Lee, J.H.; Fulp, E.; Villa, L.L.; Lazcano, E.; Papenfuss, M.R.; Abrahanmsen, M.; Slameron, J. Anic, G.M.; Rollison, D.E. & Smith, D. (2011). Incidence and clearance of genital human papillomavirus infection in men (HIM): a cohort study. *The Lancet*, Vol. 377, No. 9769, (April 2011), pp. 932-940, ISSN 0140-6736

Goldie, S.J.; Kim, J.J.; Kobus, K. Goldhaber-Fiebert, J.D.; Salomon, J.; O'Shea, M.K.H.; Bosch, F.X.; de Sanjisé, S. & Franco, E.L. (2007). Cost-effectiveness of HPV 16, 18 vaccination in Brazil. *Vaccine*, Vol. 25, No. 33, (June 2007), pp. 6257–6270, ISSN 0264-410X

Gray, R.H.; Serwadda, D.; Kong, X.; Makumbi, F.; Kigozi, G.; Gravitt, P.E.; Watya, S.; Nalugoda, F.; Ssempijja, V.; Tobian, A.A.R.; Kiwanuka, N.; Moulton, L.H.; Sewankambo, N.K.; Reynolds, S.J.; Quinn, T.C.; Iga, B.; Laeyendecker, O. & Wawer, M.J. (2010). Male circumcision decreases acquisition and increases clearance of high risk human papillomavirus in HIV-negative men: a randomized trial in Rakai, Uganda. *Journal of Infection Disease*, Vol. 201, No. 10, (October 2010), pp. 1455–1462, ISSN 0022-1899

Gregoire, L.; Cubilla, A.L.; Reuter, V.E.; Haas, G.P., & Lancaster, W.D. (1995). Preferential association of human papillomavirus with high-grade histologic variants of penile - invasive squamous cell carcinoma. *Journal National Cancer Institute*, Vol. 87, No. 22, (November 1995), pp. 1705-1709, ISSN 0027-887

Gross, G. & Pfister, H. (2004). Role of human papillomavirus in penile cancer, penile intraepithelialsquamous cell neoplasias and in genital warts. *Medical Microbiology and Immunology*, Vol. 193, No. 1, (February 2004), pp. 35-44, ISSN 1574-695X

Guerrero, D.; Guarch,R.; Ojer, A.; Casas, J.M.; Ropero, S.; Mancha, A; Pesce, C.; Lioveras, B; Garcia-Bragado, F. & Furas, A. (2008). Hypermethylation of the thrombospondin-1 gene is associated with poor prognosis in penile squamous cell carcinoma. British Journal of Urology, Vol. 102, No.6, (September 2008), pp. 747-55, ISSN 2042- 2997

Harish K. & Ravi R. (1995).The role of tobacco in penile carcinoma. *British Journal of Urology*, Vol. 75, No. 3, (March 1995), pp. 375-377, ISSN 0007-1331

Heidman, D.A.; Waterboer, T.; & Pawlita, M. (2007). Human papillomavirus 16 is the predominant type etiologically involved in penile squamous cell carcinoma. *Journal of clinical Oncology*, Vol. 25, No. 29, (October 2007), pp. 4550-4556, ISSN 2218-4333

Hernandez, B. Y.; Wilkens, L. R.; Zhu, X.; McDuffie, K.; Thompson, P.; Shvetsov, Y. B.; Ning L., & Goodman M. T. (2008). Circumcision and Human Papillomavirus Infection in Men: A Site-Specific Comparison. *Journal of Infection Disease*, Vol. 197, No. 6, (June 2008), pp. 787-794, ISSN 0022-1899

Humbey, O.; Cairey-Remonnay, S.; Guérrini, J.S.; Algros, M.P. ; Mougin, C. Bittard, H. & Aubin, F. (2003). Detection of the human papillomavirus and analysis of the TP53 polymorphism of exon 4 at codon 72 in penile squamous cell carcinomas. *European Journal of Cancer, Vol.* 39, No. 5, (March 2003), pp. 684–690, ISSN 0959-8049

IARC (2007). Human papillomaviruses, *IARC Monogr Eval Carcinog Risks Human,* Vol. 90, pp. 16–36, ISBN 92 832 1286 X

Iwasawa, A.; Kumamoto, Y.; Fujinaga, K. (1993). Detection of human papillomavirus deoxyribonucleic acid in penile carcinoma by polimerase chain reaction and in situ hybridization. *The Journal of Urology,* Vol. 149, No. 3, (March 1993), pp.59-63, ISSN 0022-5347

Jansen, K.U. & Shaw, A.R. (2004). Human papillomavirus vaccines and prevention of cervical cancer. *The Annual Review of Medicine,* Vol. 55, No. 2, (February 2004), pp. 319–31, ISSN 0066-4219

Kalantari, M.; Villa, L.L.; Calleja-Macias, I.E. & Bernard, H-U. (2008). Human Papillomavirus 16 and 18 in Penile Carcinomas: DNA Methylation, Chromosomal Recombination, and Genomic Variation. *International journal of Cancer,* Vol. 123, No. 8, (October 2008), pp. 1832–1840, ISSN 0020-7136

Kayes, O.; Ahmed, H.U.; Arya, M. & Minhas, S. (2007). Molecular and genetic pathways in penile cancer. *Lancet Oncology,* Vol. 8, No. 5, (May 2007), pp.420-429, ISSN 1470-2045

Kiyabu, M.T.; Shibata, D. ; Arnheim, N.; Martin, W.J.; & Fitzgibbons, P.L. (1989). Detection of human papillomavirus in formalin-fixed, invasive squamous carcinomas using the polymerase chain reaction. *The American Journal of Surgical Pathology,* Vol. 13, No. 3 (March 1989), pp. 221-224, ISSN 0147-5185

Koifman, L.; Vides, A.J.; Koifman, N.; Carvalho, J.P.& Ornellas, A.A. (2011). Epidemiological Aspects of Penile Cancer in Rio de Janeiro: Evaluation of 230 Cases. *International Brazilian Journal of Urology,* Vol. 37, No. 2, (March/April 2011), pp. 231-243, ISSN 1677-5538

Koushik, A.; Platt, R.W. & Franco, E.L. (2004). p53 codon 72 polymorphism and cervical neoplasia: a meta-analysis review. *Cancer Epidemiology Biomarkers & Prevention,* Vol. 13, No. 1, (January 2004), pp. 11–22, ISSN 1055-9965

Kreuter , A. Wieland, U. (2009). Human papillomavirus-associated diseases in HIV-infected men who have sex with men. *Current Opinion Infection in Diseases,* Vol. 22, No.2, (February 2009), pp.109-114, ISSN 0951-7375

Larke, N. L.; Thomas, S.L.; Silva, I.S. & Weiss, H.A. (2011). Male circumcision and penile cancer: a systematic review and meta-analysis. *Cancer Causes Control,* Vol. 22, No. 6, (June 2011), pp. 1-14, ISSN 0957-5243

Ladwing, S.M.; Rodrigues, A.R.; Horenblas, S. & Spiss, P.E. (2011). Current and future strategies in the diagnosis and management of penile cancer. *Advances in Urology,* Vol. 2011, (May 2011), 9 pages, ISSN 1687-6369

Lee, V.J.; Tay, S.K.; Teoh, Y.L. & Tok, M.Y. (2011).Cost-effectiveness of different human papillomavirus vaccines in Singapore. *BMC Public Health,* Vol. 11, (March 2011), pp. 1-11, ISSN 1471-2458

Levi, J.E., Rahal, P., Sarkis, A.S. & Villa, L.L. (1998) Human papillomavirus DNA and *p53* status in penile carcinomas. *International Journal of Cancer,* Vol. 76, No. 6, (June 1998), pp. 779–783, ISSN 0020-7136

Liegl, B. & Regauer, S (2004). Penile clear cell carcinoma: a report of 5 cases of distint entity. *American Journal of Surgical Pathology,* Vol. 28, No. 11, (November 2004) pp. 1513-1517, ISSN 0147-5185

Lont, A.P.; Kroon, B.K.; Horenblas, S. Galle, M.P.; Berkhof, J.; Meijer, C.J. & Snijders, P.J.(2006). Presence of high-risk human papillomavirus DNA in penile carcinoma predicts favorable outcome in survival. *International Journal of Cancer,* Vol. 119, No. 5, (September 2006), pp. 1078-1081, ISSN 0020-7136

Maden, C.; Sherman, K.J.; Beckmann, A.M.; Hislop, T.G.; Teh, C-Z.; Ashley, R.L. & Daling, J.R. (1993). History of circumcision, medical conditions, and sexual activity and risk of penile cancer. *Journal of The National Cancer Institute,* Vol. 85, No. 1, (January 1993), pp. 19–24, ISSN 0027-8874

Madsen, B.S.; van den Bruke, A.J.; Jensen, H.L.; Wohlfarhrt, J. & Frisch, M. (2008). Rsik factors for squamous cell carcinoma of the penis-population based case-control study in Denmark. *Cancer Epidemiology, Biomarkers and Prevention,* Vol. 17, No. 10, (October 2008), pp. 2683-2691, ISSN 1055-9965

Micali G.; Nasca, M. R.; Innocenzi, D. & Schwartz, R. A. (2006). Penile Cancer. *Journal of the American Academy of Dermatology,* Vol. 54, No. 3, (March 2006), pp. 369-391, ISSN 0190-9622

Minhas, S.; Manseck, A.; Watya, S. & Hegarty, P.K. (2010). Penile Cancer-Prevention and Premalignant Conditions. *Urology,* Vol. 76, Supp. 2A, (August 2010), pp. S24 -S35, ISSN 0090-4295

Miralles-Guri, C. Bruni, L. Cubilla, A.L. Castellsagué, X. Bosch, F.X. & de Sanjosé S. (2009). Human papillomavirus prevalence and type distribution in penile carcinoma. *Journal of Clinical Pathology,* Vol. 62, No. 10, (October 2009), pp. 870–878, ISSN 1472-4146

Moody, C.A. & Laimins, L.A. (2010). Human papillomavirus oncoproteins: pathways to transformation. *Nature Reviews - Cancer,* Vol. 10, No. 8, (august 2010), pp. 550-560, ISSN 1474-175X

Morris, B.J. & Rose BR. (2007). Cervical screening in the 21st century: the case for human papillomavirus testing of self-collected specimens. *Clinical Chemistry and Laboratory Medicine,* Vol. 45,No. 5, (May 2007), pp. 577-91, ISSN 1434-6621

Morris, B.J.; Gray, R.H.; Castellsague, X.; Bosch, F.X.; Halperin, D.T.; Waskett, J.H. & Hankin, C.A. (2011). The Strong Protective Effect of Circumcision against Cancer of the Penis. *Advances in Urology,* Vol. 2011, (May 2011), pp. 1-21, ISSN 812-368

Moscicki, AB.; Schiffman, M.; Kjaer, S. & Villa, L.L. (2006). Updating the natural history of HPV and anogenital cancer. Vol. 24, Supp. 3, (June 2006), pp. 42-51, 0264-410X

Muñoz N., Bosch F.X.; de Sanjose, S; Herrero, R.; Castellsague, X.; Shah, K.V.; Snijders, P.J. & Meijer, C.J. et al.(2003). Epidemiologic classification of human papillomavirus types associated with cervical cancer. *The New England Journal of Medicine,* Vol. 348, No. 6, (February 2003), pp.518–27, ISSN 0028-4793

Nasca, M.R.; Innocenzi, D. Micali, G. (1999). Penile cancer among patients with genital lichen sclerous. *Journal of the American Academy of Dermatology,* Vol. 41, No. 6, (June 1999), pp. 911-914, ISSN 0190-9622

Nascimento, P.S.; Ornellas, A.A.; Campos, M.M., Scheiner, M.A.; Fiedler, W. & Alves, G. (2004). Bax and bcl-2 imbalance and HPB infection in penile tumors and adjacent tissues. *Progrés en Urologie,* Vol. 14, No. 3, (April 2004), pp. 353-359, ISSN 1166-7087

Paavonen, J.; Jenkins,; D.; Bosch, F.X.; Naud, P.D.; Salmeron, J.; Wheeler, C.M.; Chow, S.; Apter, D.L.; Kitchener, H.C.,; Castellsague, X.; S De Carvalho, N. & Skinner, S.R. (2007). Efficacy of a prophylactic adjuvant bivalent L1 virus-like-particle vaccine against infection with human papillomavirus types 16 and 18 in young women: An interim analysis of a phase III double-blind, randomized controlled trial. *Lancet,* Vol. 369, No. 12, (December 2007), pp. 2161-70, ISSN 0140-6736

Palefsky, J.M. (2010). Human Papillomavirus-Related Disease in Men: Not Just a Women's Issue. *Journal of Adolescent Health,* Vol. 46, No. 2, (February 2010), pp. S12–S19, ISSN 1054-139X

Parkin, D.M.; Whelan, S.L.; Ferlay, J.; Thomas, D.B. (Ed(s).). (2003). *Cancer incidence in five continents*. IARC Scientific Publications, Vol. 8, No. 155, ISBN 92-832-2155-9

Parkin, M. & Bray, F. (2006). Chapter 2: The burden of HPV-related cancers. *Vaccine*, Vol. 24, Supp. 3, (August 2006), pp. S2/25, ISSN 0264-410X

Pascual, A.; Pariente, J.M., Godinez, R.; Sanchez-Prieto, M.; Atienzar, M.; Segura, M.& Poblet, E. (2007). High prevalence of human papillomavirus 16 in penile carcinoma. *Histology* and *Histopathology*, Vol. 22, No. 2, (February 2007), pp. 177- 183, ISSN 0213-3911.

Perceau, G.; Derancourt, C.; Clavel, C. (2003). Lichen sclerous is frequently present in penile squamous cell carcinomas but is not always associated with oncogenic human papillomavirus. *British Journal of Dermatology*, Vol. 148, No. 3, (May 2003), pp. 934-938, ISSN 1365-2133

Perera, C.L.; Bridgewater, F.H.G.; Thavaneswaran, P. & Maddern, G.J. (2010). Safety and Efficacy of Nontherapeutic Male Circumcision: A Systematic Review. *Annals of Family Medicine*, Vol. 8, No. 1, (January/February 2010), pp. 64-72. ISSN 1544-1709

Picconi, M.A.; Eijan, A.M. Distefano, A.L. (2000). human papillomavirus (HPV) DNA in penile carcinomas in Argentina: analysis of primary tumors amd lymph nodes. *Journal of Medical Virology*, Vol. 61, No. 1, (May 2000), pp. 65-69, ISSN 1096-9071

Pizzocaro, G.; Algaba, F.; Horenblas, S.; Solsona, E.; Tana, S.; Van Der Poel, H. & Watkin, N. (2010). Guidelines on Penile Cancer. *European Association of Urology*, ISBN 978-90-79754-09-0

Plummer, M. & Franceschi, S. (2002). Strategies for HPV prevention. *Virus Research*, Vol. 89, No. 2, (November 2002), pp. 285-293, ISSN 0168-1702

Poblet, E.; Alfaro, L.; Fernander-Segoviano, P.; Jimenez-Reyes, J. & Salido, E. (1999). Human papillomavirus-associated penile squamous cell carcinoma in HIV-positive patients. *American Journal of Surgical Pathology*, Vol. 23, No. 11, (November 1999) , pp. 1119-1123, ISSN 0147-5185

Pow-Sang, M. & Astigueta, J. (2009). HPV infection and the risk of penile cancer. *Journal of Andrological Sciences*, Vol. 16, (July 2009), pp. 1-6, ISSN 1120-8538

Pow-Sang, M.R.; Benavente, V.; Pow-Sang, J.E. ; Morante, C.; Meza, L.; Baker, M. & Pow-Sang, Julio M. (2002). Cancer of the Penis. *Cancer Control*, Vol. 9, No.4, (July/August 2002), pp. 305-314, ISSN 1073-2748

Pow-Sang, M.R.; Ferreira, U.; Pow-Sang, J.M., Nardi, A.C. & Destefano, V. (2010). Epidemiology and Natural History of Penile Cancer. *Urology*, Vol. 76, Supp. 2A, (August 2010), pp. S2-S6, ISSN 0090-4295

Protzel,C.; Knoedel, J.; Zimmermann, U.; Woenckhaus, C.; Poestsch, M. & Giebel, J. (2007). Expression of proliferation marker Ki67 correlates to occurrence of metastasis and prognosis, histological subtypes and HPV DNA detection in penile carcinomas. *Histology and Histopathology*, Vol. 22, No. 1,1, (November 2007), pp. 1197-1204, ISSN 1699-5848

Prowse, D.M.; Ktori, E.N, Chadrasekaran, D.; Prapa, A. & Baithun, S. (2008). Human papillomavirus associated increased in p16NK4A expression in penile lichen sclerous and squamous cell carcinoma. *British Journal of Dermatology*, Vol. 158, No. 2, (February 2008), 261-215, ISSN 0007-0963

Reis, AAS; de Paula, L.B.; de Paula, A.A.P.; da Cruz, A.D. (2010a) Clinico-epidemiological aspects associated with penile cancer. *Ciência & Saúde Coletiva*, Vol. 15, Supp. 1, (March 2011), pp. 1105-111, ISSN 1413-8123

Reis, AAS.; Silva, D.M.; Curado, M.P. & da Cruz, A.D. (2010 b). Involvement of *CYP1A1, GST, 72TP53* polymorphisms in the pathogenesis of thyroid nodules. *Genetics and Molecular Research*, Vol. 9, No. 4, (October 2010), pp. 2222-2229, ISSN 1676-5680

Reis, A.A.S.; Monteiro, C.D.; de Paula, L.B.; da Silva, R.S. & da Cruz, A.D. (2010c). Human papillomavirus and public health: cervical cancer prevention. *Ciência e Saúde Coletiva*, Vol. 15, Supp. 1, (June 2010), pp. 1060-2010, ISSN1413-8123

Rubin, M.A.; Kleter, B.; Zhou, M.; Ayala, G.; Cubilla, A.L.; Quint, W.G.V. & Pirog, E.C. (2001). Detection and Typing Human Papillomavirus DNA in Penile Carcinoma (Evidence for multiple independent pathqays of penile carcinogenesis). *American Journal of Pathology*, Vol. 159, No. 4, (April 2001), pp. 1211-1218, ISSN 0002-9440

Sakar,F.H.; Miles, M.L.; Plieth, D.H. & Crissman, J.D. (1992). Detection of human papillomavirus in squamous neoplasm of the penis. *The Journal of Urology*, Vol. 147,No. 2, (March, 1992), pp. 389-392, ISSN 0022-5347

Salazar, E.L.; Mercado, E.; & Calzada, L. (2005). Human papillomavirus HPV-16 DNA as an epitheliotropic virus that induces hyperproliferation in squamous penile tissue. *Archives of Andrology*, Vol. 51, No. 4, (July/August, 2005)pp. 327-334, ISSN 0148-5016

Salvioni, R.; Necchi, A.; Piva, L.; Colecchia, M. & Nicolai, N. (2009). Penile cancer. *Urologic Oncology. Seminars and Original Investigations*, Vol. 27, No. 6, (November/December 2009), pp. 677–685 ISSN 1078-1439

Scheiner, M.A.; Campos, M.M.; Ornellas, A.A.; Chin, E.W.; Ornellas, M.H. & Andrada-Serpa, M.J.(2008). Human Papillomavirus and Penile Cancers in Rio de Janeiro, Brazil: HPV Typing and Clinical Features. *International Brazilian Journal of Urology*, Vol. 34, No. 4, (July/August 2008), pp. 467-476, ISSN 1677-5538

Schoen, E.J. Oerhrli, M.; Colby, C.J.& Machin, G. (2000). The Highly Protective Effect of Newborn Circumcision Against Invasive Penile Cancer. *Pediatrics*, Vol. 105, No. 3, (March 2000), pp. 1-4. ISSN 0031-4005

Senba, M. Kumatori, A.; Fujita, S. Jutavijittum, P.; Yousukh, A.; Moriuchi, T.; Nakamura, T. & Toriyama, K. (2006). The prevalence of human papillomavirus genotypes in penile cancer from northern Thailand. Journal of Medical Virology, Vol. 78, No. 10, (October 2006), pp. 1341-1346, ISSN 0146-6615

Shew, M.L. & Fortenberry, J.D. (2005). HPV Infection in Adolescents: Natural History, Complications, and Indicators for Viral Typing. *Semin Pediatr Infect Dis* , Vol. 16, No. 3, (July 2005), pp. 168-174, ISSN 1045-1870

Sirera, G; Videla, S.; Herranz, P. & Corzo-Delgado, J.E. (2006). Human papillomavirus and HIV/AIDS. Vol. 24, Supp. 2, (Nov 2006), pp. 40-46, ISSN 0213-005X

Silva, R.J.C. ; Casseb, J.; Andreoli, M.A. & Villa, L.L. (2011). Persistence and Clearance of HPV From the Penis of Men Infected and Non-Infected With HIV. *Journal of Medical Virology*, Vol. 83, No. 1, (November 2011), pp. 127–131, ISSN 0146-6615

Smith, J.S.; Backes, D.M.; Bleeker, M.C.; Hudgens, M.G.; Agot, K.; Ndinya-Achola, J.O.; Hogewoning, C.J., Moses, S.; Snijders, P.J. & Smith, J.S. (2010). Male circumcision is associated with a lower prevalence of human papillomavirus-associated penile lesions among Kenyan men. *International Journal of Cancer*, Vol. 126, No. 2, (January 2010), pp. 3-32, ISSN 1097-0215

Storey A, Thomas M, Kalita A.; Harwood, C; Gardiol, D.; Mantovani, F.; Breuer, J.; Leigh, I.H.; Matlashewski, G. & Banks, L. (1998). Role of a p53 polymorphism in the development of human papillomavirus-associated cancer. Nature Vol. 393, No. 6682, (May 1998), pp. 229–34, ISSN 0028-0836

Suzuki, H. ; Sato, N.; Kodama, T. Okano, T.; Isaka, S.; Shirasawa, H.; Simizu, B. & Shimazaki J.(1994). Detection of human papillomavirus DNA and state of p53 gene in Japanese penile cancer. *Japanese Journal of Clinical Oncology,* Vol. 24, No. 1, (November, 1994), pp. 1-6, ISSN 0368-2811

Tornesello, M.L.; Duraturo, M.L.; Guida, V.; Losito, S.; Botti, G.; Pilotti, S.; Stefanon, B.; De Palo, G.; Buonaguro, L. & Buonaguro, F.M. (2008). Analysis of TP53 codon 72 polymorphism in HPV-positive and HPV-negative penile carcinoma. *Cancer Letters, Vol.* 269, No. 1, (September 2008), pp. 159–164, ISSN 0304-3835

Tseng, H-F.; Morgenstern, H.; Mack, T. & Peters, R.K. (2001). Risk factors for penile cancer: results of a population-based case-control study in Los Angeles County (United States). *Cancer Causes Control,* Vol. 12, (April 2001), pp. 267–77, ISSN 0957-5243

Van Howe, R.S. (2007). Human papillomavirus and circumcision: A meta-analysis. *Journal of Infection,* Vol. 54, No. 5 (May 2007), pp. 490-496, ISSN 0163-4453

Varma, V.A.; Sanchez-Lanier, M.; Unger, E.R.Clarck, C.; Tickman, R.; hewan-Lowe, K.; Chenggis, L. & Swan, D.C. (1991).Association of human papillomavirus with penile carcinoma: a study using polymerase chain reaction an in situ hybridization. *Human Pathology,* Vol. 22, No. 9, (September), pp. 908-913, ISSN 0046-8177

Villa, L.L & Lopes, A. (1986). Human Papillomavirus DNA sequences in penile carcinomas in Brazil. *International Journal of Cancer,* Vol. 37, No.1, (January 1986), pp.853-855, ISSN 1097-0215

Villa, L.L. (2006). Chapter 1: Biology of genital human papillomavirus. *International Journal of Gynecology and Obstetrics,* Vol. 94, Supp. 1, (January 2006), pp. S3-S7, ISSN 0020-7292

Wiener, J.S.; Effert, P.J.; Humphrey, P.A.; Yu, L.; Liu, E.T. &Walther, P.J. (1992). Prevalence of human papillomavirus tpes 16 and 18 in squamous cell carcinoma of the penis: a retrospective analysis of primary and metastatic lesions by differential polymerase chain reaction. *International Journal of Cancer,* Vol. 50, No. 5, (March, 1992), pp. 694-701, ISSN 1097-0215

Wilkin, T. & Chiasson M.A. (2004). Sexually transmitted infections in men and women, In: Principles of Gender-Specific Medicine, Legato, M.J, pp. 966-977, Elservier, Available from: http://www.sciencedirect.com/science/book/9780124409057, ISSN 978-0-12-440905-7

Wolbarst, A. (1932). Circumcision and penile cancer. *The Lancet,* Vol. 219, No. 5655, (June 1932), pp. 150–153, ISSN 0140-6736

Yanagawa, N.; Osakabe, M.; Hayashi, M. Tamura, G. & Motoyama, T. (2008). Frequent epigenetic silencing of the FHIT gene in penile cancer squamous cell carcinomas. *Virchows Archiv,* Vol. 452, No. 4, (April 2008), pp. 377-382, ISSN 0340-6075

zur Hausen, H. (2002). Papillomaviruses and cancer: from basic studies to clinical application. *Nature Reviews - Cancer,* Vol.2, No.5, (May 2002), pp. 342-350, ISSN 1474-175X

13

Human Papillomavirus in Donor Semen in Belgium

K.W.M. D'Hauwers[1], W.A.A. Tjalma[2], U. Punjabi[3] and C.E. Depuydt[4]
[1]Radboud University Nijmegen Medical Center Department of Urology Nijmegen
[2]University Hospital of Antwerp Department of Gynaecological Oncology Antwerp
[3]University Hospital of Antwerp Department of Fertility
[4]Laboratory for Molecular Pathology, Labo Lokeren Campus RIATOL, Sonic Healthcare Benelux, Antwerp
[1]Netherlands
[2,3,4]Belgium

1. Introduction

1.1 Epidemiology of HPV

Human papillomavirus (HPV) is the most common sexually transmitted infection (STI) worldwide that affects women as well as men. Around 75% of sexually active people will have an HPV infection at some point of life [1].

HPV's are small, non-enveloped DNA viruses and infect both cutaneous and mucosal squamous epithelia. They have been categorized as either low-risk types (lrHPV) or high-risk types (hrHPV) depending on their oncogenic potential [2]. Following HPV types are considered as high risk: 16, 18, 31, 33, 35, 39, 45, 51, 52, 56, 58, 59 68, 73, and 82. Types 26, 53, and 66 are considered as probable high risk (phr). The category low-risk HPV types are types 6, 11, 40, and 42. HPV type 67 is of undetermined risk. The most commonly detected types of HPV in cancers are 16 and 18 [1]. The most commonly detected HPV HPV in cancers are 16, 18 and 45.

Most HPV infections are subclinical and transient in nature. A persistent oncogenic HPV infection has been found to be a necessary but insufficient risk factor in almost all cervical cancer cases [3] and an important risk factor in a subset of penile [4], vulvar, vaginal, and anal cancers [5], anogenital warts [6], recurrent respiratory papillomatoses [7, 8], and a fraction of head, and neck tumours [9, 10]. Table 1 [11].

Men are considered to carry the virus on them, function as a reservoir and act as transmitters of the virus. HPV DNA has been detected in samples of internal and external anogenital sites.

Rintala found HPV in the vas deferens (18.5%): five of 27 vas deferens samples (of vasectomized men) contained HPV 6, 11, or 16 [12].

Svec found HPV in the epididymis: lrHPV 6 and hrHPV 16, 33, 35, 55 and 73 were detected in the epididymis of 7/17 patients, treated with epididymectomy because of nontuberculous epididymitis [13].

Site and histological type	Incidence (per 100,000)	HPV DNA range (%)
CERVIX	8-10	76-97
VULVA	0.0-3.5	
VIN3		72-100
Vulva warty-basaloid		75-100
Vulva squamous		2-23
VAGINA	0.0-1.5	
VAIN		82-100
Vagina squamous		64-91
PENIS	0.0-3.7	
PIN		90
Penis warty-basaloid		46-100
Penis squamous verrucous		31-35
ANUS	0.1-2.8 males/0.0-2.2 females	
AIN		NA
Anus squamous		>80
OROPHARYNX & TONSILS	0.3-21.5 males/0.0-2.8 females	33-72

VIN: vulvar intraepithelial neoplasia
VAIN: vaginal intraepithelial neoplasia
PIN: penile intraepithelial neoplasia
AIN: anal intraepithelial neoplasia

Table 1. Epidemiological traits of HPV and cancers.

Martorell found HPV DNA in 12 testicular biopsies of 185 infertile men (6.5%). The HVP DNA was found in Leydig cells, in Sertoli cells, and probably in germinal cells [14]. Table 2

Also the external anogenital areas have been extensively brushed to examine if these samples can be used to measure the presence of HPV DNA in a general population. Often they were combined with semen and urine samples, which are easy and painless to obtain.

Furthermore, it was assumed that HPV DNA positivity in urine of semen reflected the presence of an ''internal'' HPV reservoir.

HPV DNA is found on the foreskin, glans/coronal sulcus, penile shaft, scrotum, perianal region, urine, and urethra. Table 2

Weaver found most HPV on the foreskin [15]. Giovannelli used penile brushes (PB), urethral brushes (UB), and semen (SE). The HPV DNA detection rate in PB, UB, SE, PB and UB, and PB and SE were 88.9%, 50.0%, 33.3%, 100% and 97.2%, respectively. He concluded that the use of PB and UB appeared to be the most accurate method to screen; as an alternative to UB (which is a rather painfull swab), the use of SE with PB could be used to improve the detection rate [16]. Giuliano [17] examined penile shaft, glans penis/coronal sulcus, scrotum, urethra and semen and concluded that urethral swabs and seminal samples were adequate swabs, which contained sufficient human DNA and beta-Globin, but that HPV DNA presence was very low. She concluded that these two samples did not contribute to optimal sampling: exclusion of urethra, semen, scrotum and perinanal region resulted in a < 5% reduction in prevalence. Nielson [18] did extensive sampling of the anogenital region in healthy, heterosexual men and concluded that the more complete the sampling was, the more HPV DNA was found.

Secondly, she stated that anogenital HPV prevalence in asymptomatic men is higher than expected (previously). The penile shaft was most likely to be positive for HPV.

Author	Site	HPV DNA (%)	Types	
Rintala, 2002	Vas deferens	18.5	6, 11, 16	Post-vasectomy samples
Svec, 2003	Epididymis	41.2	6, 16, 33, 35, 55, 73	Nontuberculous epididymitis
Martorell, 2005	Testis	6.5		Testicular biopsies of infertile men
Weaver, 2004	Penile shaft	24		Men attending STD clinic
	Glans	16		
	Foreskin	28		
	Scrotum	17		
	Urine	6		
Giovannelli, 2007	Penile brushing	88.9		Partners of HPV positive women
	Urethral brushing	50.0		
	Semen	33.3		
Giuliano, 2007	Penile shaft	49.9		Heterosexual men
	Glans penis/sulcus	35.8		
	Scrotum	34.2		
	Urethra	10.1		
	Semen	5.3		

Table 2. Anogenital sites and prevalence of HPV DNA

2. HPV, semen and transport

2.1 Interaction of semen and HPV

The idea that sperm and seminal fluid could act as a vector for HPV transportation is not a new one. In 1979, epidemiological evidence had already suggested a correlation between some male penile cancers and female partner cervical carcinomas [19]. A few years later there was proof that male sexual partners of women with various benign or premalignant cervical lesions were at high risk for having penile lesions [20]. The incidence of HPV DNA in men is lower than in women, so questions rose about the possible modes of sexual transmission of HPV. Possibilities are that HPV DNA is present as free virus particles (virions) or is integrated in shed cells. Corollary questions are: 1)if the virus, once integrated in the cell's DNA, can also express certain genes: 2) if the infected sperm cell can transfer HPV DNA into an embryo or to a sexual partner.

To explore these questions Ostrow et al. (1986) examined the semen of patients with epidermodysplasia verruciformis and chronic lymphatic leukemia and found HPV 2 and HPV 5 [21]. About 95% of HPV DNA was found associated with extracts of the washes and not with the sperm pellet. They concluded that HPV DNA is not associated with the sperm itself, but is present as free HPV DNA or free virus particles. Green et al. (1989, 1991) demonstrated the presence of HPV DNA in the semen of patients with intrameatal and penile warts. They concluded that HPV DNA transmission occured from warts from which surface epithelial cells are shed during ejaculation [22, 23]. They found HPV DNA in the pellet fraction and suggested that HPV DNA is associated with cellular material since virions are supposed to be found in the supernatant fraction of the semen. More recent studies confirmed convincingly the presence of HPV DNA in semen [16, 17, 18, 24].

Question 1 was approached by Lai et al. (1996): they wanted to examine the presence and expression of HPV in human plasma and sperm cells. They examined semen of 24 randomly selected patients who attended the Fertility Clinic. Type 16 E6-E7 DNA and RNA were found in 8.3 and zero % of seminal plasma specimens, respectively, and in 25 and 8.3% of sperm cells specimens, respectively. DNA and RNA sequences of HPV type 18 were found in 33.3 and 8.3% of seminal plasma specimens and in 45.8 and 20.8% of sperm cells specimens, respectively. They suggested that HPVs not only infect human sperm cells, but also succeed in expressing certain genes in the infected sperm cells [25].

The second question was addressed by Chan et al. [26]. They developed an in vitro model that allowed sperm cells, carrying DNA fragments from HPV 16, 18, 31, and 33, from one end of an artificial reproductive tube and to come in contact with hatching mouse blastocysts at the other end of the tube. After washing the blastocysts were analyzed for the presence of foreign DNA fragments. Especially transference of DNA HPV type 18 to the blastocyst was shown. Not all DNA fragments were transferred equally. These results seemed to suggest that sperm can serve as a non-invasive gene delivery system to transport gene fragments into pre-implantation embryos. The fact that some parts of DNA were more easy to deliver, supports the assumption that a variety of factors and mechanisms are involved in transporting HPV DNA.

Pao et al. (1996) examined the take up or retaining of different regions of HPV 18 by sperm cells [27]. They collected sperm samples of 23 subfertile men and found that the oncogenic regions of the viral genome were preferentially retained: 30% (E6) and 83% (E7), vs. 17% (upstream regulatory region), 22% (E1), and 4% (L1).

In 2009, Perez-Andino et al. [28] compared the adsorption of HPV 16 to live human sperm cells in freshly ejaculated, undiluted human semen and in conditions that resemble the female genital tract. Fluorescent HPV 16 capsids were added to semen (concentration 80 microg/l) and the mixture was incubated at 37°C. Even after several hours of incubation, no HPV 16 capsids were detected on the surface of sperm. When the vaginal environment (with a more acidic pH) was mimicked, viral binding was observed on 52% (pH 8.6) and on 72% (pH 7.4) of live sperm. Their conclusion was that association of HPV16 with sperm will probably not occur in neat semen, but may happen in the female genital tract, at low pH, following the dilution of the sperm. Furthermore they found that the HPV 16 capsids bind to two specific sites at the equatorial region of the sperm head surface. They suggested that by means of competitive binding on the virus, attachment to the sperm head may be inhibited. If applicable, this would be a way of protection of sperm cells, and consequently of blastocysts, of embryos, and of sexual partners.

In 2011, Foresta et al. confirmed the binding of the virus at the equatorial region of the sperm head and demonstrated that this happened through interaction between the HPV capsid protein L1 and the receptor syndecan-1.Furthermore, they showed (using hamster egg-human sperm penetration test) that sperm transfected with HPV E6/E7 genes and sperm exposed to HPV L1 capsid protein are capable to penetrate the oocyte and transfer the virus into oocytes. Inside the oocytes, viral genes are activated and transcribed [29].

2.2 Effect of sperm washing

Fertility clinics use washing methods to clean the sperm cells from unwanted viruses. However, HPV seems resistant and sperm washing does not eliminate HPV DNA.

Olatunbosun [24] performed routine "swim up" washing of 27 semen samples that contained HPV DNA: 21 samples were from men with genital lesions, six from sperm donors without prior or current HPV infection. Dodson[30] on the other hand, separated sperm cells by percoll gradient centrifugation in a 1ml aliquot and washed four times with sterile phosphate-buffered saline. All samples, coming from men with genital lesions, still contained HPV DNA after the washing procedure (100%). In six men, without genital lesions, the procedure reduced HPV DNA below detectable levels in only two (33.3%).

Czegly [31] washed sperm cells in Percoll [Pharmacatia] or in Sperm Rinse™ [Vitrolife] and found no change in HPV status.

In 2011, Foresta and al. [32] performed semen analysis and in situ hybridization for HPV detection before and after sperm washing, discontinuous gradients, and swim-up protocols. Sperm washing centrifugation did not change the presence of HPV DNA; Ficoll density gradients and swim-ups brought about only a slight reduction.

3. HPV, semen and fertility

3.1 Effect on the sperm parameters

The actual significance of HPV infection in sperm might be poorly understood and reports are conflicting, but it is a concern for those working in the field of reproductive medicine. Recent articles mention a negative influence on the quality of the sperm and on the pregnancy outcome.

Connelly et al. [33] examined sperm samples of six subfertile patients. He found that specific sperm DNA fragmentation only occurred after exposure of the sperm to DNA of HPV types 16 and 31.These viruses caused breakage characteristics of apoptotic but not necrotic sperm. His data suggest that these viruses do adversely affect subsequent embryonic development after fertilization. HPV DNA of types 6, 11, 18, and 33 did not compromise sperm DNA integrity: apparently sperm DNA is able to resist these types, or repairing mechanisms occur.

In 1997 Lai [34] examined 24 samples of subfertile men for the presence of HPV DNA and RNA. HPV 16 DNA and RNA were found in 25% and 2% of sperm samples, respectively. HPV 18 DNA and RNA in 46% and 21%, respectively. The incidence of asthenozoospermia among patients infected with either HPV was significantly higher than in those without HPV in their sperm cells (75% vs. 8%). Performance of curvilinear velocity, straight-line velocity, and mean amplitude of lateral head displacement was significantly lower in HPV-infected specimens; the differences of linearity, beat cross frequency, and straightness were not statistically significant. Lai concluded: 1) that certain HPV-specific genes are actively transcribed; 2) that the presence of HPV in sperm cells may affect sperm motility parameters; 3) and that asthenozoospermia may be associated with sperm HPV infection.

Recent studies (2009, 2010) by Foresta and al. confirmed these findings [35, 36].

In the first study he examined 200 samples from healthy, young volunteers. Ten persons had HPV DNA positive samples, which was associated with reduced sperm motility [35].

In the second study he collected 290 sperm samples from varying populations: patients with genital warts (n=26), HPV positive partners (n=66), infertile patients (n=108), and fertile controls (n=90). HPV semen infection in these groups was as follows: 53.8%, 40.9%, 10.2%, and 2.2%. The infertile patients had a higher prevalence of HPV DNA in their sperm samples than the other groups. Comparison of sperm parameters showed a more frequent reduction of sperm motility in infected samples, especially when the infection was present in the sperm itself [36].

Rintala [37] examined sperm samples of 65 fathers-to-be; no assisted reproductive techniques (ART) were involved in the pregnancies. Ten men (15.4%) had seminal hrHPV DNA, without any affect on semen parameters such as semen volume, sperm concentration, motility and vitality of spermatozoa. No oligo- or asthenozoospermia was associated with seminal HPV DNA. However, there was a lowering of sperm pH in HPV DNA positive samples, with borderline statistical significance (7.4 vs. 7.5). Ejaculate acts as a potential alkaline buffer (pH 7.2-7.8) neutralizing vaginal acidity (pH 4.0-4.5) within seconds after ejaculation, keeping the vagina neutralized (pH 6.0-7.0) and semen motile. At pH 4.0, sperm cells are immobilized within one minute and are irreversibly immobilized and lose their vitality within 10 minutes [37].

3.2 Effect on pregnancy

Nothing is known about the exact interference of an HPV positive sperm cell, injected in the oocyte cytoplasm (like during the ICSI procedure), with embryo development. Some studies mention an influence on the pregnancy outcome, while others do not find any different rates of spontaneous abortions and major birth defects in an HPV-exposed vs. an HPV-unexposed population [38].

Perino assessed the relation ship between HPV infection in 199 infertile couples and the outcome of ART. He found a significant correlation between pregnancy loss rate and positive HPV DNA testing in the male partner of infertile couples, compared with HPV negative male partners [39].

3.3 Effect on offspring

Czegledy used six HPV positive sperm samples for in vitro fertilization (IVF) and intra-cytoplasmic sperm injection (ICSI). Three washed samples carried hrHPV 16. She tested the native sperm, the washed sperm cells, and the connected blastocysts for HPV sequences. All expectant mothers were HPV negative (negative PAP, negative colposcopy, negative HPV test). She found that (1) the washing procedures (Percoll [Pharmacatia] or Sperm Rinse™ [Vitrolife]) did not change the HPV status of the sperm cells; (2) that HPV-positive spermatozoa kept their procreative capacity (gestation); (3) that HPV positive sperm cells create healthy offspring (follow-up 5 years) [31].

3.4 (Cryo)banking

In an Italian cryobank, in 6/98 thawed samples of oncologic patients and in 2/60 samples of controls, HPV DNA was found. Seven samples carried hrHPV's 16, 18, 53 and 61. Only the sperm head was infected by the virus [40]. Besides the possible effect of the presence of the virus on the sperm parameters, or on the offspring, or on the partners, another question was if HPV-infected sperm is able to cross-contaminate cryovials and impair also the outcome of ART of other couples or infect other partners.

4. HPV, semen and cervical cancer

Cervical cancer is the second most common malignancy among sexually active women worldwide. The pivotal, though insufficient, role of persistent oncogenic HPV infection in almost all cancer cases (99.7%) is well established. Factors in the acquisition of HPV are related to sexual behavior: young age at sexual debut and multiple sexual relations. Still, it usually takes several decades between the initial HPV infection and the onset of cervical cancer.

Wang (2010) postulated that human semen may play a role in genital transmission of HPV and in cervical carcinogenesis itself, based on the following arguments [41].

- Intact genital epithelium is resistant to HPV infection. Tiny tears are necessary to make passage of HPV particles to the basal epithelial cell surface possible, and to initiate infection. Besides spermatozoa semen also contains various chemical components, which may be able to disrupt the normal architecture of cervical epithelium [42].
- Secondly, the immunosuppression of human semen allows interaction with the female and the zygotes. The cell-mediated immunity is considered as the major protection against HPV infection [43]. So, it is possible that semen-mediated immunosuppression may facilitate HPV transmission and/or may reactivate latent HPV infection.
- Chronic inflammation is generally considered a major risk factor for most cancers [44]. Prostaglandins are present in semen at 10,000-fold higher concentrations than those detected at the site of inflammation with PGE2 being the predominant type [45]. Up-regulated PGE2-synthesis is regarded as a possible promoter of cervical carcinogenesis [46]. Consequently, in sexual active women, repeated exposure of HPV infected cervical epithelial cells to high concentrations of PGE2, may be seen as a paracrine modulation of cervical carcinogenesis.
- Degradation of the extracellular matrix by matrix metalloproteinases (MMP's) is essential to tumor invasion and metastasis [47]. Semen has the capacity to stimulate the production of messenger ribonucleic acid (m-rna) for MMP-9 [48], which is correlated with the invasive behavior of cervical cancer [49].
- Furthermore, as mentioned above, HPV capsids could adsorb to spermatozoa, which are highly motile to traverse the thick mucus layer in the female genital tract [28].

However, this hypothesis is in conflict with the first results published on this issue by Nieminen et al. They did not find (dot blot DNA hybridization) any HPV DNA in the sexual partners of 27 women positive for HPV DNA [50]. The method used for the processing of the samples can be an explanation.

5. Study in the Fertility Clinic of the University Hospital of Antwerp

From the above observations, it is clear that sperm cells may be necessary co-promotors of cervical carcinogenesis and that they compromise male fertility.

Furthermore, we wanted to objectify the presence of HPV in sperm samples of subfertile men and of sperm donors.

5.1 Materials and methods

The study protocol was approved by the local Ethics Committee (UA A08 22).

Written informed consent was obtained from all couples/sperm donors.

5.2 Semen samples

Samples were obtained from 41 subfertile men and 21 sperm donors. All samples had been approved for IVF/IUI and ICSI procedures. They were submitted to real time-PCR to determine the presence of 18 HPV types.

5.3 Semen collection and analysis

Samples were collected after 3-6 days of sexual abstinence by masturbation. After liquefaction, a basic semen analysis was performed and scored according to World Health Organisation (WHO 1992) guidelines. These guidelines were adopted after successful training of lab technicians via ESHRE (European Society for Human Reproduction and Embryology) Basic Sample Analysis Courses. Quality assurance was guaranteed by applying standardized methods accompanied with regular internal and external quality controls.

5.4 Semen processing

A part of the semen sample was treated with a two-step discontinuous density gradient [51] using Puresperm® (Nidacon, International AB, Gothenburg, Sweden). Briefly, 40% and 80% Puresperm® density gradient were prepared using 1.0ml of each suspension. Semen was layered on the top of each gradient and centrifuged for 15 mins at 300g. After which the upper layer seminal plasma and the 40 - 80% interface were discarded and the remaining spermatozoa in the 80% pellet was collected from the bottom of the tube and washed once with Earle's Balanced Salt solution (EBSS, Life Technologies, Paisley, Scotland) supplemented with sodium pyruvate (0.011 g/l) and penicillin-streptomycin (50,000 units/l and 50,000 µg/l, Life Technologies, Paisley, Scotland). Samples were kept at -20°C.

5.5 DNA extraction

DNA is bound to the surface of carboxylated magnetic particles under conditions of high polyethylene glycol and salt concentrations (Magnetic Beads extraction Abott M 2000), following the manufacturer's instructions [52]. Briefly, Abbott RealTime HR HPV test procedure consists of sample preparation, reaction assembly, real-time PCR, and result reporting. During sample preparation, 0.4mL of sample is processed using the Abbott mSample Preparation SystemDNA where sample is lysed with chaotropic reagents, and DNA is captured with magnetic microparticle technology. Unbound sample components and inhibitors are washed away and the bound purified DNA is eluted and is ready for amplification. Abbott RealTime HR HPV is currently validated for use with cervical specimens collected in PreservCyt solution (Hologic Inc., Marlborough, MA, USA).

Specimens can be transported at room temperature or refrigerated, and may be stored up to 4 months at room temperature or up to 6 months refrigerated or at 10°C or colder following collection. At the completion of sample preparation, an amplification master mix is created with AmpliTaq Gold enzyme (Roche Molecular Systems, Inc. Branchburg, NJ, USA), magnesium chloride, and oligonu- cleotide reagent containing primers, probes and dNTPs. As a preparation method we used the fully automated m2000sp for medium-to-high test volume that processes up to 96 samples in a run..

5.6 Real time quantitative PCR analysis of HPV DNA

Presence of 18 different HPV geno-types was determined using TaqMan-based real-time quantitative PCR's targeting type specific sequences of viral genes: 6 E6, 11 E6, 16 E7, 18 E7, 31 E6, 33 E6, 35 E6, 39 E7, 45 E7, 51 E6, 52 E7, 53 E6, 56 E7, 58 E6, 59 E7, 66 E6, 67 L1 and 68 E7. Analytical sensitivity of the different PCR assays ranged from 1-100 copies and was calculated using standard curves for 16 type-specific PCRs constructed with plasmids containing the entire genome of the different HPV types [53]. Real-time quantitative PCR for ß-globin was always performed and was used to verify the quality of DNA in the sample and to measure the amount of input DNA [54]. The amount of ß-globin DNA (in nanograms) present in each sample was divided by the weight of 1 genome equivalent (i.e., 6.6 pg/cell) and a factor of 2 (since there are 2 copies of ß-globin DNA / cell) to obtain the number of genome equivalents in the sample. Viral loads in each specimen were expressed as the number of HPV copies / cell. The 18 HPV types we tested for were divided according to Munoz [55]

5.7 Questionnaire and screening

Standard questionnaire with questions about:

- Life style: use of tobacco, alcohol, and drugs
- Sexual history: Number of partners during the past 6 months, homosexual partners, anal sexual activities, SOI.
- Motivation to donate sperm.

Routine:

- screening for HIV, Hepatitis B, Hepatitis C, Syphilis, Chlamydia trachomatis, Neisseria gonnorhea.
- HBA1C, FSH, Testosteron, SHBG, Inhibine B

6. Results

All samples were adequate and contained sufficient beta-Globin. In the native sperm of two patients high risk HPV type 39 was found: one in a sample of a man visiting the fertility clinic, one in a sample of a sperm donor. In the gradient specimens, no HPV DNA was found.

7. Discussion

Investigation of sperm in our fertility clinic resulted in only 2 HPV DNA positive samples, out of 82. Our samples came from subfertile, but healthy men and sperm donors. Foresta [40] found a significant number of HPV DNA in thawed sperm samples from patients with testicular cancer (6.1%), when compared to the samples of controls (93.3%). The HPV types involved in the patients were 4x hrHPV, 1 medium-risk HPV, and 1 lrHPV.

Questions concerning HPV DNA in a cryobank are whether the virus can cross-contaminate other vials and if contamination has clinical consequences for the outcome of the ART, and for the health of the offspring and the receiving partner. To answer these questions, more research is needed to understand more about the exact interaction of the human papillomavirus with sperm cells and the clinical consequences of (the use of) HPV positive sperm cells.

We feel that, at this moment, routine screening of sperm for HPV, will not contribute to the safety of the procedure.

8. Overall conclusion

Research on the prevalence of HPV DNA in semen and its effect on sperm quality and pregnancy outcome is growing.

It seems that the lower pH in the vaginal environment has a double effect: it increases the capacities of the virus to adsorb to sperm cells. Consequently it affects capacities of the sperm cells in a negative way, especially the motility. Other studies mention consequent problems with embryogenic development and a worse outcome of pregnancies [39]. Therefore, it has been suggested to discourage the use of fresh semen for artificial donor insemination program, until accurate, rapid diagnostic tests are available to exclude the presence of HPV infection, and to us only frozen semen that has been appropriately screened [24].

Some author's hypothesized that the presence of HPV in semen may be a co-risk factor for women to develop, cervical cancer, later on in life. Therefore, they promote the use of condoms to prevent genital transmission of HPV and reduce the incidence of cervical cancer [41]. This advice is difficult to follow for couples with a long-lasting, monogamous sexual relationship.

The conclusions of the different studies are not unanimous and further research has to focus on the mechanisms involved, the clinical consequences, and on the prevalence of these problems.

Furthermore, the number of women vaccinated with one of the prophylactic vaccines is growing. This protection may reduce the possible risks, caused by the presence of HPV DNA in semen. Wise examined the effect of the prophylactic quadrivalent vaccine on reproductive organs and semen. He vaccinated male and female rats. All rats had a specific antibody response to the four types after each injection. There were no effects on the reproductive parameters of cohabited male rats: they had normal sperm count and sperm motility. Also the histomorphology of testis and epididymis were unchanged [56].

The vaccine will probably cause no harm to the fertility of its users, and will in addition, provide protection for the development of cervical lesions [57].

9. References

[1] Tjalma WAA, on behalf of the HERACLES/SCALEstudy group. Human papillomavirus type distribution in cervical neoplasia: results from two parallel epidemiological

studies in women with high-grade cervical intraepithelial neoplasia and invasive cervical cancer in Europe. In: IPvC 2010. Montreal, Canada, 8 February 2010. Abstract. (article submitted and expected to be in press)

[2] Munoz N, Castellsague X, de Gonzalez AB, ... Chapter 1: HPV in the etiology of human cancer. Vaccine 2006; 24S3: S1–S10

[3] Walboomers JM, Jacobs MV, Manos MM, Bosch FX, Kummer JA, Shah KV, Snijders PJ,Peto J, Meijer CJ, Munoz N. Human papillomavirus is a necessary cause of invasive cervical cancer worldwide. J Pathol. 1999; 189(1): 12-9

[4] Palefsky JM. HPV infection in men. Dis Markers 2007; 23: 261-72

[5] Carter JJ, Madeleine MM, Shera K, Schwartz SM, Cushing-Haugen KL, Wipf GC, Porter P, Daling JR, McDougall JK, Galloway DA. Human papillomavirus 16 and 18 L1 serology compared across anogenital cancer sites. Cancer Res. 2001; 61(5): 1934-40

[6] Brown DR, Schroeder JM, Bryan JT, Stoler MH, Fife KH. Detection of multiple human papillomavirus types in Condylomata acuminata lesions from otherwise healthy and immunosuppressed patients. J Clin Microbiol. 1999; 37(10): 3316-22

[7] Pou AM, Rimell FL, Jordan JA, Shoemaker DL, Johnson JT, Barua P, Post JC, Ehrlich GD. Adult respiratory papillomatosis: human papillomavirus type and viral coinfections as predictors of prognosis. Ann Otol Rhinol Laryngol. 1995; 104(10 Pt 1): 758-62

[8] Rimell FL, Shoemaker DL, Pou AM, Jordan JA, Post JC, Ehrlich GD. Pediatric respiratory papillomatosis: prognostic role of viral typing and cofactors. Laryngoscope. 1997; 107(7): 915-8

[9] Kreimer AR, Clifford GM, Boyle P, Franceschi S. Human papillomavirus types in head and neck squamous cell carcinomas worldwide: a systematic review. Cancer Epidemiol Biomarkers Prev. 2005; 14(2): 467-75

[10] Shah KV, Westra WH. Genital HPVs in the aerodigestive tract: etiologic association with a subset of oropharyngeal/tonisllar cancers and with recurrent respiratory papillomatosis. Dis Markers 2007; 23: 235-45

[11] Giuliano AR, Tortolero-Luna G, Ferrer E, Burchell AN, de Sanjose S, Kjaer SK, Munoz N, Schiffman M, Bosch FX. Epidemiology of human papillomavirus infection in men, cancers other than cervical and benign conditions. Vaccine. 2008; 26 Suppl 10: K17-28

[12] Rintala MA, Pøllänen PP, Nikkanen VP, Grénman SE, Syrjänen SM. Human papillomavirus DNA is found in the vas deferens. J Infect Dis. 2002; 185(11): 1664-7

[13] Svec A, Mikyskova I, Hes O, Tachezy R. Human papillomavirus infection of the epididymis and ductus deferens: an evaluation by nested polymerase chain reaction. Arch Pathol Lab Med 2003; 127(11): 1471-4

[14] Martorell M, Gil-Salom M, Pérez-Vallés A, Garcia JA, Rausell N, Senpere A. Presence of human papillomavirus DNA in testicular biopsies from nonobstructive azoospermic men. Arch Pathol Lab Med. 2005; 129(9): 1132-6

[15] Weaver BA, Feng Q, Holmes KK, Kiviat N, Lee SK, Meyer C, Stern M, Koutsky LA. Evaluation of genital sites and sampling techniques for detection of human papillomavirus DNA in men. J Infect Dis. 2004; 189(4): 677-85

[16] Giovannelli L, Migliore MC, Capra G, Caleca MP, Bellavia C, Perino A, Viviano E, Matranga D, Ammatuna P. Penile, urethral, and seminal sampling for diagnosis of human papillomavirus infection in men. J Clin Microbiol. 2007; 45(1): 248-51

[17] Giuliano AR, Nielson CM, Flores R, Dunne EF, Abrahamsen M, Papenfuss MR, Markowitz LE, Smith D, Harris RB. The optimal anatomic sites for sampling heterosexual men for human papillomavirus (HPV) detection: the HPV detection in men study. J Infect Dis. 2007; 196(8): 1146-52

[18] Nielson CM, Flores R, Harris RB, Abrahamsen M, Papenfuss MR, Dunne EF, Markowitz LE, Giuliano AR. Human papillomavirus prevalence and type distribution in male anogenital sites and semen. Cancer Epidemiol Biomarkers Prev. 2007; 16(6) : 1107-14

[19] Graham S, Priore R, Graham M, Browne R, Burnett W, West D. Genital cancer in wives of penile cancer patients. Cancer. 1979; 44(5): 1870-4

[20] Levine RU, Crum CP, Herman E, Silvers D, Ferenczy A, Richart RM. Cervical papillomavirus infection and intraepithelial neoplasia: a study of male sexual partners. Obstet Gynecol. 1984; 64(1): 16-20

[21] Ostrow RS, Zachow KR, Niimura M, Okagaki T, Muller S, Bender M, Faras AJ. Detection of papillomavirus DNA in human semen. Science. 1986; 231(4739): 731-3

[22] Green J, Monteiro E, Gibson P. Detection of human papillomavirus DNA in semen from patients with intrameatal penile warts. Genitourin Med. 1989; 65(6): 357-60

[23] Green J, Monteiro E, Bolton VN, Sanders P, Gibson PE. Detection of human papillomavirus DNA by PCR in semen from patients with and without penile warts. Genitourin Med. 1991; 67(3): 207-10

[24] Olatunbosun O, Deneer H, Pierson R. Human papillomavirus DNA detection in sperm using polymerase chain reaction. Obstet Gynecol. 2001; 97(3): 357-60

[25] Lai YM, Yand FP, Pao cc. Human papillomavirus deoxyribonucleid acid and ribonucleic acid in seminal plasma and sperm cells. Fertil Steril 1996; 65 (5): 1026 - 30

[26] Chan PJ, Kalugdan T, Su BC, Whitney EA, Perrott W, Tredway DR, King A. Sperm as a noninvasive gene delivery system for preimplantation embryos. Fertil Steril. 1995; 63(5): 1121-4

[27] Pao CC, Yang FP, Lai YM. Preferential retention of the E6 and E7 regions of the human papilloma virus type genome by human sperm cells. Fertil Steril 1996; 66 (4): 630-3

[28] Perez-Andino J, Buck CB, Ribbbeck K. Adsorption of human papillomavirus 16 to live human sperm. PLoS 2009; 4 (6): e5847

[29] Foresta C, Patassini C, Bertoldo A, Menegazzo M, Francavilla F, Barzon L, Ferlin A. Mechanism of human papillomavirus binding to human spermatozoa and fertilizing ability of infected spermatozoa. PLoS One. 2011; 6(3): e15036

[30] Dodson WC, Moessner J, Miller J, Legro RS, Gnatuk CL. A randomized comparison of the methods of sperm preparation for intrauterine insemination. Fertil Steril. 1998; 70(3): 574-5

[31] Czeglédy J, Szarka K. Detection of high-risk HPV DNA in semen and its association with the quality of semen. Comment on Int J STD AIDS. 2004; 15(11): 740-3.

[32] Foresta C, Pizzol D, Bertoldo A, Menegazzo M, Barzon L, Garolla A. Semen washing procedures do not eliminate human papilloma virus sperm infection in infertile patients. Fertil Steril. 2011 Apr 30.

[33] Connelly DA, Chan PJ, Patton WC, King A. Human sperm deoxyribonucleic acid fragmentation by specific types of papillomavirus. Am J Obstet Gynecol. 2001; 184(6): 1068-70

[34] Lai YM, Lee JF, Huang HY, Soong YK, Yang FP, Pao CC. The effect of human papillomavirus infection on sperm cell motility. Fertil Steril. 1997; 67(6): 1152-5

[35] Foresta C, Garolla A, Zuccarello D, Pizzol D, Moretti A, Barzon L, Palù G. Human papillomavirus found in sperm head of young adult males affects the progressive motility. Fertil Steril. 2009; 93(3): 802-6

[36] Foresta C, Pizzol D, Moretti A, Barzon L, Palù G, Garolla A. Clinical and prognostic significance of human papillomavirus DNA in the sperm or exfoliated cells of infertile patients and subjects with risk factors. Fertil Steril. 2010; 94(5): 1723-7

[37] Rintala MA, Génman SE, Pøllänen PP, Suominen JJ, Syrjänen SM. Detection of high-risk HPV DNA in semen and its association with the quality of semen. Int J STD AIDS. 2004; 15(11): 740-3

[38] Dana A, Buchanan KM, Goss MA, Seminack MM, Shields KE, Korn S, Cunningham ML, Haupt RM. Pregnancy outcomes from the pregnancy registry of a human papillomavirus type 6/11/16/18 vaccine. Obstet Gynecol. 2009; 114(6): 1170-8

[39] Perino A, Giovannelli L, Schillaci R, Ruvolo G, Fiorentino FP, Alimondi P, Cefalù E, Ammatuna P. Human papillomavirus infection in couples undergoing in vitro fertilization procedures: impact on reproductive outcomes. Fertil Steril. 2011; 95(5): 1845-8

[40] Foresta C, Ferlin A, Bertoldo A, Patassini C, Zuccarello D, Garolla A. Human papilloma virus in the sperm cryobank: an emerging problem? Int J Androl. 2011; 34(3): 242-6

[41] Wang X, Zhuang J, Wu K, Xu R, Li M, Lu Y. Human semen: The biological basis of sexual behavior to promote human papillomavirus infection and cervical cancer. Med Hypotheses 2010; 74(6): 1015-6

[42] Roberts JN, Buck CB, Thompsom CD, Kines R, Bernardo M, Choyke PL, et al. Genital transmission of HPV in a mouse model is potentiated by nonoxynol-9 and inhibited by carrageenan. Nat. Med 2007; 13(7): 857-61

[43] Stanley M. Immunobiology of HPV and HPV vaccines. Gynecol Oncol 2008; 109(Suppl.2): S15-21

[44] Baniyash M. Chronic inflammation, immunosuppression and cancer: new insights and outlooks. Semin Cancer Biol 2006; 16(1): 80-8

[45] Sales KJ, Katz AA, Millar RP, Jabbour HN. Seminal plasma activates cyclooxygenase-2 and prostaglandin E2 receptor expression and signalling in cervical adenocarcinoma cells. Mol Hum Reprod. 2002; 8(12): 1065-70

[46] Herfs M, Herman L, Hubert P, Minner F, Arafa M, Roncarati P, Henrotin Y, Boniver J, Delvenne P. High expression of PGE2 enzymatic pathways in cervical (pre)neoplastic lesions and functional consequences for antigen-presenting cells. Cancer Immunol Immunother. 2009; 58(4): 603-14

[47] Coussens LM, Fingleton B, Matrisian LM. Matrix metalloproteinase inhibitors and cancer: trials and tribulations. Science. 2002; 295(5564): 2387-92

[48] Jeremias J, Witkin SS. Effect of human seminal fluid on production of messenger ribonucleic acid for metalloproteinase 2 and metalloproteinase 9 in cervical epithelial carcinoma cells. Am J Obstet Gynecol. 1999; 181(3): 591-5

[49] Radilova H, Libra A, Holasova S, Safarova M, Viskova A, Kunc F, Buncek M. COX-1 is coupled with mPGES-1 and ABCC4 in human cervix cancer cells. Mol Cell Biochem. 2009; 330(1-2): 131-40

[50] Nieminen P, Koskimies AI, Paavonen J. Human papillomavirus DNA is not transmitted by semen. Int J STD AIDS. 1991; 2(3): 207-8
[51] Punjabi U, Gerris J, Van Bijlen J, Delbeke L, Gielis M, Buytaert Ph. Comparison between different pre-treatment techniques for sperm recovery prior to intrauterine insemination, GIFT or IVF. Hum Reprod 1990; 5: 75-83
[52] Huang S, Tang N, Mak WB, Erickson B, Salituro J, Li Y, Krumpe E, Schneider G, Yu H, Robinson J, Abravaya K. Principles and analytical performance of Abbott RealTime High Risk HPV test. J Clin Virol. 2009; 45 Suppl 1: S13-7
[53] Boulet GA, Horvath CA, Berghmans S, Moeneclaey LM, Duys IS, Arbyn M, et al. Cervical cytology biobanking: quality of DNA from archival cervical Pap-stained smears. J Clin Pathol 2008; 61(5): 637-41
[54] Depuydt CE, Benoy IH, Bailleul EJ, Vandepitte J, Vereecken AJ, Bogers JJ. Improved endocervical sampling and HPV viral load detection by Cervex-Brush Combi. Cytopathology 2006; 17(6): 374-81
[55] Munoz N. [Value of human papilloma virus testing in the diagnosis and screening of cervical neoplasia]. Med Clin (Barc) 2003; 121(12): 455-6
[56] Wise LD, Pauley CJ, Michael B, Wolf JJ. Lack of effects on male fertility from a quadrivalent HPV vaccine in Sprague-Dawley rats. Birth Defects Res B Dev Reprod Toxicol. 2010; 89(5): 376-81
[57] Joura EA, Kjaer SK, Wheeler CM, Sigurdsson K, Iversen OE, Hernandez-Avila M, Perez G, Brown DR, Koutsky LA, Tay EH, García P, Ault KA, Garland SM, Leodolter S, Olsson SE, Tang GW, Ferris DG, Paavonen J, Lehtinen M, Steben M, Bosch X, Dillner J, Kurman RJ, Majewski S, Muñoz N, Myers ER, Villa LL, Taddeo FJ, Roberts C, Tadesse A, Bryan J, Lupinacci LC, Giacoletti KE, Lu S, Vuocolo S, Hesley TM, Haupt RM, Barr E. HPV antibody levels and clinical efficacy following administration of a prophylactic quadrivalent HPV vaccine. Vaccine. 2008; 26(52): 6844-51

Permissions

The contributors of this book come from diverse backgrounds, making this book a truly international effort. This book will bring forth new frontiers with its revolutionizing research information and detailed analysis of the nascent developments around the world.

We would like to thank Dr. Davy Vanden Broeck, MSc, PhD, for lending his expertise to make the book truly unique. He has played a crucial role in the development of this book. Without his invaluable contribution this book wouldn't have been possible. He has made vital efforts to compile up to date information on the varied aspects of this subject to make this book a valuable addition to the collection of many professionals and students.

This book was conceptualized with the vision of imparting up-to-date information and advanced data in this field. To ensure the same, a matchless editorial board was set up. Every individual on the board went through rigorous rounds of assessment to prove their worth. After which they invested a large part of their time researching and compiling the most relevant data for our readers. Conferences and sessions were held from time to time between the editorial board and the contributing authors to present the data in the most comprehensible form. The editorial team has worked tirelessly to provide valuable and valid information to help people across the globe.

Every chapter published in this book has been scrutinized by our experts. Their significance has been extensively debated. The topics covered herein carry significant findings which will fuel the growth of the discipline. They may even be implemented as practical applications or may be referred to as a beginning point for another development. Chapters in this book were first published by InTech; hereby published with permission under the Creative Commons Attribution License or equivalent.

The editorial board has been involved in producing this book since its inception. They have spent rigorous hours researching and exploring the diverse topics which have resulted in the successful publishing of this book. They have passed on their knowledge of decades through this book. To expedite this challenging task, the publisher supported the team at every step. A small team of assistant editors was also appointed to further simplify the editing procedure and attain best results for the readers.

Our editorial team has been hand-picked from every corner of the world. Their multi-ethnicity adds dynamic inputs to the discussions which result in innovative outcomes. These outcomes are then further discussed with the researchers and contributors who give their valuable feedback and opinion regarding the same. The feedback is then collaborated with the researches and they are edited in a comprehensive manner to aid the understanding of the subject.

Apart from the editorial board, the designing team has also invested a significant amount of their time in understanding the subject and creating the most relevant covers. They scrutinized every image to scout for the most suitable representation of the subject and create an appropriate cover for the book.

The publishing team has been involved in this book since its early stages. They were actively engaged in every process, be it collecting the data, connecting with the contributors or procuring relevant information. The team has been an ardent support to the editorial, designing and production team. Their endless efforts to recruit the best for this project, has resulted in the accomplishment of this book. They are a veteran in the field of academics and their pool of knowledge is as vast as their experience in printing. Their expertise and guidance has proved useful at every step. Their uncompromising quality standards have made this book an exceptional effort. Their encouragement from time to time has been an inspiration for everyone.

The publisher and the editorial board hope that this book will prove to be a valuable piece of knowledge for researchers, students, practitioners and scholars across the globe.

List of Contributors

José Veríssimo Fernandes
Federal University of Rio Grande do Norte, Brazil

Thales Allyrio Araújo de Medeiros Fernandes
University of Rio Grande do Norte State, Brazil

Robert Koiss
St. Stephen's Hospital, Obstetrics & Gynecology-Gynecology-Oncology Department, Budapest, Hungary

Evanthia A. Kostopoulou and George Koukoulis
University of Thessaly, Greece

Edison Natal Fedrizzi
Department of Gynecology and Obstetrics of the Federal University of Santa Catarina, Florianópolis, Brazil
Director of HPV Project Clinical Research Center University Hospital - Federal University of Santa Catarina, Brazil

Carmen Rodríguez-Cerdeira
Department of Dermatology (CHUVI) & University of Vigo, Vigo

Silvia Díez-Moreno and E. Sánchez
Postgraduate Researcher, University of Vigo, Spanish Society of Cervical Pathology and Colposcopy, Spain

Alfonso Alba
Centre for Molecular and Cellular Studies, Lugo, Spain

Marcela Holá, Jitka Brouzdová and Karel J. Angelis
Institute of Experimental Botany AS CR, Prague, Czech Republic

Markéta Šmídková
Institute of Experimental Botany AS CR, Prague, Czech Republic
Institute of Organic Chemistry and Biochemistry, Prague, Czech Republic

Zoraya De Guglielmo Cróquer
Instituto de Oncología y Hematología, Laboratorio de Genética Molecular, Ciudad Universitaria, Calle Minerva, Los Chaguaramos, Caracas, Venezuela

Armando Rodríguez Bermúdez
Universidad Central de Venezuela, Instituto de Investigaciones Económicas y Sociales, Ciudad Universitaria, Los Chaguaramos, Caracas, Venezuela

Isabelle Bourgault-Villada
AP-HP, Hôpital Ambroise Paré, Boulogne Billancourt, UVSQ, Versailles, France
Institut Cochin, Paris, Université Paris Descartes, France

Simon Jacobelli
Institut Cochin, Paris, Université Paris Descartes, France

Márcio Campos Oliveira, Maria da Conceição Andrade and Fabrício dos Santos Menezes
State University of Feira de Santana - Bahia/State, University of Southwest Bahia, Brazil

Descamps Géraldine, Duray Anaëlle and Saussez Sven
Laboratory of Anatomy, Faculty of Medicine and Pharmacy, University of Mons, Belgium

Delvenne Philippe
Department of Pathology, CHU Sart-Tilman, University of Liège, Belgium

Lucinei Roberto Oliveira, Luciana Souza Chavasco and Ivan de Oliveira Pereira
Vale do Rio Verde University, Brazil

Andrielle Castilho-Fernandes, Alícia Greyce Turatti Pessolato, Régia Caroline Peixoto Lira, João Paulo Oliveira-Costa, Fabiana Alves Miranda, Edson Garcia Soares and Alfredo Ribeiro-Silva
Ribeirao Preto Medical School, University of Sao Paulo, Brazil

Angela Adamski da Silva Reis and Aparecido Divino da Cruz
Federal University of Goiás/Biological Sciences Institute/Department of Biochemistry and Molecular Biology Pontifical Catholic University of Goiás - Department of Biology/Núcleo de Pesquisas Replicon, Brazil

K.W.M. D'Hauwers
Radboud University Nijmegen Medical Center Department of Urology Nijmegen, Netherlands

W.A.A. Tjalma
University Hospital of Antwerp Department of Gynaecological Oncology Antwerp, Belgium

U. Punjabi
University Hospital of Antwerp Department of Fertility, Belgium

C.E. Depuydt
Laboratory for Molecular Pathology, Labo Lokeren Campus RIATOL, Sonic Healthcare, Benelux, Antwerp, Belgium